NEUROSURGICAL
OPERATIVE ATLAS

Volume 1

NEUROSURGICAL
OPERATIVE ATLAS
Volume 1

AANS PUBLICATIONS COMMITTEE

Editors

SETTI S. RENGACHARY, M.D.

Professor and Chief
Section of Neurological Surgery
University of Missouri at Kansas City
Kansas City, Missouri

ROBERT H. WILKINS, M.D.

Professor and Chief
Division of Neurosurgery
Duke University Medical Center
Durham, North Carolina

AMERICAN ASSOCIATION OF NEUROLOGICAL SURGEONS

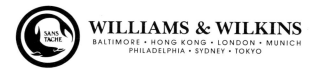

WILLIAMS & WILKINS
BALTIMORE · HONG KONG · LONDON · MUNICH
PHILADELPHIA · SYDNEY · TOKYO

Editor: Carol-Lynn Brown
Associate Editor: Marjorie Kidd Keating
Copy Editor: Janet Krejci
Designer: Dan Pfisterer
Illustration Planner: Wayne Hubbel
Production Coordinator: Raymond E. Reter

Printed in the United States of America

Library of Congress Cataloging-in-Publication Data
Neurosurgical operative atlas / AANS Publications Committee ; editors, Setti S. Rengachary, Robert H. Wilkins.
    p.   cm.
    Includes index.
    ISBN 0-683-07234-X (v. 1)
    1. Nervous system—Surgery—Atlases. I. Rengachary, Setti S.
II. Wilkins, Robert H. II. AANS Publications Committee.
    [DNLM: 1. Nervous System—surgery—atlases. WL 17 N494]
RD593.N43 1991
617.4′8′00222—dc20
DNLM/DLC
for Library of Congress   90-14551
                                 CIP

                      91 92 93 94 95
          1 2 3 4 5 6 7 8 9 10

Foreword

I am honored to write this foreword to the American Association of Neurological Surgeons' *Neurosurgical Operative Atlas*. The list of operations is impressive and covers almost every detail of neurosurgery. The authors selected to present these operations are even more impressive, representing, as they do, outstanding individuals in the United States and Canada who are respected and admired by everyone in the medical profession.

This is not the first effort the former Harvey Cushing Society has made in this field—more than 25 years ago the Board of Editors of the *Journal of Neurosurgery* agreed that it was important to publish a section, entitled *Neurosurgical Techniques*, of select operative drawings with brief explanatory text that would be published as fascicles over the ensuing years.

Most of us in neurosurgery at that time had depended on the volume devoted to the nervous system in Bancroft and Pilcher's *Surgical Treatment*, the responsibility for which had been that of Cobb Pilcher, then at Vanderbilt. Although *Surgical Treatment* was not specifically a "techniques" book, it had much technique in it and was widely used. The editorial board of the *Journal of Neurosurgery* hoped that *Neurosurgical Techniques* would serve as a more up-to-date version of that volume of *Surgical Treatment*.

Emphasis in *Neurosurgical Techniques* was given to the artists' depictions of established, safe techniques. The editors of the Journal realized that a procedure might be done sucessfully in more than one way, but at least one good and safe technique was to be described, and it was assumed that the more skilled and experienced surgeons would utilize other methods they found suitable.

The basis of the decision to focus on the drawings and to have relatively little associated text was a previous atlas, the *Atlas of Surgical Operations* (1). Many of the editors of the Journal had become familiar with this atlas during their general surgical training. Mildred Codding, who had been the artist for Harvey Cushing, had developed an effective technique of drawing the stages of operative procedures that had been and remains an effective teaching aid.

The fascicles of *Neurosurgical Techniques* in the *Journal of Neurosurgery* were to be bound together but, due to changes in publishers, this was never done. Fortunately, some of the plates were preserved and given to me, as editor of the fascicles. Three of these are shown to provide a historical perspective.

The first two figures illustrate a technique by Dr.

James Greenwood of Houston, Texas (2), who pioneered the complete removal of ependymomas in the cervical spinal cord and developed unique bipolar Bovie forceps with suction at the tips. Use of his Bovie forceps enabled him to carry out detailed dissections with magnifying lenses before the advent of the operating microscope. Figure 1 shows the spinal cord split, the tumor being removed, and a line of cleavage being developed; Figure 2 shows a further removal with the suction bipolar forceps in the field.

Figure 3 shows a cervical fusion technique (3) and is published to give due credit to Mr. George Lynch, the artist who approved of and often redrew illustrations that were published in *Neurosurgical Techniques*. Figure 3 illustrates the final stages of cervical fusion for dislocation of C-3, C-4, using bone and wire for the fusion process. This technique was used before the development of the acrylic fusion technique, which came to replace the bone grafting procedure.

As was expressed in the final paragraph of the introduction to *Neurosurgical Techniques* (4), neurosurgery was evolving rapidly, and often the procedure described had not originated with the person who wrote about it. Then, as now, surgery was a combination of new knowledge with old. Since knowledge is freely shared among surgeons nationally and internationally, original techniques and ideas are passed from teacher to student, from surgeon to surgeon, and

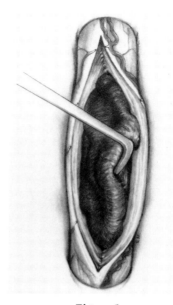

Figure 1.

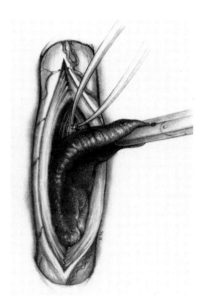

Figure 2.

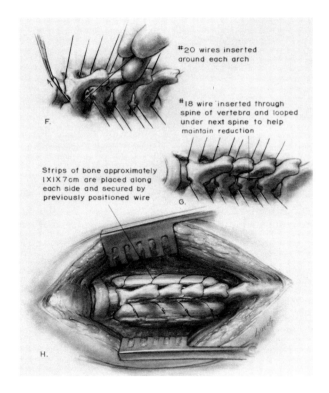

Figure 3.

altered with changing developments and experience. A procedure well-established today may seem naive or useless a few years hence. One can make valid judgments only on the basis of data that become available. Thus, it is my great pleasure to introduce this ambitious project by Dr. Wilkins and Dr. Rengachary. Not only will it update neurosurgical techniques, but it is also a further development of the effort made by the editors of the *Journal of Neurosurgery* 25 years ago. We hope it will surpass that effort.

EBEN ALEXANDER, JR.

References

1. Cutler EC, Zollinger R. Atlas of surgical operations. Illustrated by Mildred B. Codding. New York: Macmillan, 1939.
2. Greenwood J, Jr. Surgical removal of intramedullary tumors. J Neurosurg 1967;26:275–282.
3. Alexander E, Jr, Davis CH, Jr, Forsyth HF. Reduction and fusion of fracture dislocations of the cervical spine. J Neurosurg 1967;27:587–591.
4. Alexander E, Jr. Neurosurgical techniques introduction. J Neurosurg 1966;24:817–819.

Preface

Man has always had an innate urge to depict his activities in drawings, as the paintings of cave dwellers would attest. Surgical atlases perhaps represent a formalized version of such an urge; the atlases, in addition to documenting the work, have instructional value as well—being able to teach generations of trainees the craft of surgery as practiced by the masters of the trade. Although electronic images have greatly advanced the instructional process, printed artwork remains the backbone of the media for teaching.

There has been a perception among all neurosurgeons for some time that a contemporary atlas in neurosurgery is due. To fill this void, the Publications Committee of the American Association of Neurological Surgeons has undertaken the task of producing a comprehensive atlas. The atlas will be published at bimonthly intervals in the form of fascicles containing up to six operations each. To allow timely publication, topics are included in a random fashion.

The *Neurosurgical Operative Atlas,* we believe, is unique in several respects. It is comprehensive. When completed, it will contain descriptions of up to two hundred operative procedures. It is multiauthored. Given the complexity of the field and the explosive advances in techniques, it is impossible for any one individual to be skilled enough to describe the entire spectrum of techniques authoritatively. In many instances, the chosen authors are those who developed a technique originally or have used the technique so extensively as to be an authority on it. Many illustra-

tions are depicted in full color despite the high costs involved in preparing the artwork and printing. In many instances where there is more than one way to approach a problem, two different authors have been requested to write on the same subject so that the reader will benefit from knowing alternative surgical techniques.

The atlas has been possible in large measure due to the efforts and sacrifices of the contributing authors. In addition to sharing their knowledge and expertise, they have incurred large expenses in getting the artwork done; they have spent long hours with their illustrators to achieve the accurate and esthetically pleasing depiction of the procedures. One can also see the spectrum of artistic talent that made this work possible.

We thank George T. Tindall, M.D., for forming the Publications Committee; Eben Alexander, Jr., M.D., for preparing the Foreword; Carol-Lynn Brown and Majorie Keating of the Williams & Wilkins Company, and Carl H. Hauber and Gabrielle J. Loring of the American Assoiation of Neurological Surgeons for co-ordinating various phases of the project; Sherylyn Cockroft and Gloria K. Wilkins for secretarial help; members of the Publications Committee for innumerable suggestions; and Diane Abeloff for overseeing the entire artwork.

SETTI S. RENGACHARY
ROBERT H. WILKINS

Contributors

SARAH J. GASKILL, M.D.
Resident
Division of Neurosurgery
Duke University Medical Center
Durham, North Carolina

FRED H. GEISLER, M.D., PH.D.
Clinical Assistant Professor
Department of Surgery
Division of Neurosurgery
The Shock Trauma Center of the Maryland
    Institute for Emergency Medical Services
    Systems and the University of Maryland
Baltimore, Maryland
Chief of Neurosurgery
Department of Neurosurgery
Patuxent Medical Group
Columbia, Maryland

JAMES T. GOODRICH, M.D., PH.D.
Director, Division of Pediatric Neurosurgery
Leo Davidoff Department of Neurological Surgery
Albert Einstein College of Medicine
Montefiore Medical Center
Bronx, New York

CRAIG D. HALL, M.D.
Institute of Plastic and Reconstructive Surgery
Albert Einstein College of Medicine
Montefiore Medical Center
Bronx, New York

EDGAR M. HOUSEPIAN, M.D.
Professor
Department of Clinical Neurological Surgery
College of Physicians & Surgeons
Columbia University
Attending Neurosurgeon
New York Neurological Institute
Columbia-Presbyterian Medical Center
New York, New York

W. JERRY OAKES, M.D.
Assistant Professor
Division of Neurosurgery
Department of Surgery
Assistant Professor
Department of Pediatrics
Duke University Medical Center
Durham, North Carolina

JOSEPH RANSOHOFF, M.D.
Professor and Chairman
Department of Neurosurgery
New York University Medical Center
New York, New York

EDWARD TARLOV, M.D.
Department of Neurosurgery
Lahey Clinic Medical Center
Burlington, Massachusetts

ROBERT H. WILKINS, M.D.
Professor and Chief
Division of Neurosurgery
Duke University Medical Center
Durham, North Carolina

AANS Publications Committee

Contributors

JOSHUA B. BEDERSON, M.D.
Resident
Department of Neurosurgery
University of California, San Francisco
San Francisco, California

MICHAEL N. BUCCI, M.D.
Resident
Section of Neurosurgery
University of Michigan Medical Center
Ann Arbor, Michigan

EUGENE S. FLAMM, M.D.
Charles Harrison Frazier Professor and Chairman
Division of Neurosurgery
University of Pennsylvania School of Medicine
Philadelphia, Pennsylvania

SARAH J. GASKILL, M.D.
Resident
Division of Neurosurgery
Duke University Medical Center
Durham, North Carolina

PATRICK W. HITCHON, M.D.
Professor
Division of Neurosurgery
The University of Iowa Hospitals and Clinics and
    Department of Veterans Affairs Medical Center
Iowa City, Iowa

JULIAN T. HOFF, M.D.
Professor and Chair
Section of Neurosurgery
University of Michigan Medical Center
Ann Arbor, Michigan

JOHN A. JANE, M.D.
Professor and Chairman
Department of Neurosurgery
University of Virginia Health Sciences Center
Charlottesville, Virginia

MILAM E. LEAVENS, M.D.
Associate Professor and Chief
Department of Neurosurgery
The University of Texas M. D. Anderson Cancer
    Center
Houston, Texas

FREDRIC B. MEYER, M.D.
Consultant
Department of Neurosurgery
Mayo Clinic
Rochester, Minnesota

JOHN A. PERSING, M.D.
Professor
Department of Neurosurgery
Associate Professor and Vice-Chairman
Department of Plastic Surgery
University of Virginia Health Sciences Center
Charlottesville, Virginia

THORALF M. SUNDT, JR., M.D.
Professor and Chairman
Department of Neurosurgery
Mayo Clinic
Rochester, Minnesota

VINCENT C. TRAYNELIS, M.D.
Assistant Professor
Division of Neurosurgery
The University of Iowa Hospitals and Clinics and
    Department of Veterans Affairs Medical Center
Iowa City, Iowa

ROBERT H. WILKINS, M.D.
Professor and Chief
Division of Neurosurgery
Duke University Medical Center
Durham, North Carolina

CHARLES B. WILSON, M.D.
Tong-Po Kan Professor and Chairman
Department of Neurosurgery
University of California, San Francisco
San Francisco, California

RONALD F. YOUNG, M.D.
Professor and Chief
Division of Neurological Surgery
University of California, Irvine
Irvine, California

Contents

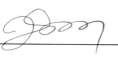

Contents

OPTIC GLIOMAS

EDGAR M. HOUSEPIAN, M.D.

INTRODUCTION

The primary indication for surgical treatment of optic glioma is disfiguring proptosis and progressive visual loss in a patient with unilateral optic nerve tumor. When indicated, tumor resection should extend from the scleral margin to the chiasm to reduce the possibility of leaving residual tumor cells in the cut stump of the optic nerve. The following section will describe in detail the important steps in performing the transcranial orbital approach required to achieve this end. Although surgical cure is a primary objective of this procedure, a secondary objective is preservation of a normal appearing globe and normal extraocular movements, thus ensuring a good cosmetic result. To achieve this end, the neurosurgeon must be familiar with the regional anatomy. Orbital exploration is somewhat alien to neurosurgery in that it does not involve the principles of intraaxial cranial surgery and there is no extraaxial space to visualize the important nerves, arteries, and veins that traverse the orbit because of their protective investment in orbital fat Thus, before describing clinical indications and surgical technique this section will briefly review orbital surgical anatomy (Figs. 1–4).

SURGICAL ANATOMY

The orbit is a pear-shaped structure with the optic canal representing the stem at the apex. The 5- to 10-mm-long optic canal enters medial to the anterior clinoid process. The lateral wall of the optic canal is formed by one of the two roots of the lesser wing of the sphenoid which also serves as the medial margin of the superior orbital fissure. In conforming to the shape of the optic nerve, the optic canal is a 4×6-mm horizontal elliptical cavity at its point of entry, is circular in its midportion, and enters the orbit as a vertical ellipse. The lateral bony margins of the orbit are formed by the greater wing of the sphenoid and the fronto-sphenoidal process of the zygomatic bone. The orbital roof (floor of the anterior cranial fossa) is formed by the frontal bone, and the orbital plate of the maxilla forms both the floor of the orbit and the roof of the maxillary sinus. The medial wall of the orbit, cov-

ered by the thin lamina papyracea, is bordered by the ethmoid and sphenoid sinuses. The frontal sinus lies in the medial portion of the superior orbital rim.

The cranial dura is redundant at the cranial end of the optic canal where it forms the falciform ligament. It then traverses the canal where the outer layer is continuous with the periorbita, while the inner layer continues as the optic nerve sheath within the orbit. The intracranial subarachnoid space is continuous with the subarachnoid space of the optic nerve, although it is partially obliterated at the annulus of Zinn were the pial surface of the optic nerve is fused to this fibrous annular band superiorly and medially.

Six of the seven extraocular muscles take their origin from the fibrous annulus of Zinn which fuses with the optic nerve dura at the apical end of the optic canal (Fig. 1). The lateral portion of the annulus of Zinn is formed by the two heads of the lateral rectus muscle. These loop widely around the superior orbital fissure forming the boundaries of the so-called oculomotor foramen.

There are two routes of entry from the cranial cavity to the orbit: the optic canal and the superior orbital fissure. The ophthalmic artery (Fig. 2) enters the orbit with the optic nerve and lies in a split layer of dura within the canal. Approximately 1 cm after entering, it gives off the central retinal artery which obliquely perforates the dura and courses to the retina within the optic nerve. The ophthalmic artery then curves medially and superiorly over the optic nerve, giving off two long posterior ciliary arteries and six or eight short posterior ciliary branches before anastomosing with the external carotid circulation. Small branches of the ophthalmic artery supply the ocular muscles at their origin near the apex of the orbit. Occlusion of the central retinal artery will result in visual loss, whereas ophthalmic artery occlusion frequently does not because of the rich external collateral supply.

The orbital veins become confluent and drain primarily through the superior orbital vein which exits through the superior orbital fissure; there is a smaller draining component through the inferior ophthalmic vein exiting through the inferior orbital fissure. The superior ophthalmic vein is the major venous drainage channel, and occlusion of this vessel along its

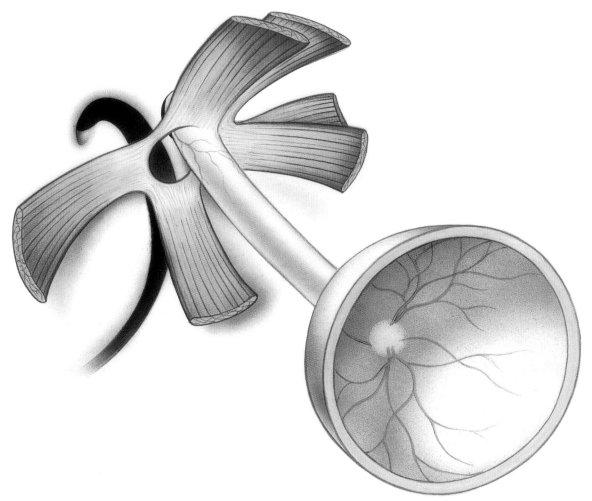

Figure 1. Six of the seven extraocular muscles take their origin from the fibrous annulus of Zinn which is fused medially with the optic nerve dura at the apical end of the optic canal. In order to remove the optic nerve in one piece from the globe to the chiasm, the annulus of Zinn must be opened and the nerve sharp-dissected from the medial dura. This necessitates sectioning of the levator origin which arises from the medial aspect of the annulus. The origin must be resutured to prevent ptosis. The two long heads of the lateral rectus muscle loop widely around the superior orbital fissure and define the oculomotor foramen. Those structures that traverse the superior orbital fissure through the oculomotor foramen thus lie directly within the muscle cone.

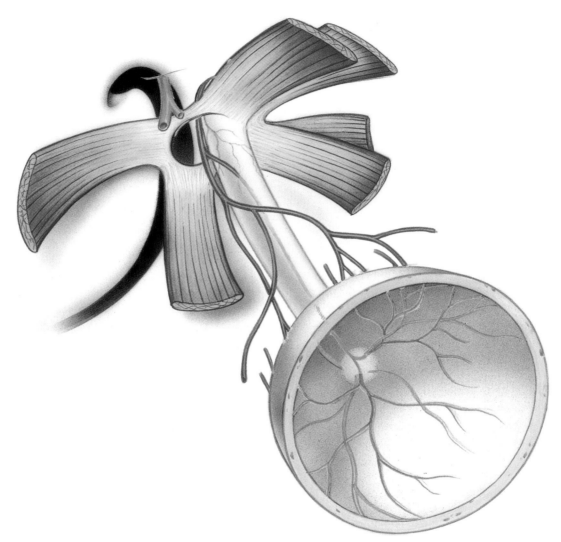

Figure 2. The ophthalmic artery enters the orbit through the optic canal and lies between the split layers of dura. The central retinal artery is given off approximately 1 cm from the point of entry of the ophthalmic artery which then loops over the optic nerve and anastomoses widely with the external carotid arterial circulation. Multiple short perforating vessels supply the retina. The major venous drainage of the orbit is through the superior orbital fissure and the cavernous sinus. There is relatively minor anastomosis with the inferior ophthalmic vein draining through the inferior orbital fissure.

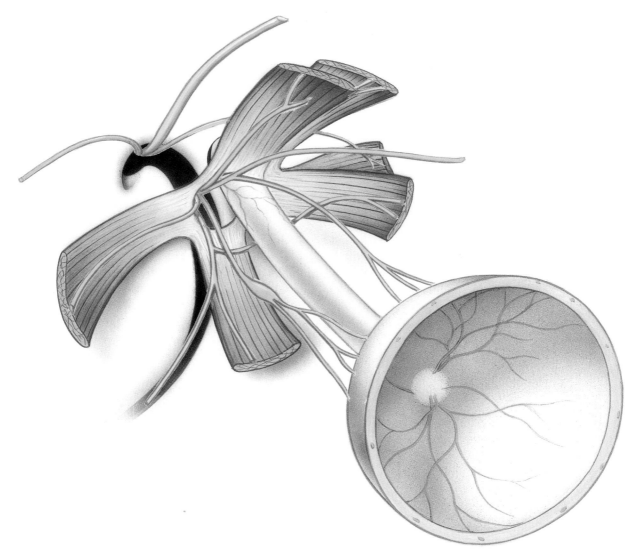

Figure 3. The fourth, first division fifth, and lacrimal nerves enter the superior orbital fissure in that order. The frontalis nerve (V1) serves as a landmark identifying the region of the levator and superior rectus muscles and is visible through the thin periorbita. The trochlear, frontalis, and lacrimal nerves lie within the orbit but are outside of the muscle cone. Those nerves that enter the orbit through the region of the oculomotor foramen lie directly within the muscle cone. The superior division of the third nerve innervates the levator and superior rectus muscles; the nasociliary nerve crosses over the optic nerve before exiting the orbit and sends branches to the laterally placed ciliary ganglion which gives off two long and several short ciliary nerves. The nasociliary nerve also directly gives off six or eight short ciliary nerves. The sixth nerve enters between the superior and inferior divisions of the third nerve and innervates the lateral rectus muscle. The inferior division of the third nerve supplies the inferior oblique and inferior rectus muscles and crosses under the optic nerve to supply the medial rectus muscle.

course or at the cavernous sinus frequently results in proptosis and chemosis.

Masses external to the periorbita may produce proptosis without affecting extraocular movement or vision, whereas tumors within the muscle cone, particularly those crowding the apex, frequently limit extraocular motility and encroach upon vision. Structures traversing the superior orbital fissure outside the oculomotor foramen will, of course, be found within the periorbita but outside the muscle cone. Thus, in order of entrance, the trochlear nerve, the frontalis branch of the fifth nerve, the lacrimal nerve, and the exiting ophthalmic vein are found within the periorbita but outside of the muscle cone (Fig. 3). Within the oculomotor foramen, in order of passage from above downward, are found the superior division of the third nerve curving upward and medially to innervate the superior rectus and levator muscles, the nasociliary branch of the ophthalmic nerve crossing forward and medial over the optic nerve, the sixth nerve innervating the lateral rectus muscle, and the inferior division of the third nerve which crosses beneath the optic nerve to reach both the medial and inferior rectus and inferior oblique muscles. The ciliary ganglion, which lies lateral to the optic nerve, receives preganglionic parasympathetic fibers from the oculomotor nerve and sends its postganglionic fibers to the sphincter of the iris and the ciliary muscle by the several long and short ciliary nerves. It is difficult to totally eradicate lesions that involve the optic canal or superior orbital fissure dura without injury to those structures which traverse them. Tumors that invade the oculomotor foramen are particularly difficult to eradicate for this reason. A review of this regional anatomy further illustrates that a direct approach to the optic nerve between the levator and medial rectus muscles can be safely achieved with the least chance of injury to the important nerve supply to any of the extraocular muscles.

One should also be cognizant of the fact that the levator muscle origin lies superior and medial to the superior rectus muscle. In view of the fusion of the annulus of Zinn with the dura of the optic nerve at this location, it is necessary to electively section the levator origin to prevent its tearing upon opening the optic nerve dura. After this attachment is sharply dissected free and the optic nerve is removed from the canal, the levator origin is resutured to the annulus.

PATIENT SELECTION

The term optic glioma as applied to all astrocytomas of the optic nerves and chiasm would better be classified into tumors affecting a single optic nerve, tumors affecting the chiasm alone or the chiasm and one or both optic nerves, and those bilateral, multicentric optic

nerve sheath gliomas affecting the optic nerves but sparing the chiasm.

Each of these presentations requires a different management plan. In addition, the differential diagnosis of tumors confined to one or more optic nerve sheaths is simply glioma versus meningioma, whereas a chiasmal glioma may be difficult to differentiate from a hypothalamic glioma. The presence or absence of neurofibromatosis is of significance but does not always differentiate glioma from meningioma. Neurofibromatosis is associated with a high proportion of single optic nerve gliomas and a very low percentage of chiasmal gliomas. In a series of 135 cases of optic glioma, 100% of those multicentric bilateral optic nerve sheath tumors were associated with neurofibromatosis. This raises the question of possibly different causation and natural history when glioma occurs with or without neurofibromatosis.

The availability of high-resolution imaging techniques further helps differentiate those orbital tumors that arise within the optic nerve from those that simply displace the optic nerve. Multicentric tumors and chiasmal involvement also can be clearly defined.

Thus, current indications for surgery in optic glioma are limited to those patients with single nerve involvement who have poor vision and disfiguring proptosis, in whom the prime object of surgery is resection of the tumor-bearing optic nerve from the globe to the chiasm, or exploration for biopsy in those cases of chiasmal glioma in which the diagnosis is in doubt. Children with multicentric optic glioma and patients with chiasmal glioma are currently followed for signs of visual change. Irradiation is recommended only if there is progressive visual loss. The rare case of exophytic chiasmal glioma has benefited from subtotal resection of tumor followed by radiotherapy.

The diagnosis of optic glioma is easy to make in a child with proptosis, pallor or gliosis of the optic nerve head, enlargement of the optic canal, and neurofibromatosis. In an older age group the differential diagnosis may be more difficult because of the prevalence of meningioma of the optic nerve. In the classical case of meningioma, there is progressive visual loss without proptosis, and optociliary shunting is pathognomonic for meningioma. Furthermore, distinctive computed tomography (CT) patterns differentiate gliomas and meningiomas. The CT appearance of the nerve in glioma is one of a massively swollen optic nerve with clear-cut margins; there may be kinking and buckling of the optic nerve as well. The common CT pattern for meningioma is a narrow, diffusely enlarged nerve with polar expansion at the apex. Unlike gliomas, there may also be calcification within the tumor. The optic nerve appears as a lucent shadow in the center of optic nerve sheath meningioma but a

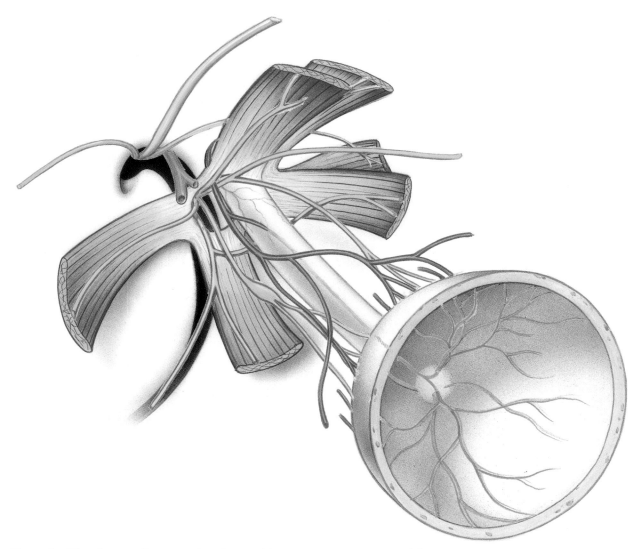

Figure 4. This drawing illustrates the relation of the extra-ocular muscles, the optic nerve and superior orbital fissure, the cranial and autonomic nerves, the course of the ophthal-mic artery, and the major venous drainage of the orbit. These very fine structures are enveloped in and protected by orbital fat.

similar appearance may occasionally be seen in gliomas associated with neurofibromatosis.

PREOPERATIVE PREPARATION

It is no longer necessary to visualize the regional circulation by angiography as part of the preoperative work-up for patients with optic glioma. There are thus no special preoperative studies or procedures required, and the anesthetic techniques used are common to all major neurosurgical procedures. Blood for replacement should be cross-matched and available but is rarely necessary. Spinal drainage is not required during the operative procedure as opening of the chiasmatic cistern readily allows free escape of cerebrospinal fluid with ventricular emptying, resulting in the development of an operating field requiring little or no retraction. An osmotic diuretic is used, however, to reduce the intraorbital pressure and to facilitate dissection within the periorbita in the presence of tumor. The patient or his family should be instructed that there is a potential for injury to one or both olfactory nerves with resulting alteration of smell and sometimes taste, especially if osmotic diuretics are used. The epidural approach to the orbit minimizes the risk of tearing the olfactory nerve. Similarly, the possibility of permanent ptosis or loss of extraocular muscle function due to injury to the third or sixth nerve must be understood preoperatively. Finally, injury to the sympathetic nerve supply or circulation to the globe may result in significant iritis which could result in the loss of the globe.

Intraoperative antibiotics and high-dose steroids are used and the latter continued for four or five days until the peak edema phase has passed.

There is no need for neurophysiological monitoring. The operating microscope is of less help in this procedure because the marked obliquity of the surgical field makes it difficult to maintain focus at higher magnifications.

In summary, the primary objective of transcranial orbital resection of optic glioma is a surgical cure; a secondary objective is maintenance of a normal appearing and moving globe to ensure a good cosmetic result.

SURGICAL TECHNIQUE

The operating table is placed in a low Fowler's position with the patient supine and the head directly midline (Fig. 5). When dealing with optic nerve tumor by the transcranial route, we prefer an osteoplastic bone flap (Fig. 6); there seems to be little advantage to elevating a free bone flap, which includes the orbital rim, because it affords no additional exposure at the apex. A coronal incision is marked and infiltrated with 1% Xylocaine with epinephrine, and the scalp and galea are incised as one. Michele clips or the equivalent are used at the

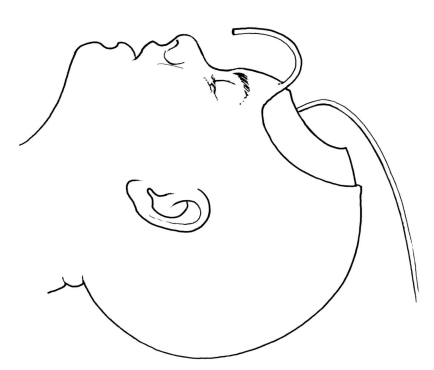

Figure 5. A coronal incision and low medial frontal flap is the preferred approach to the medial orbit.

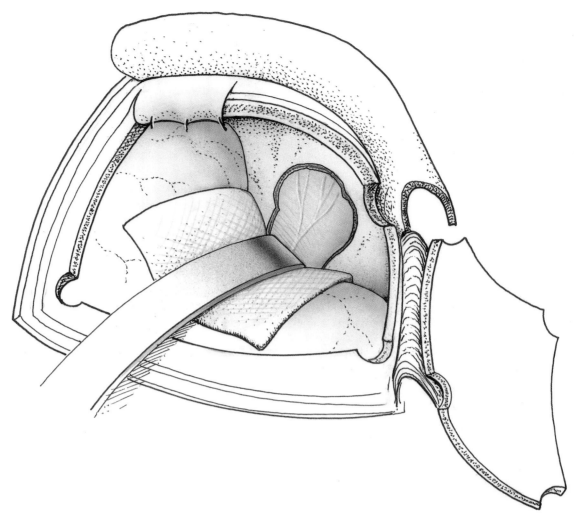

Figure 6. An osteoplastic, medial frontal flap is illustrated. It is not necessary to resect the orbital rim because it gives little additional access to the orbital apex. If the frontal sinus is entered it is exenterated, the mucosa rolled, and impacted into the ostium, and a flap of pericranium sutured to the dura for repair. The frontalis nerve is visualized through the thin periorbita after the orbit is unroofed. Prior to the epidural approach, an intradural inspection of the optic nerve allows opening of the chiasmatic cistern, release of cerebrospinal fluid with emptying of the ventricles, and the development of an adequate operative field.

scalp margin for hemostasis and the scalp and galea are reflected together over a flap roll. The subgaleal dissection is brought no closer than 1 cm from the orbital rim to minimize postoperative lid edema. Pericranium, temporalis muscle, and fascia are then incised with a cutting needle. A four-hole osteoplastic craniotomy is started with a performator and a burr and interconnected with a Gigli saw. The anterior medial trephination is made just at the top of the frontal sinus and an attempt is made to keep the mucosa intact when the sinus is unroofed. The anterior lateral trephination is made just lateral to the temporal ridge. Tenting sutures are placed posteriorly and laterally but not anteriorly, as an epidural approach will later be made to the anterior fossa. Gelfoam is placed at the dural margin.

If the frontal sinus is entered it must be carefully repaired by exenterating the mucosa and rolling and impacting it into the ostium. A small piece of muscle is placed over this, and Gelfoam is used to cover this. A flap of pericranium is then pulled downward and sutured to the dura to secure the repair.

A linear horizontal incision is made in the dura, and using a small malleable retractor the perichiasmatic cistern is visualized and entered to allow escape of cerebrospinal fluid. This is removed by suction over cottonoid and gentle retraction applied over a protective sponge (Bicol) until an adequate field is developed.

This initial intradural approach allows for both inspection of the intracranial optic nerve and identification of the site of the optic canal which is difficult to locate from the epidural approach when unroofing the orbit. If the optic nerve does not appear abnormal, sectioning of the optic nerve would be deferred until tumor pathology is proved at the time of orbital exploration. In the more usual instance where the intracranial optic nerve is grossly abnormal, it is simply cut with scissors at the chiasmal margin perpendicular to its long axis. There is no virtue in leaving a stump of optic nerve because tumor cells may remain within it.

Once these steps have been accomplished, the retractor is withdrawn and an epidural approach made along the floor of the anterior fossa. Cottonoids are used to hold the field and the retractor is advanced to the orbital apex. Orbital unroofing is started with a diamond high-speed burr and enlarged with small double-action mastoid or Leksell rongeurs and orbital micropunches. These miniaturized rongeurs are similar to Kerrison rongeurs but are scaled down in size to accommodate the eggshell-thin bone of the orbital roof and optic canal. At times it is necessary to revisualized the intradural optic nerve in order to extend the epidural orbital unroofing into the optic canal.

After the orbit and optic canal are unroofed and the periorbita exposed, the whitish frontalis nerve can be seen as the outstanding landmark showing the location of the levator and superior rectus muscles. The latter are usually blanched by orbital pathology and are difficult to visualize.

The periorbita must be incised medial to the levator and superior rectus muscle complex, following which an approach is made directly to the optic nerve through orbital fat (Fig. 7). No attempt must be made to dissect the fine structures protected by the orbital fat. Indeed, small cottonoids are used to develop and hold the surgical field at the tumor capsule; three

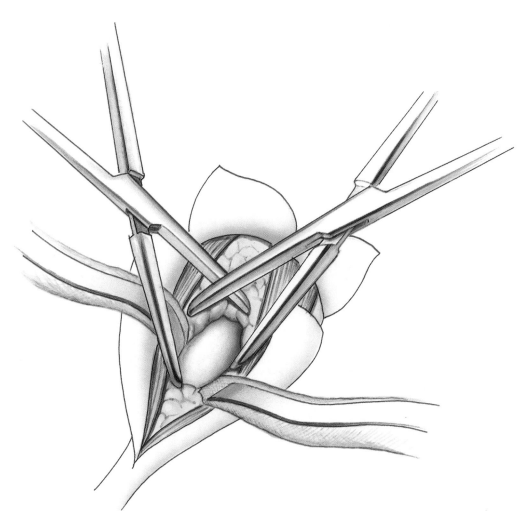

Figure 7. When the periorbita is opened medial to the frontalis nerve and levator muscle, a direct trajectory is made to the tumor-bearing optic nerve. Malleable retractors and cottonoids are used to hold the field. The fine neural structures within the orbit are protected by the orbital fat and no attempt should be made to dissect orbital fat.

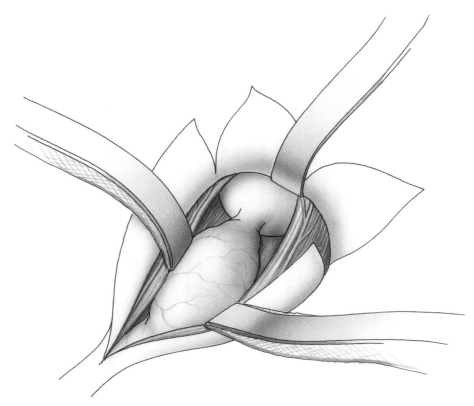

Figure 8.   Once the tumor is identified, three malleable retractors are required to hold the field.

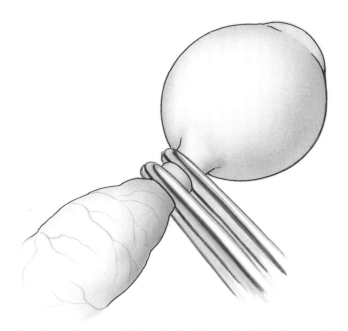

Figure 9.   The tumor-bearing optic nerve is then doubly clamped with long mosquito forceps just behind the globe.

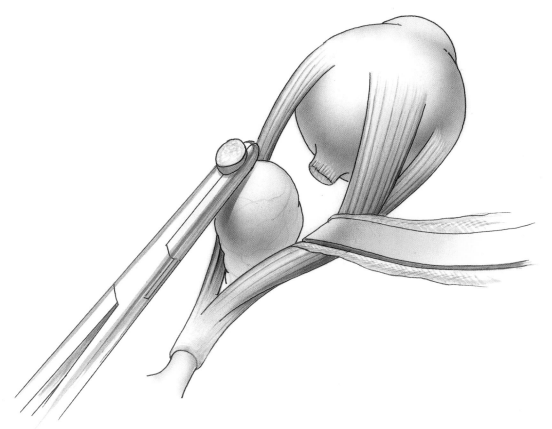

Figure 10. The optic nerve is sectioned between the forceps and the proximal clamp is left as a handle for further dissec- tion of the apical portion of the optic nerve and tumor.

narrow malleable retractors are bent to retract the levator and superior rectus muscles laterally, the medial rectus and superior oblique muscles medially, and orbital fat anteriorly toward the globe (Fig. 8).

If the tumor is large, the capsule may be incised and the tumor gutted to allow collapse and delivery through the relatively small orbital roof defect. In smaller tumors the tumor-bearing optic nerve is doubly clamped directly behind the globe and sectioned between clamps (Fig. 9). This spares injury to the sclera. The proximal clamp is then left on the cut optic nerve and is used as a handle and attention is directed toward the apical region (Fig. 10).

In young children, where the structures are small and dissection difficult, it is sufficient to section the apical optic nerve at the annulus and then to resect the optic nerve intracranially at the cranial end of the optic canal and remove the tumor in two pieces. The intracanalicular portion may be simply coagulated over a nerve hook without fear of recurrence. This is entirely *unacceptable* technique when dealing with optic nerve sheath meningioma because the intracanalicular residual may recur.

In order to remove the optic nerve bearing tumor in one piece from the globe to the chiasmal margin, it is necessary to continue the linear periorbital incision through the canalicular dura (Fig. 11A); in so doing, the levator origin is sectioned because of its medial origin at the annulus (Fig. 11B). The optic nerve is then sharp-dissected from its tether at the annulus of Zinn and the specimen is removed in one piece. If there is bleeding from the ophthalmic artery at the optic canal it is simply bipolar coagulated.

It is imperative that the levator origin be reattached to the annulus with a fine figure of eight suture (5-0 or 6-0) (Fig. 11C). The fourth nerve may or may not be visualized but cannot be spared, and, as indicated, there is little functional or cosmetic consequence of fourth nerve section in a blind eye. By sweeping orbital fat directly on the tumor capsule and protecting it with cottonoids, the medial approach to the optic nerve is relatively safe and affords access without injury to the nerve supply to the levator or superior rectus muscles above or the inferior and medial rectus muscles below the optic nerve.

The cruciate incision in the periorbita is closed with one or several fine sutures and Gelfoam is placed over the roof defect. Although perhaps not mandatory,

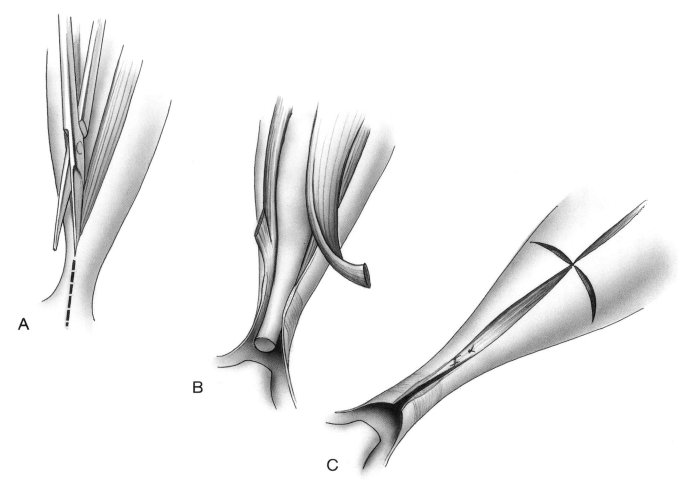

Figure 11. A, the periorbital incision is carried directly through the apical dura, annulus of Zinn, and intracanalicular dura. If not already sectioned at the chiasm, the optic nerve is once again visualized intradurally and sectioned with long fine scissors close to the chiasm. **B,** in doing so, the origin of the levator muscle is sectioned. At this point the entire nerve may be sharp-dissected free from the region of the annulus and removed as one specimen. **C,** once the tumor has been removed, the levator muscle must be sutured to its origin at the annulus and the periorbita closed with one or more fine sutures.

titanium mesh screen is used to bridge this defect to prevent the possibility of pulsating proptosis. This does not interfere with magnetic resonance imaging or CT scanning. It is extremely important that the orbital roof defect be simply bridged and not totally covered, and that the mesh must be bent to reform the *arched* roof of the orbit. Any *flat* repair, as with acrylic, will reduce the orbital volume and result in postoperative proptosis. The orbital bridge need not be sutured in place; it is simply covered with Gelfoam. The reexpanding brain will reposition the dura against it and hold it in place. The dura is then closed in a watertight fashion using 4-0 silk. Gelfoam is placed over the dural suture line, a single epidural Hemovac drain is placed through a posterior trephination, and separate bilateral subgaleal drains are placed through separate stab wounds at the temporal regions bilaterally. Titanium mesh buttons are used to cover the medial-most trephinations. If the temporalis muscle and fascia are meticulously closed at the temporal ridge, no artificial covering is needed for the anterolateral trephination. The pericranium is usually closed with interrupted 3-0 Vicryl; 3-0 Vicryl is also used to close the galea and interrupted 4-0 silk is used to close the scalp. A firm dressing is applied and should not be removed for four or five days to prevent the collection of subgaleal fluid in the frontal region.

After a head dressing is applied it is wise to perform a temporary tarsorrhaphy to allow the placement of a separate pressure dressing over the eye. Should there be marked swelling or postoperative hemorrhage within the orbit, the cornea under pressure is endangered unless the lids are closed in this fashion. The pressure dressing, which should be removed and replaced each day, is maintained until the third or fourth day. Once swelling has subsided, the temporary tarsorrhaphy may be removed. Perioperative and postoperative anticonvulsant therapy is used for three or four months after this exploratory procedure.

SUMMARY

When optic nerve resection is indicated for tumor, the transcranial approach should be the primary approach to avoid leaving residual tumor at the apex and within the optic canal. The primary objective of transcranial orbital exploration for optic nerve glioma is resection of tumor with maintenance of the globe and with an excellent cosmetic result. Complications may be minimized by being familiar with the regional anatomy, by approaching the optic nerve between the levator and superior oblique muscles, by avoidance of dissection of orbital fat and its contents, by developing the field directly on the tumor capsule in the orbit, and by sectioning and resuturing the origin of the levator muscle when the annulus of Zinn must be opened to remove the tumor in one specimen from globe to chiasm.

FIBROUS DYSPLASIA INVOLVING THE CRANIOFACIAL SKELETON

JAMES T. GOODRICH, M.D., PH.D.
CRAIG D. HALL, M.D.

INTRODUCTION

This chapter will deal with fibrous dysplasia of the craniofacial complex, in particular the forehead, orbital rim, lateral and medial orbital walls, the orbital roof, and the optic foramen. The discussion will involve the "worst case scenario," assuming that, if the surgeon can handle this type of case, the simpler cases will be easier to treat.

Fibrous dysplasia can involve the calvarium and any of the upper facial bones. Its etiology is unknown but the pathology involves a replacement of normal bone with a fibro-osseous matrix. The surgical principle involves removing all of the dysplastic bone (or as much as possible) and replacing it with normal calvarial bone harvested from other parts of the head. Fibrous dysplasia can be of a simple type called monostotic, where only one bone unit is involved, or polyostotic, where two or more bones are involved. In this chapter we will deal with the more complicated polyostotic type.

The most common presenting complaints in fibrous dysplasia of the craniofacial complex are proptosis (Figs. 1 and 2), diplopia and headaches, and, in severe cases, progressive blindness due to optic nerve compression.

An x-ray film of the skull will show a sclerotic mass expanding the calvarial and orbital bones. The radiologists typically describe a "ground glass" appearance. There will also be sclerosis or even a cystic appearance to the bone. It is not uncommon to see complete obliteration of the frontal and nasal sinuses. The proptosis is secondary to the orbital fibrous dysplasia compressing the globe and forcing the eye forward. As a result of this, an early presenting complaint can be diplopia.

The principle behind the surgical treatment of fibrous dysplasia of the craniofacial complex is threefold: 1) Since neural compression is common, particularly of the optic nerve, decompression of the nerve is

essential. 2) Removal of *all* dysplastic bone is essential, as any residual can form a new dysplastic center. 3) Use of the patient's own bone for grafts to achieve a satisfactory cosmetic result is preferred.

At the Montefiore Medical Center we have elected to do the reconstruction with calvarial bone which is membranous, because we have found that this significantly lessens the risk of resorption which occasionally occurs with rib (endochrondral bone) grafts placed in the craniofacial region. Another advantage of using calvarial bone is the reduction in operative exposure. This technique also avoids the complications that can occur with rib harvesting, such as pneumothorax and chest wall pain.

PREOPERATIVE EVALUATION

All patients should have x-ray films of the skull in the routine views to document the extent of dysplastic involvement of the skull and surrounding orbital and nasal structures. Computed tomography scanning with bone windows in the axial and coronal views is also performed. If three-dimensional reconstruction is available, it can be extremely helpful in determining preoperatively the amount of bony removal that will be required. We have not found magnetic resonance imaging to be helpful, so we do not use it routinely.

If the optic nerve is compressed, we routinely do visual acuity and visual field testing to have baseline values. Damage to the optic apparatus and to the nerves supplying the extraocular muscles are the most significant complications to be avoided. Subtle damage may already have occurred preoperatively, and it is best to document this prior to any surgical intervention.

Since an extensive resection can involve the frontal and paranasal sinuses we culture the nasal passageways to look for virulent organisms. If any are detected, the patient is placed on an appropriate antibiotic coverage 24 hours before surgery. We routinely start an anti-staphylococcal antibiotic at the time of

15

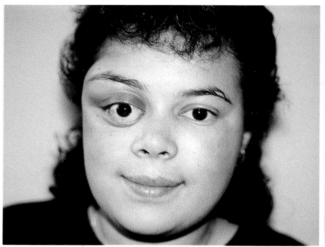 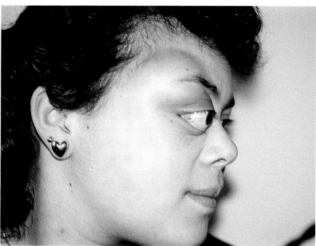

Figures 1 and 2. Frontal and lateral view of a patient with orbital proptosis secondary to fibrous dysplasia. Typical proptosis is evident with fibrous dysplasia involving the right orbital unit including rim, lateral, and medial walls. As a result, the eye is pushed forward and downward. Interestingly, the only visual symptom was double vision; the visual acuity was normal.

anesthetic induction in the operating room. Because the surgical manipulations are extradural, we do not routinely use anticonvulsant medications.

PREPARATION FOR OPERATION

Fibrous dysplastic bone can be and usually is, highly vascular. As a result, the blood loss in these procedures can be quite high. We routinely plan for a blood loss of 3 to 5 units. If the family is cooperative, we ask for pedigree blood donations from the family members one week in advance. If available, a "cell saver" unit can rescue up to 50% of the patient's lost blood volume. Because of the risk of extensive blood loss, all patients require at least two large-bore intravenous lines of 16 gauge or larger. If there is any history of cardiac or pulmonary problems, we routinely put in a central venous pressure line. An arterial line is mandatory for monitoring blood gases, hematocrit, electrolytes, etc. during the procedure. We request an osmostic diuresis, usually with mannitol (0.5 g/kg), at the time of anesthetic induction. A spinal drainage system is placed in the lumbar region to assist in cerebrospinal fluid (CSF) withdrawal and brain relaxation. Because of the extensive exposure and brain relaxation that will be needed (remembering that surgical exposure back to the optic foramen is often necessary), every effort at relaxation must be done to reduce retraction pressure on the frontal lobes. A simple removal of 35 to 50 ml of CSF can cause a dramatic relaxation of the frontal lobes.

The use of steroids is always an issue in these types of cases. On our service we do not routinely use steroids as part of our preoperative management. If there is evidence of postoperative brain or optic nerve edema, the patient will be placed on dexamethasone at that time.

OPERATIVE POSITIONING

The patient is placed in the supine position with the head resting on a cerebellar (horseshoe) headrest (Fig. 3). The head is placed in a slightly extended, brow-up position. Rigid fixation devices like a Mayfield clamp are specifically avoided, as the surgeon will need to move the head (usually never more than 10 to 15 degrees); this flexibility can prove to be very useful.

We also reverse the table so that the head of the patient is at the foot end of the operating table. This allows the surgeon and his assistant to sit with their knees comfortably under the table and not obstructed by the table pedestal or foot unit.

Anesthesia equipment is placed on the side opposite the lesion and parallel to the table. Routine orotracheal intubation is performed. All lines are run off to the side of the anesthesia unit. The operating surgeon is placed at the head of the patient with the assistant to the side. The nurse comes in over the patient's abdomen but is positioned no higher than the mid-thoracic region. This allows the surgeon to be able to move around to see the patient's face fully for cosmetic evaluation. For this reason we also avoid the use of bulky overhead tables, such as the Fallon table.

All of the patients have bilateral tarsorrhaphies prior to formal draping. This prevents unintentional injury to the globe and cornea.

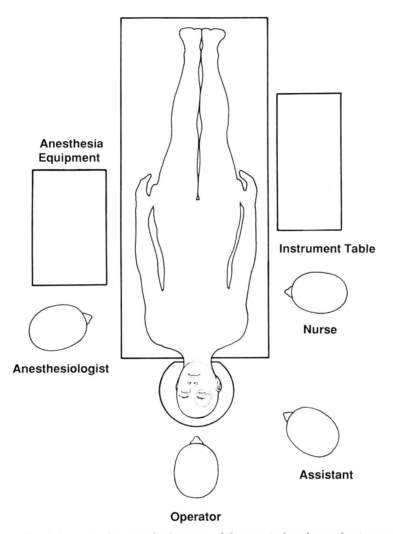

Figure 3. Schematic showing the location of the surgical and anesthesia teams.

SURGICAL DRAPING TECHNIQUES

The head is fully shaved and draped for a bicoronal incision. In addition, both eyes with their tarsorrhaphies must be visible. The facial drape is placed over the nose and nares, but well below the lower orbital rim. This allows the eyes to be visualized during the reconstruction. The rest of the draping can be done according to the surgeon's preference. An important additional point is to keep the drapes reasonably loose, so that the head can be moved.

We routinely run all our suction lines, cautery cords, etc. past the foot of the patient. As both surgeons are sitting, this allows easy mobility of the chair; i.e., they are not rolling over the cords and tubes.

Because the operative site is usually copiously irrigated during the procedure, it is important to have waterproof outer drapes. Some of the newer drapes have large plastic bags for fluid collection; we have found these to be quite useful.

OPERATIVE TECHNIQUE

Skin Incision

Because an extensive exposure of the calvarium and orbits is required, we routinely use a bicoronal incision from tragus to tragus. The incision must be well behind the hairline, both for cosmetic closure and to allow for a large pericranial flap that can be used in the subsequent repair.

Flap Elevation

A full thickness flap is turned following the standard subgaleal plane. It is important to leave the pericranium intact. This is then elevated as a second, separate layer. The flaps are carried down to the orbital rim to the level of the supraorbital nerve and artery. These are frequently encased in a small notch of bone. This notch can be opened with a small Kerrison rongeur or osteotome. It is easier to elevate the artery and nerve with the pericranial layer. It is important to preserve these structures or there will be anesthesia in the forehead postoperatively. The flap must also expose the entire belly of the temporalis muscle and the zygomatic arch. In the midportion of the face the nasal suture should be fully exposed. Using the small periosteal dissector or a Penfield dissector it is possible to come under the orbital rim and dissect it safely back approximately 1 to 2 cm. The temporalis muscle has to be elevated as a unit. Starting at its squamosal insertion, it is elevated using a Bovie electrocautery with a fine needle tip. The dissection is carried out in such a fashion that the temporalis muscle will be elevated from the zygoma back to the ear, fully exposing the pterional "keyhole."

Craniotomy

The craniotomy is carried out to incorporate all of the dysplastic bone in the removal. It is easiest to do the frontal craniotomy by first taking out a forehead bone flap that encompasses as much of the forehead dysplasia as possible (labeled A in Fig. 4). This provides the window which will allow exposure to the orbital roof and walls. We prefer to use a high-speed drill system with a craniotome (e.g., Midas Rex with a B-1 footplate) as this gives a speedy bone removal, thereby decreasing blood loss. We next elevate the frontal lobe with gentle retraction to see how far into the orbital roof the dysplastic bone extends. Then, by further dissecting under the orbital roof, the dysplastic portion can be completely visualized (Fig. 5). There is usually extensive blood supply crossing these planes, so the bleeding can be quite copious. Keep plenty of Avitine and Gelfoam available for packing in these spaces to control the oozing. Once the limits of the dysplastic bone have been determined and the brain is adequately relaxed and retracted, we proceed with the bone resection. Using a combination of osteotomes and a small cutting burr, like the Midas Rex C-1 attachment, the roof is removed as a unit (Fig. 5). It is helpful to have the assistant place a malleable retractor under the orbital roof. This will prevent the drill or osteotome from damaging the orbital contents. On occasion, the dysplasia can go back to the clinoids and orbital foramen. In these cases, the entire roof must be removed (Fig. 5). A small diamond burr on a high-speed drill unit is the best method for removing this part of the bone. It allows the surgeon to remove the bone without injury to the underlying structures. Once this is completed, attention is turned to the lateral orbital wall and zygoma (labeled B in Fig. 4). This portion of the procedure can be done quite easily. The only important points are to have adequate exposure of the zygomatic arch and a good dissection of the orbit. The lateral canthal ligament must be sectioned and then reattached at the end of the procedure. Doing this prior to the medial part will allow easy mobilization of the eye and surrounding structures with minimal trauma.

Next, attention is turned to the most difficult phase—resecting the medial nasal structures (labeled C in Fig. 4). By removing the orbital roof and lateral orbital wall, the surgeon now has some mobility and freedom in moving the eye. If the dysplastic bone involves the nasal bone and medial orbital wall, the medial canthal ligament must be cut. The assistant then retracts the eye laterally, and the bone is removed with an osteotome and fine cutting burr. The frontal sinuses are usually occluded with bone, which can complicate matters. If the sinuses are not occluded, the frontal sinus can be entered and used as an operating space within which to work. Once all the dysplastic bone is removed, the reconstruction is started.

Calvarial Bone Harvesting

By using a bicoronal skin flap, a large amount of normal calvarial bone is exposed. Once the surgeon has resected the dysplastic bone and determined how much bone is needed to reconstruct the defect, a craniotomy is performed on the opposite calvarium (labeled *D* in Fig. 4). Remember that the most useful

bone is over the convexity, where the diploë is well formed. In the squamosal area, the bone thins out and is hard to split. The bone is taken to a sterile table set up next to the operating field. Using a combination of small osteotomes, a fine cutting tip like a Midas Rex C-1, and a reciprocating saw, the bone is split along the diploic space. Copious irrigation is essential, because the bone must not be allowed to heat up; this would lead to dead bone and subsequent necrosis. Once the bone has been split, the inner table of the

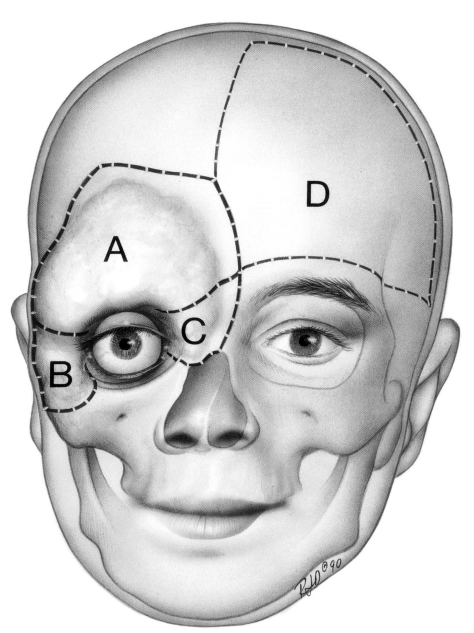

Figure 4. Frontal view showing four-piece bone removal. **A,** frontal bone maximally involved with fibrous dysplasia; **B,** lateral orbital wall; **C,** medial orbital wall. The orbital wall roof which is also removed is not shown in this drawing. **D,** graft from the opposite calvarium.

calvarium is placed back in the harvest site. The outer table, because of its smooth contours, is used as the reconstructing bone.

Craniofacial Reconstruction

The reconstruction is done in the reverse order from the resection. The medial orbital wall is constructed

first and wired or plated into position (labeled *C* in Fig. 6). The nasal bone and cribriform plate are usually the most solid structures to work with. The medial canthal ligament also has to be reattached, which can be done easily through a small drill hole. Next, a piece of bone is fashioned to form the orbital roof. This is an important structure which must be solidly placed (Fig.

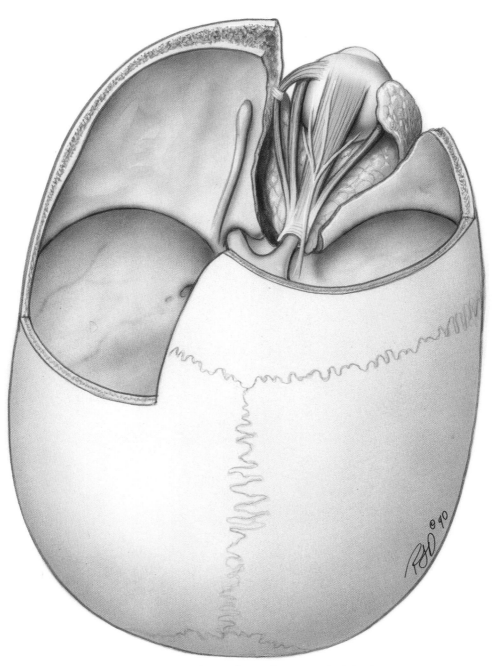

Figure 5.   Schematic drawing showing the frontal fossa after removal of the dysplastic orbital roof and decompression of the optic nerve.

8). If it is not, subsequent proptosis of the eye can occur due to downward pressure of the frontal lobe. The bone used to reconstruct the lateral orbital wall is attached to the roof with either wires or miniplates (labeled *A* in Fig. 6). The squamosal portion of the temporal bone can also act as an excellent place to anchor this bone. The orbital rim is then fashioned and attached medially to the nasal unit and opposite orbital rim (labeled *B* in Fig. 6). This is the key cosmetic unit and must be perfectly placed to avoid facial asymmetry. The rest of the craniotomy is then closed in a mosaic fashion using the remaining pieces of bone. Miniplates have proved to be extremely useful in stabilizing these various bone units.

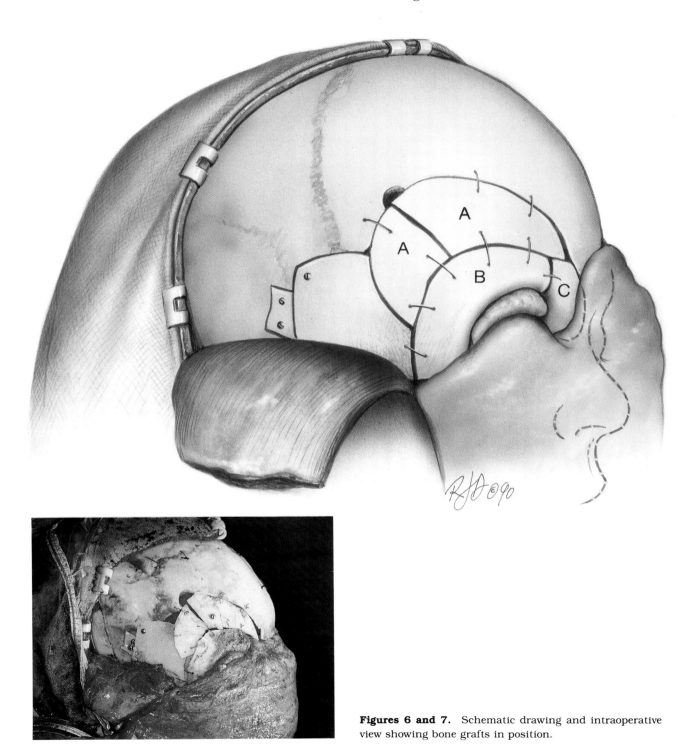

Figures 6 and 7.   Schematic drawing and intraoperative view showing bone grafts in position.

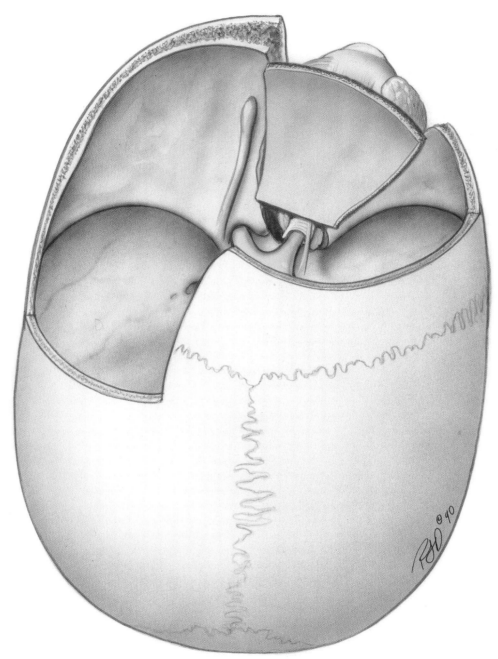

Figure 8. Schematic drawing showing the split thickness calvarial bone graft in position in the orbital
roof region.

Repair of Frontal Sinus

One of the most devastating postoperative complications is infection arising from the sinus. If the frontal sinus is not obliterated by dysplasic bone, it must be cleaned and exenterated of mucosal lining. We routinely cover the sinus with the pericranial flap to isolate it from the epidural space. The same principle applies to the other paranasal sinuses if they are violated.

Pericranial Tissue

The pericranial tissue is a most useful repair structure. It not only provides additional vascularity to the bone but it also helps smooth out the rough contours of the bone that has been harvested and used as grafts. Therefore, we make every effort to use this structure and place it back into its natural anatomical position.

Temporalis Muscle

To prevent a postoperative depressed concavity over the temporal unit, the temporalis muscle is laid back into position. Sometimes a relaxing incision must be made posteriorly to allow the muscle to be advanced forward to cover the keyhole and to be reattached to the zygoma. This is critical or there will be a significant depression over this region postoperatively.

Closure

The closure is done in a routine fashion. Hemostasis must be meticulous because of the amount of dead space that can form. A drain to light suction is placed for at least 24 to 48 hours. A fluid collection next to sinus spaces can lead to a devastating postoperative infection. Scalp closure is done in a routine fashion closing both the subgaleal and skin layers.

POSTOPERATIVE CARE

We routinely place the patients on antibiotics to cover skin organisms and possible nasal contaminants for at least 72 hours. The risk of osteomyelitis is high and can be quite devastating to the patient, so every attempt must be made to avoid it. There may be significant periorbital swelling postoperatively; ice packs are applied to the eye and periorbital regions for symptomatic relief. If there is significant swelling at the end of the operation, we ordinarily leave the tarsorrhaphy in place for about two days. Intensive care for at least 48 hours is mandatory with close monitoring for hemodynamic changes from excessive blood loss and for the development of an epidural hematoma.

The surgeon must always be attentive to postoperative CSF leaks. If any dural tears have occurred they must be repaired meticulously. Should a postoperative CSF leak occur, then placement of a lumbar CSF drain may be necessary to divert the fluid. These usually need to be left in place for five to seven days. However, close attention to dural tears and verifying dural integrity by asking the anesthesiologist to perform Valsalva's maneuver at the end of the case should prevent this problem from occurring.

DEPRESSED SKULL FRACTURE IN ADULTS

FRED H. GEISLER, M.D., PH.D.

DEFINITION

Depressed skull fractures may occur after head trauma. By definition, a depressed skull fracture is a fracture in which the outer table of one or more of the fracture edges is below the level of the inner table of the surrounding intact skull. The greatest bone depression can occur either at the interface of the fracture with the intact skull or near the center of several fracture fragments that are displaced inward. A depressed fracture results when the impact energy is applied over a small contact area. Typical examples include: assaults with a hammer, club, or pipe; sports injuries caused by a hockey stick, golf club, or golf ball; or a motor vehicle accident in which the victim's head strikes either the interior of the car or an object outside the car as he/she is thrown from the vehicle.

PREOPERATIVE EVALUATION

Many patients with depressed skull fractures experience initial loss of consciousness and varying degrees of neurologic deficit. Recovery is determined by the extent of the brain injury. However, one quarter of the patients experience neither loss of consciousness nor neurologic deficit and another quarter experience only a brief loss of consciousness. The diagnosis of a depressed skull fracture is often made on routine skull films by noting either an area of double density (indicative of overlying bone fragments) or the presence of comminuted or circular fractures. However, the full extent and the depth of the fractured fragments are rarely appreciated on these studies. Physical examination of patients with depressed skull fractures is difficult because of scalp mobility and swelling. Scalp mobility can result in nonalignment of the scalp laceration and the depressed skull fracture. Traumatic scalp swelling obscures the step-off at the bony edges, preventing accurate assessment of the extent of skull deformity for the first few days.

A computed tomographic (CT) head scan is the diagnostic method of choice. When the image display

windows are adjusted to optimize bony detail, they display the position, extent, and number of fractures as well as the presence and depth of depression. With the imaging windows set to optimize intracranial contents, the same CT scan also allows an assessment of the underlying brain for contusion or hematoma from superficial penetration of bone fragments, small bone fragments or foreign bodies within the brain substance, and other traumatic intracranial lesions. Occasionally, coronal CT images through fractures near the vertex of the head or extending into the skull base are used to supplement the standard CT images because the depth of a depression is more accurately measured on CT images perpendicular to the depression. Differences between the amount of dural laceration and cortical damage among similar CT scan images occur because the position of the brain, bone fragments, and remaining intact skull at the time of the scan may differ from the actual maximal depth of the fragments at the time of impact. The brain, for example, may undergo linear or rotational movement and the skull can deform temporarily during the impact. Immediately after the injury, the depressed bone fragments tend to rebound partially or spring back as the deformed skull attempts to resume its anatomic shape. Also, only crude estimates of the sharpness of the bone edges can be made from the CT images because the limit of resolution is 1 mm.

RATIONALE FOR SURGICAL TREATMENT

Although a focal neurologic deficit from the altered cortex directly under a depressed bone fracture occasionally improves after elevation of the bone fragments (presumably by increasing local cortical blood flow), this procedure usually produces no neurologic change, implying that cortical damage is inflicted at the time of impact. The brain dysfunction generally undergoes a neurologic recovery phase of several weeks to months, similar to that following a stroke or a head injury without a depressed fracture. The incidence of epilepsy following a depressed skull fracture is apparently determined by the cortical damage at the

25

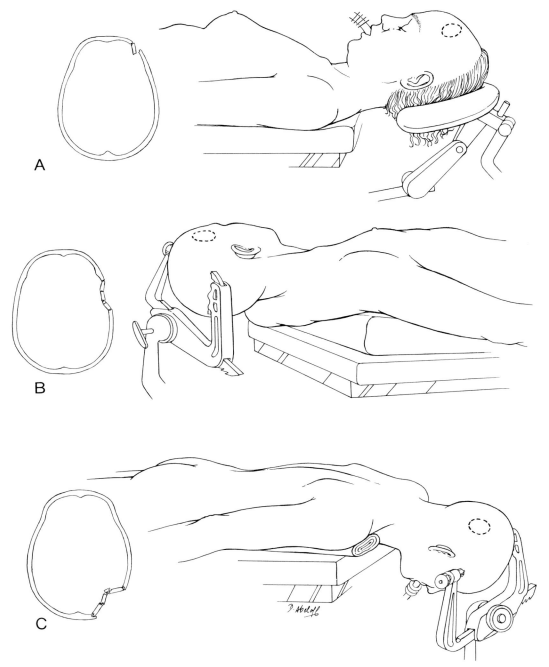

Figure 1. Three different positions used in the management of patients with depressed skull fractures are illustrated along with a diagrammatic representation of CT images through the depressed skull fracture. The position is individualized for each patient with the majority of the surgical area at or near the horizontal plane. The skin incision and location of the midline are marked before draping. **A,** a patient with an anterior frontal depressed skull fracture positioned supine in the horseshoe head holder with the neck flexed 10 degrees in preparation for a bicoronal scalp incision. **B,** a patient with a posterior frontal depressed skull fracture held in the three-point pin skull holder positioned with the head rotated to place the majority of the depressed skull fracture near the horizontal plane. Note the pad under the patient's right shoulder to lessen the rotation of the neck and possible cerebral venous outflow impairment. **C,** a patient with a posterior parietal/occipital depressed skull fracture held in the three-point pin skull holder in the prone position. A 10- to 15-degree rotation of the head can be used to place the surgical area exactly in the horizontal plane. If the neck is rotated, reference to the skin mark at the midline prevents inadvertent extension of the exploration to encroach or cross the midline.

time of impact since it is not altered by the elevation of the fragments. Thus, the treatment of depressed skull fractures is based not on initiating neurologic recovery or preventing epilepsy but, rather, on correction of a cosmetic deformity as well as on prevention of infection in open fractures. The treatment of an individual depressed skull fracture depends on the presence or absence of: 1) cosmetic deformity and its extent; 2) scalp laceration; 3) dural laceration; 4) contusion or laceration of the underlying brain; 5) extension of the fracture over a venous or paranasal sinus; and 6) coexistence of other traumatic intracranial lesions, including epidural, subdural, and intracerebral hematomas, cerebral contusions, midline shift, and ventricular compression.

In closed depressed fractures, the indication for surgery is usually cosmetic, with the procedure performed on an elective basis in the first few days after the trauma when the patient is cleared for elective anesthesia. The location of the depression, thickness of the scalp, and patient's body image perspective are critical to the surgical decision. The forehead is the area where the greatest cosmetic deformity occurs. Depressions of 3 mm or more result in deformities for which most patients request correction. When the orbital rim is involved or the scalp is thin, repair of smaller depressions is often requested. Exploration is more urgent in a patient with a large closed depressed fracture where the radiologic appearance suggests dural laceration, brain penetration, mass effect, or underlying epidural, subdural, or intracerebral hematoma. The hematoma is evacuated, the dura is repaired, and the bone fragments are replaced and wired in anatomic position.

A compound depressed fracture represents a neurosurgical emergency because of the risk of bacterial infection of the contents of the cranial cavity. The initial surgery is performed within 24 hours and usually within the first 12 hours after the accident. The major objectives of the surgery are to: 1) remove contaminated bone fragments and foreign material (hair, cloth, dirt, etc.) in the scalp wound, between the bone fragments, and in the cortex; 2) debride devitalized scalp, dura, and brain; and 3) provide a watertight closure of the dura. Removing devitalized tissues and contaminated material is essential to reduce the incidence of infection. Often foreign material or hair wedged between bone fragments is not visualized through the overlying scalp incision. Thus, simple wound irrigation and closure may be inadequate for the debridement of the foreign material. Dural closure is essential to prevent the leakage of cerebrospinal fluid from the wound and brain herniation into the fracture area. Dural closure also acts as a bacterial barrier, preventing the intracranial spread of infection from the scalp. Cosmetic correction is performed during the initial surgery only if considered safe; otherwise, a cranial defect is left and the cosmetic repair is performed later. The major reasons to postpone the cosmetic repair are preclusion of additional anesthesia by major head injury or multitrauma, gross contamination of wounds where the bone fragments cannot be adequately cleaned, and a surgical delay of more than 24 hours. Both the final neurologic deficit and the incidence of epilepsy are decreased by this management plan because it reduces the potential for intracranial infection and intracerebral hematoma.

OTHER PREOPERATIVE CONSIDERATIONS

Preoperatively, patients receive a single dose of steroids (methylprednisolone sodium succinate, 250 mg, I.V.); no antibiotics are used in open fractures, whereas one dose of a prophylactic antibiotic (such as nafcillin sodium, 1 g, I.V., or vancomycin hydrochloride, 500 mg, I.V.) is used just prior to skin incision in closed fractures. Grossly contaminated material in the scalp wounds and representative bone fragments recovered from the cortex are sent for culture in appropriate medium. The culture results are used to guide antibiotic therapy if an infection occurs following thorough debridement and irrigation during the surgery.

SURGICAL TECHNIQUE

The patient's head is held in place either by the Mayfield three-point head holder or the Mayfield horseshoe. When using the three-point head holder, the surgeon must avoid applying the pins at the fracture sites. If a pin is positioned into a fracture line, it will not only be mechanically unstable but may even extend the fracture or cause displacement of fragments as the head holder is applied. The patient is positioned with the depression in a horizontal plane. Thus, patients with depressions on the forehead are positioned supine, whereas those with depressions in the occipital area are positioned prone (Fig. 1). The draping should allow for extension of the incision if additional exposure is required during the exploration. An example of the surgical treatment of an open depressed skull fracture with intact dura and a bone cranioplasty is shown in Figure 2, A–E, and with dural penetration and cortical laceration in Figure 3, A–K.

In an elective elevation of a closed depressed fracture for cosmetic improvement, the surgeon can use one of several standard scalp incisions behind the hairline. The exact size and placement is determined by: 1) exposing the intact skull for at least 2 cm circumferentially around the depressed fragment, including the larger inner table splinters; and 2) planning to

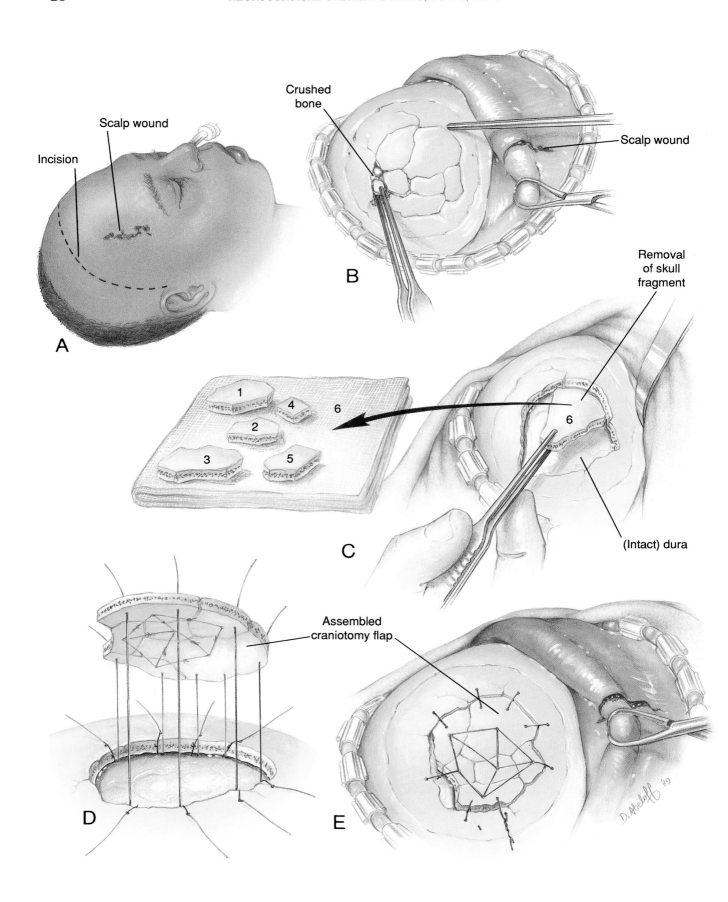

Incision

Scalp wound

A

Crushed bone

Scalp wound

B

Removal of skull fragment

6

(Intact) dura

C

1
4
2
6
3
5

D

Assembled craniotomy flap

E

D. Abeloff '89

Figure 2. The treatment of an open depressed skull fracture with intact dura is shown here. In this example, the large bone fragments were reassembled and used in a bone cranioplasty. **A,** a right frontal scalp wound with an underlying depressed fracture is present. The location of the bicoronal scalp incision is noted in the figure. **B,** note the continuation of the scalp wound on the inside of the scalp flap and multiple small pieces of fractured bone in the superior-posterior area of the depressed skull fracture being debrided in this example. **C,** the large bone fragments are removed using gentle force in an outward direction without angulation. Angulation of the fragments or the application of force while removing them can lever them into or pull them through the dura or cortex. A sharp fragment of inner table not in the visual field can cause either a new or extension of the original dural or cortical laceration if not removed gently. Note that the large fragments are numbered and kept in relative position so that they can be easily reassembled in their anatomic position. If the fragments cannot be easily removed or if no portion of the fracture exposes the dura after the loose fragments are debrided, then a burr hole and circumferential slot craniectomy technique is used, as illustrated in Figure 3. **D,** the bone fragments are reassembled and firmly wired together in anatomic position to form a bone cranioplasty. These wire twists are all bent flat against the inner table. Note the dural tacking sutures circumferentially fixing the dura to the intact skull. The bone assembly is fixed to the skull with circumferential wires. **E,** the wires fixing the bone assembly to the skull are twisted and bent to lie between the bone assembly and the intact skull. The positions of the twisted wires prevent all sharp ends from inadvertently poking the inner aspect of the scalp in normal relative scalp and skull motion with its unpleasant sensation. At this point, the scalp laceration is debrided to normal appearing and vascularized edges and then the galeal layer is sutured from inside. The scalp incision is closed in two layers. Finally, the superficial portion of the scalp laceration is further debrided if necessary and closed with cutaneous sutures.

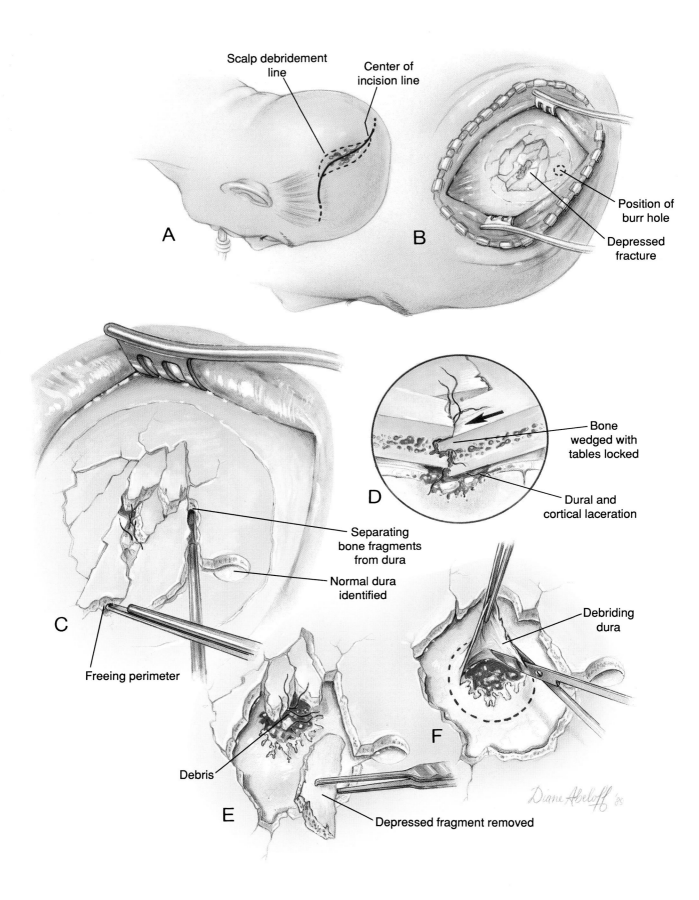

Scalp debridement line

Center of incision line

Position of burr hole

Depressed fracture

A

B

Separating bone fragments from dura

Normal dura identified

Bone wedged with tables locked

Dural and cortical laceration

D

Freeing perimeter

C

Debris

Depressed fragment removed

E

Debriding dura

F

Diane Abeloff '88

Figure 3. This illustrates the treatment of an open depressed skull fracture with dural penetration and brain laceration treated with surgical intervention that includes dural and cortical debridement, dural repair with a graft, and craniectomy. **A,** the scalp debridement lines are centered on the scalp closure line to provide both adequate initial debridement and to allow wound closure after scalp mobilization with minimal tension. **B,** an initial burr hole is placed slightly beyond the edge of the depressed skull fracture to expose normal dura and allow identification of the normal anatomic relationship of inner table contacting dura. **C,** the burr hole is enlarged toward the edge of the depressed skull fracture and then extended into a slot craniectomy starting circumferentially in both directions around the edge of the depressed skull fracture as visualized on the outer table. Note the separation of the bone fragments from the dura as the slot craniectomy is proceeding. This prevents inadvertent dural laceration or debridement with the Kerrison punch at the edge of the craniectomy. The central impacted bone fragments are sequentially unlocked by this procedure. **D,** the bone fragments are locked together in this example because the hard outer table of one fragment was impacted into the soft diploic space of adjacent fragments. Note hair wedged between the bone fragments. The sharp edge of a fracture fragment has lacerated the underlying dura and cortical surface. **E,** the depressed fragments that have been unlocked are removed with a gently outward nontwisting motion. **F,** the dura is debrided to remove shredded and contaminated dura near the dural laceration. Note the small blood clot coating the cortical surface indicating an underlying cortical laceration.

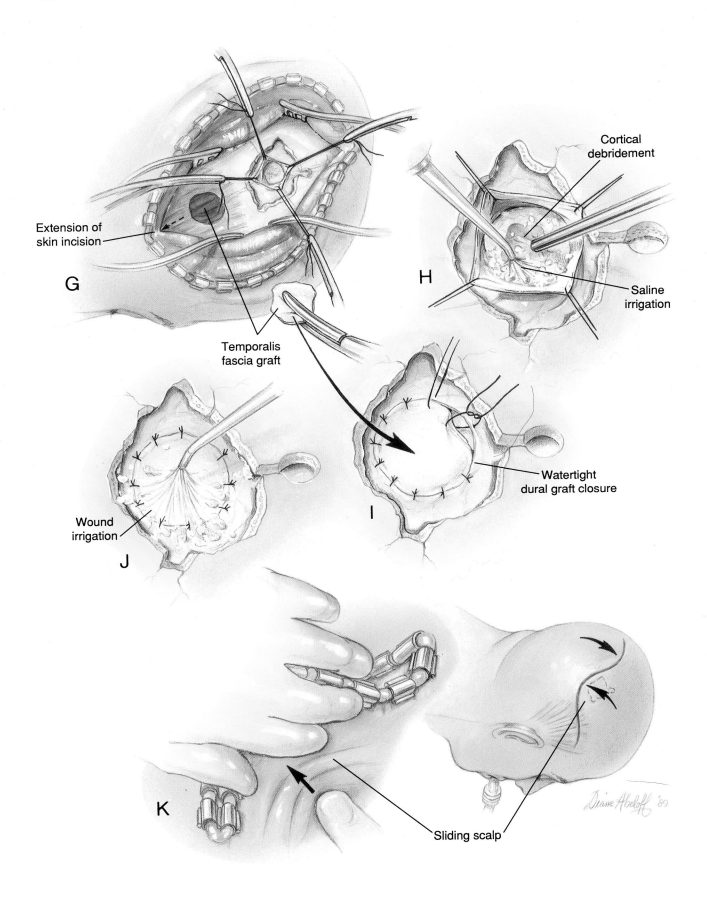

Extension of skin incision

G

Cortical debridement

H

Saline irrigation

Temporalis fascia graft

Wound irrigation

J

I

Watertight dural graft closure

K

Sliding scalp

Diane Abeloff '89

Figure 3. (*continued*) **G,** the inferior end of the scalp incision is extended to expose the temporalis fascia for harvesting a portion as a dural graft. **H,** the pulped and contaminated cerebral cortex is debrided gently with normal saline irrigation and suction. Hemostasis is obtained with bipolar coagulation on the cortex. **I,** the dura is closed watertight with interrupted or running dural sutures. **J,** after dural closure, the wound is copiously irrigated with antibiotic solution. **K,** the scalp wound is closed by manually sliding the skin edges together to eliminate the gap produced by the scalp debridement and then by sewing in two layers with galeal and cutaneous sutures.

provide pericranium or temporal fascia for a dural graft in case it is needed to repair the dura. The curvilinear "S" incision (Fig. 3A) and the flap (Fig. 2, A and B) are the two varieties of scalp incisions. The S incision is useful in 1- to 6-cm diameter depressions behind the hairline because it is easily extended should more exposure be required. A flap incision must be made of adequate size initially because it cannot be enlarged without adding a "T" to the incision, with its potential healing problems. In cases in which an underlying intracranial lesion requires surgical attention, a large frontotemporal-parietal scalp flap is made that allows exposure of both the intracranial lesion and the depressed skull fracture.

The scalp laceration associated with a compound depressed skull fracture is usually stellate or contains an area of contused/devitalized tissue. These areas require debridement to normal scalp to prevent breakdown of the covering over the depressed fracture site. If a breakdown occurs, it usually cannot be treated with local care measures; removal of the bone, skin debridement/rotation, and delayed cranioplasty may often be necessary. The skin flap is planned with consideration of scalp closure strategy after debridement. The S incision allows local debridement by increasing the width of its center and then sliding the two sides together (Fig. 3, A and K). Either the flap incision has to be very large to allow for debridement and suturing in its center (for example, a bicoronal skin flap for a forehead laceration with the debridement and repair of the forehead scalp (as shown in Fig. 2, A and B), or else the debrided area must be on one of the edges so that the two sides of the incision can be slid together. When intact, the pericranium is carefully opened and saved for harvest later as a dura graft or closure over the fracture site for an additional barrier protecting the bone cranioplasty and the brain from a scalp infection. However, if the pericranium is shredded and or contaminated, then it is debrided.

Once the depressed skull fracture is exposed with a margin of 2 cm circumferentially around it, a decision as to how to remove the bone fragments is made based on 1) how firmly the bone chips are wedged together and with the surrounding skull and 2) the amount of angulation or twisting necessary to remove the individual fragments. The surgeon must consider the likelihood that the visualized fragments are only the top portion of a far larger fragment with razor-sharp edges already in or directly on top of the cortex.

Occasionally, the fragments are loose and are easily removed from the wound in a straight linear fashion outward from the brain (Fig. 2, B and C). These fragments are not wedged in place and do not tamponade vessels since they contain no compressive forces. More commonly, however, the bone fragments are wedged

firmly in place as a result of the mechanical configuration of the diploic bone of the skull: the outer table locks either into the diploic space or under the inner table; the inner table can lock under itself (Fig. 3D). The diploic layer is soft and compressible when compared to the cortical tables. During the impact, the diploic layer adjacent to the fracture edges undergoes compression and remodeling, filling the spaces between the locked tables and firmly fixing them in place. In most cases, a burr hole to establish the normal skull/dura relationship (Fig. 3C) is made just adjacent to the depressed area in the outer table away from the areas shown on the CT to have radial splinters of fractures in the inner table and also away from the venous sinuses. The burr hole is then extended into a small slot craniectomy with a Kerrison punch (2- or 3-mm, 40- or 90-degree upbiting). To accomplish this, the dura is first stripped from the skull for a few millimeters in the direction of the planned slot craniectomy using a smooth dissector such as a Penfield No. 3 or No. 4. Then the overlying bone is removed with the Kerrison punch, taking care not to inadvertently place the lower jaw of the Kerrison punch into the subdural space and debride dura (Fig. 3C). The skull/dural interface is carefully followed to the edge of the fracture of the outer table. Occasionally, the skull/dural relationship is initially visualized between fracture fragments and the strip craniectomy can be started there. The outer table limit of the fracture is then followed circumferentially in both directions with a Kerrison punch. As this circumferential, thin, ring-shaped craniectomy cut is being completed, pieces of the fractured bone will become separated from the other pieces and the intact skull, allowing atraumatic removal. When the circumferential cut has been completed with the Kerrison punch where needed and all bone fragments in the center of the depressed fracture have been removed, the skull edges are all inspected for remaining splinters of the inner table and dural lacerations. Remaining splinters of bone under the skull edge are debrided with a Kerrison punch, reaching under the edge. Care is taken to preserve the largest possible fragments of bone and to note carefully the interrelationship of the fragments if a repair of the cranial defect is to be performed at the initial procedure (Fig. 2C). This procedure is not necessary if the operative goal is to leave a craniectomy, planning a delayed secondary cosmetic repair; in these cases, the depressed fragments can be reduced in size for atraumatic removal with a rongeur (Leksell or Smith-Petersen) or a Kerrison punch.

Depressed skull fractures located over a venous sinus or extending into the frontal air sinus require special handling. The surgical elevation of fractures over a venous sinus may involve massive blood loss if a depressed fragment has been plugging a sinus tear. Unless grossly contaminated with foreign material, presenting as a major cosmetic deformity, or causing intracranial hypertension secondary to sinus occlusion, such fractures are managed with scalp debridement and copious irrigation, followed by serial postoperative CT scans for signs of brain abscess for at least a year. If this fracture requires debridement and elevation, then four burr holes (two proximal and two distal, one on each side of the sinus) are made with the fracture area in the center of the rectangle and then connected with a cranial saw. The entire craniotomy flap with the depressed fracture within is then elevated. Massive bleeding can occur with this elevation until proximal and distal control of the sinus is obtained. If the fracture involves the frontal sinus, the sinus is cranialized by first stripping its mucous membrane completely and removing the posterior wall of the sinus and then plugging the ostium with the remaining mucous membrane and applying cautery. Bone chips harvested from intact noncontaminated skull in the periphery of the surgical field or a muscle graft from the temporalis muscle are then laid over the ostium.

After the bone fragments have been completely removed, the dura is fully inspected. If the dura is intact, it is not opened unless the CT scan indicated an intracerebral or subdural lesion requiring further operative therapy. Shredded dura is debrided (Fig. 3F). Small dural lacerations are enlarged to allow inspection of the cortex. Superficial hematomas on the cortex and debris are removed with gentle irrigation and suction. Brain that has been pulped by the indriven fragments is removed with gentle suction until normal brain is exposed and the fragments and debris are removed (Fig. 3H). Gentle irrigation with normal saline via a 10-ml syringe with a No. 18 angiocatheter with the tip positioned in the depth of a cortical laceration can often deliver deep bone chips and debris, minimizing the amount of cortical resection. Bipolar coagulation is used for hemostasis. The dura is then closed water-tight using 4-0 silk or braided nylon (Nurolon) suture with a dural graft, if necessary, of pericranium or temporal fascia. After the dura is closed, the wound is irrigated with copious quantities of bacitracin (50,000 units in 1 liter of normal saline irrigation). This antibiotic irrigation is used for mechanical debridement of the skull and scalp before scalp closure.

In most cases, the large bone fragments are saved for the cranioplasty at the end of the operation (Fig. 2, C, D, and E). These fragments are first washed in 10% povidone-iodine (Betadine) solution to remove hair, dirt, foreign debris, and devitalized tissue and are then rinsed thoroughly in normal saline. They are then reassembled into the shape of the skull before the fracture to resemble a craniotomy flap. They are wired together with stainless steel wire (3-0, No. 24, or No. 26 monofilament surgical suture) with the twists on the inside of the bone and flush with the inner table. Dural tacking sutures of 4-0 silk or braided nylon are used to hold the dura to the skull edges. In larger repairs a central dural tacking suture is also used. This is inserted by first making a single pass through the dura directly below two holes in the bone assembly. The two ends of this central dural stitch are then passed through these two holes and tied to fix the center of the dura to the bone assembly after it has been secured in final position. The reconstructed craniotomy flap is now wired into place at several circumferential points. The scalp is closed with absorbable suture (2-0 Polyglactin 910) in the galea layer and skin staples or 3-0 nylon suture to close the cutaneous layer. A Jackson-Pratt drain is used in the subgaleal space for 24 hours in those cases where fracture lines or contused scalp does not allow complete hemostasis with cautery to be obtained before closure. Postoperative x-ray films of the skull and a CT scan of the head with both soft tissue and bone imaging display windows are obtained as a base line for comparison with the same studies obtained several months or years later which are used for the assessment of bone incorporation/absorption and the cranial shape.

CERVICAL HEMILAMINECTOMY FOR EXCISION OF A HERNIATED DISC

ROBERT H. WILKINS, M.D.
SARAH J. GASKILL, M.D.

INTRODUCTION

A cervical disc herniation usually occurs in a posterolateral direction, compressing the ipsilateral exiting nerve root (Fig. 1). The most commonly affected cervical disc is the one between the C-6 and C-7 vertebrae, and this C6-7 disc herniation compresses the C-7 nerve root.

The patient with a suspected cervical disc herniation usually presents with pain in the neck that extends into one upper extremity in a radicular fashion. Loss of neurological function appropriate to the affected nerve root may also be present. Such a patient is managed first by rest, analgesics, a muscle relaxant, and/or cervical traction. The usual criteria for proceeding with further diagnostic tests and therapy are: 1) absence of improvement with the measures just mentioned, 2) significant weakness or marked hypesthesia in an important area (e.g., the dominant thumb and index finger), or 3) evidence of myelopathy.

PREOPERATIVE CONSIDERATIONS

Plain x-ray films of the cervical spine are helpful in assessing the presence and degree of cervical spondylosis and in identifying another cause of neck and arm pain such as a metastatic carcinoma. In our opinion, magnetic resonance imaging is not as sensitive in the identification of a cervical disc herniation as is cervical myelography followed by computed tomography scanning, so we ordinarily obtain the latter studies to verify the clinical diagnosis.

The usual posterolateral cervical disc herniation can be exposed either through an anterior approach, which involves removing the intervertebral disc, or through a posterior approach, which involves removing lateral portions of two adjacent laminae and the medial portion of the facet joint. If a disc herniation has occurred with a direct posterior (central) vector, and is causing myelopathy, the anterior approach is preferred because the surgeon can remove the herniated disc without manipulating the spinal cord (and possibly increasing the myelopathy). However, for the more common posterolateral disc herniation that is causing a radiculopathy and no myelopathy, we prefer the posterior approach because of its simplicity: it does not involve risk of injury to the anterior structures of the neck, such as the esophagus and the ipsilateral recurrent laryngeal nerve; it does not involve bone grafting or a second surgical incision; and, in our hands, it takes less time than an anterior cervical discectomy and the patient recovers more quickly.

The posterior approach to a cervical herniated disc through a partial hemilaminectomy can be performed with the patient in a prone, lateral, or sitting position. We prefer the sitting position because there is less venous congestion, the anatomical alignment of the spine is easy for the surgeon to visualize mentally after the patient is draped, and the blood and irrigation solution run out of the exposure rather than pooling within it. However, when the sitting position is used, we think that Doppler monitoring should be performed for venous air embolism and that an intra-atrial catheter should be placed before the operation is begun, to permit the aspiration of any air that might enter the right atrium through the venous system. In actuality, venous air embolism seldom occurs during operations for cervical disc herniation, although it is common during posterior fossa operations in the sitting position. We may be overly cautious in using the Doppler monitor and the intra-atrial catheter.

SURGICAL TECHNIQUE

The patient usually arrives in the anesthesia induction room wearing elastic antiembolism stockings which were ordered the previous day as part of the routine preoperative orders. If not, the patient's lower extremities are wrapped with elastic wraps to prevent the pooling (and thrombosis) of venous blood in the lower extremities during the operation and in the immediate postoperative period. A restraining strap is placed across the patient to prevent a fall off the oper-

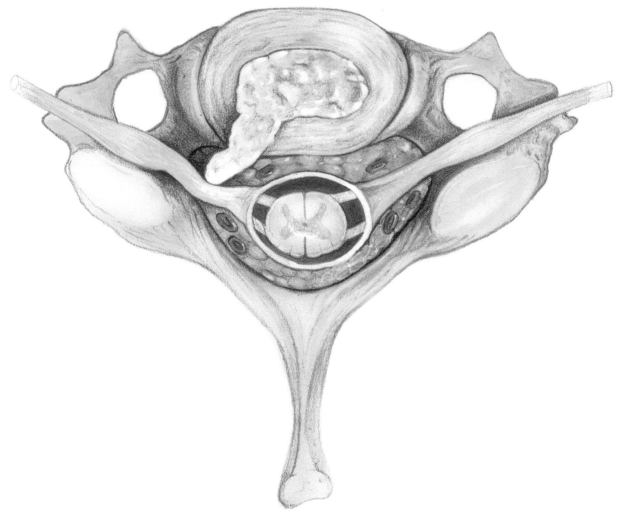

Figure 1. Posterolaterally herniated cervical disc compressing a nerve root.

ating table. A catheter is inserted into an upper extremity vein and intravenous fluids are begun. Prophylactic antibiotics are also given. We follow the Malis regimen, giving 1 g of vancomycin intravenously in 250 ml of 5% dextrose in distilled water or in 0.25 N saline over at least one hour and giving 80 mg of tobramycin intramuscularly. In addition, streptomycin is added to the irrigating fluid used during the operation, at a concentration of 50 μg/ml.

An intra-atrial catheter is inserted, usually via the basilic or cephalic vein. When these veins cannot be used successfully, the catheter is inserted via the internal jugular vein. Its position is verified by a portable x-ray film of the chest. A vascular catheter is also placed in the radial artery to permit the direct monitoring of arterial blood pressure. A urinary catheter is usually not inserted because of the relatively short duration of the operation.

After the induction of anesthesia, the patient's eyes are protected by ophthalmic ointment and eyelid tapes or adhesive plastic eyelid covers. A three-point head clamp is applied, and the operating table is adjusted such that the patient comes into a sitting position, with a bolster under the buttocks. Pillows are placed beneath the knees so the hips and knees are each flexed to about 100 to 120 degrees. The patient's arms are usually placed in the lap, and the head clamp is fixed to the table with the patient's head in straight alignment and flexed somewhat forward. The normal headrest is removed from the table to expose the posterior surface of the neck and upper thorax. Care is taken to prevent direct pressure against any superficial nerve, such as the ulnar nerve at the elbow and the common peroneal nerve at the knee.

The posterior surface of the neck is prepared with antiseptic solutions and dried. The spinous processes

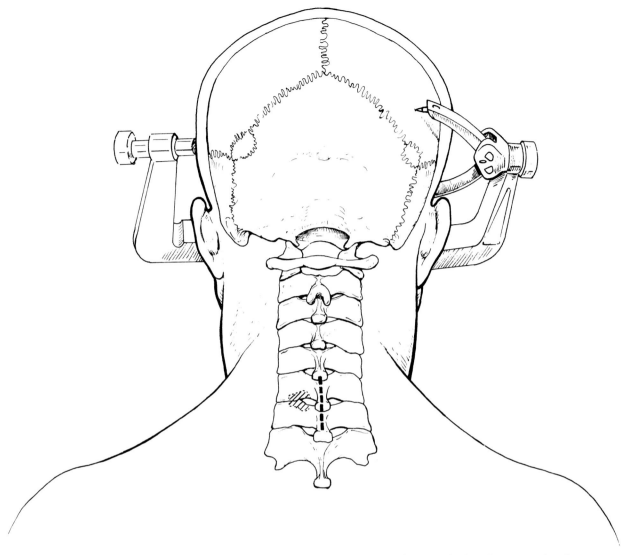

Figure 2. The skin incision (*dotted line*) used to expose a herniated disc between the C-6 and C-7 vertebrae.

are palpated by the surgeon to aid in planning the incision. The spinous process of the seventh cervical vertebra is ordinarily the most prominent, which can be verified on the lateral x-ray film that was made during the patient's diagnostic workup. The line of the proposed incision is marked on the skin (Fig. 2). The operative area is then draped as a sterile field, using, along with the towels and drapes, an adhesive transparent plastic skin covering. Just before the operation is begun, a portable x-ray machine is positioned on the same side of the table as the anesthesiologist, to permit a lateral localization film to be made after the ipsilateral laminae are exposed.

The incision is carried through the skin and subcutaneous tissues down to the posterior aspects of the spinous processes. The fascia is divided along the side of the spinous processes with cutting cautery, and the ipsilateral paravertebral muscles are stripped away from the spines and laminae by subperiosteal dissection using a periosteal elevator. Adherent muscle strands and tendons are divided with curved Mayo scissors. A Williams or Scoville retractor is then inserted to maintain the exposure of the laminae and the facet joint (Fig. 3A).

A metallic marker, such as a No. 4 Penfield dissector, is placed at the facet joint and a lateral x-ray film is made to verify the level. If the marked joint is the correct one, the surgeon proceeds; otherwise the surgeon enlarges the exposure to arrive at the proper facet joint.

With a cup curette, soft tissue is removed from the lateral aspects of the appropriate laminae and from the facet joint. The inferior edge of the superior lamina is exposed in this way, and a portion of it is removed

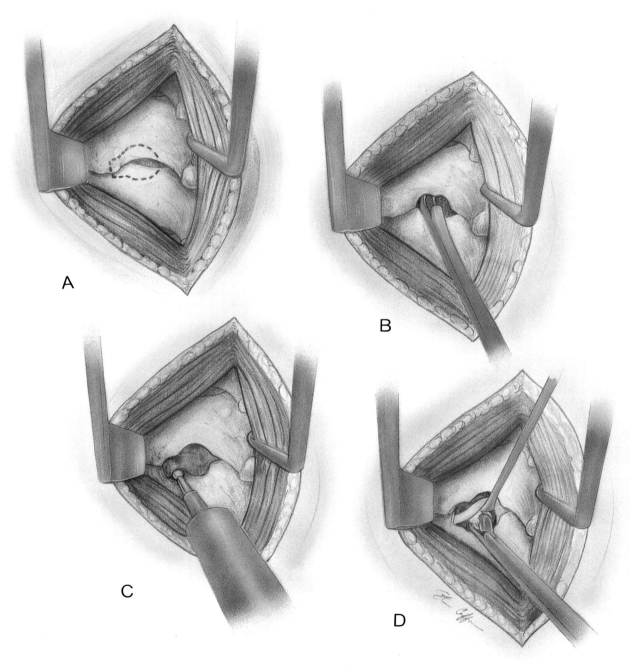

Figure 3.   **A,** the paravertebral muscles have been stripped away from the laminae and spinous processes of C-6 and C-7 and a self-retaining retractor has been inserted. The area within the *dotted keyhole line* represents the extent of bone removal. **B,** a portion of the inferior edge of the superior lamina is removed with Kerrison rongeurs. **C,** the medial aspect of the facet joint is drilled away using a diamond burr. **D,** herniated disc material is removed from under the axilla of the C-7 nerve root.

with Kerrison rongeurs (Fig. 3B). The superior rim of the inferior lamina is removed laterally in similar fashion.

The medial aspect of the facet joint is removed along the exiting nerve root, to expose its posterior surface. This can be done with a small Kerrison rongeur, but if the nerve root is already compressed within the intervertebral foramen it may be compressed further by the insertion of the footplate of the rongeur. Thus, it is safer to expose the nerve root with a diamond burr (Fig. 3C), using constant irrigation during the drilling to avoid thermal injury to the nerve. The bone is drilled down to a thin remaining shell, which is then removed with a small cup curette.

The ligamentum flavum is removed to expose the lateral aspect of the dura mater within the spinal canal and the medial aspect of the nerve root. The epidural veins may be coagulated with bipolar current (with care taken to avoid thermal or electrical injury to the nerve root and spinal cord) or may be compressed temporarily by cottonoid pledgets with radiopaque markers (having attached strings that extend out of the wound as a reminder to the surgeon to remove them before the closure).

The disc herniation is usually best approached under the axilla of the nerve root (Fig. 3D). With gentle superomedial retraction by an instrument such as a No. 4 Penfield dissector, the herniated disc material is exposed. If the posterior longitudinal ligament is still intact over the disc protrusion, it should be incised with a No. 11 scalpel blade. The disc herniation is removed with a small pituitary rongeur. Additional disc fragments can sometimes be squeezed into view by pressing forward on the posterior longitudinal ligament with a blunt nerve hook or small dissector. These fragments are then removed as well. The disc space itself is not entered. Before closure, the area anterior to the nerve root and the adjacent dura mater is palpated with a blunt nerve hook or a small dissector to verify that all obtainable disc fragments have been removed and that the nerve root has been decompressed (i.e., is slack). The surgeon must be careful to avoid vigorous or prolonged manipulation of the nerve root, which may injure the root and result in unnecessary postoperative pain or neurological dysfunction. Occasionally the disc herniation is best approached at the shoulder of the nerve root rather than the axilla; the steps in exposure and removal of the disc fragments are essentially the same. With either route the surgeon must be certain that the protruding material is the disc herniation. At times, the nerve root will be found to be in two parallel parts; the risk is that the surgeon may retract one part and incise the other, thinking it is the disc herniation.

We usually cover the exposed dura and nerve root with absorbable gelatin sponge, but this step can be omitted. The muscles are reapproximated to the interspinous ligament or ligaments with interrupted sutures, and the fascia is closed with similar sutures. After closure of the subcutaneous tissues and skin, a sterile dressing is applied and the patient's head holder is detached from its support. The operating table is flattened to bring the patient again into a supine position. The head holder is removed from the patient's head, and the pin puncture sites are covered with an antibiotic ointment. The anesthetic is reversed. The eye covers are removed. The patient is extubated and sent to the recovery room. The intra-arterial and intravenous catheters and the leg wraps or stockings are removed subsequently, as appropriate.

POSTOPERATIVE COURSE

After the anesthetic has worn off, the patient may be out of bed as comfort permits. Medication is given as needed to provide adequate pain relief. We ordinarily do not recommend the use of a cervical collar. The patient is encouraged to begin restoring the range of neck movement to normal. An exercise program is initiated to reverse any residual upper extremity weakness. The patient is discharged from the hospital when sufficient comfort has been achieved, usually on about the fifth postoperative day. The skin sutures are removed before discharge. The patient increases activity gradually at home and returns in one month for reevaluation. Ordinarily, the patient is released to return to work at that time.

LATERAL SPHENOID WING MENINGIOMA

JOSEPH RANSOHOFF, M.D.

PATIENT SELECTION

A lateral sphenoid wing meningioma may grow to a large size before it causes any neurological symptoms. This tumor bridges the sphenoid wing and can grow symmetrically in the anterior and middle fossae or more toward one or the other. As the tumor enlarges it gradually displaces the adjacent cortex and at the same time the knee of the middle cerebral artery and only rarely surrounds or encases this vessel. The blood supply to these tumors is mainly from the extracranial circulation, including middle meningeal and superficial temporal arteries.

The symptomatology may be unilateral headaches, often misinterpreted as migraine, with radiation to the forehead and homolateral eye, and seizures which may be of the focal motor or the partial complex type. Very late in the course of the disease, signs of increased intracranial pressure and/or intellectual deterioration may occur.

The decision to undertake surgical removal of the lateral sphenoid wing meningioma is based on the size of the tumor, the patient's age, the patient's general medical condition, the presence or absence of cerebral edema, and shift of intracranial structures. Whereas there is no alternative method of management other than surgical excision and the use of anticonvulsants to control seizures, relatively small tumors in patients over age 70 can be safely observed with serial computed tomography (CT) or magnetic resonance imaging (MRI) scans. The risks of surgical intervention are postoperative hemorrhage and medical complications which in a healthy individual should be no more than 5%. The specific risk in these tumors relates to potential damage to the middle cerebral artery with subsequent neurologic deficit. Radiation therapy in these globular tumors is not indicated except for en plaque residual tumor following surgery. The value of "radiosurgery," either with gamma knife or modified linear accelerator, in small tumors in poor-risk patients remains to be evaluated.

DIAGNOSTIC EVALUATION AND PREOPERATIVE CONSIDERATIONS

CT and MRI scans without and with contrast enhancement are clearly the major diagnostic tools in the initial evaluation of these patients prior to surgery. The enhanced MRI study will not only demonstrate the bulk of the tumor but also the degree of dural involvement which may extend beyond the limits of the globular mass and can be of great importance in planning for a total surgical removal. Furthermore, the displacement and/or involvement of the middle cerebral artery can generally be seen on the MRI scan and gives a clear indication as to the surgical risks related to damage of this vessel.

Cerebral angiography is of great assistance in carrying out surgery in view of the fact that the major blood supply to this tumor arises almost solely from the extracranial circulation (Fig. 1A), which lends itself ideally to superselective catheterization and preoperative embolization (Fig. 1B). A postembolization MRI scan as well as a postembolization CT scan can demonstrate the degree of blood supply of the tumor arising from the intracranial circulation and aid in operative planning as well as in detailing the potential risks to the patient and family (Fig. 2, A and B).

Corticosteroids are used in the perioperative period and are instituted the night before surgery unless, of course, the patient has required longer term use of steroids for control of cerebral edema; 125 mg of Solu-Medrol is administered intravenously the night before surgery, the morning of surgery, and every 6 hours thereafter for 24 to 48 hours depending on the patient's condition. Thereafter, a rapid or slow steroid taper is appropriate, depending on the patient's postoperative status. Anticonvulsants (either phenobarbital or Dilantin) are administered preoperatively even in those patients who have not had seizures, with appropriate blood levels being ascertained prior to the initiation of surgery. It seems that Dilantin is poorly tolerated by the elderly patient, and therefore we have tended in more recent times toward the increased use of phenobarbital. If the patient has partial complex

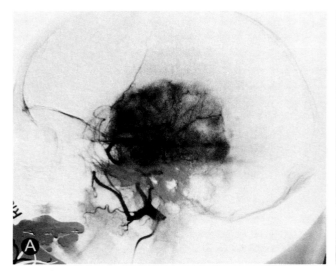

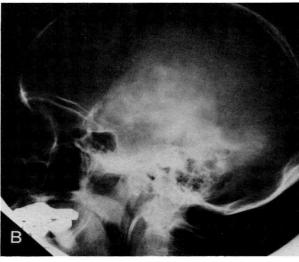

Figure 1. **A,** lateral selective external angiogram prior to embolization. **B,** lateral x-ray film of the skull after emboliza- tion showing the cast of the tumor produced by Gelfoam powder emboli impregnated with Conray.

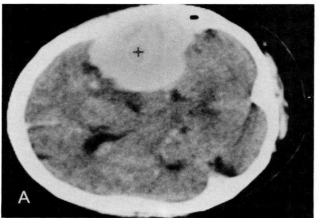

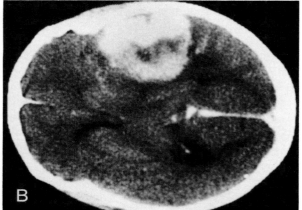

Figure 2. **A,** contrast-enhanced CT prior to embolization. **B,** contrast-enhanced CT after embolization showing tumor necrosis.

seizures, phenobarbital may be replaced with Tegretol in the postoperative period.

SURGICAL TECHNIQUE

There are no special precautions in terms of anesthetic technique in the management of these tumors. Mannitol (250 ml of a 20% solution) is administered intravenously over a period of 15 to 20 minutes as the skin incision is being made. An indwelling urinary catheter is essential. Pneumatic compression boots can be used in an effort to prevent postoperative pulmonary embolism. These must be applied in the operating room once a patient has been anesthetized but should not be used if the patient has been at bed rest for a significant period of time prior to surgery. They are then continued until the patient is fully ambulatory.

Skin Incision and Bone Flap

After induction, the patient's head is shaved and a Faulkner-type incision is marked on the scalp (Fig. 4A). For right-sided incisions a shoulder roll is placed beneath the right shoulder and the head turned toward the left side. The Mayfield three-pin head holder is applied in such a way that the sprocket for attachment to the operating table will be directed perpendicular to the floor when the patient's head is turned 60 degrees to the left of midline. A single pin of the head holder is placed ipsilateral to the skin incision and this should penetrate the skull approximately 4 cm posterior to the external auditory meatus. The head is then secured to the operating table using the Mayfield table clamp so that the head is elevated above the heart level, rotated 60 degrees, and slightly extended, and the operating table is slightly flexed (Fig. 3). After the skin is cleansed, the incision is marked on the scalp using a No. 10 blade starting at the level of the zygoma a few millimeters anterior to the tragus and is extended superiorly behind the hairline curving anteriorly to end 3 cm lateral to the midline. The posterior limb of the incision is modified to accommodate tumors which extend more posteriorly into the temporal fossa. Following draping and infiltration of the planned incision line with 1% lidocaine containing epinephrine, the incision is started at the zygoma and carried down through the galea to the areolar connective tissue overlying the temporalis fascia. Care is taken in this region to identify the superficial temporal artery and, if necessary, to dissect it using Metzenbaum scissors in order to retract it anteriorly with the reflected scalp flap. Occasionally, it becomes necessary to sacrifice the posterior branch of this artery. Above the superior temporal line the incision is carried down to the periosteum and, following the application of Raney clips to control bleeding, the skin is reflected anteriorly using an elevator to dissect through the subgaleal connective tissue. A sponge roll is used to support the base of the scalp flap while it is retracted toward the base and held using skin hooks (Fig. 4B). The periosteum over the superior temporal line is then incised along its superior margin using a No. 10 blade

and the periosteum is stripped from the outer table of the bone and reflected anteriorly. Using a Bovie electrocautery, the temporalis muscle and fascia are incised beginning at the level of the zygoma, extending superiorly to end at the zygomatic process of the frontal bone. This frees a large portion of the temporalis muscle to be reflected posteriorly away from the area of craniotomy, thus avoiding injury to the frontalis branch of the facial nerve. In this way this branch of the facial nerve is carried anteriorly and inferiorly with the remaining portion of the temporal muscle and fascia (Fig. 4C). A Bovie electrocautery is used to separate the remaining temporal muscle from the temporal crest and, most importantly, from the zygomatic process of the frontal bone anteriorly.

With the bisected temporalis muscle reflected anteriorly and posteriorly away from the pterion, two burr holes are placed, one just superior to the zygoma near the floor of the middle fossa and the second just posterior and inferior to the frontal process of the zygoma which is the floor of the frontal fossa. A craniotome is used to develop a cranial opening beginning with the temporal burr hole and extending anteriorly until the sphenoid ridge is encountered. The craniotome is then withdrawn and redirected through the frontal burr hole and again a cranial groove developed posteriorly until the sphenoid wing is encountered. Following stripping of the dura from the inner table of the calvarium, the craniotome is then directed from the temporal burr hole superiorly to develop a cranial flap which extends a few centimeters superior to the superior temporal line and anteriorly onto the supraorbital rim and floor of the frontal fossa. The resulting cranial

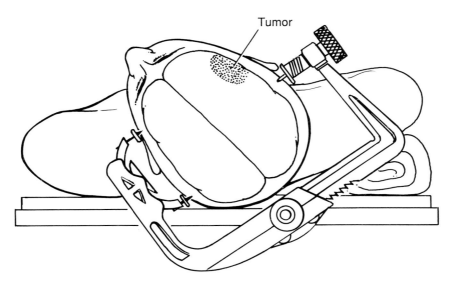

Figure 3. Patient position on the operating table.

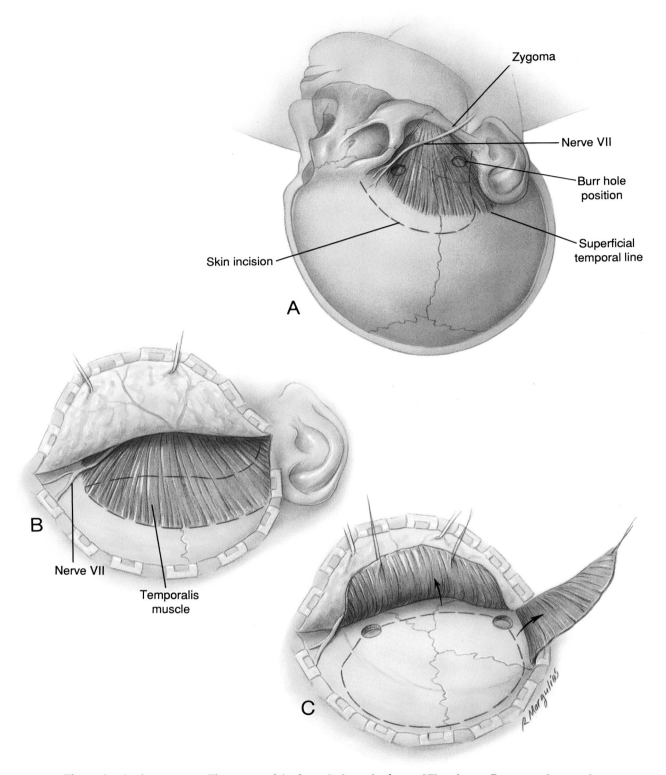

Figure 4. **A,** skin incision. The course of the frontalis branch of nerve VII is shown. **B,** temporalis muscle incision outlined. **C,** temporalis flap elevated and bone flap outlined.

flap will be hinged on the sphenoid wing, and this is fractured as the cranial flap is lifted from the intact dura. Then, the dura is dissected from the remaining sphenoid wing and small bony keel. Removal of this bone using a Leksell rongeur alternating with dural stripping results in a flattened greater wing of the sphenoid and allows unobstructed work in the region of the dura of the pterion extending from the lateral portion of the middle and frontal fossae. The dura is then tacked to the surrounding perimeter of the cranial opening.

Once the dura has been exposed, the ultrasound localizer should be used to demonstrate the location of the meningioma in relationship to the bone flap and exposed dura so that additional removal of bone can be completed as necessary. The dural incision is usually initiated parallel to the floor of the frontal fossa allowing sufficient margin of dura, i.e., 2 to 3 cm, in order to permit tenting of the dura to the adjacent muscle at the base, a technique that provides for good hemostasis (Fig. 5A). The dura is then opened over the middle fossa and finally the incision is carried across the area of the sphenoid wing using the closed Metzenbaum scissors to dissect it from the adjacent tumor. Here will be encountered a good deal of blood supply to the tumor from the middle meningeal artery which will be coagulated with the bipolar cautery. Thereafter, depending upon the height of the tumor, the dura is opened in a semicircular fashion, retracted toward the vertex, and held in place with traction sutures. Again the ultrasonic localizer can be used to be certain that the entire tumor, which may be partially buried under a shelf of cortex, is accessible through the operative exposure.

Tumor Removal

Utilizing the general principle of all meningioma surgery, that is, initially to devascularize the tumor from its dural attachment, the surgeon approaches along the base of the anterior fossa and coagulates the dural attachment along the sphenoid wing. At this point, the surgeon also observes the relationship of the tumor to the adjacent brain and the extent of the arachnoidal plane which can be developed between the tumor and the brain. This initial dissection can be aided with the use of the operating microscope. If necessary, a resection of the lateral inferior portion of the frontal lobe can be carried out with the use of suction and the bipolar cautery. Elective resection of noncritical brain tissue is far preferable to vigorous retraction as the latter will inevitably lead to significant postoperative edema (Fig. 5A). Once the total anterior aspect of the tumor has been demonstrated to its most medial extent, a self-retaining retractor can be used to hold the exposure.

Then attention is focused on the middle fossa aspect of the tumor. There may be significant blood supply to the tumor arising from the lateral aspect of the middle fossa dura. Once again, elective resection of the anterior aspect of the temporal lobe, if necessary, is far preferable to vigorous retraction. Having exposed both the temporal as well as frontal aspects of the tumor, the surgeon then proceeds along the "knife edge" of the sphenoid wing, devascularizing the tumor in this area. These tumors almost always displace the knee of the middle cerebral artery and adjacent branches medially (Fig. 5B) but not the venous drainage to the dura at the lateral aspect of the sphenoid wing; these veins must be divided carefully in order to provide good exposure of the tumor.

If the tumor is large, one can consider debulking before attempting to dissect the superior aspect of the capsule from the adjacent brain and middle cerebral artery. If the tumor has been successfully embolized, it is often sufficiently necrotic to be easily debulked with simple suction. The ultrasonic aspirator is also of great value in carrying out this maneuver (Fig. 5B). As one debulks the tumor, small arterial branches within the tumor itself will come into the suction apparatus and periodically should be coagulated. In large tumors, the most medial aspect of the attachment of the tumor to the dural base will not yet have been fully visualized and care must be taken not to violate the medial aspect of the capsule. Here, once again, the ultrasonic localizer can be of value in determining the amount of tumor which has been removed and the amount which remains medially and superiorly. Proceeding in this fashion, a small amount of tumor may be left attached at the dural base which will be attended to later as the important aspect of the operative procedure now is to remove the major bulk of the tumor from the intracranial cavity.

As the superior and medial aspects of the tumor capsule are dissected from the adjacent brain, the operating microscope should be used. Depending on the vectors of growth, the middle cerebral artery may be displaced directly medially or somewhat posteriorly. Review of the angiography at this time can assist in the localization of this vessel. As the tumor capsule is retracted laterally and inferiorly the adjacent brain and arachnoid plane are exposed and cottonoids should be placed in this plane of dissection; it is important not to place one cottonoid on top of the next, but rather replace each as the dissection proceeds in the depth of the wound. Once the main trunk of the middle cerebral artery has been identified at the most superior aspect of the tumor capsule, one proceeds with careful microsurgical technique to peel the vessel off the tumor capsule (Fig. 5C). Often a major vessel will have indented the tumor, so to speak, and whereas initially one may have the impression that the vessel is encased in tumor, meticulous dissection may

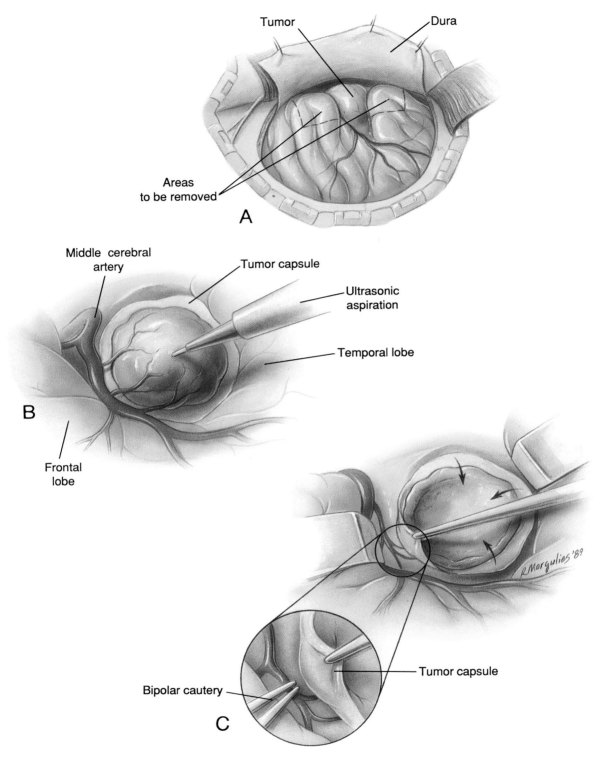

Figure 5. A, dura reflected and tumor partially exposed. *Dotted lines* indicate areas of frontal and temporal lobes for elective resection, if needed. **B,** relationship of the middle cerebral artery to the tumor. Ultrasonic aspirator on the tumor for debulking. **C,** tumor debulked. Dissection of the capsule from the middle cerebral artery and adjacent brain. A bipolar cautery is used to coagulate small branches feeding the tumor.

achieve a total removal of the tumor from this area without damaging the vessel. If necessary, however, a small fragment of capsule may remain attached to the middle cerebral artery to be reexamined once the major portion of the tumor has been removed. The appearance of cerebrospinal fluid welling up from the medial aspect of the capsule will indicate proximity to the base of the tumor. With progressive debulking and retraction of the capsule, always identifying the major arterial vessels, a complete gross removal of the tumor can usually be achieved.

After removing the bulk of the tumor there will be a good view of the base of the skull and adjacent sphenoid wing. It is important to remove the entire dural attachment as recurrence of meningiomas occurs almost always from the dural involvement at the base of the skull. Not only is visual examination important, but also an intraoperative review of the gadolinium-enhanced MRI scan will show the operator the extent of dural involvement. The CO_2 laser can be very effective in vaporizing the dura down to the bare bone and probably is the preferred method of removing the dural base of the tumor. The CO_2 laser can be either hand-held or manipulated through the operating microscope. Adjacent brain structures should be protected with cottonoid patties. If the lateral aspect of the sphenoid wing itself is invaded with tumor, this should be removed either with a high-speed air drill or with rongeurs. If a small amount of meningioma has been allowed to remain adjacent to the main trunk of the middle cerebral artery, this area should be inspected before removal of the brain retractors. Any tumor that cannot be dissected finally from this major vessel should be gently coagulated with the bipolar cautery. The wound should be thoroughly irrigated to evaluate any areas of venous oozing from the cerebral structures. It is our practice to then coat the entire exposed area with a thin layer of oxidized cellulose. The superior dural flap should then be placed over the exposed brain and wherever possible closed both frontally and temporally. The area that cannot be completely closed can be covered with a pledget of collagen film. Whereas this substance has not been generally utilized in neurosurgical procedures, we have found it to be very effective as a dural replacement. It does not require suturing to the adjacent dural edges and fully protects the underlying brain and adheres nicely to the dural surface. The collagen film is placed over the area as it comes from the sterile package and then is flooded with irrigating solution covered with a large cottonoid patty and suction applied. When the patty is removed the film will have fallen into place and the edges can be gently tucked in, in this instance along the base of skull both in the frontal and middle fossae.

Closure

The bone flap is inspected for any involvement by meningioma which should be removed with the high-speed drill. If a large area of bone flap has been removed, this can be replaced with stainless steel or titanium screen. The bone flap is wired in place and the closure carried out in routine fashion. A subgaleal Jackson-Pratt drain is placed and a head dressing applied, being careful to protect the exposed ear from compression.

COMPLICATIONS

In the postoperative period the two major complications to be avoided are seizures and hematoma formation. Both Dilantin and phenobarbital should be used intraoperatively; postoperatively, however, one drug or the other should be discontinued. If the patient had been on anticonvulsant therapy for preoperative seizures, that regime should be continued at the time of discharge. Steroids should be tapered rapidly over a period of three to seven days. If the patient's postoperative course is satisfactory, a noncontrast CT scan should be obtained 48 hours postoperatively to rule out any intracranial hematoma and to assess the degree of brain edema. The latter can serve as a guide to the program of steroid withdrawal.

It is important, however, to consider a postoperative CT scan prior to extubation if there has been any damage to the middle cerebral artery or any degree of brain swelling at the completion of the operative exposure. Long-term follow-up should include a repeat MRI scan with gadolinium enhancement three months postoperatively and, if this is entirely negative, a further MRI scan in one year to confirm total removal. If residual tumor is known to remain at the base of the skull or small fragments are attached to the critical cranial vessels, similar studies should be considered at somewhat more frequent intervals. Consideration of postoperative radiation therapy to the base of the skull can be important if any evidence of residual tumor or regrowth can be demonstrated.

SELECTIVE MICROSURGICAL VESTIBULAR NERVE SECTION FOR INTRACTABLE MÉNIÈRE'S SYNDROME

EDWARD TARLOV, M.D.

INTRODUCTION

Intractable Ménière's syndrome is found in a small proportion of patients with complaints of dizziness. Fluctuating hearing loss, tinnitus, and bouts of violent vertigo characterize the disorder. Vertigo is often the most disabling feature of the disorder. Most patients with Ménière's syndrome are managed by otolaryngologists. Diuretics, salt restriction, and vestibular sedatives are ordinarily the initial treatments of choice. In the years since Prosper Ménière first described the disorder, a variety of surgical treatments have been used when medical measures have failed. Endolymphatic shunting operations carried out in an effort to relieve tinnitus and hearing loss have been disappointing for relief of vertigo. Labyrinthine destructive procedures that can relieve vertigo will invariably abolish hearing, a disadvantage since the disorder may become bilateral in about 20% of instances. Selective microsurgical vestibular nerve section can relieve the vertigo with preservation of hearing. This is an excellent operation for sufferers of Ménière's disease who are not totally deaf in the affected ear and who are refractory to medical management.

The diagnosis of true Ménière's syndrome is not common among the whole spectrum of patients with complaints of dizziness. Strict clinical criteria for diagnosis should be used. In most instances the onset is between ages 30 and 60, with the young and very old rarely being affected. The recurring attacks usually increase in frequency. Ultimately, there is almost always a permanent hearing loss in untreated cases, and vertigo may continue after deafness is complete. The incidence of the disorder has been estimated at 1:100,000 population.

Vertigo is the first symptom in the majority of patients and can be the most disabling feature of the disease. Tinnitus is almost always present and may be the most reliable indicator of which labyrinth is in-

volved in unilateral cases. The stage of fluctuating hearing loss may last from a few weeks to several years before it becomes fixed. Fluctuations of deafness usually correspond with bouts of vertigo. A premonitory aura with fullness in the head or affected ear is common. Drop attacks ("the otolithic crisis of Tumarkin") occasionally occur as a result of loss of tonic influences of the otoliths. In severe attacks the patient may be thrown to the ground or, if seated as when dining, may suddenly become disoriented with respect to gravity. Nystagmus may accompany the attacks, but its direction is not of localizing value.

Electronystagmography with caloric testing is usually abnormal and may demonstrate canal paresis with diminished responses to warm and cold water or air on the affected side. Occasionally, directional preponderance or spontaneous nystagmus to the side opposite the diseased labyrinth occurs. On audiological testing the majority of cases show low-frequency perceptive hearing loss with fairly good discrimination, loudness recruitment, and negative tone decay found on impedance audiometry. Brainstem auditory-evoked response testing demonstrates normal latencies.

The most important differential diagnosis is that of acoustic neuroma. The latter tends not to cause severe vertigo as in Ménière's disease. The loss of vestibular function is usually slow, producing mild ataxia rather than paroxysmal disturbances. Magnetic resonance imaging with gadolinium in suspicious cases is helpful in excluding the possibility of an acoustic neuroma. Brainstem auditory-evoked response testing can identify an eighth nerve lesion but is, of course, not specific for its nature.

Pathological examination of the temporal bones in patients who died following operation has shown dilation of the endolymph spaces at the expense of the perilymph spaces. This is thought to cause symptoms because it is necessary to have equal perilymph and endolymph pressures for normal cochlear and vestibular function. The situation is analogous to hydrocephalus or glaucoma in that there is an accumulation of an excess endolymph most probably due to deficient reabsorption.

Because of the relatively high incidence of bilateral involvement, efforts at preserving existing hearing or improving hearing have considerable potential value. Nevertheless, destruction of the labyrinth has continued as a standard otological operation when hearing preservation is not a consideration. This may be performed as a transmastoid or a permeatal procedure. It results in a total loss of hearing and is not a desirable form of treatment in patients with unilateral Ménière's syndrome if there is useful hearing in the affected ear or if there is loss of hearing on the other side from other causes. It is also not desirable in bilateral Ménière's syndrome if both ears are affected early in the disease, if one labyrinth has been destroyed before disease appears in the other ear, or if hearing is poor in one ear and is rapidly failing in the other.

A variety of operations to relieve the excess pressure of endolymph have been carried out, principally aimed at preserving or improving hearing and relieving tinnitus. The idea of creating a fistula from the endolymphatic sac to the mastoid cavity or to the subarachnoid space has produced a standard series of shunting alternatives. Controversy about the efficacy of these procedures has existed. Medical labyrinthectomy with streptomycin is indicated in the occasional instances in which there is no labyrinthine function on the opposite side. It would be most accurate to say that at this time the value of shunting procedures alone for Ménière's syndrome is unproven. Because the procedure can be combined with vestibular nerve section and because the latter relieves the most disabling symptom, however, the shunting procedures seem worthy of further trials.

Because the endolymph pressure is usually lower than the cerebrospinal fluid (CSF) pressure, the precise physiological mechanisms involved in any benefit from shunting the endolymph to the subarachnoid space are unknown.

The pioneer neurosurgeons had broad experience with vestibular nerve section in this disorder, and the operation proved to be quite reliable. Dandy refined the operation to the extent that only two deaths occurred among his 587 cases. Vertigo was relieved entirely in 90%. Five percent were unchanged, and 5% were worse. In the majority of these 587 cases the entire eighth nerve bundle was sectioned with total loss of auditory as well as vestibular function. Fifty-four of Dandy's patients had facial paralysis, of whom 17 had permanent facial paralysis. Of 95 patients in whom only the vestibular portion of the nerve was sectioned, 9 had improved hearing, 27 had un-changed hearing, 46 were worse, and 13 were totally deaf. The experience of Olivecrona was similar. Falconer in a later era was able to preserve hearing on the operated side to some degree in his eight patients. The microsurgical technique described herein permits consistent postoperative hearing preservation.

GENERAL INDICATIONS FOR SURGERY IN MÉNIÈRE'S SYNDROME AND CHOICE OF OPERATION

Since Ménière's syndrome is primarily treated by otologists, most of the operations in recent years have been carried out as otological services. When hearing on the affected side is absent and the patient is mainly troubled by severe whirling attacks, labyrinthectomy is indicated. Labyrinthectomy may be carried out via a transmastoid or permeatal approach. This operation is effective in eliminating vertigo. The imbalance following labyrinthectomy is usually short-lived, and good compensation for this usually occurs without significant residual imbalance.

When hearing loss is the major symptom and the major therapeutic effort is to be aimed at preserving hearing, with the vertigo as a minor component, an endolymphatic shunting procedure is indicated.

The operation described here is indicated when hearing preservation is a consideration and when the vertiginous attacks are severe. The morbidity of the operation has been quite low, and it has proved thus far to be very effective for control of whirling vertigo, with this most disabling symptom having been eliminated in almost all cases.

We have carried out this procedure as a combined neurosurgical-otological operation. The vestibular nerve can safely be exposed via three routes: an extradural approach along the floor of the middle fossa, in the cerebellopontine angle or medial internal auditory canal, and in the most lateral portion of the canal where the superior and inferior vestibular nerves are separate. Theoretical considerations might make it desirable to section only the superior vestibular nerve in order to reduce postoperative imbalance. Our experience, however, has been that postoperative imbalance from section of the entire vestibular nerve is minimal. The middle fossa approach requires some degree of retraction on the temporal lobe. For these reasons we have not employed the middle fossa exposure of the vestibular nerve, and the exposure of the vestibular nerve in the internal auditory canal carries a risk to hearing. Accordingly, we have favored section of the vestibular nerve in the posterior fossa itself.

It may be worthwhile to review the relative advantages and disadvantages and our experiences with the approach anterior to the sigmoid sinus compared with the exposure that we now use routinely, posterior

to the sigmoid sinus. In our initial cases, we used an otological exposure through the mastoid anterior to the sigmoid sinus.

The mastoid is burred away, exposing the sigmoid sinus. The large mastoid emissary vein is skeletonized in this approach, and a wide bony removal over the sigmoid sinus is carried out. As the operation is carried out in the supine position, we have never had difficulties with air embolization or with handling of the sigmoid sinus in any way. The wide bony removal over the sigmoid permits gentle downward extradural retraction of the sigmoid and cerebellar hemisphere to facilitate a less tangential angle of visualization of the vestibular bundle as it passes into the internal auditory meatus. Depending on the shape of the lateral wall of the posterior fossa, which is somewhat variable, exposure of the dura anterior to the sigmoid sinus is nearly tangential to the dura, a factor that makes a tight dural closure somewhat more difficult. The dural opening is bounded anteriorly by the internal auditory meatus and posteriorly by the sigmoid sinus. An opening is made in this small dural area. In an individual with a short muscular neck or one with a thick mastoid, there is little leeway to alter or vary the surgeon's line of visualization of the intradural structures. The exposure of the eighth nerve bundle, although adequate to section the vestibular nerve, is quite limited. For orientation, it is helpful to gain a view of the trigeminal nerve superiorly and the ninth, tenth, and eleventh nerves inferiorly. We have not encountered any difficulties requiring hemostatic control of adjacent vessels, but the exposure anterior to the sigmoid sinus would be somewhat limited to accomplish this if necessary. Positive identification of the eighth nerve complex, by confirmation of its proximity to the flocculus, visualization of the fifth nerve rostrally and the ninth, tenth, and eleventh nerve complex below, and identification of the bony internal auditory meatus, is facilitated by the wider exposure through the posterior fossa. We have preferred the posterior approach, since dural closure of the very thin, tangentially exposed dura anterior to the sigmoid sinus is difficult. With the anterior approach we have had several CSF leaks, a not infrequent problem in transmastoid or translabyrinthine exposure of the posterior fossa. Accordingly, we have since modified the operation in the manner described below and have found the exposure posterior to the sigmoid sinus to be more simple and expeditious. In addition, the retrosigmoid approach gives a wide view of the posterior fossa. In the supine position with the head turned contralaterally, it is quite striking how little cerebellar retraction is necessary once CSF has been aspirated. The structures behind the endolymphatic sac are clearly seen from within the dura when the procedure is carried out in this manner. Morbidity has been minimal, and dural closure over a patch graft has never been a problem.

POSITION

We formerly considered the advantages of the sitting position virtually indispensable in posterior fossa surgery. During development of our own microsurgical approaches to tic douloureux, particularly in the elderly, it became clear to us that the cerebellopontine angle can be safely and widely exposed in the supine position. The view obtained once the surgeon becomes familiar with the use of this position is virtually identical to that obtained in the sitting position except that the surgical field is rotated 90 degrees. The sitting position has many advantages, especially for large cerebellopontine angle tumors. Nevertheless, we have been using the supine position increasingly for routine cranial nerve surgery in the posterior fossa, including surgery for tic douloureux, small acoustic neuromas, and this operation for Ménière's syndrome. The hazards of the sitting position, principally relating to hypotension and air embolism, are eliminated without losing most of the advantages of the sitting position. The head of the operating table is slightly elevated, a step that markedly reduces venous pressure. The neck is rotated contralaterally and is moderately flexed. Two fingers can be inserted beneath the chin when the neck is in proper position. When CSF has been aspirated from the cisterna magna, almost no cerebellar retraction is necessary. No arterial or central venous line is necessary. Figure 1 demonstrates the patient's head position from the surgeon's viewpoint. The surgeon is seated behind the patient's head. The operating microscope is brought in from the surgeon's left to permit easy access by the scrub nurse to his right hand.

SURGICAL TECHNIQUE

The overall orientation in the supine position from the surgeon's viewpoint is demonstrated in Figure 1A. We prefer a Mayfield three-point head fixation unit that allows the use of the Leyla Yasargil self-retaining retractor system. A paramedian incision about 1 cm posterior to mastoid prominence is used as indicated. Minimal hair shaving is necessary. A small laterally placed craniectomy is carried out. This extends over the junction between the transverse and sigmoid sinuses. The dura is opened inferiorly at first. Ordinarily, the cerebellar hemisphere is somewhat full at this stage. With a cottonoid over the cerebellar hemisphere, CSF is aspirated from the convexity subarachnoid space as shown in Figure 2A, to obtain a slack cerebellum as shown in Figure 2B. The force of gravity provides most of the necessary cerebellar re-

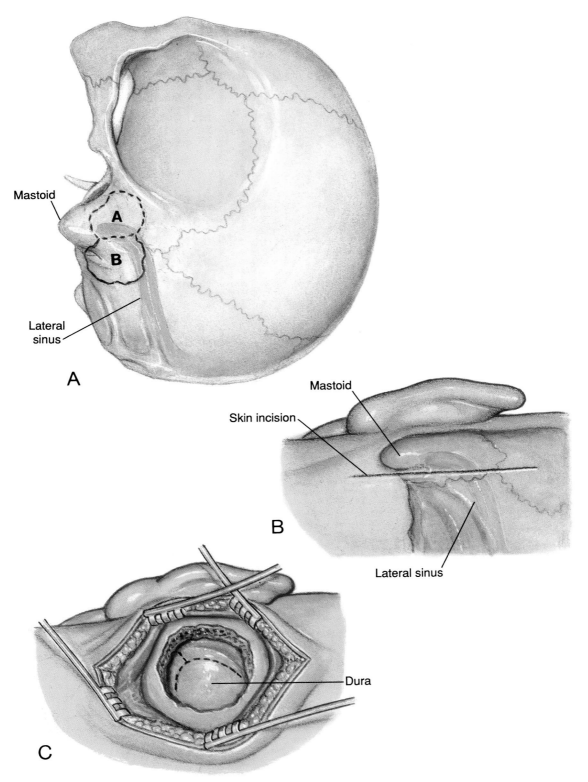

Figure 1. **A,** position of head turned to right with patient supine. In our early experience the opening as made at *area A* to bring us down to dura anterior to the sigmoid sinus. We have since changed the procedure to make our opening posterior to the sigmoid sinus (*area B*). **B,** the skin incision. **C,** dural exposure posterior to the sigmoid sinus. (**A:** Modified from Tarlov EC. Microsurgical vestibular nerve section for intractable Ménière's syndrome: Technique and results. Clin Neurosurg 1986;33:667–684. **B** and **C:** Modified from Tarlov EC, Oliver P. Selective vestibular nerve section combined with endolymphatic sac to subarachnoid shunt for intractable Ménière's syndrome: Surgical technique. Contemp Neurosurg 1983;4(26):1–8.)

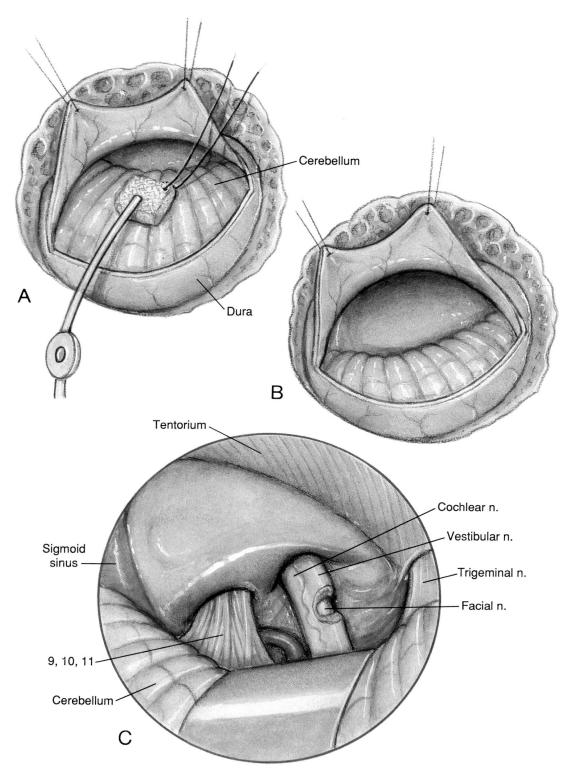

Figure 2. **A,** showing aspiration of CSF from surface subarachnoid space over cerebellar hemisphere. **B,** slack exposure resulting from CSF aspiration. Minimal retraction and changing the angle of visualization results in the view in **C. C,** lower cranial nerves in view and vestibular portion of vestibulocochlear nerve sectioned. The retractor's function is largely to protect the cerebellar hemisphere. (**B** and **C**: Modified from Tarlov EC, Oliver P. Selective vestibular nerve section combined with endolymphatic sac to subarachnoid shunt for intractable Ménière's syndrome: Surgical technique. Contemp Neurosurg 1983;4(26):1–8.)

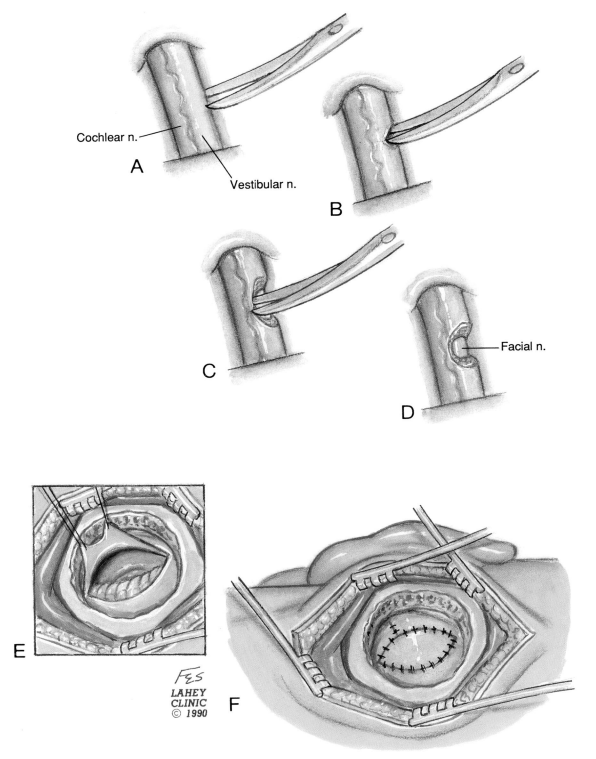

Figure 3. **A, B, C,** and **D,** distraction of cut vestibular nerve to expose facial nerve without manipulation of cochlear nerve. **E,** slack exposure prior to closure. **F,** dural closure over patch graft. (Redrawn in color from Tarlov EC. Microsurgical vestibular nerve section for intractable Ménière's syndrome: Technique and results. Clin Neurosurg 1986;33:667–684.)

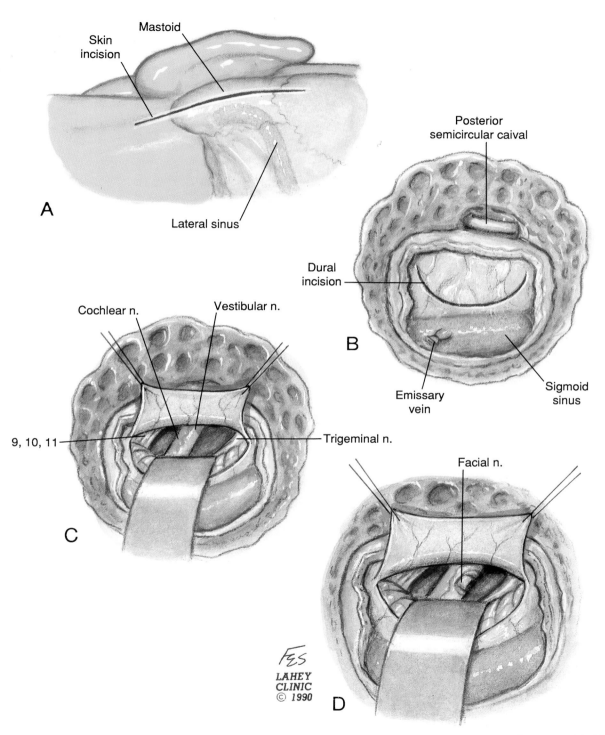

Figure 4. **A,** prior technique no longer used, demonstrating incision over mastoid. **B,** dural opening anterior to sigmoid sinus. **C,** limited exposure of vestibulocochlear bundle. **D,** section of vestibular bundle. (Modified from Tarlov EC. Microsurgical vestibular nerve section for intractable Ménière's syndrome: Technique and results. Clin Neurosurg 1986;33:667–684.)

traction from here on. Petrosal veins are identified at this point, the arachnoid is swept medially off their junction with the petrosal sinus, and the veins are coagulated. They are then divided with curved microscissors, leaving the usual cuff adjacent to the petrosal sinus for safety. The retractor is then used to place the arachnoid over the internal auditory meatus on a slight stretch. The retractor's function here is largely to protect the cerebellar hemisphere; as the redundant arachnoid forms a cistern at this point, the arachnoid can be swept medially and left intact over much of the cerebellopontine angle cistern system.

On a number of occasions, tortuous vessels in the region of the eighth nerve complex have been observed. We have not infrequently seen these during the course of operations for tic douloureux, in patients without eighth nerve signs or symptoms. Although it has been suggested that vascular cross-compression may be a causative factor in Ménière's syndrome, no causative relationship between such vessels and the symptoms of Ménière's syndrome has, in our opinion, ever been proven, and we would not consider it presently advisable to carry out vascular decompression in severely symptomatic patients with Ménière's syndrome, although the microvascular decompression operation has, we believe, proven its value in the treatment of tic douloureux. Once the retractor has been correctly positioned a wide view of the eighth nerve complex from the internal auditory meatus to the brainstem is obtained. The vestibular portion of the eighth nerve occupies the superior 50% of the combined bundle. It is usually slightly more gray than the more inferiorly lying cochlear division. At the level of the internal auditory meatus a plane of cleavage between the vestibular and cochlear divisions may be visible. Gently depressing the vestibular portion of the nerve inferiorly allows visualization of the facial nerve lying anterosuperiorly. Vessels coursing along the eighth nerve bundle must be preserved if hearing preservation is to be accomplished. Frequently there are few or no vessels to contend with, but it is occasionally necessary to carefully dissect around a small vessel, separating it from the nerve sharply if it courses across the vestibular nerve itself. A clear plane of cleavage between the vestibular and cochlear portions cannot always be visualized. When this is the case, we section the superior 50% of the combined cochlear and vestibular bundle. No manipulation of the cochlear portion is carried out. Following such sections, no postoperative vestibular function on this side has been demonstrable postoperatively. As the cochlear nerve and its blood supply are delicate, no manipulation of the cochlear nerve is carried out. The view obtained once the vestibular nerve has been sectioned is indicated in Figures 2C and 3D.

In an effort to determine its value in guiding the surgeon to preserve cochlear nerve function, we have used intraoperative brainstem auditory evoked response testing. With the availability of facilities for this testing, the procedure itself is simple enough. A special microphone is placed on the ipsilateral ear. Once the appropriate scalp leads have been placed, satisfactory intraoperative tracings can be obtained. Even with rapid averaging techniques the time delay necessary for the interpretation does not permit immediate feedback to the surgeon carrying out his manipulations. Accordingly, the test may demonstrate that some surgical manipulation previously carried out has caused a change in the evoked response latency. This information would only be helpful to the surgeon if it were available during the course of each movement, which it is not. Thus, although the procedure is technically feasible, we have not found it helpful in preserving cochlear function.

A pericranial graft taken in the initial phase of the procedure is used in the dural closure. The muscles, subcutaneous tissues, and skin are then closed in layers, and a small dressing is applied. Steroid preparation and postoperative treatment for several days have reduced the side effects of the procedure. Postoperative vertigo seems to be proportional to preoperative vestibular function as determined by electronystagmography, as would be expected. Patients with the most severe vestibular impairment preoperatively have been the least disturbed in the early postoperative period. Patients have all been discharged within one week and have minimal residual ataxia in one month.

With this approach, CSF leakage has not been a problem. Our earlier transmastoid exposures did lead to CSF leakage, and reclosure of the wound was necessary on several occasions in view of the thinness of the dura anterior to the sigmoid sinus and its oblique angle in relation to the surgeon's view (Fig. 4). No facial weakness or any other unwanted effect outside the eighth nerve system has occurred.

The procedure can be carried out in the manner described without producing loss of hearing. Among 50 patients operated upon so far we have operated several times on the only hearing ear and on several patients with normal hearing preoperatively and postoperatively.

All of the patients have had relief from their whirling attacks of dizziness thus far, and, as this is the most disabling feature of the disorder, this fact is worthy of note. The procedure appears to be promising in the surgical treatment of intractable Ménière's syndrome when relief of vertigo with hearing preservation is desired.

CHIARI MALFORMATIONS AND SYRINGOHYDROMYELIA IN CHILDREN

W. JERRY OAKES, M.D.

INTRODUCTION

Chiari malformations, or hindbrain hernias, are being diagnosed and operated upon with increasing frequency. For the purposes of this chapter, two separate entities will be discussed. The Chiari I malformation is characterized by caudal descent of the cerebellar tonsils. The brain stem and neocortex are typically not involved and the patient does not suffer from a myelomeningocele. Syringomyelia is commonly but not invariably present. The Chiari II malformation is almost always seen in conjunction with spina bifida and is a more severe form of hindbrain herniation. The neocortex and brain stem are dysmorphic and the cerebellar vermis (not the tonsils) is displaced into the cervical spine. Accompanying the vermis are dysmorphic and elongated aspects of the medulla and lower pons as well as the lower aspect of the fourth ventricle. Again, syringomyelia is commonly associated with this lesion. Not discussed in this chapter is the rare Chiari III malformation.

CHIARI I MALFORMATION

With the advent of magnetic resonance imaging (MRI) the detection of caudal displacement of the cerebellar tonsils and the presence of an associated syrinx has become safe and accurate. Typically the tonsils are at least 3 mm below the plane of the foramen magnum. They lose the rounded appearance of their caudal pole and become pointed or "peg-like." This is associated with obliteration of the subarachnoid space at the craniocervical junction with the impaction of tissues into this confined region. When all of the above criteria are not met, the situation should be judged in connection with the clinical symptomatology of the patient. The presence of syringomyelia or other developmental anomalies will assist in the interpretation of the intradural findings at the craniocervical junction.

Patients with a symptomatic Chiari I malformation are generally offered operative intervention. The more severe the neurological deficit the stronger the case for

intervention. When occipital pain is the only symptom and no neurological signs are present, the degree of disability from the discomfort should be carefully weighed against the risks of the procedure, prior to the implementation of surgical intervention. When syringomyelia is present, I generally favor intervention even with minimal symptoms. Intracranial pressure should be normalized prior to consideration of craniocervical decompression. Approximately 10% of patients with Chiari I malformation will have hypertensive hydrocephalus and ventriculoperitoneal shunt insertion should precede other considerations. Flexion and extension views of the cervical spine are also important to resolve questions of spinal stability and other bony anomalies. If significant basilar invagination is present, this issue should be addressed prior to a posterior procedure which may add to spinal instability. It should be emphasized that computed tomography of the brain without the use of subarachnoid contrast is notoriously poor in its ability to detect the presence of a significant Chiari malformation.

Once a candidate for surgery has been appropriately chosen, the patient is prepared with preoperative corticosteroids and a broad spectrum antibiotic. The patient is positioned prone (Fig. 1) in a pin-type head holder with the neck flexed. The head of the table is elevated somewhat, but no central venous access is mandatory since lowering the head will eliminate the gradient for air embolization. A chest Doppler monitor is used for the detection of air embolization and to monitor slight changes in the patient's pulse. Patients are not allowed to breathe spontaneously. This significantly lowers the likelihood of serious pulmonary complications postoperatively. Muscle relaxants are allowed to become fully effective during the induction of anesthesia to avoid the Valsalva maneuver during placement of the endotracheal tube. A severe Valsalva maneuver has been associated with progression of symptoms in some patients.

The skin incision is made from a point 2 cm below the external occipital protuberance to the midportion of the spinous process of C-2 (Fig. 2A). It is quite

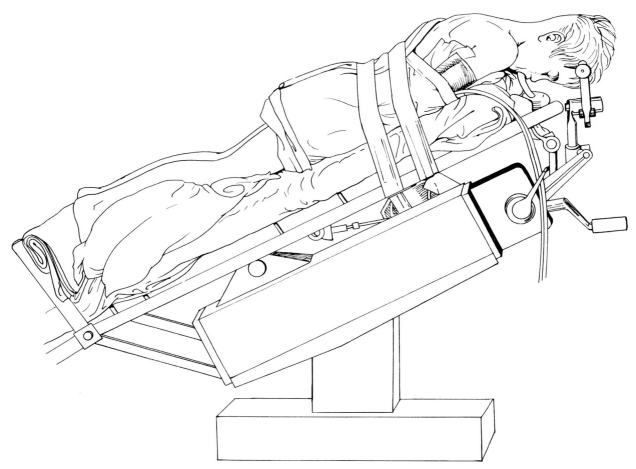

Figure 1. Optimal positioning of a patient for exposing a Chiari malformation.

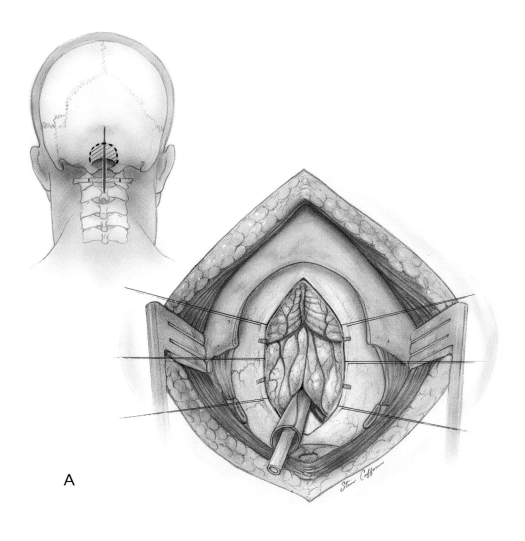

A

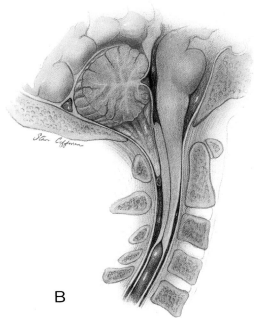

B

Figure 2. **A,** operative exposure of a Chiari I malformation. A stent has been placed through the fourth ventricular outlet. **B,** Chiari I malformation associated with syringomyelia; midline sagittal section.

unusual for the tonsilar tissue to descend below the level of the upper portion of C-2 (Fig. 2B), and by not removing the important muscular attachments at C-2 the postoperative pain is significantly decreased and the likelihood of postoperative spinal deformity seen in conjunction with syringomyelia is substantially lessened. The avascular midline plane of the occipital musculature is divided with monopolar current. No incision transecting muscle is necessary in this procedure since the plane dividing the left and right muscular bundles completely separates these two groups. A small amount of fat will mark this natural cleavage plane. Again using the monopolar current, the muscle insertion immediately above the foramen magnum is separated from the occipital bone and the posterior arch of C-1. The arch of C-1 itself is removed as well as the occipital bone immediately above this (Fig. 2A). There is no need for lateral exposure and bone laterally situated is left intact. This minimizes risk to the vertebral veins and arteries. The bone edges are waxed and the dura is opened in the midline. Initially, the dura over C-1 is opened. Care is taken as the incision is extended across the circular sinus near the foramen magnum. This sinus can be formidable and should not be approached nonchalantly. With the dura retracted laterally, the arachnoid is opened in the midline. The subarachnoid adhesions are lysed with a sharp instrument and are not simply torn. The arachnoid edge is then clipped to the dural edge with metal clips.

The tonsils, which can be recognized by their vertical folia, are separated in the midline to expose the floor of the fourth ventricle. Care is taken to free the caudal loop of the posterior inferior cerebellar artery and avoid damage to this vessel or the branches. Again adhesions are cut rather than torn. On separating the cerebellar tonsils, a veil of arachnoid is sometimes encountered. This veil should be opened widely. Obstruction to cerebrospinal fluid flow can also occur from the posterior inferior cerebellar arteries. These vessels may approximate in the midline and be adherent to one another. They should be separated and mobilized laterally with great care. Options at this point differ but I prefer to place a stent (Fig. 2A). This is composed of a short length of ventricular catheter (3 to 5 cm), and on the outer surface of the catheter a section of soft drainage tube is sewn in place. The tip of the ventricular catheter is removed leaving an open hollow conduit. The stent has two lumens, one within the ventricular catheter and a second between the catheter and the drain. This stent is then carefully placed with one end of the tube lying in the midportion of the fourth ventricle and the other in the cervical subarachnoid space distal to the lower margin of the cerebellar tonsils. Care is taken to position this stent

in the subarachnoid space, not the subdural space. The stent is held in position with a fine suture sewn to an avascular portion of the medial aspect of the pia over the tonsil. Closure is then accomplished with a generous dural graft, either of cadaveric origin or harvested from the nuchal ligament. A central dural tack-up suture is used to further expand the subarachnoid space in this area. Closure is with absorbable suture which is known to react minimally in the subarachnoid space.

Following the operation, patients may experience some nausea and vomiting as well as hiccups. These are almost always self-limited. Neurological deficits which are well-established prior to the operation are unlikely to reverse following operative manipulation. Long-standing pain and temperature loss is very unlikely to return. Hand and arm weakness with fasciculations and loss of muscle bulk may improve functionally but will not normalize. A particular problem exists when pain is a major component of the presentation. Children and adolescents infrequently have a major problem with pain. Adults, however, may be quite discouraged by the persistence of discomfort in the neck, shoulders, and/or arms. Pain may very well persist despite a physiologically successful operation with obliteration of the syrinx cavity. This limitation of surgical intervention should be carefully explained to the patient prior to surgery. Mild scoliosis (less than 35 degrees) may improve or simply stabilize, whereas more severe spinal deformity may well progress despite adequate treatment. With the advent of MRI scanning the status of syringohydromyelia can be assessed easily. If a sizable syrinx persists months to years after craniocervical decompression *and* symptoms attributable to this lesion are serious or progressive, consideration can be given to a laminectomy over the lower aspect of the syrinx and the placement of a syrinx to subarachnoid shunt or to a syrinx to peritoneal shunt. If a syrinx to subarachnoid shunt is chosen, placement of the distal catheter in the free subarachnoid space is an important technical maneuver. Catheters can easily be mistakenly placed in the subdural space without benefit to the patient.

CHIARI II MALFORMATION
Children with a myelomeningocele may develop symptoms referable to their hindbrain hernia. Symptoms and signs are generally age-specific, with infants developing lower cranial nerve disturbances (difficulty with swallowing, weak cry, inspiratory wheeze, aspiration pneumonia, absent gag, and opisthotonos) and older children more commonly developing progressive upper extremity spasticity. Ataxia of the trunk or appendages is recognized much less often. Since some degree of hindbrain herniation is present in the vast

majority of spina bifida patients, MRI evidence of hindbrain herniation must be accompanied by progressive or severe symptomatology to warrant operative intervention. Many patients will remain clinically stable for long periods despite significant deformity. As many as one-third of patients will develop difficulty with phonation, swallowing, or apnea by age three years. If the "asymptomatic" remainder were followed for a longer period or if less serious symptoms were considered significant this one in three figure would undoubtedly be higher. Because the symptoms of the Chiari II malformation are frequently life threatening, symptomatic Chiari II malformation is the leading cause of death in the treated myelomeningocele population today. When treated conservatively, as many as 10 to 15% of all patients will die from the malformation by the age of three years.

The decision for surgical intervention is controversial. Because there is a significant likelihood of stabilization or actual improvement with conservative care, some would argue against operative intervention. This is supported to some degree by autopsy material that demonstrates hypoplasia or aplasia of vital lower cranial nerve nuclei. Against this, however, is the experience of numerous surgeons who have seen dramatic improvement in many patients following decompression. In addition, objective evidence of physiologic functioning has been reported to improve with both brain stem evoked responses and CO_2 curve following operation. With these conflicting pieces of evidence one can quickly appreciate the surgeon's dilemma.

With increasing experience, my willingness to operatively intervene is increasing. This is due to the relatively low incidence of operative complications and the clear improvement demonstrated by some patients. Poor results are more commonly due to a delay in offering operative intervention. Once serious difficulties are clinically evident with breathing, swallowing, or phonation, the situation may very well be irreversible. In that case, the best that operation can be expected to do is to maintain the poor level of lower cranial nerve function seen immediately prior to operation. Problems with aspiration pneumonia, apnea, and other life-threatening difficulties may very well persist.

The solution to this problem does not seem to be a continuation of a conservative approach, accepting a 10 to 15% mortality. Rather, an earlier identification of patients at high risk for serious problems, and offering this group intervention, seems to be a more logical option. Being able to detect this high-risk group prior to the development of irreversible life-threatening problems is a key provision.

If serious problems with phonation, swallowing, or breathing are detected and normal intracranial pres-

sure is present, urgent intervention is appropriate when full support of the child is proposed. It is also important to emphasize that normalization of intracranial pressure is a prerequisite to consideration of craniocervical decompression. Patients with questionable shunt function are well served to first have their shunt revised. If progressive or serious symptoms persist after adequate shunt revision, decompression of the craniocervical junction can be contemplated. Again, the MRI has made the diagnostic evaluation of this group of patients almost risk-free and quite precise.

As with the Chiari I patients, corticosteroids and a broad spectrum antibiotic are given preoperatively. Steroids are not a substitute for a needed craniocervical decompression. The anesthetic management and positioning of the patient are similar to those for the Chiari I patient. Of some difference, however, is the fact that decompression should extend to the level of the caudally displaced posterior fossa tissue. This is frequently below the level of C-4. By removing this additional bone and displacing the musculature, the risks of cervical deformity are substantially increased even if the laminectomy is kept quite medial away from the facets. Since the lower portion of the fourth ventricle is usually not within the posterior fossa, the occiput may need to be removed minimally if at all (Fig. 3B). If it is elected to open the dura over the posterior fossa, great care is necessary. The transverse sinus in the patient with spina bifida is frequently placed very near if not at the level of the foramen magnum (Fig. 3B). An unknowing opening of the dura and sinus in this area may well lead to an operative disaster. The elasticity of the tissues of the cervical spine is pronounced. In removing the laminal arch of small infants, each bite with the rongeur needs to be crisp and clean. Undue distortion of the spinal cord may occur if this principle is not followed. It is important to study the preoperative MRI for the position of the fourth ventricle, the cerebellar vermis, and the possibility of a medullary kink. The position of all these structures is critical to the intradural exploration.

Once the dura is opened, finding the caudal extent of the fourth ventricle can be difficult (Fig. 3A). Intraoperative ultrasound may be of help in localizing this structure. The choroid plexus usually maintains its embryonic extraventricular position, marking the caudal end of the fourth ventricle. When present, this is a reliable intraoperative marker. Unfortunately, dense adhesions and neovascularity at points of compression or traction may be found, especially near C-1, and this may make dissection treacherous. The fourth ventricle may be covered by vermis with its horizontal folia or the choroid plexus may simply lie within the displaced ventricle.

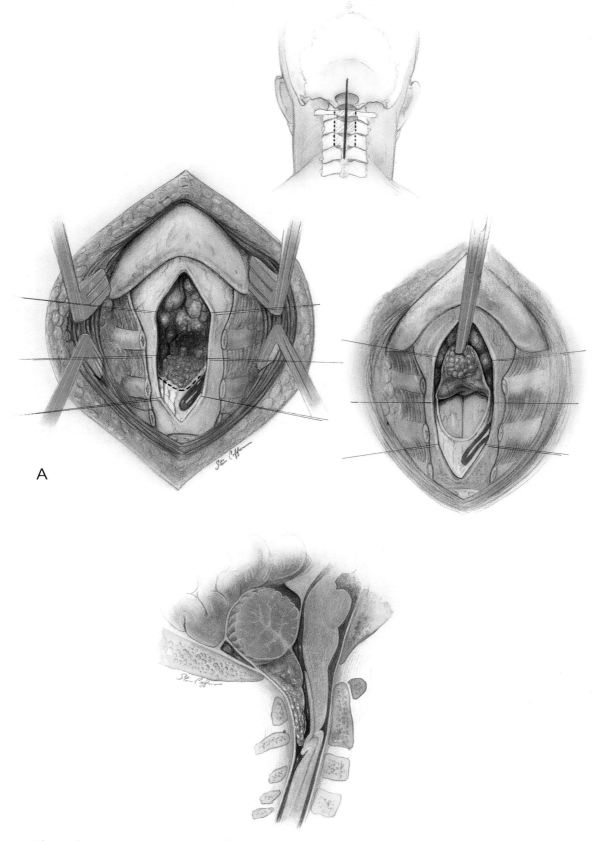

Figure 3. A, operative exposure of a Chiari II malformation. **B,** Chiari II malformation: midline sagittal section.

If the purpose of the intradural manipulation is to open the foramen of Magendie and provide free egress of cerebrospinal fluid from the fourth ventricle, this can be accomplished by the placement of a stent as with the Chiari I malformation patients. It is necessary to find and open the tissue widely over the caudal aspect of the fourth ventricle. It may happen that several planes of dissection are developed before the floor of the fourth can be adequately appreciated. It is important during the exploration of each of these avenues that vascular and neural tissues be preserved and that natural planes be developed so that no irreparable damage to the delicate tissues of the lower brainstem occurs. The caudal aspect of a medullary kink can easily be mistaken for the appropriate target. This dissection is one of the most difficult in pediatric neurosurgery. Errors or simple tissue manipulation may convert a tenuous portion of the medulla or lower pons to permanently damaged tissue. The surgeon should always bear in mind the risk-benefit ratio for each of his actions, and this particular area is unforgiving of even small excesses of manipulation. Grafting of the dura and closure are similar to the previous description.

In addition to the avoidance of problems with infection, hemorrhage, and increased neurological deficit, patient selection and the timing of intervention are critical to the successful outcome of decompressing a patient with a Chiari II malformation. Despite what was thought to be appropriate and timely intervention, an alarmingly high percentage of patients with lower cranial nerve abnormalities treated surgically eventually progress. This raises the question of whether the current strict selection criteria are too restrictive and whether less symptomatic infants should be considered for decompression. This area of speculation remains in dispute.

CAROTID BODY TUMORS

FREDRIC B. MEYER, M.D.
THORALF M. SUNDT, JR., M.D.

CLINICAL PRESENTATION

The most common presenting symptom in a patient with a carotid body tumor is a palpable neck mass. This may be detected either by the patient or by the physician during a routine examination. Other symptoms often include hoarseness, dysphagia, stridor, or, possibly, tongue weakness.

On examination, the neck mass is located below the angle of the jaw and is often laterally mobile but vertically fixed because of its attachment to the adventitia of the carotid artery. Although most of these masses have a transmittable pulse, an audible bruit is infrequent. The incidence of cranial nerve involvement has been estimated at 20% and usually includes the vagus and hypoglossal nerves. Rarely, a patient may also present with a Horner's syndrome. The stridor and dysphagia may be secondary to either vagus involvement or compression of the pharynx by the adjacent tumor. In either situation, these specific findings are most suggestive of a large tumor extending to the base of the skull.

In any patient with a carotid body tumor and hypertension, it is important to consider catecholamine secretion by the tumor or the possibility of multicentricity including a pheochromocytoma elsewhere. Therefore, on preoperative evaluation, it is important to consider the possibility of excess catecholamine production which would have significant anesthetic implications.

The differential diagnosis includes a branchial cleft cyst, carotid artery aneurysm, primary or metastatic carcinoma, adenopathy, nerve sheath tumor, and glomus jugulare tumor. All suspicious neck masses should be evaluated by radiological imaging studies. Injudicious local biopsy may result in uncontrollable hemorrhage.

DIAGNOSIS

The best diagnostic test at present for evaluating the anatomic pathology is a transfemoral cerebral angiogram. The presence of an enhancing oval mass widening the angle of the carotid bifurcation with displacement of both the internal and external carotid arteries is essentially pathognomonic of a carotid body tumor. Although the blood supply is primarily from the bifurcation and external carotid artery, contribution from the internal carotid artery, vertebral artery, and thyrocervical trunk can occur. On angiography it is important to note the cephalic extent of the tumor blush to help plan surgical exposure. Bilateral carotid angiography is important to evaluate the potential for collateral cerebral blood flow and to identify possible multicentric paragangliomas of the contralateral carotid body and glomus jugulare.

Contrasted enhanced computed tomography (CT) and magnetic resonance imaging are useful to demonstrate the lateral and medial extent of the tumor. This is especially important in noting the displacement of the pharynx. However, it may be difficult to determine whether the mass is an aneurysm as opposed to a carotid body tumor on these diagnostic studies. Ultrasonography has also been advocated as a noninvasive diagnostic test in patients with a strong family history or a history of a contralateral carotid body tumor.

NATURAL HISTORY AND SURGICAL SELECTION

The malignancy potential of carotid body tumors has been reported to range from 2.6 to 50%. The pathological criteria for malignancy are based on the standard criteria of cellular atypia and mitoses, local invasion, and dissemination. However, unique for these tumors is that the histological appearance does not correlate strongly with the potential for malignancy. Currently, the metastatic rate for carotid body tumors is approximately 5%. Although metastatic spread occurs most commonly to the regional lymph nodes, metastases to the brachial plexus, cerebellum, lungs, bone, abdomen, pancreas, thyroid, kidney, and breast have been reported. Metastases should not be confused with multicentricity of paragangliomas at other sites in the body.

Carotid body tumors will grow relentlessly if not resected. Several retrospective studies have reported a mortality rate of approximately 8% in untreated cases.

Although some authors have reported palliation with radiation therapy alone, it is generally agreed that radiation is not an acceptable primary treatment. In addition, some authors have recommended radiation therapy for incomplete resections, although there is no convincing evidence to demonstrate that this is effective. The morbidity associated with unresected tumors is significant and includes progressive lower cranial nerve palsies, dysphagia, airway obstruction, and extension to the skull base with infiltration of the central nervous system. Accordingly, in an otherwise medically healthy patient, complete surgical removal is the recommended treatment of choice.

Epidemiological studies have demonstrated that there are two forms of this disease. First, there is the more common sporadic form in which there is a 5% incidence of bilateral carotid body tumors. The second, less common, form is a familial disease with an autosomal dominant transmission. Within this second group, there is a 32% incidence of bilateral tumors. Therefore, if a positive family history is obtained in the initial evaluation of a patient, early examination of other family members is strongly recommended because the ease of resection is based on the size of the tumor. When patients who have undergone resection of a carotid body tumor on one side develop a contralateral tumor, surgical resection is recommended only if 10th nerve function is intact on the previously operated side. Otherwise the risk of bilateral 10th nerve palsies with a high potential for repeated aspiration would be unacceptably great. In that specific instance it would be most prudent to observe the tumor through noninvasive means such as ultrasound or CT scanning.

SURGICAL TECHNIQUE
The surgical approach advocated here emphasizes six fundamental concepts:

1) The preservation of cerebral blood flow during and after the operation is critical. Therefore, all patients are monitored with intraoperative electroencephalography. Furthermore, patients with large tumors in whom temporary carotid artery occlusion may be required have intraoperative baseline occlusion xenon-133 cerebral blood flow studies. Trial balloon occlusion of the internal carotid artery during the preoperative angiographic assessment may also be of benefit.

2) Distal exposure of large tumors at the base of the skull is obtained by mobilization of the parotid gland. This approach facilitates identification of the lower cranial nerves cephalad to the tumor and aids in their preservation.

3) These tumors are dissected in the capsular-adventitial plane as opposed to the subadventitial plane which has been advocated by some surgeons. This plane is developed by using bipolar coagulation and magnification. This minimizes the risk of arterial wall injury and untimely hemorrhage.

4) Great effort is taken to maintain the integrity of the external carotid artery since it is a potential source of collateral flow.

5) Although some authors recommend the routine use of a shunt in large tumors, shunts are only used when the electroencephalogram and cerebral blood flow studies demonstrate insufficient perfusion during carotid artery occlusion. This minimizes the risks associated with a shunt and avoids an unnecessary arteriotomy. In most cases, meticulous dissection eliminates the need for either a temporary carotid artery occlusion or shunt placement.

6) Since exposure is critical in successful removal of these tumors, a longitudinal incision is used extending from the ear to the suprasternal notch along the anterior sternocleidomastoid muscle. Although cosmetically less appealing than the horizontal incision advocated by some surgeons, it permits excellent exposure of both the distal and proximal carotid arteries. In addition, the ipsilateral leg is prepared and draped for surgery in case a saphenous vein graft is required.

The patient is intubated with a wire endotracheal tube. It is important to have not only an arterial line for monitoring of blood pressure but also good venous access in case a rapid transfusion is required. As indicated in Figure 1, the patient is positioned in a similar manner to that used for a carotid endarterectomy. The ipsilateral cervical region is draped extending from the clavicle up to the face both anterior and posterior to the ear. The lower part of the incision is similar to that used in a routine carotid endarterectomy and parallels the anterior border of the sternocleidomastoid muscle, ending several centimeters superior and lateral to the suprasternal notch. The cervical segment of the incision runs along the anterior border of the sternocleidomastoid muscle and ascends to a point just behind the lobe of the ear. In the lower quarter of the postauricular sulcus, it drops to the bottom of the ear, skirts the earlobe, and then ascends in a pretragal skin crease to the superior border of the zygoma. After the proximal common carotid artery is identified and vascular loops are placed around it, the parotid gland is then mobilized prior to further dissection of the tumor.

The superficial cervical fascia is incised and the posterior border of the parotid gland is exposed and elevated. The anterior-inferior surface of the auricular cartilage is followed deep to its "pointer," the triangular projection of cartilage at its medial limit. The temporoparotid fascia is incised between the mastoid process and the posterior margin of the parotid gland, and the facial nerve is found adjacent to the fascia. A finger placed on the mastoid tip and directed ante-

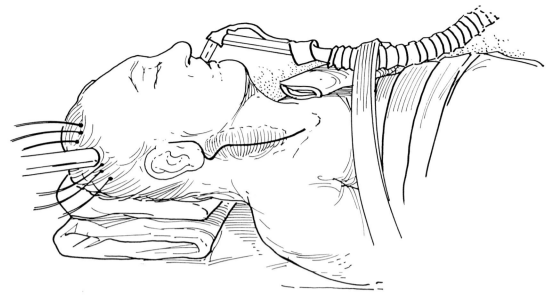

Figure 1. The skin incision is located along the anterior border of the sternocleidomastoid muscle but then extends to in front of the ear to facilitate parotid mobilization. The probe adjacent to the parietal boss is for intraoperative cerebral blood flow monitoring. The scalp has been wired with electrodes for continuous intraoperative electroencephalographic monitoring. (Copyrighted by Mayo Foundation.)

riorly, the cartilaginous "pointer," and the palpable junction of the external auditory meatus (the tympanomastoid suture) all point to the main trunk of the 7th nerve. Once the main trunk is identified, the lower division and marginal mandibular nerve which form the upper limit of the deep dissection can be traced forward by sharp dissection and elevated safely using mobilized parotid tissue as a "bundle." The posterior belly of the digastric muscle is followed to its point of insertion in the mastoid groove and divided there. The stylohyoid muscle lies superior and parallel to the digastric muscle and should also be divided, exposing the deeper stylomandibular ligament which must also be resected for adequate distal exposure of the internal carotid artery.

Although this relationship between nerves and muscles is referred to by anatomists as a "retroparotid fossa," the tissue is in fact densely bound by deep, thick cervical fascia; until this fascia is divided it is not possible to elevate or mobilize the parotid gland superiorly and thus it is not possible to expose and isolate the distal internal carotid artery. For high exposure it is usually necessary to identify the origin of the 7th nerve, but seldom is it necessary to trace this nerve distally into the parotid gland itself. The use of fishhooks as retractors rather than heavy self-retaining retractors often avoids damage to the marginal mandibular branch of the facial nerve.

After mobilization of the parotid gland and exposure of the distal internal carotid artery, the proximal common carotid artery is followed distally by dissection of the deep fascia anterior to the sternocleidomastoid muscle. This dissection is carefully extended cephalad to the bifurcation where the caudal limits of the tumor are usually encountered. At this point vascular tapes are then placed around the internal and external carotid arteries prior to further dissection of the tumor. Baseline and occlusion xenon-133 cerebral blood flow studies and electroencephalography are performed. It is important to know the potential for collateral blood flow ahead of time in case the carotid artery must be quickly occluded for hemostasis.

As depicted in Figure 2, the common facial vein is often incorporated into the tumor capsule and must be ligated along with veins draining into it from the surrounding tissue. The tumor is then isolated along its medial and lateral borders. The proper plane of dissection is identified between the lower pole of the tumor and the common carotid artery using bipolar forceps under magnification. Since the tumor's main blood supply is from the carotid bifurcation and external carotid artery, the dissection delineates this attachment first (Fig. 3). Usually there is an areolar plane between the tumor and artery except for its subadventitial attachment at the bifurcation. With the use of bipolar cautery, the multiple perforating arteries arising from the vasa vasorum are coagulated and divided (Fig. 3). The tumor is usually fed by large proximal branches of the external carotid artery,

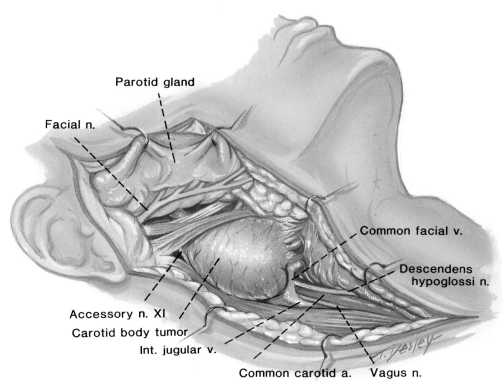

Figure 2. The parotid gland has already been mobilized and the rostral extent of the tumor delineated. The common facial vein is often incorporated into the tumor and must be ligated. Note that fishhooks are used to retract both the skin and the parotid gland to prevent cranial nerve injury. (Copyrighted by Mayo Foundation.)

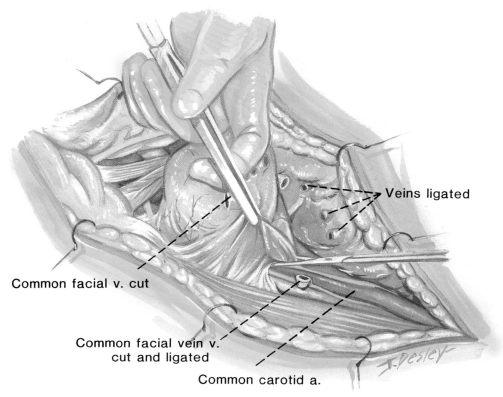

Veins ligated

Common facial v. cut

Common facial vein v.
cut and ligated

Common carotid a.

Figure 3. After dissection of the medial and lateral borders of the tumor from the surrounding tissue, its attachment to the common carotid and external carotid arteries is attacked with bipolar cautery. Not depicted in these diagrams are the vascular loops which have been placed around the common carotid artery and its major divisions for quick hemostasis if necessary. (Copyrighted by Mayo Foundation.)

which must be ligated individually (Fig. 4). The same is true for feeding arteries from the vertebral artery and thyrocervical trunk which develop in very large lesions. The tumor is grasped with forceps and rotated superolaterally to expose the tumor-carotid artery interface. By dissecting in the periadventitial layer close to the arteries, the risks of injuring the superior and recurrent laryngeal nerves can be minimized.

It should be noted that we have encountered, on several occasions during routine carotid endarterectomies, an anteriorly located aberrant vagus nerve. Furthermore, in two cases of carotid body tumors, the vagus nerve was actually incorporated within the tumor bed and had to be carefully dissected out. Identification of the vagus nerve in reference to the tumor is greatly facilitated by mobilization of the parotid

gland. The other cranial nerve which can be injured at this point in the dissection is the hypoglossal nerve. Usually the tumor displaces the hypoglossal nerve superiorly. Again, identification of the nerve in the submandibular region is important for its preservation. The mandibular branch of the facial nerve can also be injured by excessive retraction under the angle of the jaw, but the prior parotid mobilization usually provides sufficient room. In tumors with a large lateral extension, the spinal accessory nerve should be identified and protected.

After dissection and ligation of the feeding arteries from the common and external carotid arteries, the lateral and superior poles of the tumor are further mobilized (Fig. 5). Laterally and somewhat posteriorly it is common for the tumor to derive a large share of its

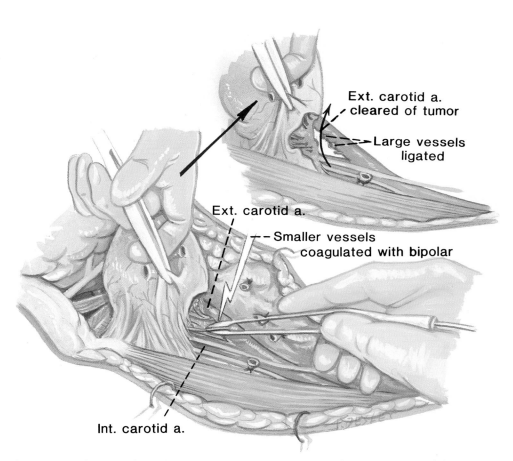

Ext. carotid a. cleared of tumor

Large vessels ligated

Ext. carotid a.

Smaller vessels coagulated with bipolar

Int. carotid a.

Figure 4. The tumor is dissected from the arteries in an areolar plane between the capsule and the adventitia. Only the tumor's origin from the adventitia is removed in a subadventitial plane. Bipolar cautery is essential to coagulate the multiple perforating vessels of the vasa vasorum without injury to the parent artery. (Copyrighted by Mayo Foundation.)

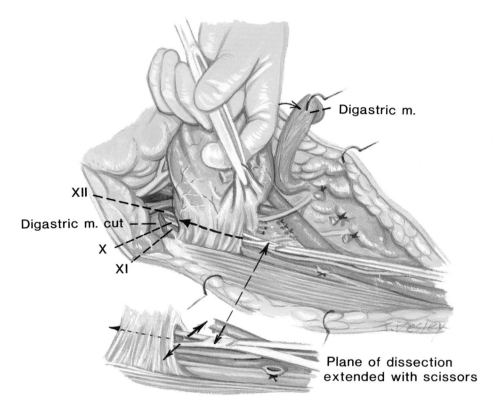

Digastric m.

XII

Digastric m. cut

X

XI

Plane of dissection
extended with scissors

Figure 5. The superior and lateral poles of the tumor are further mobilized after the main blood supply to the tumor has been ligated. (Copyrighted by Mayo Foundation.)

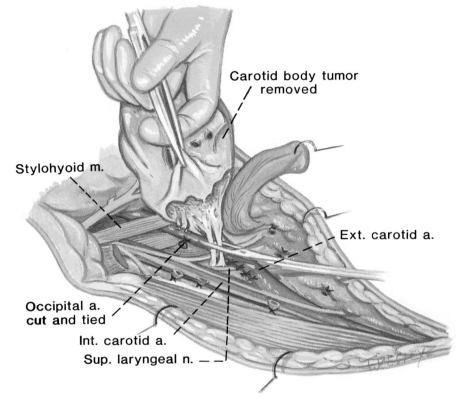

Carotid body tumor removed

Stylohyoid m.

Ext. carotid a.

Occipital a. cut and tied

Int. carotid a.

Sup. laryngeal n.

Figure 6. As a last step, the posterior wall of the tumor is dissected from the carotid artery complex and the cranial nerves. Rotation of the tumor improves exposure of this interface and facilitates protection of the superior laryngeal nerve. After tumor removal, adequate hemostasis is obtained and the wound is closed in multiple layers over one drain placed between the carotid artery and sternocleidomastoid muscle. (Copyrighted by Mayo Foundation.)

blood supply from the carotid sheath. These vessels are quite large but can be usually controlled with bipolar coagulation. This approach leaves the medial posterior attachment between the internal and external carotid arteries for last. In this manner, better visualization of the vagus nerve and its very important branch, the superior laryngeal nerve, is achieved. As the tumor is elevated from its bed, the superior laryngeal nerve is dissected away from the tumor capsule (Fig. 6).

After excision of the tumor, the arteries are carefully inspected for any arterial wall injury, and cerebral blood flow is again measured. If blood flow is low, or if a segment of the artery appears suspicious, the artery is occluded and a local arteriotomy is made. The appropriate arterial repair and, if necessary, endarterectomy are performed with a saphenous vein patch graft repair. The occasional massive carotid body tumor may extend up to and erode the foramen lacerum and petrous bone. Tumors that extend into the posterior fossa need to be approached through a combined neck dissection and suboccipital craniectomy similar to that utilized in removal of the glomus jugulare tumor. However, remnants of tumor left within the foramen lacerum are probably unresectable.

POSTOPERATIVE COMPLICATIONS

The major morbidity associated with carotid body tumor resection is lower cranial nerve palsies, specifically injury to branches of the vagus nerve including the superior and recurrent laryngeal nerves. Rarely, the hypoglossal nerve may be injured along with the sympathetic chain. In our experience, cranial nerve palsies occurred only in tumors which were greater than 5 cm in length. Documentation of damage to the superior laryngeal nerve is difficult unless electromyography of the cricothyroid muscle is performed. Clinically, these patients present with difficulty in swallowing and possibly aspiration. The proximity of the superior laryngeal nerve to the recurrent laryngeal nerve means that, if there is injury to one, both are usually involved. However, hoarseness alone implies recurrent laryngeal nerve injury which can be documented on pharyngeal examination. Evidence for superior laryngeal nerve injury includes difficulty with swallowing or aspiration. If there is injury of the recurrent laryngeal nerve, Teflon injection of the paralyzed vocal cord achieves good palliative relief. If injury to the superior laryngeal nerve leads to persistent aspiration, then a percutaneous gastrostomy may ultimately be required.

OLFACTORY GROOVE MENINGIOMAS

JOSHUA B. BEDERSON, M.D.
CHARLES B. WILSON, M.D.

INTRODUCTION

Meningiomas arising near the midline of the anterior cranial fossa may be divided according to their specific origin from the anterior falx, cribriform plate, medial orbital roof, ethmoid region, planum sphenoidale, tuberculum sellae, diaphragma sellae, or anterior clinoid processes. Based on similarities between the symptoms, signs, and operative approaches, traditionally these tumors have been separated into two groups, the olfactory groove meningiomas and the suprasellar meningiomas. Olfactory groove meningiomas characteristically attain a large size prior to diagnosis, unlike the suprasellar meningiomas, which arise closer to the optic chiasm and cause much earlier compression of the visual pathways.

CLINICAL PRESENTATION

As with other meningiomas, women are affected more frequently than men. The incidence is very low prior to age 30, and peaks in the fifth and sixth decades. The clinical course spans a range of months to years, lasting longer than 3 years in one-fourth of patients. The clinical presentation involves visual loss, frontal lobe dysfunction, headache, anosmia, or seizures, either alone or in combination. Focal motor deficits are rarely noticed by the patient, although on careful neurological examination abnormalities may be detected in nearly one-third of patients. Similarly, anosmia is an uncommon presenting complaint, but it is almost universally detected on examination. Unilateral sparing of smell is rare, but when present it is important to document so that an attempt can be made during surgery to preserve this function.

RADIOLOGICAL STUDIES

High quality preoperative radiographic examination is essential. This should include magnetic resonance imaging (MRI) with gadolinium enhancement. Sagittal MRI reveals the relationships between the tumor and the anterior visual pathways, sellar contents, ven-

tricular system, and the anterior cerebral arteries (Fig. 1A). In tumors with bilateral extension, which is usual, sagittal or coronal MRI indicates the volume of tumor on each side, contributing information essential for preoperative planning (Fig. 1B). The extent of peritumoral edema and mass effect, the degree of bony involvement, and the configuration of the frontonasal sinuses are all carefully noted. When MRI is unavailable, late generation computed tomography (CT) is obtained without and with intravenous contrast administration, and should include direct coronal imaging. Although bilateral cerebral angiograms demonstrate the relationships between the tumor and the anterior cerebral artery branches, comparable information can be obtained on a high-field strength MRI scanner, and for this reason cerebral angiography is redundant. Depending on the precise origin along the subfrontal dura, the primary blood supply comes from branches of the anterior or posterior ethmoidal arteries. Capsular arteries are recruited from the pial circulation. Preoperative embolization is precluded because only very rarely does the tumor receive any contribution from the external carotid circulation.

PREOPERATIVE PREPARATION

Rare contraindications to surgery can be found in elderly patients whose asymptomatic tumors are discovered incidentally during workup of unrelated medical problems. However, there are currently no effective alternatives to surgery. Unless medical problems, primarily cardiopulmonary, pose an unacceptable risk, removal is advised. The potential risks of surgery should be explained to patient and family and include, but are not limited to, stroke due to damage to anterior cerebral arterial branches, visual loss, frontal lobe retraction injury, postoperative hemorrhage, cerebrospinal fluid fistula, frontonasal sinus infection, meningitis, and tumor recurrence.

Careful preoperative medical evaluation of cardiac, pulmonary, and renal status is performed. All patients are treated preoperatively with dexamethasone and an anticonvulsant. Prior to surgery, 1 autologous unit of fibrin adhesive and 2 units of packed red blood cells

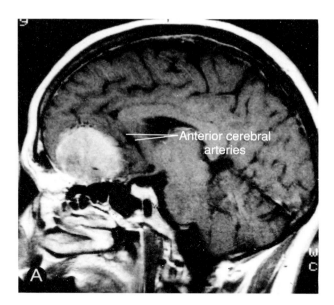

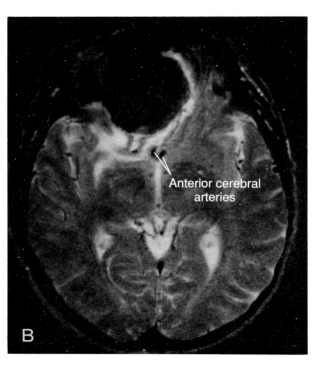

Figure 1. **A,** sagittal MRI showing the relationship between an olfactory groove meningioma and the anterior cerebral arteries, anterior visual pathways, sellar contents, and the ventricular system. **B,** a T2 weighted axial MRI showing peritumoral edema and dorsal displacement of the anterior cerebral arteries. In addition, the volume of the tumor on each side of the midline is indicated, which helps in preoperative planning.

are reserved in the blood bank. Arterial pressure is monitored by a radial artery catheter. Large-bore intravenous access is obtained, and a urinary bladder catheter is inserted. All patients are fitted with sequential compression stockings. Preoperative prophylactic intravenous antibiotics are administered prior to the skin incision, and should include both Gram-positive and Gram-negative coverage. Dexamethasone, 20 mg, is administered intravenously.

Because intracranial pressure (ICP) is often elevated in patients with larger tumors, induction of general endotracheal anesthesia includes a period of preintubation mask hyperventilation after administration of a narcotic or thiopental. Hypotension is rigorously avoided due to the risk of decreasing cerebral perfusion in the presence of increased ICP. Nasotracheal intubation is inadvisable due to the risks caused by tumor involvement of the cribriform and ethmoidal regions. After intubation, controlled hyperventilation is used to keep the PCO_2 initially between 28 and 30 mm Hg. If further reduction of ICP is needed during exposure, the PCO_2 can be dropped below 25 mm Hg. Mannitol, 500 ml of a 20% solution, is administered intravenously at the time of the skin incision.

SURGICAL TECHNIQUE

Positioning
The patient is placed in the supine position, with the operating table gently flexed and all pressure points carefully protected. The head is elevated above the heart, facing straight up, slightly extended, and placed in three-point skeletal fixation (Fig. 2).

Operative Technique
In planning the operation, several features of olfactory groove meningiomas are important: their usual bilaterality, frequently large size, broad dural attachment through which most of the blood supply is derived, and intimate relationships to the anterior cerebral arteries and, in the largest tumors, the anterior visual pathways.

A coronal skin incision is used (Fig. 3A) and scalp hemostasis is obtained by the application of compressive plastic clips. Dissection is carried out in the subgaleal areolar plane, leaving the underlying pericranium intact. The scalp is reflected and retracted anteriorly to the supraorbital ridge over rolled sponges (Fig. 3B). The posterior scalp flap is gently reflected

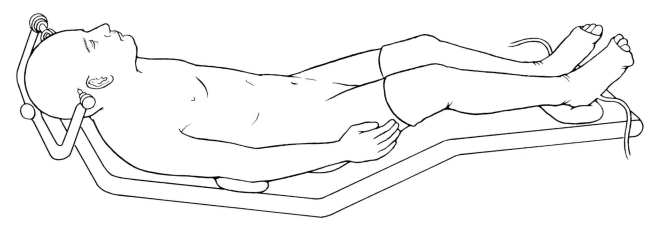

Figure 2. Operative positioning of a patient for removal of an olfactory groove meningioma.

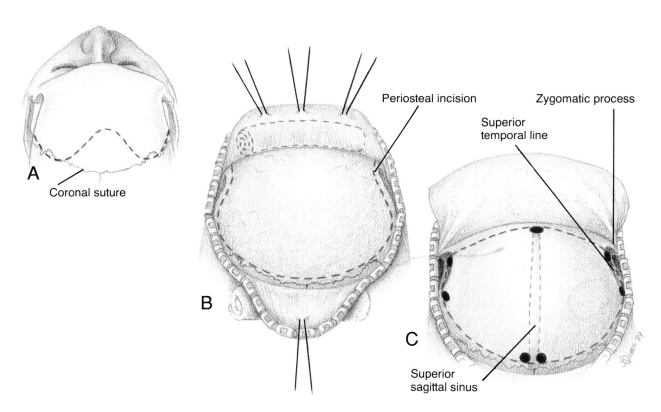

Figure 3. **A,** coronal skin incision. **B,** retraction of the anterior and posterior scalp flaps; the *dashed line* represents the line of periosteal incision. **C,** location of burr holes and outline of the bone flap.

back to expose the coronal suture. The pericranium is then incised posteriorly along the coronal suture and bilaterally along the superior temporal lines to the supraorbital ridge. It is elevated from the bone, leaving its anterior attachment intact. Although a periosteal elevator can be used, we have found it helpful to elevate the pericranium by firmly sweeping it forward with a dry sponge. Preservation of the intact pericranium is important for later closure of the frontonasal sinus and for repair of dural defects over the ethmoid sinus. Exposed tissues are covered with a moist sponge.

Although a unilateral subfrontal approach has been used by others, we prefer a bifrontal craniotomy. A free bone flap or osteoplastic bone flap can be used. The goal of this exposure is to open directly onto the orbital roofs, so that there is no overhanging frontal bone and brain retraction can be minimized. Bilateral burr holes are placed in the "key holes" just behind the zygomatic process of the frontal bone, inferior to the temporal line. When using an osteoplastic bone flap, and for a right-handed surgeon using a free bone flap, a third burr hole is made over the right anterior temporal fossa. This provides the base for an osteoplastic flap and the access for later exposure of the optic chiasm. The fourth burr hole is made over the left posterior frontal lobe. A single midline anterior burr hole (the fifth) is made just above the nasion, so that its inferior aspect is at the midline floor of the anterior fossa. With few exceptions, the frontal sinus will be entered. The sixth and seventh burr holes are made on either side of the superior sagittal sinus just anterior to the coronal suture (Fig. 3C). The bone is cut using the air craniotome posteriorly and the hand-held Gigli saw for the supraorbital cuts. This allows the latter cuts to be flush with the orbital roof. The osteoplastic flap is reflected laterally and covered with a moist sponge. The free flap is stored in saline-soaked sponges. The commonly used antibiotic solutions may be cytotoxic and should not be used for storage of the bone flap. Bleeding from the sagittal sinus is controlled with thrombin-soaked Gelfoam, and epidural hemostasis is obtained by placement of epidural tackup sutures. At this time, wire holes can be made in the bone edge and in corresponding points along the bone flap.

The frontal sinuses are nearly always entered. They are denuded of mucosa, including that portion of the sinuses within the reflected bone flap. The frontal sinuses have a variable anatomy and may extend posteriorly along the orbital roof to the planum sphenoidale, or laterally to the edge of the orbit. All the mucosa must be removed in order to avoid subsequent formation of a mucocele. The nasofrontal ostia are plugged with muscle, and the sinuses are filled with Gelfoam soaked in antibiotic solution and packed with bone wax (Fig. 4). Later, the sinuses will be covered with a pericranial flap, but this should be delayed until after the tumor has been removed. It is sometimes necessary to resect much of the subfrontal dura (to which pericranium would normally be sewn) when it is involved by tumor, and it may be necessary to use part of the pericranial flap to repair the dural defects. In some cases the frontal sinuses are small and despite opening into them the mucosa remains intact. In this setting the mucosa can be left in situ, carefully displaced toward the ostia, and covered with Gelfoam and pericranium.

Transverse dural incisions are made over each frontal lobe just above the anterior edge of the craniotomy and are carried to the edge of the sagittal sinus. Using self-retaining retractors and protecting the brain with moist cottonoid strips, the frontal lobes are retracted laterally and the sagittal sinus is doubly ligated with 3-0 silk sutures placed under direct vision through the convexity dura on each side and through the falx just beneath the sinus (Fig. 5). These are left uncut for later reapproximation of the dura. The sagittal sinus and falx are then incised. Larger tumors may incorporate the free edge of the falx, but it can be cut above the tumor to mobilize the convexity dura.

The frontal lobes are gently retracted posterolaterally, exposing the rostral pole of the tumor near the midline. With the exception of cortical veins, vascular attachments between the frontal lobes and the tumor capsule are bipolar coagulated and divided, and an incision is made in the base of the tumor at its junction with the anterior dura (Fig. 6). Every effort is made to preserve the cortical vessels by "sweeping" or "brushing" them off the tumor capsule. The anterior aspect of the tumor capsule is then entered, and piecemeal removal of the tumor can begin at its most rostral dural attachment. Because bilateral frontal lobe retraction constitutes a major insult to the brain, any further brain retraction is focused on the right frontal lobe. Most of the tumor decompression can be safely accomplished from this side, reserving further left frontal lobe retraction for dissection of the plane between tumor and brain (see below). All tumor removal is performed under the operating microscope.

The Cavitron ultrasonic aspirator or cutting cautery loop is passed along the base of the tumor in the plane of the orbital roof and is then swept upward through the overhanging tumor. Simultaneously, this separates the base of the tumor from the floor of the frontal fossa and interrupts the tumor's major blood supply (Fig. 7). All attachments of tumor to dura and bone are removed along the floor of the anterior fossa. The exposed feeding arteries entering the sessile base of the tumor are coagulated or their foramina packed with bone wax. Subsequent internal tumor decom-

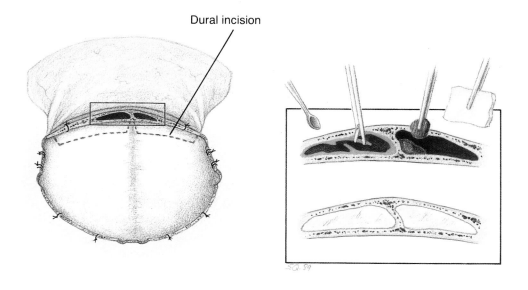

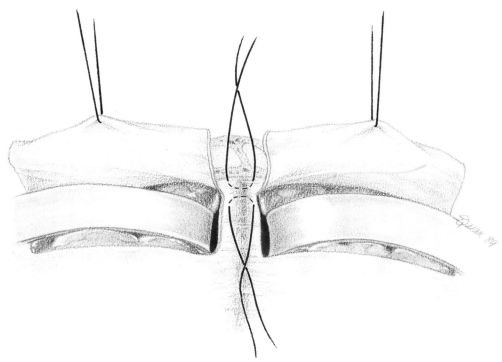

Figure 5. Technique of ligation of the superior sagittal sinus.

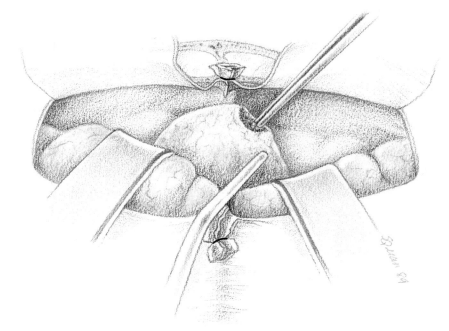

Figure 6. Gentle retraction of frontal lobes exposing the olfactory groove meningioma; piecemeal removal of the tumor is begun.

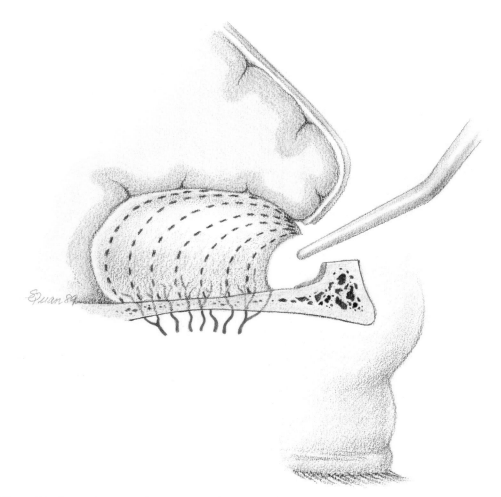

Figure 7. Sagittal section depicting the dissection of the tumor from the floor of the frontal fossa.

pression can proceed with relatively little bleeding if undercutting precedes removal of the overhanging tumor. Piecemeal tumor removal is continued in this manner with little or no additional frontal lobe retraction until only a shell of tumor remains. As the posterior portion of the capsule is approached, great care is taken to watch for embedded branches of the anterior cerebral arteries.

As the tumor's periphery is approached from within, the capsule becomes pliable and tends to collapse inward and forward. To minimize brain retraction the tumor is gently mobilized forward (rather than retracting the frontal lobes posteriorly) by use of retention sutures or heavy forceps gently applied to the tumor capsule. The surface of the frontal lobe is gently brushed away from the tumor with moist cottonoid strips as the capsule is mobilized (Fig. 8). With the exception of invasive meningiomas, this plane is well-defined. At this stage it is necessary to advance the brain retractors into the plane between tumor and frontal lobe. If internal decompression and anterior

mobilization of the capsule have been achieved, this can be done with minimal additional retraction pressure on the brain.

As the posterior part of the tumor capsule is dissected, major branches of the anterior cerebral arteries are identified and spared. Some knowledge of their orientation will have been obtained from the MRI scans, and these should be available in the operating room. Small branches may be embedded within the tumor and if they cannot be dissected free they should be divided to avoid avulsion from the pericallosal artery. At this stage it is sometimes possible to identify uninvolved dura of the medial sphenoid wing behind the tumor and, working medially, to expose the right anterior clinoid process, internal carotid artery, and optic nerve. With large tumors that overhang these structures it may be necessary to use the right-sided exposure obtained during the opening to work down the sphenoid wing from the right side. This can be facilitated by temporarily rotating the operating table to the left. Large tumors compress the optic nerves

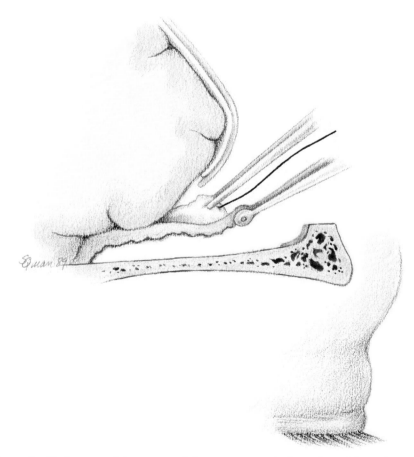

Figure 8.   Technique of separation of the tumor capsule from the subfrontal cortex.

and chiasm, and the capsule must be reflected anteriorly using gentle dissection to separate it from the depressed chiasmal complex (Fig. 9A).

With the optic nerves and chiasm and carotid arteries protected by cottonoid strips, the remaining tumor along with its entire dural attachment is removed (Fig. 9B). This may require following the tumor into the ethmoid or sphenoid sinuses. Hyperostotic bone should be removed with an air drill. The extent of bone removal is determined by the age of the patient, the vascularity of the bone, and the involvement of the paranasal sinuses.

Closure

Exposed bone is packed with bone wax and any dural defect over the sphenoid and ethmoid sinuses is covered with a pericranial graft. The pericranial graft can be free or, when the anterior dura has been removed, it can be left attached. This has the advantage of simultaneously covering the previously packed frontonasal sinuses. If an extensive bone defect has been created, it is packed with a graft of adipose tissue or muscle prior to closure of the overlying dural defect. The covered floor of the frontal fossa is then sealed with autologous fibrin adhesive.

Hemostasis in the friable tumor bed may be the most demanding part of the procedure. The retractor blades are removed one at a time, and the underlying protective cottonoids are floated off with direct irrigation. Bipolar coagulation is used to occlude the thinwalled veins on the surface of the compressed brain. The irrigating solution should remain clear after Valsalva's maneuver. The brain cavity is then lined with a sheet of Surgicel.

The dura is first reapproximated using the sagittal sinus sutures and then closed in a watertight fashion if possible. If the dura has been torn extensively during reflection of the bone flap, it may be necessary to repair the defect with a pericranial patch graft. If it has not been done already, the pericranium is reflected over the packed frontal sinuses and sewn to the dura. Epidural hemostasis is obtained using tack-up sutures, bone wax, bipolar coagulation, and either Gelfoam or Surgicel. The dura is tacked up to the surrounding bone if not already done, and the intervals between tack-up sutures are gently packed with strips of Surgicel. All dural bleeding points are coagulated and the sagittal sinus is covered with a strip of Gelfoam if any oozing persists. In the case of an osteoplastic flap, the bone flap is waxed. The undersurface of the detached temporalis muscle is inspected and any bleeding points coagulated. The bone flap is replaced and wired to the surrounding skull with 28-gauge stainless steel wire. The anterior wires are tightened first to minimize the cosmetic defect caused by the gap between bone flap and skull. The anterior and midline burr holes are covered with titanium wire mesh or filled with methylmethacrylate cement. The incisions into the temporalis muscle are closed. The scalp flap is inspected and any bleeding points coagulated. The galea is closed, beginning with a single suture joining the flaps in the exact midline. Raney clips are removed and large bleeding vessels coagulated as they are encountered. The skin is closed with vertical mattress nylon sutures.

POSTOPERATIVE CARE

Of primary concern in the postoperative period is brain edema. Although no important cortical draining veins are interrupted by this procedure as a rule, frontal lobe retraction may cause significant brain edema. Swelling may begin soon after surgery and is maximal 2–3 days later. Dexamethasone, 16–24 mg/day, is administered and can be increased temporarily if edema worsens. Serum osmolarity is measured every 6 hours and 50 g of mannitol is administered intravenously to maintain an osmolarity between 285 and 300. Modest restriction of free water intake is maintained for 3 days.

Unlike masses in other locations, postoperative frontal fossa hematomas may not cause focal neurological deficits until brain stem herniation is imminent. Therefore a high index of suspicion should be maintained, and any deterioration in mental status must be investigated. New postoperative visual or motor deficits, depressed mental status, or any deterioration of neurologic status in the postoperative period should prompt a CT scan.

Compression of the hypothalamus or pituitary stalk by tumor and surrounding edema may lead to transient postoperative diabetes insipidus. Strict recording of intake, output, daily weight, and serum electrolytes is routine. Urine output greater than 200 ml/hour in combination with a urine specific gravity less than 1.005 may be sufficient to institute treatment with aqueous vasopressin, administered subcutaneously, and titrated to reduce urine output and maintain normal serum electrolytes and osmolarity.

If cerebrospinal fluid (CSF) rhinorrhea occurs it is treated initially by lumbar subarachnoid CSF drainage via a closed system. In the immediate postoperative period while brain swelling is maximal, great care must be taken not to precipitate rostrocaudal brain stem herniation by this treatment. The leak will stop during drainage, which is continued for 4 days. After this period, the drain is clamped and evidence of further leakage is sought. If there is any question as to the existence or location of a CSF leak, labeled cotton pledgets are placed bilaterally in the superior nasal cavity under direct vision. Radionuclide is injected

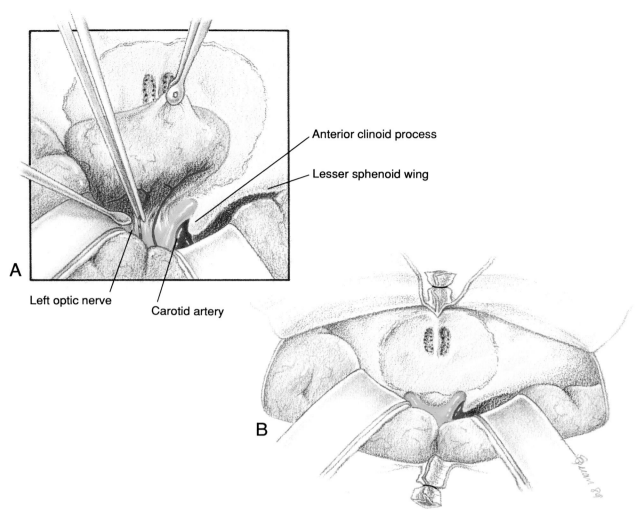

Anterior clinoid process

Lesser sphenoid wing

A

Left optic nerve

Carotid artery

B

Figure 9. **A,** separation of the tumor capsule from the optic nerves and chiasm. **B,** view of the floor of the anterior cranial fossa after complete removal of the tumor along with its dural attachment.

into the subarachnoid space and the cotton pledgets examined 24 hours later for evidence of radioactivity. Differential activity in the pledgets can direct subsequent transnasal or, rarely, subfrontal reparative procedures to the proper location.

Late postoperative bone flap infections are rare, but transgression of the frontonasal sinuses may create a predisposition for this complication. Removal of the bone flap may be required, followed by a course of antibiotic therapy and delayed cranioplasty.

Tumor recurrence is rare following complete excision of a true olfactory groove meningioma. When it does occur, reoperation is generally indicated. If complete excision is not possible, or in rare cases of invasive meningioma, postoperative radiotherapy is indicated.

CEREBRAL ANEURYSMS AT THE BIFURCATION OF THE INTERNAL CAROTID ARTERY

EUGENE S. FLAMM, M.D.

INTRODUCTION

This chapter will focus on the operative management of patients with aneurysms arising in the region of the bifurcation of the supraclinoid internal carotid artery. These comprise approximately 5% of all intracranial aneurysms. Of our 40 patients with aneurysms of the bifurcation of the internal carotid artery, 70% were Grades I–III, 10% were Grades IV and V, and 20% had unruptured aneurysms. There is no specific clinical presentation that increases the probability of finding an aneurysm in this location. The special surgical considerations for this aneurysm concern the local anatomy, particularly the arrangement of the perforating arteries near the bifurcation of the carotid artery and the path of the anterior choroidal artery in relation to the aneurysm. Although there are many similarities in the management of all patients with subarachnoid hemorrhage (SAH) from aneurysms, specific details of this location will be stressed.

SELECTION OF PATIENTS AND TIMING OF SURGERY

All patients with SAH from aneurysms at the carotid bifurcation are considered for surgery regardless of age. Some consideration must be made for the neurologic grade of the patient. In those patients who are Grades I–III and alert, surgery is carried out on the earliest regular operating day. In the past two years we have abandoned the idea that surgery must be performed within the first three days after SAH or else delayed until two weeks. At the present time, we will operate on any day after SAH if the patient is alert and does not have significant vasospasm on angiography or increasing velocities as measured by transcranial Doppler ultrasonography.

OPERATIVE INDICATIONS

In patients who have had a SAH, there is little to contraindicate surgery of a ruptured aneurysm of the carotid bifurcation provided that the medical and neurological condition of the patient will permit surgery to be performed safely. The indications for surgery of an unruptured aneurysm in this location are similar to those for other locations. Because of the position of this aneurysm deep in the medial sylvian fissure, there is an increased tendency for intracerebral hemorrhage, and, for this reason, surgery prior to SAH may be even more appropriate with this aneurysm location.

PREOPERATIVE PREPARATION

The preoperative care of patients with SAH is as important to their overall outcome as the actual surgical procedure. The major steps, once the diagnosis of a SAH is made, include determining the neurologic status of the patient, localizing the site of the aneurysm, and embarking on a course that will prepare the patient for surgical obliteration of the aneurysm.

Timing of Angiography

We prefer to carry out angiography soon after the patient is admitted. This is done not on an emergency basis but when the full neuroradiologic team is available. Although a second study prior to delayed surgery is necessary, the first angiogram provides an early diagnosis which is of obvious importance for managing the patient.

Preoperative Observation

All patients are cared for in a specialized neurosurgical intensive care unit. General issues of management deal with control of the patient's blood pressure, sedation and relief of headache, and fluid balance. A goal for blood pressure is at the patient's norm prior to SAH. Care is taken to avoid hypotensive levels, particularly in patients with a previous history of hypertension.

Fluids

No attempt is made to restrict fluid intake in patients with SAH. The usual daily intake is 2500–3000 ml/day either orally or intravenously. This is regulated by use of a central venous pressure maintained between 8 and 10 cm H_2O. Colloid is liberally used to maintain blood pressure and central venous pressure in the desired ranges. The is particularly important in patients who develop cerebral vasospasm either with or without clinical signs of ischemia.

Anticonvulsants

All patients with SAH are placed on phenytoin as soon as the diagnosis has been made. This is continued postoperatively for three to six months even in patients who have never had a seizure.

Corticosteroids

Corticosteroids are not used routinely during the preoperative period unless there is evidence of increased intracranial pressure. In preparation for surgery patients are started on methylprednisolone 12 hours prior to surgery. An intravenous dose of 250 mg every six hours is given; this is continued at this level during the first three postoperative days and then tapered over the next four to five days. While on steroids, patients receive antacids or histamine blockers.

SURGICAL TECHNIQUE

Anesthetic Techniques and Aids to Exposure

To maximize the exposure of the circle of Willis and reduce the amount of retraction required, several adjuncts are utilized. An intravenous infusion of 20% mannitol (0.5–1.0 g/kg) is begun at the time of the skin incision. Patients also receive furosemide (40 mg) on call to the operating room. Another important adjunct is spinal drainage. A catheter introduced through a Touhey needle is inserted into the lumbar subarachnoid space after induction of anesthesia. The drainage is not opened at this time. When the dura has been exposed and tented the spinal drainage is begun. This delay prevents stripping away of the dura which may cause epidural bleeding that is difficult to control. Furthermore it is easier to open the leaves of the arachnoid in the sylvian fissure if there is some cerebrospinal fluid (CSF) present. In addition to the relaxation of the brain and reduction of the need for retraction that this method provides, it facilitates the microdissection since the surgeon can work in a drier field and does not constantly have to remove CSF while working on the aneurysm. Spinal drainage is

avoided in patients with moderate amounts of atrophy since intracranial access to CSF is easy. The risk of excessive removal with subsequent collapse of the brain is thus avoided.

The final step to achieve a slack brain is to maintain the $Paco_2$ in the range of 25–30 mg Hg before the dura is opened; thereafter Pco_2 is kept between 30 and 35 mg Hg.

Operative Positioning

All intracranial microsurgery should be performed with the head secured by skull fixation. This is necessary to reduce any movement of the head which will interfere with the microdissection that is carried out at $\times 16$–20 magnification. A system that permits this as well as the attachment of self-retaining retractors and other adjuncts is particularly helpful.

The head is turned to a full lateral position and the vertex is dropped slightly toward the floor. The zygoma is almost parallel with the floor. This permits better direct visualization of the region of the optic nerve and carotid artery and reduces any obstruction to vision by the temporalis muscle or floor of the anterior cranial fossa. A folded sheet or shoulder roll should be placed beneath the ipsilateral shoulder to reduce the amount of stretch placed on the carotid artery, jugular vein, and brachial plexus (Fig. 1A).

Draping

Skin towels are sutured or stapled to all areas in front of the hairline. Towel clips are never used. This reduces the chance of damage to the skin and facilitates the reflection of the scalp flap.

Skin Incision

As shown in Figure 1B, a curvilinear incision at or just behind the hairline is used. It extends from the level of the zygoma, 1 cm in front of the tragus, to a point between the midline and pupillary line. The incision line may be infiltrated with local anesthetic but epinephrine is not used. Care is taken to preserve the superficial temporal artery although this is not always possible. The pterional craniotomy is the same for virtually all aneurysms of the carotid circulation and upper basilar artery.

Operative Procedure

Although aneurysms at the distal end of the internal carotid artery are among the less frequent aneurysms of the anterior circulation, they can be a most challenging problem because of the size that they may attain, the increased likelihood of intraoperative rupture, and the involvement of several major vessels, namely the anterior and middle cerebral arteries, the

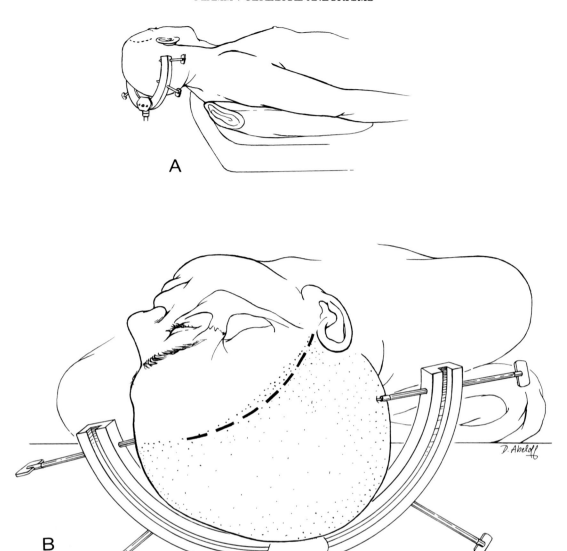

Figure 1. **A,** overall view of the patient positioned for a right pterional craniotomy. The head is turned fully to the left and the right shoulder is elevated. **B,** detail of the incision line which is behind the hairline and is only slightly curved.

anterior choroidal, as well as the internal carotid artery itself.

The temporalis fascia is incised with a scalpel; this permits closure as a separate layer which reduces postoperative swelling in the area. The scalp flap is reflected inferiorly in a single layer using the cutting cautery to separate the temporalis muscle from the skull. The bony landmarks that are utilized are the zygomatic process of the frontal bone, the lateral margin of the supraorbital ridge, and the zygoma. The muscle is reflected downward until these structures are visualized or, in the case of the zygoma, easily palpated (Fig. 2A).

A single burr hole is placed in the temporal region. From this hole a free bone flap measuring 5 × 4 cm is created with the craniotome. An initial cut is made from the burr hole to the sphenoid wing as far as is possible. The craniotome is then returned to the burr hole and the remainder of the flap created; it is usually necessary to crack the bone at the sphenoid wing by elevating the flap. It is essential that the bony opening be flush with the floor of the frontal fossa (Fig. 2B). A

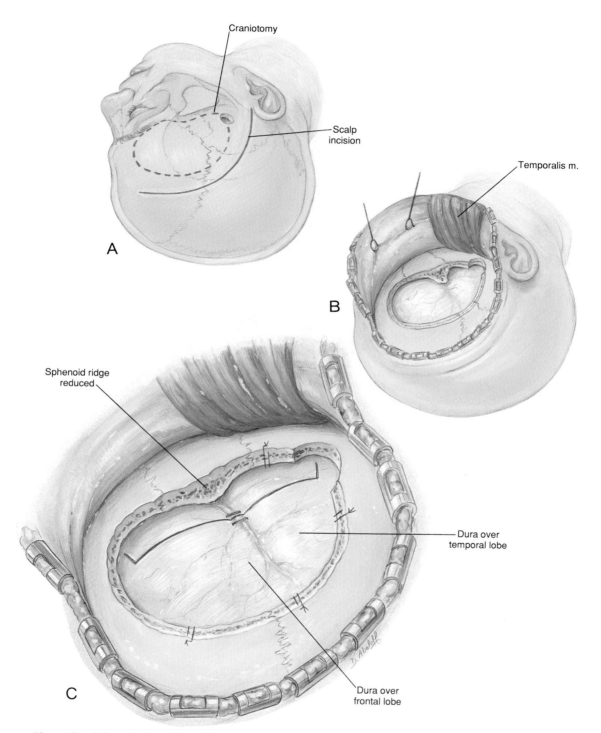

Figure 2. A, burr hole and bone flap superimposed within the scalp flap. **B,** bone flap removed. **C,** bony opening after reduction of the sphenoid wing. Dural incision is indicated.

minor variation is made when a left- or right-sided exposure is used. For a right-handed surgeon, a left-sided craniotomy should have 1–2 cm more frontal exposure to permit the free introduction of instruments without coming into contact with the margin of the flap. This is less of a problem when the exposure is on the right side because instruments in the surgeon's right hand will cross the temporal lobe.

The lateral aspect of the sphenoid wing is then rongeured away so that it will offer no obstruction to the line of vision. It is not necessary to drill this away because 1.5 cm of the wing can easily be removed with rongeurs. After dural tenting sutures have been placed the spinal drainage is opened.

A linear dural incision is made along the base of the exposure, 2 cm from the craniotomy margin. Care is taken not to coagulate the dura so that a good dural closure can be performed. If necessary, the middle meningeal artery is secured with small titanium clips (Fig. 2C).

It is difficult to describe all the nuances of the dissection techniques used in aneurysm surgery. The first step is the identification of the optic nerve. Once this has been seen the exposure is maintained with a self-retaining retractor. The landmarks for identifying the optic nerve are the olfactory tract and the sphenoid wing. The nerve is found at the point of intersection of these two structures (Fig. 3A). A second self-retaining retractor is placed on the medial edge of the temporal lobe. At times it is advisable to coagulate and divide some of the temporal bridging veins before any retraction is carried out.

The operating microscope is now brought into use and the dissection proceeds at increasing magnifications as the carotid artery and aneurysm are exposed. The first step of the microdissection is to divide various arachnoid connections. This frees the aneurysm from any undue traction and increases the room in which to operate within the subarachnoid space. The arachnoid between the frontal lobe and optic nerve is first divided. This plane is extended laterally into the medial portion of the sylvian fissure. As the arachnoid is divided additional retraction increases the exposure of the carotid artery. Once this arachnoid is opened the dissection can proceed along the carotid toward the point of origin of the aneurysm (Fig. 3B).

Even before these planes are well-established the surgeon should develop a mental picture of the location of the neck. Should rupture occur before the dissection has been completed, it is helpful to have a good idea of where the neck is so that a rapid and accurate dissection and application of the clip can be carried out while bleeding is controlled by the suction.

A specific detail of importance when operating upon carotid bifurcation aneurysms is to identify both the anterior cerebral and middle cerebral arteries before beginning the dissection of the neck of the aneurysm. The dissection of the neck should begin by working along the respective A1 and M1 segments back toward the aneurysm rather than starting the dissection directly at the neck (Fig. 3C). In my experience this reduces the risk of intraoperative rupture of the aneurysm by reducing the manipulation of the dome itself.

A watertight closure of the dura should also be attempted. The bone flap must be securely fastened to provide for a good cosmetic result. It is advisable to tie the superior frontal bone flap suture first so that this area gets the best approximation of the bone edges.

A subgaleal drain with a closed vacuum system is placed beneath the scalp flap for 24 hours. This reduces the periorbital swelling that may develop.

Vascular Considerations

Posterior Communicating and Anterior Choroidal Arteries

The relationship of several branches of the carotid, middle cerebral, and anterior cerebral arteries to an aneurysm of the carotid bifurcation must be considered during the dissection and when the clip is applied. One must be certain not to overlook a relationship between the aneurysm and branches of the posterior communicating and anterior choroidal arteries. Although these arteries arise proximal to the bifurcation of the carotid artery, their course posteriorly may carry them very close to the neck or fundus of an aneurysm at the top of the carotid artery (Fig. 3D). This must be remembered when placing a clip across the neck of the aneurysm; the blades that pass deep to the carotid artery must not occlude these other vessels as they pass through the subarachnoid space behind the carotid artery. The artery should be located before the clip is applied so that it is not included in the clip as it passes deep to the aneurysm. This is a small but important detail of this aneurysm location that should be stressed.

Recurrent Artery of Heubner

By virtue of its recurrent nature, the artery of Heubner courses laterally past the region of the carotid bifurcation. It is essential that any relationship between the aneurysm and this vessel be delineated to avoid compromising this very important artery.

Lenticulostriate Vessels

Although the lenticulostriate arteries that arise from the A1 and M1 segments, respectively, are usually not in the immediate vicinity of the carotid bifurcation, their position must be confirmed in each case to be certain that they are not compromised by the dissec-

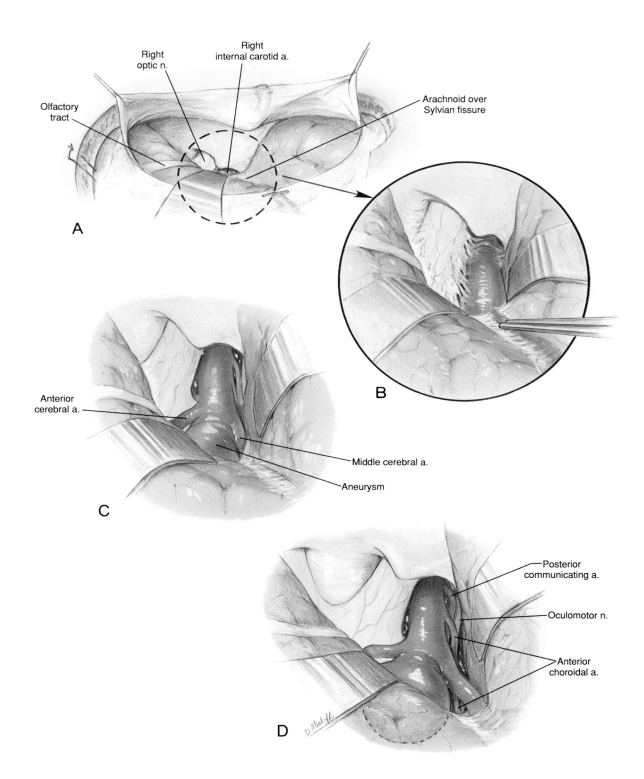

Olfactory tract

Right optic n.

Right internal carotid a.

Arachnoid over Sylvian fissure

A

B

Anterior cerebral a.

Middle cerebral a.

Aneurysm

C

Posterior communicating a.

Oculomotor n.

Anterior choroidal a.

D

Figure 3. **A,** initial view through the microscope to indicate the relationship of the olfactory tract, optic nerve, carotid artery, and sphenoid wing. **B,** exposure of the proximal supraclinoid carotid artery. Note the placement of the retractors to facilitate the opening of the sylvian fissure. **C,** identification and dissection of both the anterior and middle cerebral arteries as well as the aneurysm neck. **D,** final dissection in preparation for application of the clip. Note the relationship of the branches of the carotid artery to the neck of the aneurysm.

tion or the clip. Occasionally, a very distinct vessel of 100–200 μm may be found in close association with the neck of the aneurysm.

Clip Application

The selection of the appropriate clip should begin early in the course of the dissection so that the surgeon has a good idea which clips and clip appliers will be best suited for the particular aneurysm. It is important to remember that the neck of an aneurysm becomes wider than the initial diameter when it is compressed. It is important to have a clip long enough to account for this increase.

Although smaller carotid aneurysms can usually be safely clipped by placing the clip at right angles with the parent vessel, it is often better to apply the clip so that the blades are parallel with the parent vessels (Fig. 4, *A* and *B*). This is particularly important when dealing with larger thick-walled aneurysms. Failure to do this increases the chances of compromising the lumen of the vessel or producing a kink in the parent vessel.

An additional problem encountered with carotid aneurysms, especially larger ones, is the tension within the aneurysm. This often prevents the clip from closing completely; there is also an increased chance of rupture if the clip does not completely obliterate the aneurysm when it is applied. Several techniques are available to reduce the tension within the aneurysm. Temporary occlusion of the internal carotid artery in the neck dramatically reduces the pressure in the supraclinoid carotid artery and within the aneurysm. This is utilized for large aneurysms arising from the proximal supraclinoid carotid artery. For aneurysms at the bifurcation of the carotid artery, temporary clips can be applied directly to the supraclinoid carotid artery. They must be positioned so that the working space necessary to clip the aneurysm is not compromised.

Another technique that has been helpful with large thick-walled aneurysms is suction decompression. A 21-gauge scalp vein needle with the flanges removed is connected to the operating room suction (Fig. 4C). By puncturing the dome of the aneurysm where it is thick, blood can be suctioned through the aneurysm and the intraluminal tension reduced. Although this may not cause a thick walled aneurysm to collapse, the aneurysm becomes softer and more pliable. The clip can then be closed down easily and more safely. Blood loss has not been more than 100 ml when this technique has been employed.

In almost all cases the aneurysm should be punctured and opened after it has been clipped. Only in this way can the surgeon be certain that the goal of obliterating the aneurysm has been achieved. It is surprising how often an aneurysm may bleed when this is done after a seemingly perfect clip application. The only exception to this procedure is when no further adjustment of the clip is safe or possible. While this occurs with some of the larger ophthalmic region aneurysms, it should not pose a problem for the distal carotid aneurysms. In cases where the aneurysm is not punctured, a postoperative angiogram is used to ensure complete obliteration of the aneurysm.

Intraoperative Neurophysiologic Monitoring

We have come to rely on intraoperative monitoring for most aneurysms. When dealing with aneurysms of the carotid bifurcation, particularly when temporary occlusion of the carotid artery is anticipated, we utilize both quantitative electroencephalography (EEG) and somatosensory evoked potentials (SEP). Electrodes for stimulation and recording these parameters are applied before the patient is draped. Oftentimes the nature of the aneurysm is such that no departure can be made from the procedure even when changes in EEG and SEP are noted. They should, however, be used to alert the surgeon of the need for possible readjustment of the retractor position or pressure. Changes in these neurophysiologic guidelines are also helpful to determine the advisability of continuing temporary occlusion of the carotid artery.

Specialized Instrumentation

Operating Microscope

The usual arrangement for the operating microscope is the Contraves mount for the Zeiss microscope. The preferred objective lens is 300 mm; this allows ample room to work between the lens and point of focus. It is essential to be able to focus the microscope without using one's hands; this allows the surgeon to keep both hands in the field at all times and make minor adjustments of the focus as the dissection proceeds. This is particularly important when the arachnoid is being dissected from the neck of the aneurysm. The surgeon should be seated, and the surgeon should be free to move and change positions, as well as to shift the microscope, with minimal effort.

Instrumentation

Fairly rigid, moderately heavy bipolar forceps with different tip sizes and angulations are used. By using heavier stainless steel, rather than titanium instruments, it is possible to use them both for dissection and coagulation. The lighter instruments do not have sufficient spring to be used in a spreading fashion to divide the arachnoid and do not provide enough proprioceptive feedback to the surgeon.

A variety of sharp arachnoid knives is an important

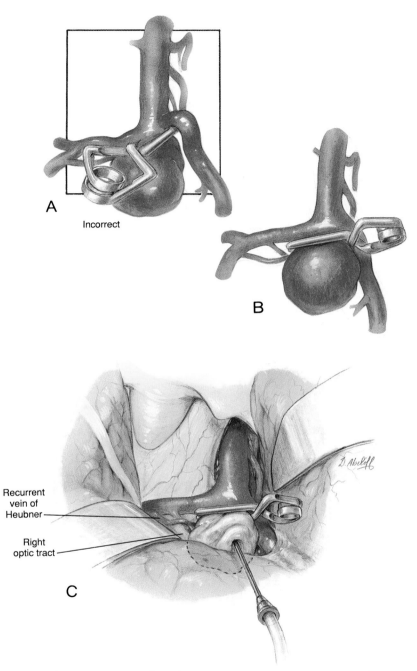

Recurrent
vein of
Heubner

Right
optic tract

Figure 4. **A,** incorrect clip placement may result in distortion of the carotid bifurcation. **B,** placement of the clip parallel to the bifurcation of the carotid artery preserves the normal anatomical relationships and normal flow patterns. **C,** final view of occluded aneurysm with suction decompression to facilitate clipping and ensure complete obliteration.

part of the equipment needed. These can be used effectively in places where scissors cannot; small disposable knives such as the Beaver blades can be used to good advantage for this purpose. Less traction is transmitted to the aneurysm if the arachnoid is divided sharply rather than tearing it with forceps.

An adequate array of microsurgical instruments is necessary. In addition to the standard instruments, a group of dissectors with varying curved and straight tips, both on bayonet and straight handles, are helpful for retracting vessels and the aneurysm itself. A No. 7 vented Frazier-type suction tip is used on the left side with a vacuum of 100 mm Hg. A larger tip is kept on the right side for the first assistant in the event of rupture of the aneurysm.

Although it is not appropriate to discuss all of the details of aneurysm clips here, certain points should be stressed. Several suitable clips should be selected and loaded by the surgeon before the dura is opened. My own preference is for larger clips that will fit the aneurysm. In the past few years I have relied on a full complement of Sugita-type clips.

The use of a self-retaining system for brain retractors is essential for all microsurgery and particularly for surgery of aneurysms. Since the operative exposure is small, there is usually insufficient room for the hands of an assistant on a brain retractor. Furthermore, the retraction must be gentle and precise; this can only be achieved with mechanically secured retractors. For aneurysms of the carotid bifurcation, a minimum of two self-retaining retractors are needed to part the lips of the sylvian fissure.

POSTOPERATIVE MANAGEMENT AND COMPLICATIONS

The goals of postoperative care are to maintain adequate cerebral perfusion, to reduce any postoperative cerebral swelling and increase in intracranial pressure, and to prevent the occurrence of seizures. These aims can be accomplished by continuing the preoperative medical regimen of corticosteroids, anticonvulsants, and fluids.

Upon transfer to the recovery room, blood pressure is maintained at normal to slightly elevated levels. Central venous pressure is maintained at 6–8 cm H_2O by administering colloid and/or whole blood. Corticosteroids, in our practice 250 mg of methylprednisolone every six hours, are maintained at this level for three days and then tapered over the next five days. Levels of anticonvulsants are determined initially after surgery and during the postoperative period.

Since most aneurysms have been opened intraoperatively we do not routinely perform postoperative angiography. If there is any change in the patient's neurologic condition or if the aneurysm was not opened at surgery, angiography is carried out.

At present all patients are being managed with a dihydropyridine calcium channel blocker to reduce the incidence of cerebral vasospasm and delayed ischemia. The efficacy of this regimen is monitored with transcranial Doppler measurements and follow up angiography when indicated by neurologic deterioration. We prefer to document the occurrence of vasospasm rather than presume that it is the cause of any neurologic deterioration.

TREATMENT OF UNILATERAL OR BILATERAL CORONAL SYNOSTOSIS

JOHN A. PERSING, M.D.
JOHN A. JANE, M.D.

INTRODUCTION

Synostosis of the coronal suture may involve all or just a part of the suture. Different degrees of involvement of the suture result in distinctly different skull shapes.

The patient with partial or unilateral coronal synostosis is characterized by ridging of the prematurely fused half of the coronal suture, flattening of the ipsilateral frontal and parietal bones, bulging of the ipsilateral squamous portion of the temporal bone, and bulging of the contralateral frontal and parietal bones. Radiographically, in addition to sutural sclerosis, the harlequin abnormality (relative elevation of the greater wing of the sphenoid bone ipsilateral to the fused suture) is present. Basal computed tomographic (CT) scanning demonstrates narrowing of the sphenopetrosal angle, ipsilateral to the fused coronal suture, and deviation of the anterior cranial base from the midline toward the side of the fused coronal suture.

The patient with bilateral coronal synostosis, however, characteristically has ridging of the coronal suture bilaterally, flattening of the caudal portion of the frontal bones and supraorbital ridges, and bulging of the cephalad portions of the frontal bones. The occiput is flattened, and the squamous portion of the temporal bone is excessively prominent. The vertex of the skull is more anteriorly situated than normal. The skull frequently takes on a turribrachycephalic, or "tower shaped," appearance.

The diagnosis of bilateral coronal synostosis is usually made clinically but is supported radiographically showing "sclerosis" of the coronal suture, associated with the bilateral harlequin deformity of the greater wing of the sphenoid in the orbits. CT scanning is supportive in demonstrating bony fusion across the sutural margins and a narrowed sphenopetrosal angle bilaterally.

Because the shapes with differing suture involvement are so disparate, so are the operative treatments. The treatments for unilateral and bilateral coronal synostosis will be addressed separately.

UNILATERAL CORONAL SYNOSTOSIS

Preoperative preparation includes autologous or designated blood donation for patient use perioperatively, and prophylactic antibiotics to be used intraoperatively, extending 24 hours postoperatively. No steroids, anticonvulsants, or lumbar cistern drains are used.

Anesthetic monitoring technique includes arterial and central venous lines, Foley catheter, and O_2 monitor for blood loss (and replacement); and Doppler, end-tidal CO_2, and nitrogen monitors for venous air embolism. The child's trunk and extremities are wrapped circumferentially around with soft cotton, and all irrigation fluids are warmed intraoperatively to preserve body heat.

The timing of surgery in patients with coronal synostosis, optimally, is within the first few weeks of life. This is done in order to reduce the potential effects of increased intracranial pressure on brain growth and to take advantage of the ameliorative effect on skull shape by the remaining normal growth of the brain. Bone remodeling techniques are also easier in the younger child.

Distinction is made between the child who is less than 1 year of age with respect to bone remodeling techniques versus the child who is older than 1 year of age, as the bone becomes much more brittle with increasing age.

The patient is placed supine on the operating table on a padded headrest. Only minimal hair (maximum width, 1 cm) is clipper-prepared at the time of surgery. Remaining hair anterior to the intended incision line, if long enough, is covered with masking tape or aluminum foil following braiding. The face is prepared into the field to be able to judge orbital and frontal symmetry intraoperatively. The bifrontal region is exposed by a bicoronal incision extending to the tragal region bilaterally. Dissection of the anterior scalp flap is in the supraperiosteal plane to reduce blood loss.

Burr holes are placed bilaterally at the pterion, and parasagittally posterior to the coronal suture (Fig. 1). Alternatively, if the anterior fontanel is patent, entry to

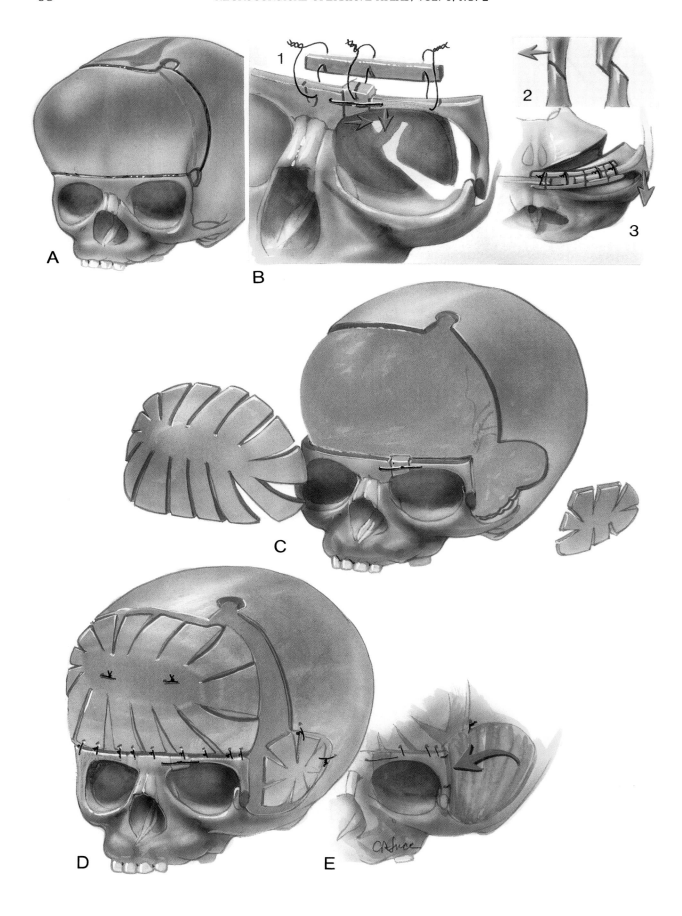

Figure 1. A, unilateral coronal synostosis. Bifrontal craniotomy is performed removing both the hypoplastic and protuberant frontal bone. Further removal of the basal extension of the involved coronal suture (*blue dashes*) into the cranial base is performed by rongeur. **B,** *1,* the shortened mediolateral axis of the supraorbital rim is augmented by an interposition bone graft (*yellow*), supported posteriorly by an additional bone graft along the supraorbital rim. The whole rim is then replaced inferiorly to equal the supraorbital rim height on the opposite side. *2,* the zygomatic process of the frontal bone is cut obliquely and the supraorbital rim and lateral wall of the orbit moved anteriorly to increase the su-perolateral projection of the orbital rim (*3*). **C,** the frontal bone undergoes radial osteotomy and is reshaped to achieve symmetrical frontal contour. The squamous portion of the temporal bone ipsilateral to the fused suture is removed, and radial osteotomies are performed to allow bone remodeling. **D,** the squamous portion of the temporal bone is returned in place and secured posteriorly and inferiorly. The frontal bone is secured to the advanced orbital rim. A segment of anterior parietal bone is removed to create a neocoronal suture. **E,** the temporalis muscle is advanced forward and attached to the lateral portion of the orbital rim and frontal bone.

the epidural space may be gained at the fontanel's margin, in place of a separate burr hole. A bifrontal craniotomy, incorporating the coronal suture, is performed, avoiding placement of a burr hole in the region of the glabella. In young patients, a bifrontal craniotomy yielding a solid single bone segment may not be possible as the metopic suture is patent. This patency allows the two frontal bone segments to be independently mobile. However, the periosteum, left intact by supraperiosteal dissection, aids to tether the bones and keep them in relative alignment.

The greater wing of the sphenoid bone which is thickened and displaced superiorly, ipsilateral to the fused coronal suture, is rongeured away to the level of the lateral supraorbital fissure. This removes the lateral aspect of the abnormal basal portion of the "coronal ring" (e.g., the frontosphenoid suture). The orbit ipsilateral to the fused suture is shortened mediolaterally. The superior orbital rim then is augmented by interposition and supporting bone grafts placed following osteotomies to the roof and lateral orbital wall (Fig. 1B). As the superior rim also is often displaced cephalad compared to the contralateral side, it is positioned caudad to equal the height of the opposite orbital rim.

The orbital rim is advanced to a slightly overcorrected position and not tethered to the cranial base or the posterior body of the zygoma. Instead, bone grafts, harvested from the parietal region, are inserted posterior to the advanced orbital rim to wedge it forward. They are secured to the rim only by suture or wire. The dura is plicated in the frontal region contralateral to the fused coronal suture to achieve frontal symmetry. Radially oriented osteotomies are placed into the center of the convex "contralateral" (to the fused coronal suture) frontal bone and the flattened "ipsilateral" frontal and parietal bones (Fig. 1C). This bone is remodeled by selective fractures using the Tessier rib bender to achieve the desired, symmetrically convex, form. The squamous portion of the temporal bone ipsilateral to the fused suture is removed by osteotomy and cut radially to allow contouring with the mallet and Tessier rib bender. The temporal bone is attached by wire suture to the surrounding bone anteriorly, inferiorly, and posteriorly to prevent recurrence of the temporal bulging. The frontal bone plate is attached to the orbital rims superiorly and laterally but is not attached posteriorly to the parietal bone. A rim of parietal bone approximately 5–10 mm wide is excised to create, in effect, a "neo"-coronal suture (Fig. 1D). The temporalis muscle is reflected anteriorly to fill in the gap between the orbital rim, which has been advanced, and the squamous portion of the temporal bone (Fig. 1E). The scalp flap is then closed in two layers (galea and skin).

"LATE" UNILATERAL CORONAL SYNOSTOSIS

In the patient with unilateral coronal synostosis treated after 1 year of age, the correction of skull irregularities is initially much the same as in the child less than 1 year of age. Burr holes are placed in the pterion region bilaterally and the parasagittal region medially behind the hairline. No burr holes are placed in the glabella region; the frontal bone is fractured forward here following weakening osteotomy of the outer table of the skull with a side-cutting air-driven drill bit. A bifrontal craniotomy is performed, leaving 5 mm of frontal bone height cephalad to the apex of the orbital rim. The dura is plicated in the frontal region contralateral to the fused suture in the area of excess frontal prominence. An osteotomy of the orbital rim ipsilateral to the fused suture is performed as described earlier. This orbital rim is advanced to a slightly overcorrected position compared to the contralateral side. The hollow, immediately posterior to the advanced orbital rim, is filled in with bone chips harvested from the parietal bone region, either as split or full segment cranial bone grafts.

The bulging in the squamous portion of the temporal bone is addressed by elevating this bone by craniotomy and radially cutting it. Kerfs or endocranial grooves through the inner table of the skull are oriented transverse to the radial osteotomies, on the concave surface of the bone. The dura is plicated locally and the bone is flattened by mallet and returned into place. A major distinction is now made from the younger patient (less than 1 year of age) in the frontal bone remodeling (Fig. 2). The frontal bone is cut into vertically oriented "slats" of bone. The periosteum is allowed to remain on the external surface of the bone to aid in bone alignment if fracture of the more brittle bone occurs during reshaping. Kerfs, or bone-weakening channels, are placed transverse to the long axis of the bone "slats" endocranially, to allow more accurate remodeling of the bone and achievement of frontal symmetry. The newly shaped "frontal bone" is attached to the supraorbital margin and to the more posteriorly located temporal and parietal bones if the child is older than 3 years of age. A gap is allowed to remain posteriorly (creating a neocoronal suture) if the child is between 1 and 3 years of age. The scalp is then closed. The nasal radix deviation is ordinarily not surgically corrected in infancy.

BILATERAL CORONAL SYNOSTOSIS

The patient with bilateral coronal synostosis is prepared for surgery similar to the patient with unilateral coronal synostosis, including arterial pressure and air embolus monitoring. One major difference, however, relates to operative positioning.

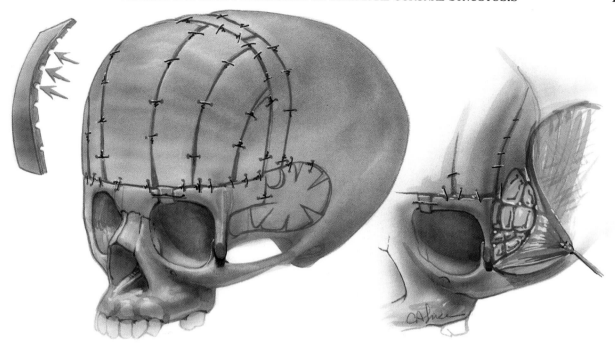

Figure 2. Late unilateral coronal synostosis. A bifrontal craniotomy is performed, but contrary to the younger patient, only a minimal amount of the lateral wing of the sphenoid is removed. The frontal bone is cut into vertically oriented slats. The undersurface of each slat receives kerfs (*green arrows*) oriented transversely and is remodeled to achieve a symmetrical form. The orbital rims are advanced by orbital osteotomy with bone grafts inserted to lengthen the mediolateral axis of the superior orbit. Additional bone grafts are placed in the region of the pterion anteriorly to prevent postoperative hollowing (*inset*).

The patient is placed in a modified prone position in order to correct both the frontal and occipital abnormalities associated with bilateral coronal synostosis. Before placing the patient in this position, however, it is important to assess the stability of the cervical spine and the craniovertebral junction by preoperative lateral cervical spine roentgenograms in flexion and extension. Positioning the patient on the operating table is greatly aided by a vacuum-stiffened bean bag to mold to the upper body and neck. The face and arms must be padded with large amounts of cushioning foam to prevent pressure sores and compression nerve palsies.

The approach for the child in infancy under the age of 1 begins with a supraperiosteal dissection of anterior and posterior scalp flaps to expose the frontal, parietal, and occipital regions. A transversely oriented periosteal incision is placed 1 cm above the orbital rims, and an incontinuity, subperiosteal, and subperiorbital dissection is completed. The temporalis muscle is elevated out of the temporal fossa, and the occipital musculature, from the nuchal line in the occipital bone cephalad to the level of the superior rim of the foramen magnum caudad, is likewise elevated subperiosteally. The skull abnormalities are then reassessed. If there is an absolute elevation of the height of the skull associated with shortening of the skull anteroposteriorly, accompanied by periorbital hypoplasia, as is ordinarily the case, the procedure proceeds as follows: Burr holes are placed in the pterion regions bilaterally, and parasagittally in the anterior parietal bone just posterior to the coronal suture (Fig. 3, *A* and *B*). Similarly, a biparieto-occipital bone graft is outlined with multiple burr holes adjacent to the sagittal and transverse sinuses. If the metopic or sagittal sutures are widely patent and preclude elevation of the frontal or parieto-occipital bones as a single piece, separate frontal or parieto-occipital bone grafts should be elevated on each half of the skull. Once the bone is elevated both frontally and parieto-occipitally (Fig. 3C), further dissection epidurally may be carried out below the level of the transverse sinus to allow the surgeon to fracture outward (posteriorly) the occipital bone. These outfractures or "barrel staves" increase the "bony capacity" by enlarging the perimeter of the skull locally, allowing later brain and dural displacement in this region as the height of the skull is reduced. Barrel stave osteotomies in the occipital bone in the midline and paramedian regions are longer than those placed further laterally, to achieve elonga-

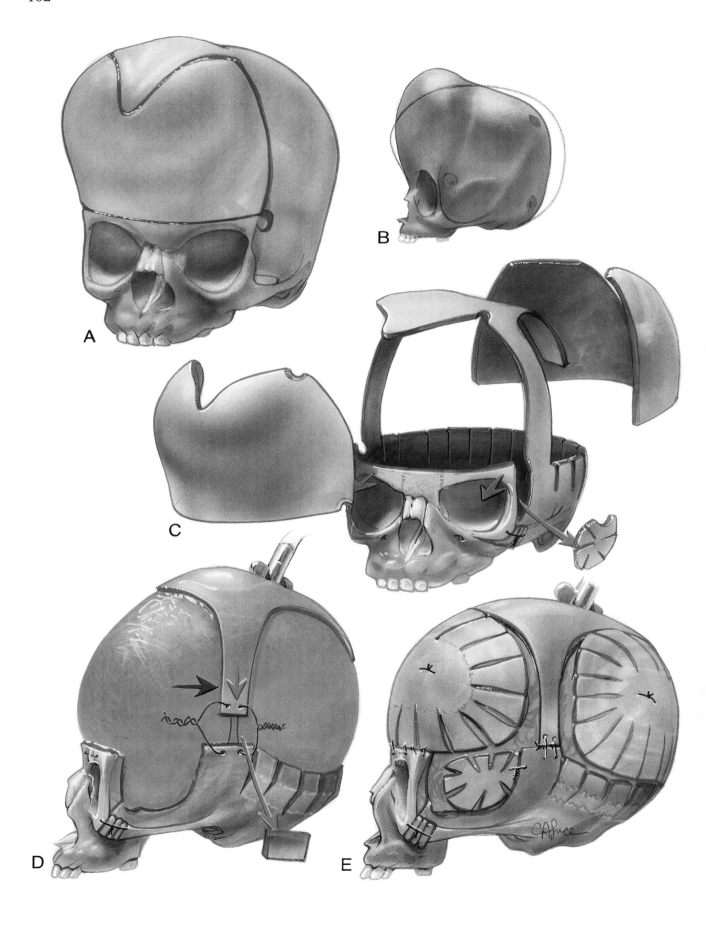

Figure 3. **A,** bilateral coronal synostosis. The skull in bilateral coronal synostosis demonstrates flattening occipitally and bulging frontally with an anteriorly displaced skull vertex. **B,** burr holes are placed as indicated on the lateral view of the skull. **C,** a bifrontal graft is elevated. A biparieto-occipital bone graft is developed posteriorly leaving a bony bridge between the two hemicrania across the occiput. The remaining occipital bone undergoes barrel stave osteotomy. An osteotomy in the orbital roof, lateral wall, and floor mobilizes the orbital rim in the form of the letter "C." The orbital rims are advanced and secured with parietal bone grafts inserted into an oblique osteotomy in the zygoma. **D,** the vertex of the skull is shifted posteriorly by severing the parietal bone struts, removing a segment of bone, and relocating the strut posteriorly (*blue arrow*). This reduces the prominence of the frontal "bossing." The basal and parietal bone segments are cinched together while the intracranial pressure is monitored. **E,** the frontal and temporal bone grafts are reattached to the basal skull, but the parieto-occipital bone graft is allowed to "float" with attachments only to the underlying dura.

tion of the anteroposterior axis of the skull without further widening of the parieto-occiput. The occipital bone barrel staves are fractured posteriorly, at the base of the skull, and then inwardly at their distal margin so they do not create a pressure point on the overlying scalp.

In the lateral sphenoid region, the thickened and abnormally elevated superior portion of the greater wing of the sphenoid bone is removed by rongeur to the level of the lateral supraorbital fissure. With this bone removal, the basal extension of the coronal suture, the lateral frontosphenoid suture, is removed. "C"-shaped orbital osteotomies (superior, lateral, and inferior orbital wall osteotomy to the level of the inferior orbital foramen) are performed in both orbits to increase orbital rim projection bilaterally. The advanced orbital rims are held forward by parietal bone grafts which are wedged in the osteotomy site in the body of the zygoma and secured to the rim anteriorly. A craniotomy is performed to remove the abnormally convex squamous portion of the temporal bone. The bone is reshaped by a combination of radial osteotomies into the center of the convexity and controlled fractures of the bone segments with the Tessier rib bender. The dura is plicated locally, and the temporal bone returned, to be secured to the surrounding base of the skull posteriorly and inferiorly.

At this point, two parietal bone struts remain, extending from the vertex of the skull to the basal portion of the temporal and parietal bones. These two cephalocaudally oriented struts of bone are severed at their caudal interface with the more basal skull and are shifted posteriorly approximately 1–2 cm (Fig. 3D). The shift is performed in order to reduce the bulging contour of the dura in the superior frontal region and replace posteriorly the elevated vertex point which has become displaced anteriorly. If further contouring of the dura is needed, dural plication sutures are placed at this time.

In order to safely reduce the height of the skull, a twist drill hole is placed in the right paramedian parietal bone and a pressure transducer is inserted to measure intracranial pressure (ICP) (Fig. 3E). Wire and nylon sutures are passed through drill holes in the lateral bone struts and the basal skull. The wire is slowly cinched down over the course of 30–60 minutes, and the intracranial pressure is continuously monitored under conditions of normocapnia and normotension. Presently, we recommend that while the vertex of the skull is being cinched down, cerebral perfusion pressure of approximately 60 mm Hg be maintained. During the initial stages of the height reduction, however, the intracranial pressure may be elevated (>20 mm Hg) for short periods. If the surgeon does not observe a rapid reduction in intracranial pressure over the course of 1–2 minutes, then a smaller increment in reduction of the cranial vault height is necessary over a longer period of time. Ultimately, the same degree of height reduction may be achieved, but it may take longer to do so. Caution must be exercised during this maneuver to prevent brain injury.

While the incremental cinching-down process is being achieved, the frontal and parietal bone are remodeled to give the contour desired. Radially oriented osteotomies in the frontal and parieto-occipital bones allow for reshaping by a series of controlled fractures with the mallet and the Tessier rib bender. After completing the reshaping of the frontal bone, it is attached with wire sutures to the orbital rim. The posterior aspect of the frontal bone is not secured with wire and is allowed to "float free." The parieto-occipital bone segment adjacent to the barrel staves in the occipital bone is shortened to allow a gap of approximately 5–10 mm between the bone edges. This is done in order to encourage further displacement of the neurocranial capsule posteriorly, postoperatively. The parieto-occipital bone graft is attached to the surrounding dura, but is not fixed to bone posteriorly to further aid this posterior displacement process.

The temporalis muscle is advanced forward to attach to the lateral portion of the supraorbital rim and the scalp incision closed. No drains are used. A postoperative skull molding cap is routinely used as an additional guide to aid skull shape normalization for an additional 2–3 months.

"LATE" BILATERAL CORONAL SYNOSTOSIS

The patient who is older than 1 year of age is treated similarly in terms of positioning and craniotomy lines to the child less than 1 year of age. The difference is that the bone at 1 year of age is more difficult to reshape, fracturing more readily, by the methods employed at less than 1 year of age. Therefore, the operative technique is modified as follows.

Following bifrontal and biparieto-occipital craniotomy, the orbital rims are advanced forward in the shape of the letter "C" bilaterally. Bone grafts are wedged in at the osteotomy site in the zygoma and secured by transosseous wires. Barrel stave osteotomies are performed in the parieto-occipital region; the staves are fractured posteriorly to elongate the anteroposterior axis of the skull. The squamous portion of the temporal bone is removed by craniotomy. The remaining cephalocaudally oriented parietal bone struts extending from the vertex of the skull are severed, and an intracranial pressure monitor is inserted in the right parietal bone. The parietal bone struts are displaced posteriorly approximately 1 cm, and the height of the skull is slowly reduced by cinching down on the wire loops in the basal parietal and

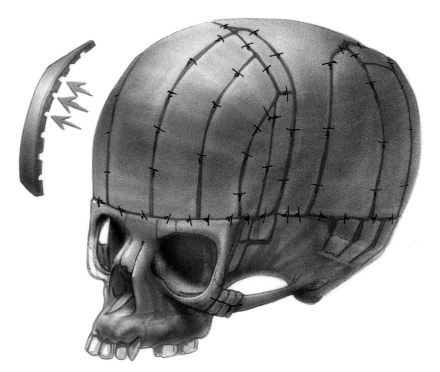

Figure 4. Late bilateral coronal synostosis. Bifrontal and biparieto-occipital bone grafts are elevated. The orbits undergo "C"-shaped orbital rim osteotomy and advancement. Occipital barrel staves are developed. The parietal bone struts are shifted posteriorly and shortened to reduce the frontal contour projection. The frontal bone and parieto-occipital bone are split into vertically oriented slats and undergo remodeling aided by kerfs (*green arrows*) placed on the endocranial surface of the bone.

temporal bones. We have observed that it requires a longer time for intracranial pressure reductions to occur in older children when compared to similar incremental reduction in vault height in younger children, perhaps due to thickened dura with increasing age or scarring of the dura from previous surgery. Therefore, smaller increments of adjustment should be anticipated over a given time period. The cerebral perfusion pressure should be maintained at approximately 60 mm Hg, under conditions of normocapnia and normotension. The frontal and parieto-occipital bones are then cut into vertically oriented "slats," approximately 2 cm wide, leaving the periosteum attached to the external surface of the skull bone (Fig. 4). Transversely oriented kerfs are placed through the inner table of the skull (concave surface of the bone), and controlled fractures are performed on the "slats" for reshaping. The individual bone segments are wired or sutured with long-acting absorbable suture to give the desired form. The temporal bone, because of its thinness, ordinarily can be molded by radially oriented osteotomies and kerfs on the inner table of the skull, without cutting the bone into "slats." This allows easier fixation to the basal skull, posteriorly and inferiorly. Bone chips from the parietal region are used to fill

in the temporal hollow behind the advanced orbital rim, and the temporalis muscle is transferred anteriorly and attached to the supralateral orbital rim.

Patients who are older than 3 years of age may have the bone fixed in a slightly overcorrected position to allow for further brain growth, yet still provide the stability necessary for reconstruction of the skull. In the child between 1 and 3 years of age, the brain is still growing rapidly, and provision must be made for this by allowing greater room for growth by not fixing the remodeled bone, particularly in the anteroposterior axis, while still employing the bone remodeling techniques for the older child. Skull molding caps are generally not used postoperatively in patients undergoing this procedure who are older than 1 year of age.

The complications associated with this procedure are few, but the possibility of cerebral infarction or mortality is still present. Blood loss and hypothermia are the immediate intraoperative concerns, and greater blood loss should be expected with osteotomies of the basal vault bone. Postoperatively as well, diffuse oozing from all the osteotomy lines needs to be anticipated and frequent checks of the blood count should be taken. If intravenous fluid loading is not given at the initiation of the operative procedure, venous air embolism may occur. Lastly, the major concern with the reduction in skull height is the possibility of cerebral herniation. If the skull height is reduced with the provision for ICP monitoring, and the guidelines for reduction are met as described earlier, the risk is small and no negative neurologic sequelae have yet been noted in our cases.

CONVEXITY MENINGIOMA

SARAH J. GASKILL, M.D.
ROBERT H. WILKINS, M.D.

INTRODUCTION

The convexity meningioma arises from the meninges over the cerebral convexity, and as it grows it indents the underlying brain. Its main blood supply ordinarily comes from regional meningeal arteries such as the anterior branch of the middle meningeal artery shown in Figure 1. At times the convexity meningioma may grow through the dura mater into the overlying calvarium; hyperostosis of the overlying bone is a typical response. When that growth pattern occurs, the tumor may also receive some of its blood supply through scalp vessels such as the superficial temporal artery. In rare instances, the meningioma grows completely through the calvarium and produces a second continuous mass beneath the scalp.

PATIENT SELECTION

The mere presence of a convexity meningioma is not justification for its removal. For example, a small asymptomatic tumor that has been discovered by accident in an elderly woman can be followed by serial computed tomography (CT) or magnetic resonance imaging (MRI) examinations, and if it remains asymptomatic and does not increase significantly in size, it does not require surgical excision. On the other hand, surgical treatment is appropriate in an otherwise healthy patient with a reasonably long life expectancy, especially if the tumor is of moderate or large size, if it has been shown by serial CT or MRI studies to be increasing in size, or if it is producing symptoms.

SURGICAL TECHNIQUE

In designing an operation to remove a convexity meningioma, the surgeon should try to interrupt as much of the blood supply as possible early in the operation. Ordinarily this is done as the scalp flap is reflected and the dura mater is opened. In the unusual circumstance of a very vascular lesion, preoperative embolization of the tumor should be considered.

Because a convexity meningioma is ordinarily a benign tumor that is easily accessible, every effort should be made to obtain a cure by a complete tumor removal. This dictates the removal not only of the main tumor, but also of any portion of the dura mater and bone thought to be invaded by the tumor. Therefore, the surgeon should plan for dural grafting, which is usually necessary, and cranioplasty, which is also required at times.

The operation may be performed with the patient in a supine, lateral, prone, or semi-sitting position, depending on the specific location of the lesion. In general, the head should be positioned so the region of the tumor is most prominent. The proposed cranial opening should be centered on the tumor and should be larger than the tumor to permit its removal.

For the ordinary convexity meningioma, we prefer to use a scalp flap that is based anteriorly, laterally, or posteriorly and is turned down away from the superior sagittal sinus (Fig. 2A). A free bone flap (i.e., not hinged on the temporalis muscle or other soft tissue)

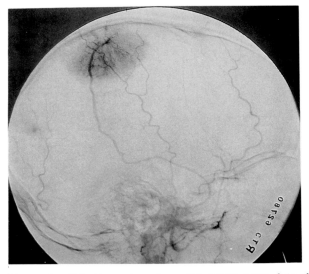

Figure 1. Selective external carotid arteriogram, lateral view. The tumor blush of a convexity meningioma is demonstrated. The principal source of blood supply to the meningioma is the anterior branch of the middle meningeal artery.

is then created in one of several ways. Several burr holes can be made and connected with a high-speed drill, craniotome, Gigli saw, or rongeurs (Fig. 2A); or a single perforation can be made and the bone flap formed with a high-speed drill or craniotome. The latter technique is faster and there are fewer irregularities in the skull when the bone flap is replaced at the end of the operation. However, the dura mater is more likely to be cut flush with the bone edge (especially in an elderly individual in whom the dura mater is thin and is very adherent to the calvarium), making it more difficult to close in watertight fashion at the end of the operation.

Depending on the vascularity of the tumor, there may be excessive bleeding from the bone edges along the line of separation around the craniotomy flap. This can be minimized by rapidly separating the bone flap from the underlying dura mater. This may be done by using two periosteal elevators inserted into the bony opening at some distance apart, to pry the bone flap away from the dura. A third instrument such as a No. 2 Penfield dissector is then used simultaneously or subsequently to separate the bone flap from the underlying dura and tumor (Fig. 2, B and C). The surface of the dura is covered temporarily with absorbable gelatin sponge and cottonoid strips to control bleeding

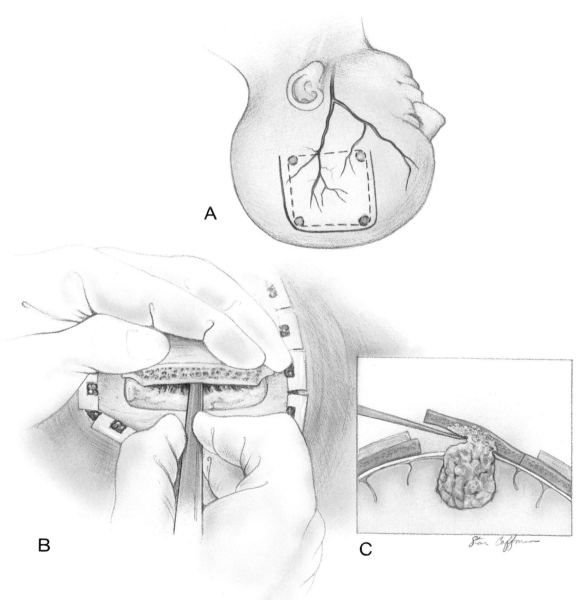

Figure 2. Scalp and cranial flap for removal of a convexity meningioma. **A,** outlines of typical scalp and bone flaps for removal of a convexity meningioma. **B** and **C,** elevation of the bone flap and separation of the underlying dura mater and tumor from the inner table of the skull.

from this source, and bone wax is spread into the exposed diploic spaces of the calvarium around the periphery of the bony opening to stop bleeding from that source (Fig. 3).

Periodic drill holes are made through the bone edge around the cranial defect and heavy nonabsorbable sutures are inserted for use during the closure (Fig. 3). Cottonoid strips are placed between these sutures and the skin edge to prevent possible bacterial contamination. The dura is then opened circumferentially around the tumor, with a margin of uninvolved dura at least 1 cm in width (Fig. 4). As the dura is opened, meningeal vessels are sealed shut with bipolar coagulation. Hemostatic clips may be used, but will cause some degree of artifact on postoperative CT and MRI

examinations. The dura mater is then tacked up around the periphery of the bony opening using interrupted 3-0 nonabsorbable sutures (Fig. 4, inset). A brain spoon or similar shield is inserted during this suturing to prevent needle injury to the underlying brain. At the previously mentioned drill holes, the dura is tacked to the bone. Between these it is tacked to adjacent soft tissue such as the periosteum or temporalis fascia.

If it is small, the meningioma and its attached dura are gradually separated from the adjacent and underlying cerebral cortex and are removed en bloc (Fig. 5). If it is larger, and especially if a portion of the cortex overlies the equator of the tumor, the center of the meningioma can be removed by various instruments

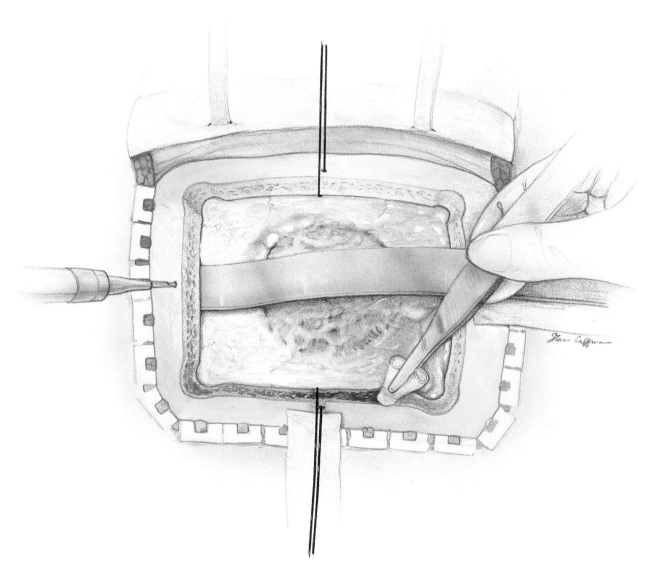

Figure 3.   Application of wax to the bone edges for hemostasis and a technique of creation of drill holes for anchoring the bone flap.

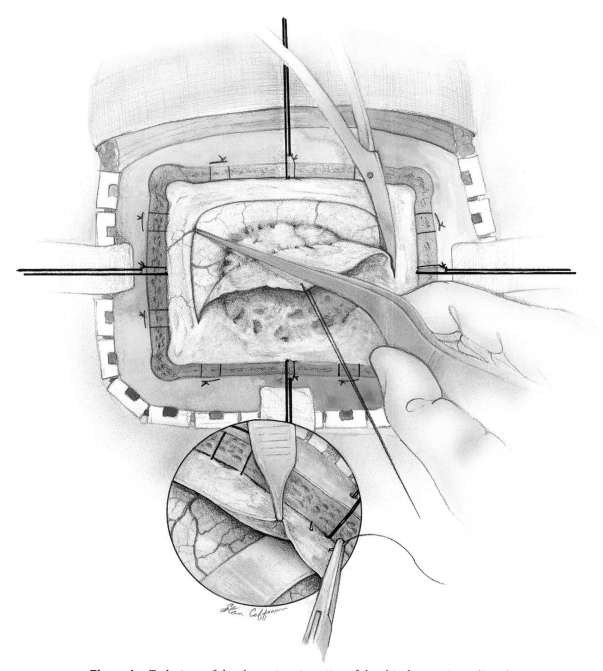

Figure 4. Technique of dural opening; insertion of dural tack-up sutures (*inset*).

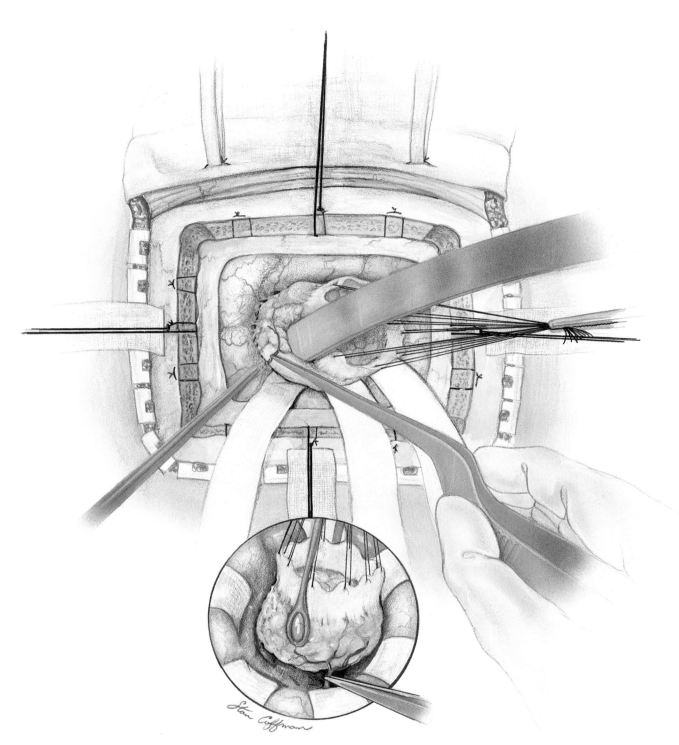

Figure 5. Technique of removal of a meningioma en bloc. Bipolar coagulation of vascular feeders to the tumor (*inset*).

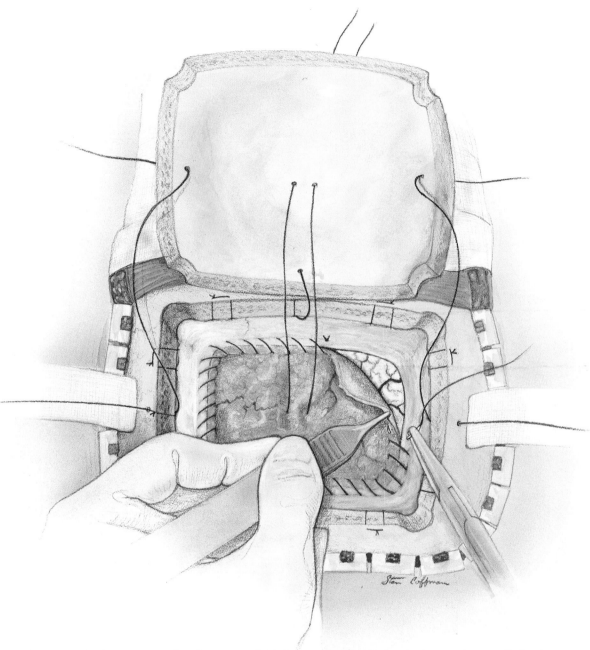

Figure 6.   The dura mater is closed in watertight fashion using a graft of periosteum or temporalis fascia.
As the bone flap is replaced, the dura is tacked up to it.

(depending on its consistency) such as bipolar cautery, suction, cutting loop cautery, ultrasonic aspiration, and laser vaporization. This reduces the bulk of the tumor and permits the separation of its external surface from the brain without excessive brain retraction.

In either case, the separation of the tumor from the brain is done gradually around its circumference and then beneath it as the tumor is retracted away from that portion of the cortex receiving the surgeon's attention (Fig. 5). The surgeon coagulates and divides all vessels that bridge between the cortex and the tumor but tries to leave the intrinsic cortical vessels intact. At all times the surgeon should attempt to minimize the damage done to the cortex by the process of separation; however, some damage almost always occurs, and the surgeon should warn the patient preoperatively that a temporary or permanent neurologic deficit, appropriate to the location and size of the tumor, might result. We find it helpful to insert a cottonoid strip between the tumor and cortex at each location after the separation has been made (Fig. 5). Thus, when the surgeon has completed the separation around the periphery of the meningioma, a circumferential series of cottonoid strips is in place. The tumor is then lifted out of its bed and any remaining attachments are coagulated and divided (Fig. 5, *inset*).

After hemostasis has been achieved, the defect left by the tumor removal is filled with warm irrigation solution and the wound is closed in anatomical layers. A fascial graft ordinarily can be obtained from the exposed periosteum or temporalis fascia to be sewn circumferentially in watertight fashion to fill the dural defect (Fig. 6). If not, fascia lata or a dural substitute can be used. If a small portion of the bone flap appears to be involved by tumor, it should be removed before the flap is replaced; if the majority is involved, the entire flap may need to be sent to the pathology laboratory. As the bone flap is sutured back into position, the underlying dura and dural graft are tacked up to its center (Fig. 6). Any residual bony defects can be filled with methyl methacrylate or some other cranioplasty material. The scalp is closed in two layers and a compressive head dressing is applied.

OCCIPITAL LOBECTOMY

MILAM E. LEAVENS, M.D.

INTRODUCTION

Occipital lobectomy is a useful procedure that may be partial or complete, depending on the patient's pathologic condition and the extent of involvement of the occipital lobe and adjacent brain. Gliomas, arteriovenous malformations, metastatic tumors, and, less often, meningiomas are the usual indications for performing a lobectomy.

The boundaries and important anatomical features of the occipital lobe and adjacent brain are shown in Figure 1. The occipital lobe has roughly a pyramid shape, with four triangular sides. The relationship of these external features of the occipital lobe to the cranial sutures, dural sinuses, ear, mastoid bone, and vein of Labbé is shown in Figure 2. Placement of the bone flap is based on these anatomical features so that the exposure is adequate for performing the lobectomy while avoiding injury to the dural sinuses and avoiding opening of the mastoid air cells.

SURGICAL TECHNIQUE

The anesthesia used is continuous Sufenta (sufentanil citrate) opioid infusion with Norcuron (vecuronium) muscle relaxant, and a small amount of Forane (isoflurane, USP) inhalation agent. The patient is placed in the lateral position, supported by a bean bag and axillary roll, with the head in a three-quarters position on a doughnut (Fig. 1C) or in a three-pin fixation head holder. This is followed by routine preparation of the skin and draping. The patient is infused intravenously with an antibiotic, usually 1 g of Ancef (cefazolin sodium) during the operation and then postoperatively every 6 hours for 24 hours. The patient also receives intravenously a single maintenance dose of 300 mg of phenytoin and 4–6 mg of dexamethasone every 4 hours. The $PaCO_2$ is kept between 25 and 30 mg Hg, and, if needed to further control intracranial pressure, 0.5 to 1 g/kg of mannitol is given intravenously.

The scalp incision and flap, position of the bone flap, and dural incision for a right-sided lobectomy are shown in Figures 1 and 2. The occipital pole is adjacent to the torcular herophili and is near the inion.

The parieto-occipital fissure is near the lambdoid suture plane at the midline. The lambdoid suture is 6.5 cm from the inion.

Incision and Exposure

Part of the skin incision is in the midline extending from just above the inion to beyond the parieto-occipital fissure. The length of the midline scalp incision will vary, depending on whether the lobectomy is to include part or all of the occipital lobe in either hemisphere, or the occipital lobe and posterior temporal and parietal lobes in the nondominant hemisphere. The upper end of the midline scalp incision continues laterally, extending over the upper mastoid region, but it may end more anteriorly above the ear if a larger bone flap is needed. The combined scalp, occipital muscle, and periosteum are dissected off the calvarium in one layer.

Identifying the middle of the inion, visualizing the sagittal suture, and knowing the position of the upper mastoid bone, are vital to locating the superior sagittal and transverse sinuses and placing the burr holes properly. The venous sinuses are about 0.75 cm wide. Burr holes 1 and 2 (Fig. 2) are placed 1.5 cm lateral to the midline. Burr hole 2 is placed 2 cm from the inion. Burr hole 3 is on a plane through the middle of the mastoid bone and 5.5 cm from the tip of the mastoid. The bone cut between burr holes 2 and 3 is above the transverse sinus and mastoid bone. The position of the remaining burr holes depends on the size of the tumor and the amount of exposure required. A rim of temporalis fascia may be left attached to the free bone flap and resutured during closure. During the formation of the bone flap a suction trap is used to collect bone dust, which is used during the closure.

Dural tack-up and wire holes are placed in the calvarium and bone flap. Dural tack-up sutures are used but left untied until the time of closure. Intraoperative ultrasound is invaluable in locating the gross boundaries of the intracerebral lesion. The dura is opened with a T incision. The base of the dural flaps is along the dural sinuses. A view of the exposed brain after opening the dura is shown in Figure 2. The point marking the 75% distance from the nasion to the inion and the point on the upper lateral margin of the

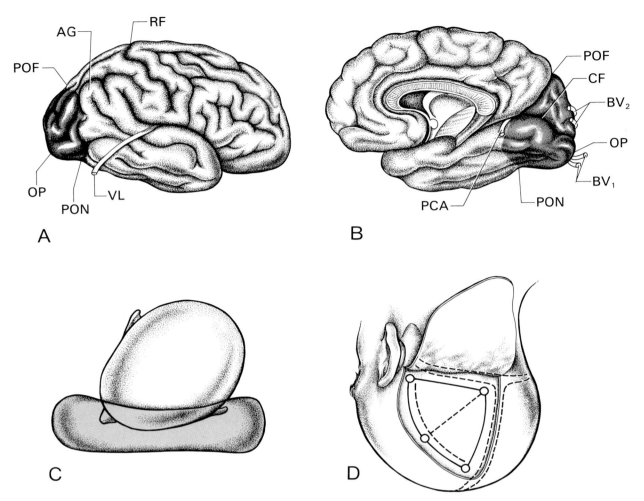

Figure 1. **A** and **B,** lateral and medial surfaces of the occipital lobe. **C,** head position. **D,** scalp incision and flap, position of the bone flap, dural incision. *RF,* rolandic fissure; *AG,* angular gyrus; *POF,* parieto-occipital fissure; *OP,* occipital pole; *PON,* preoccipital notch; *VL,* vein of Labbé; *CF,* calcarine fissure; *BV₂,* bridging veins to superior sagittal sinus; *BV₁,* bridging veins from occipital pole to torcular herophili; *PCA,* posterior cerebral artery.

orbit are useful. When they are connected, the resulting line marks the plane of the sylvian fissure. The supramarginal gyrus, which is anterior to the angular gyrus, will be on the turned-up distal end of the sylvian fissure.

Shown in Figure 2 is the angular gyrus with its surprisingly close position to the occipital pole and the midline, which is a position of considerable significance to planning an occipital lobectomy on the dominant hemisphere. The location of the angular gyrus has been measured to be 35 ± 4 mm from the occipital pole and 24 ± 2 mm from the midline. On a fresh cadaver brain the location of the angular gyrus in the two hemispheres measured 35 and 43 mm from the occipital pole and 27 and 25 mm from the midline. The intact, functioning angular gyrus may be resected in the nondominant hemisphere but should not be resected in the dominant hemisphere because of the morbidity of persistent postoperative dysphasia. Localization of speech in the temporal and parietal lobes in the language-dominant hemisphere is very variable. Rarely does speech representation extend into the occipital lobe. It is reasonable, however, to perform an occipital lobectomy in the dominant hemisphere if that procedure is needed to excise a neoplasm or an arteriovenous malformation, although it is not advisable to extend the cortical resection beyond the occipital lobe without first localizing the posterior extent of speech localization by stimulation mapping techniques. Well-demarcated occipital tumors extending anteriorly in the dominant hemisphere may be removed without use of such techniques. After the occipital lobectomy, the tumor that remains anteriorly is carefully removed, preserving the brain adjacent to it,

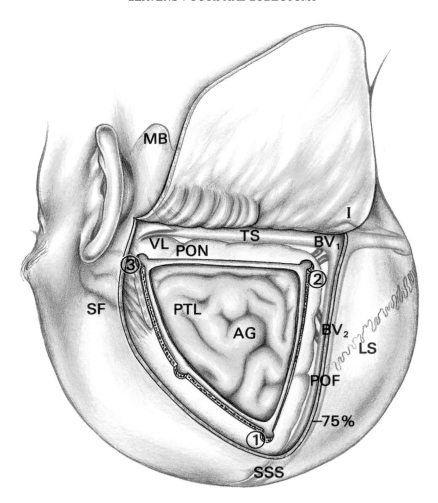

Figure 2. Exposed occipital lobe shown with adjacent brain and vascular anatomy. *1*, *2*, and *3* (*circled*), burr holes 1, 2, and 3; *MB*, mastoid bone; *SF*, sylvian fissure; *LS*, lambdoid suture; *TS*, transverse sinus; *PTL*, posterior temporal lobe; *SSS*, superior sagittal sinus; *75%*, point on skull at 75% distance from nasion to inion; *I*, inion. For additional abbreviations, see the legend to Figure 1.

using a bipolar cautery, suction, laser, and the Cavitron ultrasonic aspirator (CUSA) with little or no brain retraction.

The preoccipital notch, the most lateral border of the occipital lobe, is 6 cm from the occipital pole adjacent to the lateral aspect of the transverse sinus and near the vital vein of Labbé at its termination into the transverse sinus. Because occlusion of this vein may result in a devastating hemorrhagic infarction of the brain, it should be identified and preserved during the lobectomy. An exception would be its sacrifice in order to remove tumors that have infiltrated the adjacent temporal and parietal lobes in the nondominant hemisphere.

Lobectomy

The initial steps in performing the lobectomy after exposure of the cortex is retraction to identify, coagulate, and divide medial bridging veins (Fig. 3) and then, with similar retraction, to locate the occipital pole. The occipital pole bridging veins are preserved until the resection is completed. Measurements are made from the occipital pole to mark the I_1 (first incision posterior to the angular gyrus) cortical incision for a resection limited to the occipital lobe. The approximate distances from the occipital pole to the preoccipital notch of 6 cm, to the angular gyrus of 3.5 cm, and to the parieto-occipital fissure of 4.5 cm are measurements used to avoid injuring the angular gyrus while making the I_1 incision.

The I_2 (second incision anterior to the angular gyrus) cortical incision in the nondominant hemisphere includes part of the posterior parietal and temporal lobes and will be determined by the size and

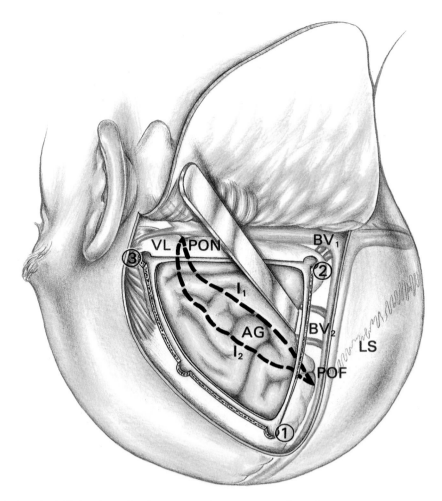

Figure 3. Retracted occipital lobe shows bridging veins. I_1 (first incision posterior to the angular gyrus) marks the plane of the occipital lobe resection. I_2 (second incision anterior to the angular gyrus (nondominant hemisphere)) marks the position of the neoplasm or arteriovenous malformation (Fig. 3). The vein of Labbé is identified so it can be protected and preserved.

incision for a larger resection in the nondominant hemisphere. For additional abbreviations, see the legends to Figures 1 and 2.

The cortical incision is made using bipolar cautery, suction, and scissors to coagulate and divide the pia mater and cortical vessels. Retraction is confined to the occipital lobe being resected. With the aid of a headlight, loupes, and retraction, the incision through the white matter is slowly advanced, as are the incisions through the pia mater of the occipital lobe and cortical tissue adjacent to the falx and the tentorium cerebelli. The branches of the posterior cerebral artery in the parieto-occipital fissure and the calcarine fissure are identified, coagulated, and divided. If there is an occipital ventricular horn it will also be divided. Hemostasis should be maintained and blood should not be allowed to pool in the ventricle or subdural space. After the occipital lobe has been dis-

connected from the brain, the bridging veins connecting it to the torcular herophili are coagulated and divided. The specimen is removed, leaving the cavity shown in Figure 4. Hemostasis must be absolute before closure and is obtained by bipolar cautery, with Surgicel (oxidized cellulose) placed, where needed, on the cut surface of the brain, and by filling the cavity temporarily with saline-soaked cotton balls.

Closure and Technical Points

The dura is closed with continuous 4-0 Neurolon. Before closure of the dura is complete, air is removed from the lobectomy site by filling the cavity with saline solution.

Illustrated in Figure 5 are advantageous techniques for making the scalp incision, securing the bone flap, and bandaging the patient. Figure 5A illustrates the method of using the unipolar cutting and

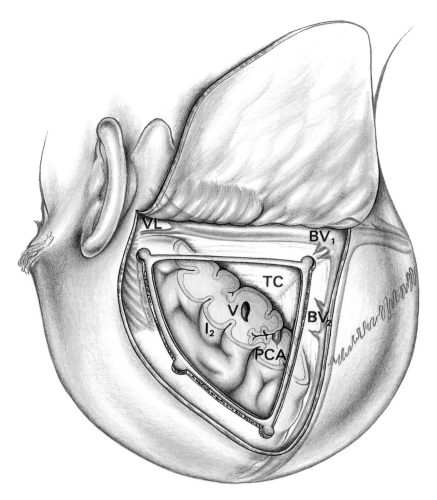

Figure 4. View of the intracranial cavity after I₂ incision and resection of the occipital lobe and part of the temporal and parietal lobes in the nondominant hemisphere. *TC*, tentorium cerebelli; *V*, ventricle. For additional abbreviations, see the legends to Figures 1–3.

coagulating machine (Neomed or Bard) with a straight, small electrode blade with a ⅞-inch insulated shank (ME 2280, American V. Mueller).

The Neomed is set at 20 cutting and 20 coagulation, with fine adjustments made as needed. The initial millimeter incision is done with a No. 15 steel knife blade; the rest of the incision of the scalp and pericranium is done with the electrosurgical unit. Steady, moderately fast 2–3-mm deep cuts (Fig. 5A-2) are used, retracting the wound edges as the cuts are made and keeping the blood sucked away. Small bleeding sites from the skin edges and subcutaneous fat are controlled with the unipolar cautery coagulation current (Fig. 5A-3). This is done lightly and briefly. In some patients, bipolar cautery may be needed to control bleeding from larger vessels. Infiltration of the scalp with 1% lidocaine with 1/100,000 epinephrine is not mandatory but may be used before making the

scalp incision to add to hemostasis. With proper application of this technique, the patient will lose only a few milliliters of blood. Hemostats and scalp clips are not needed for hemostasis. The wounds heal well and look no different from those made without the electrosurgical cutting blade. Some surgeons produce a satisfactory scalp wound using an electrosurgical machine alone without using a steel knife initially.

Craniotomy bone flaps cut with power tools are relatively small considering the bone opening they have to fill. If not sutured back into place with care, they may eventually become depressed. To avoid this, the bone flap is rotated so that it touches the calvarium at three or four places (Fig. 5B). In those places it is firmly secured to the calvarium with 26-gauge stainless steel wire. These wire sutures are twisted tightly and cut, leaving 4–5-mm lengths that are forced into the outside wire holes. Each wire is tapped

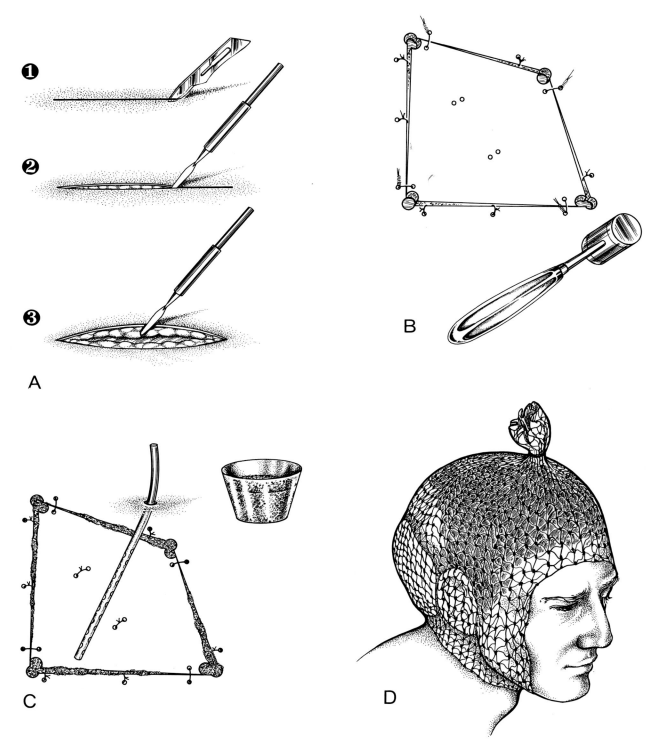

Figure 5. **A,** optional scalp incision technique using a steel knife blade in combination with the unipolar electrosurgical cutting and coagulation current. **B,** method of rotating and fixing the bone flap in place with 26-gauge stainless steel wire. **C,** craniotomy bone defects shown filled with bone dust; the use of a subgaleal drain is illustrated. **D,** dressing is held in place with No. 7 Surg-O-Flex tubular elasticized net bandage.

flat on the skull using the handle of a periosteal elevator or a small mallet. To foster healing of the wound so that the bone flap becomes firmly fixed in place and without scalp depression over defects in the skull, the burr holes and empty spaces around the flap are filled with bone dust (Fig. 5C), which is washed free of blood before it is applied. Reopening the wound months or years later reveals the bone flap held firmly in place by the wire sutures, the bone dust permeated by fibrous tissue, and, in some patients, new bone formation.

After hemostasis of the scalp is achieved, and to prevent the development of a significant postoperative subgaleal hematoma, the galea is sutured firmly to each of the wire sutures and to each dural tack-up suture hole in the calvarium using 3-0 Vicryl suture. The dura, galea, and bone flap are sutured together using 3-0 Vicryl sutures through one or two pairs of holes placed in the bone flap. In large craniotomy wounds or wounds that are not perfectly dry, a Davol medium $\frac{1}{8}$-inch drain with enclosed suction is used in the subgaleal space for 12 to 24 hours (Fig. 5C).

The galea is closed with interrupted 3-0 Vicryl, and the scalp is closed with continuous 4-0 nylon or with staples. A transfusion is rarely required for this operative procedure.

The wound is covered with bacitracin ointment, Adaptic dressing, 4 × 4-inch sponges, and abdominal pads. In small and moderate-sized craniotomy wounds, the dressing is held in place with a "ski cap" made from No. 7 tubular elasticized net bandage (Fig. 5D). For patients with large craniotomies and those who require a subgaleal drain, a standard pressure-roll bandage is used.

COMPLICATIONS

Perioperative mortality is 1% or less. A postoperative complete homonymous hemianopsia is expected. Injury to the angular gyrus in the dominant hemisphere will result in dysphasia manifested by dyslexia, dysgraphia, and acalculia. Failure to close the dura properly and seal opened mastoid air cells with muscle or pericranium sutured firmly in place may result in a cerebrospinal fluid fistula, meningitis, or brain abscess.

Intracranial pressure may remain elevated postoperatively if the neoplasm has not been completely excised or if blood has been allowed to collect and remain in the ventricle and subdural space. Concavity of the scalp over burr holes and over a depressed bone flap occurs if the bone flap has not been properly secured and burr holes filled in or covered.

SPINAL MENINGIOMAS

MICHAEL N. BUCCI, M.D.
JULIAN T. HOFF, M.D.

INTRODUCTION

Meningiomas are the second most common tumor of the spinal canal, accounting for 20% of intraspinal neoplasms. Most of the tumors are intradural and extramedullary in location. Two-thirds occur in the thoracic spine; 80% are in women. The duration of symptoms is variable. Root pain, segmental motor changes, and spasticity are common early findings.

PREOPERATIVE CONSIDERATIONS

Myelography and postmyelography computed tomography usually demonstrate the typical "crescent-shaped" appearance of an intradural extramedullary lesion. Magnetic resonance imaging is now the diagnostic procedure of choice, which demonstrates these lesions in multiple planes (Fig. 1).

Preoperative preparation usually consists of dexamethasone (10 mg, by mouth or intravenously) at midnight and on call to the operating room. Concurrent administration of either antacids or a H_2 receptor blocker is also advisable. Preoperative antibiotic prophylaxis is optional, usually consisting of either 1 g of nafcillin or cephalothin intravenously.

SURGICAL TECHNIQUE

The operation is usually performed with general anesthesia; however, spinal anesthesia may be considered in high-risk patients with low thoracic or lumbar lesions. Central venous access and arterial pressure monitoring are helpful, but not essential.

The operation is performed with the patient in the prone position. All pressure points are well-padded. A comfortable head rest is essential. For patients with upper thoracic or cervical tumors, three-point skull fixation with the cervical spine in neutral position is best.

Prior to preparation and draping, anterior-posterior roentgenograms are obtained in patients with thoracic meningiomas in order to best localize the lesion. Alternatively, the patient may be taken to the radiology department prior to surgery where fluoroscopy can be employed to localize these lesions relative to surface anatomy. Although intraoperative evoked

potential monitoring may be beneficial in some cases, intradural extramedullary tumors can be resected safely without this additional monitoring.

After preparation and draping, a midline incision is employed and the fascia is incised down to the spinous processes. The muscular attachments are stripped bilaterally in the subperiosteal plane, exposing the laminae out to the facet joints (Fig. 2A). The spinous processes and laminae are carefully removed using either bone rongeurs, a high-speed air drill, or both. Enough bone is removed both above and below the tumor to permit an adequate dural opening (Fig. 2B).

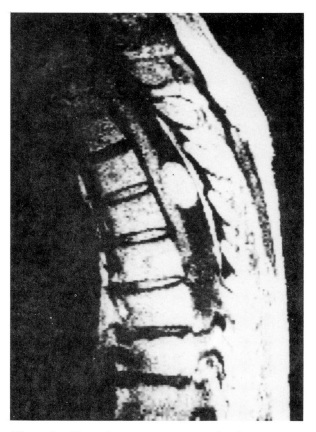

Figure 1. Magnetic resonance image of a thoracic meningioma, T2 weighting, with a paramagnetic contrast agent administered. Note the clear definition of this intradural extramedullary lesion.

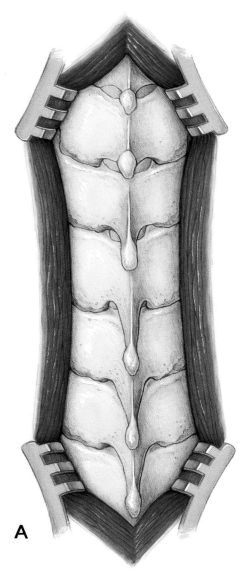

A

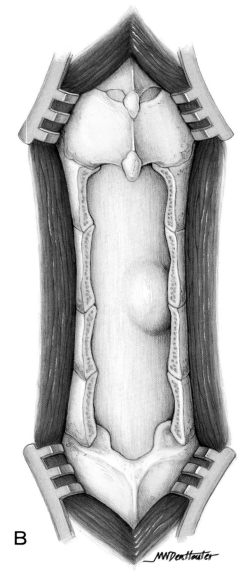

B

Figure 2. **A,** thoracic spine, posterior elements, with muscular attachments stripped in the subperiosteal plane. **B,** decompressive thoracic laminectomy exposing the dorsal dura. Enough bone is removed both above and below the tumor to permit safe removal.

At this point, the operating microscope is brought into the field. The dura is opened in the midline, taking care to preserve the arachnoid intact. A microdissector is then used to separate the dura and arachnoid. Dural tack-up sutures are placed and cottonoid pledgets are laid over the exposed dura. Tension on the sutures provides better exposure and relative hemostasis from the epidural space (Fig. 3A). The tumor is usually visible beneath the arachnoid.

If the tumor is located dorsally, the arachnoid is carefully opened by sharp dissection (Figs. 3B and 4).

The arachnoid edges are secured to the dura with clips. If the tumor is ventrally located, an additional arachnoid layer may be present lateral to the exposed spinal cord.

The tumor is best debulked prior to dissection of the tumor-cord interface. Bipolar coagulation and piecemeal removal using an ultrasonic surgical aspirator or cutting bipolar coagulator minimize spinal cord manipulation, providing a safe and gentle method for removal (Fig. 3C). The plane between tumor and spinal cord is usually well-developed and

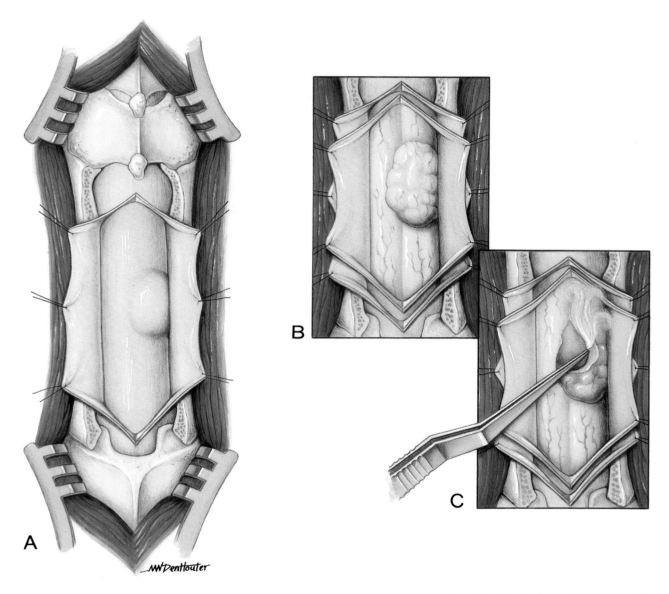

Figure 3. **A,** illustration of the dural opening, exposing an intact arachnoid layer overlying the tumor. **B,** arachnoid opening reveals the extramedullary neoplasm causing spinal cord compression. A well-developed plane exists between the lesion and the spinal cord. **C,** illustration of piecemeal tumor removal using bipolar electrocautery.

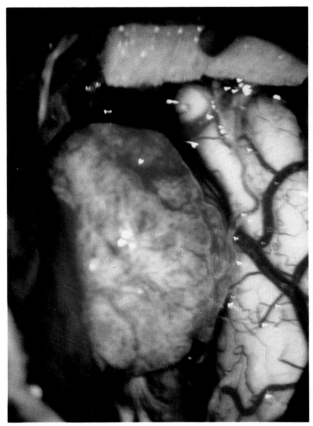

Figure 4. Intraoperative photograph of a cervical (C1-2) meningioma prior to resection. Note the extramedullary location.

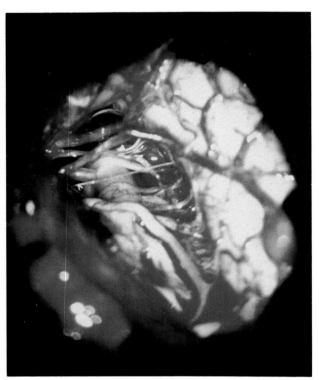

Figure 5. Intraoperative photograph of the cervical spinal cord following resection of a meningioma. Note the vertebral artery located ventral to the spinal and spinal accessory nerve rootlets.

easy to delineate after central debulking. The tumor edges fold in, allowing circumferential arachnoid dissection and eventual delivery of the tumor capsule (Fig. 5).

For ventrally located tumors, division of the dentate ligaments and possibly of selected dorsal rootlets facilitates both tumor exposure and removal.

Meticulous hemostasis is essential prior to dural closure. A watertight closure follows. Muscle, fascia, and subcutaneous tissue are closed in layers. The skin is generally closed with a subcuticular suture, and then Steri-strips are placed. Drains are not used.

The major postoperative complications include infection, cerebrospinal fluid leakage, and increased neurologic deficit. Perioperative antibiotic prophylaxis, careful wound closure, and dexamethasone administration lessen these risks.

PERCUTANEOUS TRIGEMINAL GLYCEROL RHIZOTOMY

RONALD F. YOUNG, M.D.

PATIENT SELECTION

Patients are generally selected for any form of surgical therapy of trigeminal neuralgia based on previous failure of pharmacological treatment. The diagnostic criteria for trigeminal neuralgia are: 1) sharp, knife-like pain of duration from a fraction of a second up to several seconds to one minute; 2) pain confined within one or more of the major peripheral divisions of the trigeminal nerve; and 3) the presence of trigger zones from which innocuous stimuli trigger the patient's characteristic pain.

Ablative procedures such as percutaneous glycerol rhizotomy (PGR) should not be utilized for patients with atypical facial pain. However, some patients present with histories somewhat atypical for trigeminal neuralgia with generally longer-lasting pain and sometimes a constant ache between pains. The latter is particularly true of patients treated with carbamazepine. Patients who lack trigger phenomena and whose pain extends beyond the trigeminal distribution should not be considered for percutaneous trigeminal rhizolysis.

Patients with recurrent trigeminal neuralgia after previous surgical procedures such as microvascular decompression or radiofrequency rhizolysis may be treated successfully with PGR as may patients who develop trigeminal neuralgia as a consequence of multiple sclerosis. The procedure is most appropriate for patients with pain in the second division alone, the second division and the first division, the second and the third division, or all three divisions. Patients with exclusively third division trigeminal neuralgia respond poorly to percutaneous glycerol rhizolysis. The exact reason for the failures in such patients is unclear, but PGR produces maximal sensory changes in the second and first divisions and minimal or no change in the third division.

There are few, if any, absolute contraindications to surgery. Patients with hypertension require appropriate medical therapy preoperatively and intraoperatively.

PREOPERATIVE PREPARATION

A preoperative cerebral imaging study, preferably a magnetic resonance scan or computed tomographic scan with intravenous contrast, is recommended to exclude structural lesions as the cause of the patient's trigeminal neuralgia. Recommended preoperative laboratory studies include a complete blood count, screening of electrolyte levels, and assessment of clotting ability utilizing the prothrombin time and the partial thromboplastin time. X-ray films of the chest are obtained for patients over the age of 40 or with a previous history of pulmonary disease, and an electrocardiogram is obtained for patients over the age of 40 or with a previous history of cardiovascular disease.

Preparation of the patient for the procedure includes insertion of an intravenous line for administration of intravenous sedation. Blood pressure is monitored every five minutes with an automatic sphygmomanometer. I have not monitored arterial blood pressure by an indwelling catheter except in a rare patient such as an individual with an unruptured intracranial aneurysm. The patient is prepared for the procedure with intravenous midazolam, a short-acting benzodiazepine, and fentanyl, an opiate analgesic. Dosages are adjusted according to the patient's body size, age, and previous drug utilization. The parasympatholytic agent glycopyrrolate is also administered to prevent bradycardia which may accompany penetration of the foramen ovale. A broad spectrum antibiotic such as cefazolin is administered intravenously about 30 minutes prior to beginning the procedure in an attempt to prevent a rare case of meningitis following PGR.

OPERATIVE PROCEDURE

The procedure is carried out with the patient in the supine position. The head is rotated approximately 15° away from the side of the patient's pain (Fig. 1). The skin of the side of the face around the angle of the mouth is prepared with suitable topical antiseptic. Sterile drapes are then applied across the upper chest. Beginning at a point about 2.5 cm lateral to the angle of the mouth on the side of the patient's pain, the skin

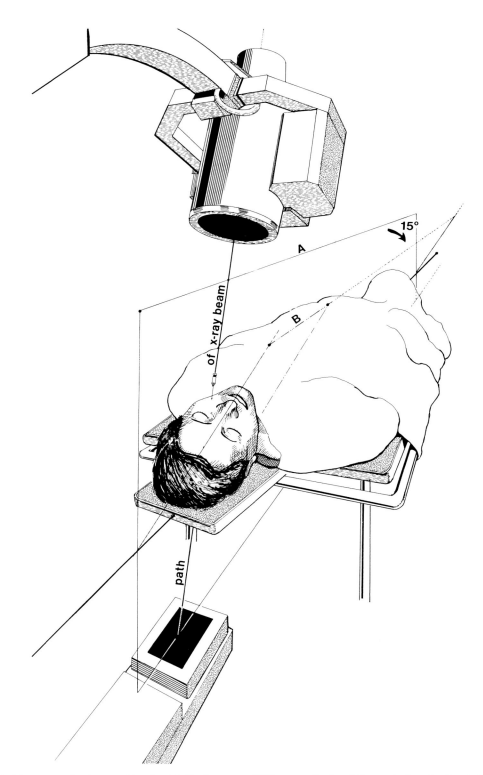

Figure 1. Angled fluoroscopic view used to identify the foramen ovale and place the needle for PGR. *Plane A* represents the mid-sagittal plane which is rotated 15° (*plane B*) away from the side of pain. The fluoroscopic beam is then angled 40° from vertical and the central ray is directed about 2–3 cm lateral to the angle of the mouth. The foramen ovale is then seen as in Figure 2.

and deep tissues are infiltrated with approximately 2–3 ml of 1% Xylocaine solution. The anesthetic agent is introduced first by raising a small skin wheal with a 25-gauge needle and then with use of a 22-gauge, 1.5-inch needle. Care should be taken that the oral mucosa is not penetrated with the needle used to introduce the local anesthetic.

A C-arm fluoroscopy unit is employed and the beam is angled about 40° from vertical and the central ray of the beam is directed at a point about 2.5 cm lateral to the angle of the mouth on the side of the patient's pain (Fig. 1). The foramen ovale is then identified by a brief fluoroscopic view. Hyperextension of the patient's neck is unnecessary, but slight changes in the angle of the fluoroscopic beam may be required in order to place the foramen ovale in an "en face" position. In addition, slight rotations of the head greater than or less than the original 15° may be required to place the foramen ovale in the central portion of the fluoroscopic image. Using this technique, the foramen ovale appears on the edge of the shadow of the petrous bone midway between the ramus of the mandible laterally and the maxilla medially (Fig. 2).

When the foramen ovale has been identified, the needle which will be used for glycerol injection is introduced at a point about 2.5 cm lateral to the angle of the mouth on the side of the patient's pain. When the pain is on the left side, the needle is grasped in the right

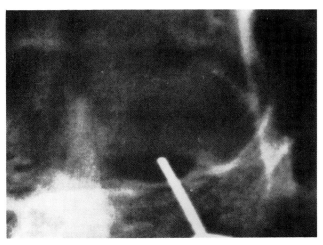

Figure 3. Correct position for needle puncture of the right foramen ovale just medial to the midpoint of the foramen. Satisfactory punctures may be made more medial but not more lateral to this point. (From Young RF. J Neurosurg 1988; 69:39–45. With permission.)

hand and the index finger of the left hand is placed inside the patient's mouth. When the patient's pain is on the right side, the needle is grasped in the left hand and the right index finger is placed within the oral cavity. The technique of insertion of the needle is the so-called "Härtel technique." As the needle is introduced, the gloved finger inside of the mouth prevents penetration of the oral mucosa. As soon as the tip of the needle passes the pterygoid plate, the position is viewed briefly fluoroscopically. The needle direction is then changed as required and advanced incrementally under intermittent fluoroscopic viewing.

The key to successful instillation of glycerol into the retrogasserian cistern is accurate puncture of the foramen ovale. The ideal point for puncture of the foramen ovale is in the center of the medial half of the foramen (Figs. 3 and 4). Punctures in the lateral half of the foramen may result in the needle tip being placed beneath the temporal lobe or in the temporal lobe (Fig. 5). When the needle is placed along the medial edge of the foramen ovale, the needle may enter the cavernous sinus. If the needle is placed too close to the anterior or posterior edges of the foramen ovale, extradural or subdural placement of the needle tip rather than subarachnoid placement is likely. As the needle tip enters the foramen ovale, slight contraction of the masseter muscle frequently occurs and the patient may experience a brief twinge of pain. In addition, firm resistance is felt as the foramen is penetrated. As soon as the foramen is penetrated, no attempt is made to advance the needle further at this point.

The patient's head is then rotated until it is in the neutral position and the C-arm fluoroscope is changed

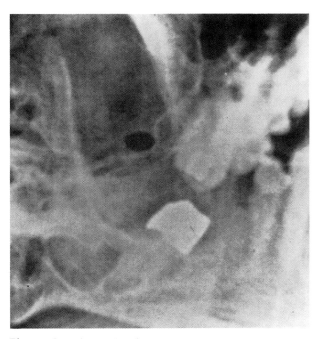

Figure 2. The right foramen ovale as viewed fluoroscopically, as demonstrated in Figure 1. The ramus of the mandible is lateral and the maxilla medial. The foramen appears on the edge of the shadow of the petrous bone. (From Young RF. J Neurosurg 1988; 69:39–45. With permission.)

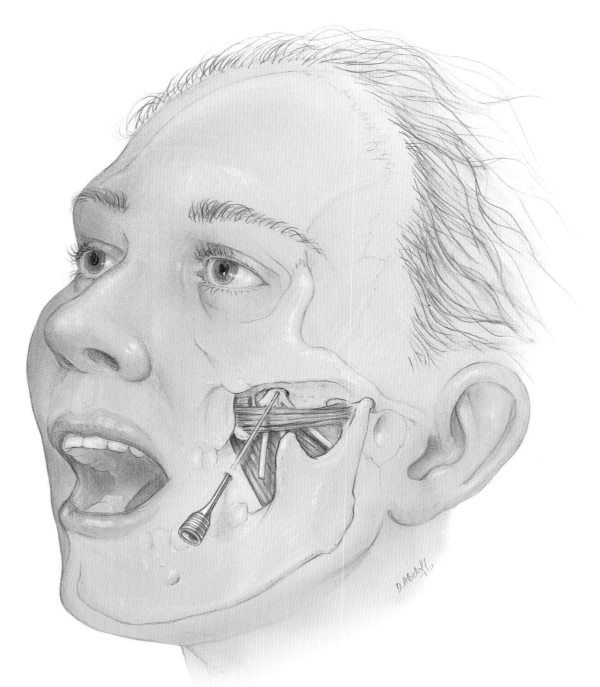

Figure 4. Cutaway anatomical view of needle puncture of the left foramen ovale. The needle is in the medial half of the foramen and midway between the anterior and posterior borders. The mandibular division is seen exiting from the skull via the foramen. Since the needle passes through the nerve, contraction of the masseter muscle with jaw closure often accompanies puncture of the foramen.

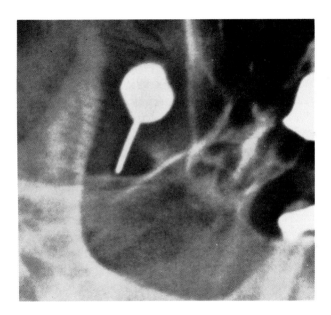

Figure 5. Incorrect puncture of the right foramen ovale. The needle is too lateral. Punctures at this point may yield cerebrospinal fluid from the subarachnoid space beneath the temporal lobe. Glycerol should not be injected at this point. The needle should be withdrawn and the foramen repunctured. (From Young RF. J Neurosurg 1988; 69:39–45. With permission.)

to the lateral view (Fig. 6). The depth of the needle is then ascertained (Figs. 7 and 8). The needle is slowly advanced and the stylet is removed intermittently to ascertain flow of spinal fluid. The needle is advanced only 1–2 mm incrementally. As soon as cerebrospinal fluid flow is obtained, further advancement of the needle is stopped. If the needle tip passes posterior to the shadow of the clivus without obtaining spinal fluid, then the needle is again slowly withdrawn and rotated slightly during the withdrawal, again observing for cerebrospinal fluid flow. If cerebrospinal fluid (CSF) flow is not obtained, the needle is withdrawn from the foramen ovale, the patient's head is again rotated 15°, and the angled fluoroscopic view is utilized for repuncture of the foramen ovale. A second or perhaps at most a third attempt to obtain cerebrospinal fluid flow is made utilizing the same technique with slight differences in the point of repuncture of the foramen ovale. Surprisingly, a second puncture in a relatively similar position to the first may give cerebrospinal fluid flow when the first puncture did not.

If cerebrospinal fluid flow is not obtained, a decision must be made as to how to proceed. Preoperative discussion with the patient concerning this decision is essential. Two possibilities present themselves. The first includes an injection of glycerol even though cere-

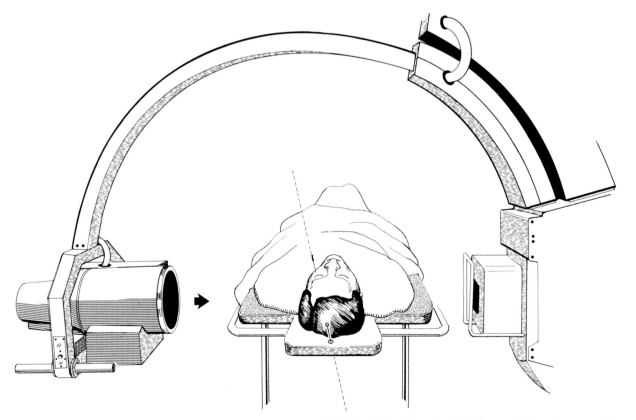

Figure 6. Lateral fluoroscopic view used to assess needle depth. The head is placed in the neutral position and the fluoroscopic beam is horizontal.

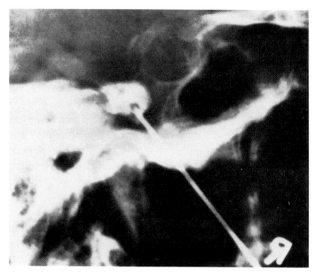

Figure 7. Metrizamide trigeminal cisternogram viewed with a lateral fluoroscopic beam as in Figure 6. The needle is positioned low in the cistern in good position for glycerol injection for pain in the mandibular division, mandibular and maxillary division, or all three divisions. A slight needle advancement would be ideal for maxillary division pain alone or a combination of maxillary and ophthalmic division pain. (From Young RF. J Neurosurg 1988; 69:39–45. With permission.)

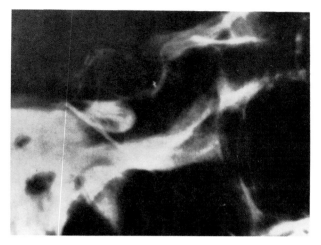

Figure 8. Metrizamide trigeminal cisternogram demonstrating an excessively posterior position of the needle tip not recommended for glycerol injection. The needle enters the cistern very posteriorly suggesting that the foramen ovale was punctured near the posterior rim. Repeat puncture of the cistern is recommended from this position before glycerol is injected. Compare the needle position to that shown in Figure 7. (From Young RF. J Neurosurg 1988; 69:39–45. With permission.)

brospinal fluid is not obtained. In this instance, the likelihood for successful amelioration of the patient's pain is probably at most 50%. The second alternative, which is my preference, is to proceed with radiofrequency trigeminal rhizotomy at this point. I use a needle which allows both glycerol injection through a Luer locking hub as well as radiofrequency rhizolysis using a thermistor radiofrequency heating probe.

Other authors have recommended a retrogasserian cisternogram using water-soluble contrast material injected through the needle to confirm that the needle tip is within the cistern as well as to estimate the volume of the cistern (Figs. 7 and 8). My experience suggests that cisternography is not helpful and may indeed be counterproductive. In order to carry out cisternography, the patient must be placed in the sitting position to fill the cistern and avoid the contrast material running into the posterior fossa. The cistern must be emptied by placing the patient supine and then PGR must be carried out with the patient sitting again. These manipulations risk dislodging the needle tip from the cistern. Furthermore, if CSF is obtained and the needle is correctly placed in the foramen ovale as previously described, the needle tip will be in the cistern. If CSF is not obtained, there is little value in injecting contrast material. The technique described

for penetrating the foramen ovale is the only one which will reliably place the needle tip in the cistern. Radiographic techniques which employ submentovertex or anteroposterior and lateral views only cannot ensure that the foramen ovale is correctly punctured.

If clear cerebrospinal fluid is obtained after puncture of the foramen ovale, then the patient is brought into the sitting position and the head is flexed so that the orbitomeatal line is angled slightly below the horizontal. The lateral fluoroscopic view is used to ascertain that the needle position has not changed. In elderly patients with slack facial tissues, it is possible for significant accidental withdrawal of the needle to occur as the patient is brought into the sitting position. Occasionally, it may be necessary to hold the needle in place while the patient is moved and at all times during glycerol injection, but generally this is not required. When the depth of the needle has been confirmed to be the same as in the supine position and when cerebrospinal fluid flow is confirmed, the patient is ready for glycerol instillation.

Sterile anhydrous glycerol is used. The glycerol is prepared by the hospital pharmacy in 2-ml ampules, and 1 ml of glycerol is drawn into a 1-ml tuberculin syringe using an 18-gauge needle. The 18-gauge needle is removed and the tuberculin syringe containing the glycerol is attached to the needle in the foramen ovale after removal of the stylet. The glycerol is injected slowly, in increments of 0.05 ml or approximately 1 drop. The hub and barrel of the needle generally contain a volume of about 0.1 ml of cerebrospinal fluid, and therefore I make an initial total injection of approximately 0.15 ml of which only 0.05 ml is actually injected because of the dead space just mentioned. Within 30 to 60 seconds, the patient will usually describe sensations of tingling, pins and needles, or burning in the distribution of the branch of the trigeminal nerve closest to the needle tip. Most commonly, the patient describes the feeling of paresthesias around the upper lip and angle of the mouth. Further glycerol is injected to a minimum volume of about 0.15 ml actual injected volume. About five minutes after the initial injection, testing of the patient's facial sensation is begun with a pin and the corneal reflex is monitored intermittently. If little or no analgesia is obtained, further glycerol is injected in 0.05-ml aliquots and facial sensation is tested further. When the patient notices a significant decrease in sharpness of the pin, usually at least a 50% decrease compared with the normal side, the injection is terminated. If the corneal reflex is decreased or the patient complains of paresthesias and burning in the eye and the trigeminal neuralgia pain is not within the first trigeminal division, no further glycerol is injected. The final total volume of glycerol varies from approximately 0.15 ml to about 0.55 ml, with an average of about 0.35 to 0.4 ml. At the conclusion of the procedure, the needle is withdrawn and pressure is applied over the injection site. The patient is maintained in the sitting position with the head flexed forward as previously described for approximately one hour. The patient may be transferred from the radiology suite to a recovery area as soon as the needle is withdrawn.

SPECIALIZED INSTRUMENTATION

A portable C-arm fluoroscopy unit with television reproduction of the enhanced image is essential. A simple 20- or 22-gauge, 3.5-inch spinal needle may be used for this procedure, but, as previously described, I use a needle which may be utilized either for glycerol injection or for radiofrequency rhizotomy. If cerebrospinal fluid flow is not obtained from the needle or if pain is located exclusively within the third trigeminal division, I prefer the radiofrequency technique.

COMPLICATIONS

In my experience, virtually all patients who will experience long-term relief of trigeminal neuralgia experience at least some alteration in facial sensation. About two-thirds of patients experience analgesia of a more significant degree such that pain sensation is reduced by 50% or more compared with the normal side. Reduction or absence of the corneal reflex occurs in 5–10% of patients in whom the pain does not involve the ophthalmic division. Unlike the corneal reflex changes which occur with radiofrequency rhizolysis, there is rarely a complete absence of the corneal reflex. There may be regions of the cornea from which the reflex cannot be obtained, but a careful examination will usually reveal some areas of the cornea from which the reflex can still be obtained. I have not experienced in my own patients nor have I seen any patient suffering from neuroparalytic keratitis or blindness following PGR of the trigeminal nerve.

I have likewise not seen any patient of my own who has experienced anesthesia dolorosa after PGR but I have seen one patient in whom anesthesia dolorosa resulted after three different attempts at glycerol rhizotomy. Weakness of the muscles of mastication is likewise an unusual complication with glycerol rhizotomy. I have never observed paresis of cranial nerves other than the trigeminal, nor inadvertent puncture of foramina other than the foramen ovale with this technique. Rarely a large hematoma may form rapidly in the tissues of the cheek which prevents the needle tip from reaching the cistern. In such patients, pressure is applied manually, an ice pack is used, and the procedure is delayed until the hematoma resolves.

In my opinion, the key to the avoidance of complications is the incremental injection of glycerol with intermittent monitoring of facial sensation. In rare cases, despite apparent perfect placement of the needle within the retrogasserian cistern and despite the flow of cerebrospinal fluid, the patient experiences little or no immediate alteration in sensation upon glycerol instillation. In such patients, I usually instill a total volume of about 0.35 ml. Surprisingly, in a few such patients, a slow onset of facial analgesia has developed over a period of 30–90 minutes.

Using the needle placement technique described here, accidental puncture of any foramen other than the foramen ovale should not occur. Likewise, accidental placement of the needle beneath the temporal lobe or in the temporal lobe should not occur.

Occasionally the patient may experience a burst of repetitive typical trigeminal neuralgic pains which may last for as long as several hours. For this reason, patients are monitored in the postoperative recovery room for at least two hours following withdrawal of the needle, and intravenous narcotics are used in the instance of a shower of repetitive pains. The vast majority of patients experience complete relief of trigeminal neuralgia within one to two hours. An occasional patient will experience relief of pain over 24 hours or more. I have not seen patients who have persisted with trigeminal neuralgia for 24 to 48 hours after glycerol rhizotomy in whom the pain has eventually resolved, unlike the experience reported by others.

LUMBAR HEMILAMINECTOMY FOR EXCISION OF A HERNIATED DISC

PATRICK W. HITCHON, M.D.
VINCENT C. TRAYNELIS, M.D.

PATIENT SELECTION

Traditionally, a patient who presents with low back pain radiating into one lower extremity is thought to harbor a unilateral lumbar herniated intervertebral disc provided other lesions have been ruled out. Other conditions that can mimic a herniated disc include primary or metastatic tumors of the spine, pelvis, or retroperitoneum, spondylolisthesis, and spinal infections, to mention a few. It is to be emphasized that the majority of patients with a herniated disc, with or without radiculopathy, improve with bedrest.

Plain roentgenograms of the lumbar spine rule out fractures, lytic or blastic lesions, or spondylolisthesis. Magnetic resonance imaging (MRI) has been gaining favor in the past 2–3 years as a noninvasive potentially diagnostic study. The value of MRI lies in its noninvasive feature, although its potential in identifying herniated discs is restricted to relatively large lesions. Where MRI is unavailable, a plain computed tomographic (CT) scan can be helpful. Should the above studies be nonconfirmatory, and the patient is considered a surgical candidate, the most reliable study is that of lumbar myelography with a water-soluble contrast agent, followed by CT. Myelography need only be performed when the patient is considered for surgical treatment after failure of conservative therapy.

All nonsteroidal anti-inflammatory medications, phenothiazines, and antidepressants are discontinued 1 week prior to surgery. Routine blood work, including platelet count, prothrombin time, and partial thromboplastin time are mandatory. All patients undergo x-ray films of the chest and an electrocardiogram, and those with a history of angina pectoris or those over 65 years of age have a consultation with a cardiologist. Typing and screening of the patient's blood without cross-matching is sufficient.

SURGICAL TECHNIQUE

Positioning

A number of devices are available for positioning of the patient undergoing lumbar disc surgery. They include foam laminectomy rolls, the Wilson frame, and the Cloward frame. The choice of a device is based on its performance in reducing intra-abdominal pressure and flexing the lumbar spine, its ease of application, and the distribution of body weight to obviate pressure sores. We have adopted the Cloward frame, which satisfies most of the above criteria. The lateral decubitus position is reserved for obese patients or those for whom the prone position is contraindicated, such as patients with a prominent transplanted kidney. All patients are transported to the operating room wearing thigh-high antithromboembolic hose. General anesthesia is induced and the patient is then positioned on the Cloward frame with straps across the thighs and with the head turned to one side (Fig. 1).

Once intravenous fluids have been started, the first dose of a 2-day course of prophylactic cefazolin sodium is administered. The skin is shaved and an adhesive plastic drape is applied to both buttocks to exclude the perineum from the surgical field. The lumbar region is scrubbed with Betadine soap for 10 minutes and then painted with a 10% solution of povidone-iodine followed by isopropyl alcohol. With a sterile marking pen the proposed surgical incision is outlined on the patient's spine, using the iliac crests and spinous processes as landmarks. Plain x-ray films and/or myelographic studies should be posted on a viewbox in the operating room. Once the proposed incision is marked, the surgical field is draped using first a plain or iodinated adhesive plastic sheet, then towels, and, finally, cloth or disposable sheets. Sutures or staples are applied on the corners to fix the drapes. Traditionally, the authors have preferred to infiltrate a proposed incision with 1% Xylocaine with 1/200,000 epinephrine for hemostasis.

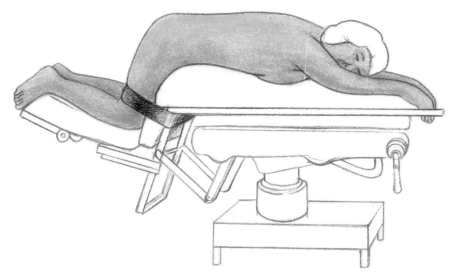

Figure 1. The patient is positioned prone on the Cloward frame with the hips flexed and the arms extended. The abdo- men is suspended within the frame, reducing intra-abdomi- nal pressure.

Incision and Exposure

The skin incision for a single level hemilaminectomy may be 2–3 inches long, depending on the patient's weight. The greater the retraction necessary, the longer the incision. For simplicity, this chapter will address removal of an L4–5 herniated disc on the right side, with the surgeon standing on the ip- silateral side and the assistant on the opposite side.

The skin incision is carried down to the fascia with a scalpel. Bleeding points are controlled with bipolar coagulation. At this point, with an Allis clamp applied to a spinous process as a marker, a lateral x-ray study is obtained to confirm the level. A self-retaining Adson retractor is utilized to expose the underlying fascia. With the electrocautery, the fascia is incised and the paraspinal muscles dissected away from the spinous processes and laminae in the subperiosteal plane. Manual retraction of the muscle is performed either with a Cushing or Cobb periosteal elevator. To prevent potential interlaminar slippage of the instrument, the largest elevator is preferred. To achieve nontraumatic dissection with minimal blood loss, the cutting cur- rent has been found to be most useful in exposing the leading and trailing edges of the laminae all the way laterally to the facet joint. Inadvertent entrance into the facet joint is to be avoided in order to reduce the chances of developing postsurgical arthritis. The lami- nae are polished using an elevator and a 4 × 8-inch sponge folded upon itself to measure 2 × 8 inches. One sponge is used per level. This process is repeated for improved exposure. All sponges should be marked with a radiopaque thread. It is important for both the surgeon and scrub nurse to keep count of the sponges to avoid unnecessary delays of wound closure in case of a miscount.

Once the sponges have been withdrawn, a 1¼- inch Taylor retractor is inserted to maintain exposure. The shortest possible retractor should be used so as not to interfere with the surgical procedure. The pointed tip of the retractor is engaged lateral to the facet joint and 2–3 pounds of weight are suspended from the proximal end to maintain its position (Fig. 2). Excessive weight is unnecessary and may predis- pose to the dislodgement of the retractor and injury to the facet joint.

Hemilaminectomy and Discectomy

The caudal edge of the L4 lamina is now removed a distance of 1–1.5 cm rostrally using a Leksell rongeur. Bleeding from the underlying cancellous bone is con- trolled with bone wax. An angled curette is utilized to free the ligamentum flavum from the undersurface of the L4 lamina. This dissection is necessary to facili- tate insertion of the 40° Kerrison footplate for the com- pletion of the partial hemilaminectomy of the caudal edge of L4. An oval window is created that extends laterally to the facet joint and measures 2 × 1.5 cm. From here on the operation requires magnification with loupes, or a microscope if two surgeons are in- volved. Using a No. 15 blade, the ligamentum flavum is incised as far medially as is possible, parallel to its fibers. This opening should be sufficient to advance a half-inch cottonoid into the epidural space. The cot- tonoid displaces the thecal sac away from the ligamen-

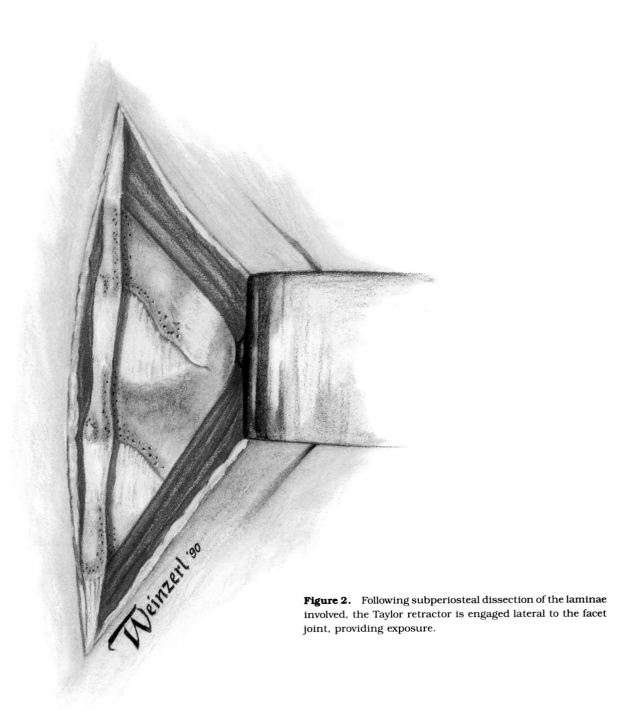

Figure 2. Following subperiosteal dissection of the laminae involved, the Taylor retractor is engaged lateral to the facet joint, providing exposure.

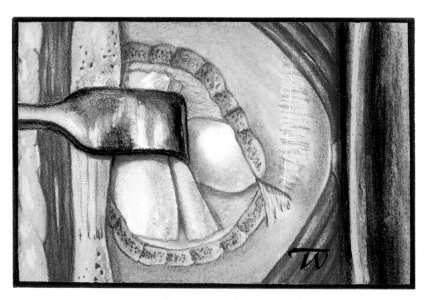

Figure 3. Following laminotomy and dissection of the epidural space, the affected root is retracted medially, exposing the herniated disc beneath. The laminotomy extends laterally to the facet joint.

tum flavum, thereby reducing the chance of injury to the thecal sac. The ligamentum flavum is then grasped by a Cushing forceps or Allis clamp and is pulled laterally. With the cottonoid in place, the ligamentum flavum is further incised to the facet joint. A Scoville curette completes the excision of the ligamentum flavum by cutting it between the sharp edge of the curette and the facet joint. Following removal of the ligamentum flavum, a small laminotomy of the rostral edge of L5 will further improve exposure. Inspection of the epidural space reveals fat and epidural veins. Gently the epidural vessels may be coagulated and the space lateral to the L5 nerve root dissected in search of the herniated disc. If accomplished hastily, this dissection may result in an excessive amount of blood loss. Bipolar coagulation is performed with low current to prevent sparking and potential injury to the L5 nerve root.

Once the nerve root and thecal sac are identified, the D'Errico or Love root retractor is applied against the L5 nerve root which is then retracted medially by the assistant (Fig. 3). Retraction of the nerve root may be quite difficult with a chronic herniated disc because of adhesions and scarring between the fragment and the affected root. On the other hand, if the herniation is only weeks old, this retraction may be quite simple. In the presence of scarring, a No. 4 Penfield or Church scissors may be needed to free up the nerve root from the adhesions. In case of persistent bleeding from the epidural veins, a ¼-inch cottonoid may be inserted rostrally and another caudally for tamponade.

With the nerve root retracted, the herniated disc comes into view. If a free fragment exists within the canal, this extruded portion may be removed using a straight pituitary forceps. Occasionally, the herniation may be subligamentous; if so, a small incision into the posterior longitudinal ligament is sufficient for the disc herniation to deliver itself. Once the herniated fragment has been excised, attention is then directed to the annulus. This annulus harbors a degenerated disc and, furthermore, is defective, having allowed a disc fragment to herniate. It is our belief that such a disc is pathologic and is likely to result in recurrent herniations. A vigorous disc exenteration, performed unilaterally, reduces the incidence of such a postoperative complication.

With the root still retracted, the annulus is incised with a No. 15 blade. The medial vertical incision is performed first and then the annulus is incised laterally both rostrally and caudally adjacent to the endplates of L4 and L5, respectively. The sharp edge of the blade should at no time be directed medially toward the nerve root or thecal sac. Finally, the lateral edge of this window is incised and the window is removed, allowing access to the disc space. The disc exenteration that is performed henceforth depends, to a great extent, on the size of the window created. A No. 1 or 2 straight curette is initially utilized to enlarge the window. The angled Cone curettes, starting with the medium and proceeding to the large, are advanced into the disc space to the level of the elbow on the curette (Fig. 4). This prevents penetration of the annulus anteriorly and possible vascular injury. The end-plates of

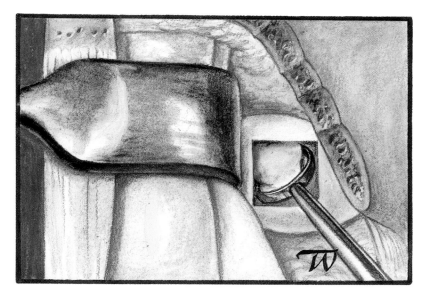

Figure 4. Following removal of the free fragment or the subligamentous component, a window is incised in the annulus. The window should be large enough to allow the introduction of the Cone curettes for further disc exenteration. The curette is to be manipulated so that the cutting edge remains within the disc space.

L4 and L5 are scraped, fragmenting the disc material and cartilage which is subsequently removed with pituitary forceps. Disc removal cannot be accomplished with the forceps alone. Undue vigor with the Cone curettes may result in penetration of the end-plates and entry into the cancellous vertebral body. This results in bleeding that can be controlled only with bone wax applied with a dissector, and/or Avitene. The disc is removed with a sweeping motion of the curette from medial to lateral, and from ventral to dorsal. Forceful irrigation into the disc space can often yield retained fragments that have not yet delivered themselves. Once the removal is thought to be complete, careful inspection of the L5 nerve root is performed medially and along its course toward the neural foramen. A right-angled dural separator may be advanced ventral and medial to the nerve root for the identification of retained fragments. The separator should be rotated such that these fragments are swept out lateral to the nerve root. A malleable bent probe is now advanced along the nerve root toward the neural foramen, both dorsally and ventrally, in search of residual disc fragments. Following inspection, the wound is irrigated and all cottonoids are removed. Large wads of Gelfoam or Surgicel should not be left in the epidural space, and are removed. If bleeding persists, Avitene may be applied and the excess removed by irrigation.

In the presence of sufficient subcutaneous adipose tissue, a fat graft measuring approximately 1.5×2 cm may be easily harvested unilaterally and applied over the nerve root. By preventing adhesions between the spinal muscles and the nerve root, this fat graft may facilitate future dissection, if necessary. The Taylor retractor is now removed and bleeding points from the muscle coagulated. Drains are not used.

Closure

The fascia is approximated using 2-0 Vicryl, which is an absorbable suture material. Sutures in the muscle are not necessary. The fascial closure usually provides sufficient obliteration of dead space and good apposition of the muscle against the laminae and spinous processes. The subcutaneous tissue may be approximated with 3-0 Vicryl; staples or 3-0 nylon in a vertical mattress suture are used for skin closure. A dressing is applied consisting of two sponges secured into position with an elastic-type adhesive tape. An excessively thick dressing is unnecessary and may be uncomfortable when the patient lies on his back.

POSTOPERATIVE CARE

Postoperatively the patient is allowed activity as tolerated. On the first postoperative day the patient is expected to start sitting up for meals and to begin walking. Postoperative analgesia is provided with meperidine hydrochloride, 100 mg, and Vistaril, 25 mg, intramuscularly every 3–4 hours as necessary. These medications may be switched to the oral route at the patient's request. Should the patient develop lumbar muscle spasms, a muscle relaxant, such as diazepam in 5–10-mg doses intramuscularly, may be prescribed as necessary. Patient-controlled analgesia pumps or thoracolumbar immobilizers are not warranted for this type of surgery. By 5–7 days postoperatively, the patient is able to ambulate independently and may be discharged home. Prior to release from the hospital, physical therapy consultation is sought to guide the patient in nonstrenuous exercises that are to be continued at home. Skin sutures may be removed 7–10 days postoperatively. The patient is generally unable to return to employment until after a 6-week postoperative examination. At that time, x-ray films may be obtained if deemed necessary by the physician. Lifting in excess of 30 pounds is not recommended for up to 3 months from surgery. A compromise can usually be achieved by the patient and his employer. If satisfied with the outcome of surgery, the surgeon may discharge the patient with instruction to return should the need arise.

COMPLICATIONS

An early but rare postoperative complication within the first 2 days of operation is cauda equina compression by an epidural hematoma. This demands immediate evacuation following diagnosis if reversal of neurological deficit is to be achieved. A resurgence of back pain, with or without radiculopathy, and an elevated erythrocyte sedimentation rate, days or weeks postoperatively, is pathognomonic of discitis. In the case of aseptic discitis, radiologic studies will show sclerosis of the adjacent end-plates rather than loss of cortical margins. Treatment usually consists of bedrest, bracing, and nonsteroidal anti-inflammatory drugs. The presence of fever, chills, and leukocytosis suggest a bacterial wound infection. If the CT scan or MRI shows an abscess in the subcutaneous tissues overlying the laminae, open surgical drainage, packing, and administration of intravenous antibiotics are indicated. With purulent discitis and osteomyelitis, plain roentgenograms may show destructive changes of the end-plates if the condition has been present for at least 3 weeks. A needle aspiration of the disc space and identification of the organism is necessary to guide the subsequent antibiotic treatment regimen. A generally cited overall complication rate with hemilaminectomy and discectomy is less than 5%. In the absence of a complication, the surgical treatment for lumbar herniated disc is one of the most rewarding in neurosurgery.

Contributors

RICHARD P. ANDERSON, M.D.
Chief Resident
Department of Neurosurgery
West Virginia University Hospitals
Morgantown, West Virginia

EHUD ARBIT, M.D.
Associate Attending Surgeon
Neurosurgery Service
Department of Surgery
Memorial Sloan-Kettering Cancer Center
New York, New York

KIM J. BURCHIEL, M.D.
Professor and Head
Division of Neurosurgery
Oregon Health Sciences University
Portland, Oregon

RALPH B. CLOWARD, M.D.
Clinical Professor
Department of Neurosurgery
John A. Burns School of Medicine
University of Hawaii
Honolulu, Hawaii

SARAH J. GASKILL, M.D.
Resident
Division of Neurosurgery
Duke University Medical Center
Durham, North Carolina

DAVID J. GOWER, M.D.
Assistant Professor
Division of Neurosurgery
University of Oklahoma Health Sciences Center
Oklahoma City, Oklahoma

HAROLD J. HOFFMAN, M.D.
Professor of Surgery
Division of Neurosurgery
University of Toronto
Chief of Neurosurgery
The Hospital for Sick Children
Toronto, Ontario, Canada

HOWARD H. KAUFMAN, M.D.
Professor and Chairman
Department of Neurosurgery
West Virginia University Hospitals
Morgantown, West Virginia

PHYO KIM, M.D.
Resident
Department of Neurologic Surgery
Mayo Clinic/Mayo Medical School
Rochester, Minnesota

ARTHUR E. MARLIN, M.D.
Chief, Pediatric Neurosurgery
Vice Chairman, Pediatric Surgery
Santa Rosa Children's Hospital
San Antonio, Texas

DENNIS E. McDONNELL, M.D.
Associate Professor
Department of Surgery
Section of Neurosurgery
Medical College of Georgia
Augusta, Georgia

ARNOLD H. MENEZES, M.D.
Professor and Vice Chairman
Division of Neurosurgery
The University of Iowa Hospitals and Clinics
Iowa City, Iowa

BURTON M. ONOFRIO, M.D.
Professor
Department of Neurologic Surgery
Mayo Clinic/Mayo Medical School
Rochester, Minnesota

JOHN A. PERSING, M.D.
Professor
Department of Neurosurgery
Associate Professor and Vice-Chairman
Department of Plastic Surgery
University of Virginia Health Sciences Center
Charlottesville, Virginia

JOSEPH H. PIATT, JR., M.D.
Head, Pediatric Neurosurgery Section
Division of Neurosurgery
Oregon Health Sciences University
Portland, Oregon

SYDNEY S. SCHOCHET, M.D.
Professor of Pathology, Neurology, and Neurosurgery
Department of Pathology (Neuropathology)
West Virginia University Hospitals
Morgantown, West Virginia

JATIN SHAH, M.D.
Attending Surgeon
Head and Neck Service
Department of Surgery
Memorial Sloan-Kettering Cancer Center
Professor
Cornell University Medical College
New York, New York

Contents

TRANSORAL SURGERY FOR CRANIOVERTEBRAL JUNCTION ANOMALIES

ARNOLD H. MENEZES, M.D.

INTRODUCTION AND PATIENT SELECTION

Abnormalities at the craniovertebral junction have been recorded for several centuries. But, it is only in the past four decades that antemortem recognition of these lesions has stimulated surgical therapy. Several approaches to the anterior craniovertebral junction have been developed. The transoral-transpalatal-pharyngeal route is most frequently used for decompression of this area. Advances in neurodiagnostic imaging and microsurgical instrumentation have expanded the use of this approach.

The bony abnormalities of the craniovertebral junction may be divided into reducible and irreducible categories. Primary treatment for reducible craniovertebral junction (CVJ) lesions is stabilization. Surgical decompression of the cervicomedullary junction is performed when irreducible pathology is encountered. Should the lesion be ventrally situated, a transoral-pharyngeal decompression is required. In dorsal compression, a posterior approach is used. If instability exists following either situation, a posterior fixation is necessary. Thus, the factors that influence the surgical approach to lesions of the craniovertebral junction are: 1) reducibility, 2) the direction of encroachment, and 3) the type of lesion.

These factors are assessed with plain x-ray films, polytomography, and myelography with computed tomography. Dynamic studies determine anteroposterior stability in the flexed and extended positions and vertical stability under traction. Magnetic resonance imaging, including a dynamic study, is currently the procedure of choice (Fig. 1, A and B).

Mere identification of a ventrally placed lesion at the craniovertebral junction is not an indication for an anterior transoral approach. The main indication for the transoral operation is irreducible ventral compression of the cervicomedullary junction, whether it is from bone, granulation tissue, or abscess. The exposure obtained is from the clivus to the C2-C3 interspace (Fig. 2). Bony tumors and chordomas have been approached in a similar manner. Primary intradural tumors such as schwannomas and meningiomas are best approached via the dorsal route because they reside within the subarachnoid space. However, should this not be possible, a ventral transoral operative approach may be necessary. On occasion, midline vertebral basilar artery aneurysms have been clipped via this route.

PREOPERATIVE PREPARATION

A magnetic resonance imaging (MRI)-compatible halo is used for cervical traction and stabilization prior to the transoral procedure. A high caloric intake is advised. Oropharyngeal cultures are obtained three days prior to the operation. No antibiotics are used unless pathologic flora are present.

The entrance to the oral cavity must provide a working distance of 2.5 to 3 cm between the upper and lower teeth. This span may not be available in patients afflicted with rheumatoid arthritis with involvement of the temporomandibular joints. In such a circumstance, a median mandibular split with midline glossotomy may be necessary to gain access into the oral cavity.

Evaluation of lower cranial nerve and brain stem function is extremely important. Difficulty in swallowing, tracheal aspiration, or repeated upper respiratory infections would mandate a tracheostomy at the start of the operative procedure. A tracheostomy maintains a safe open airway should obstruction from lingual swelling occur early in the postoperative convalescence.

Sensory evoked responses and brain stem latencies from median nerve stimulation are assessed before surgery to allow for comparison during the operation. Custom-built teeth guards for the upper and lower dentition are obtained via impressions taken a few days prior to surgery. They protect the teeth during

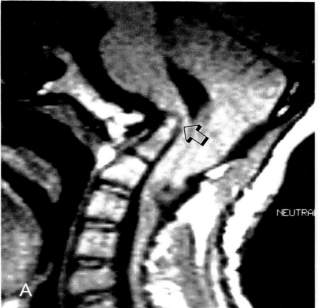 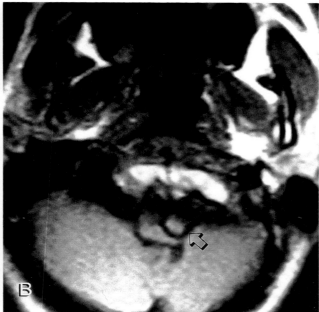

Figure 1. **A,** midsagittal T1-weighted MRI of the cranio004-vertebral junction. There is assimilation of the atlas and severe basilar invagination. The odontoid process invades the medulla oblongata (*open arrow*). **B,** axial T1-weighted MRI made 15 mm above the plane of the foramen magnum. The odontoid process grossly indents the medulla (*open arrow*).

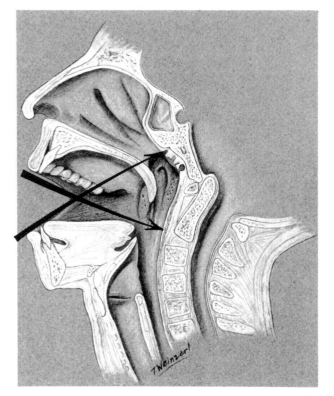

Figure 2. Illustration of the rostrocaudal exposure (*between arrows*) obtained via the transoral operation.

surgery when the self-retaining Dingman mouth retractor is used.

SURGICAL TECHNIQUE

Anesthesia
The patient is brought sedated to the operating room with halo traction set at 5–7 pounds. Topical oropharyngeal and nasopharyngeal anesthesia is used and supplemented with bilateral superior laryngeal nerve blocks to facilitate an awake fiberoptic oropharyngeal intubation with the patient in the best position judged from preoperative dynamic studies. Following this, the patient is positioned appropriately for the operative procedure and examined awake to check the neurologic status. General anesthesia is then administered. Nasopharyngeal intubation is to be avoided since it disrupts the integrity of the high naso-oropharyngeal mucosa. The patient is positioned supine with the head resting on a Mayfield headholder and traction is maintained throughout the entire operative procedure. In circumstances where the bony anomaly or tumor has been recognized to violate the dura and the subarachnoid space, a lumbar spinal subarachnoid drain is installed.

Operative Procedure
A tracheostomy is performed when the operation involves the high nasopharynx and the craniocervical junction. Operative procedures at the level of atlas and

axis may not require a tracheostomy. In the latter circumstance, an armored endotracheal tube is secured to an incisor tooth in the midline and held in place by the Dingman self-retaining tongue retractor during the operation. A tracheostomy is essential when the operative procedure involves the clivus and there is brain stem dysfunction. When the operation is limited to the upper cervical spine, the soft palate is drawn up into the high nasopharynx via sutures attached to soft rubber tubing passed through the nostrils and then withdrawn. The abdomen is prepared for possible harvesting of fascia and fat grafts, should this be necessary after intradural exploration.

A gauze pack occludes the laryngopharynx. The oral cavity, nasopharynx, and oropharynx are cleansed first with 10% povidone-iodine solution, then with hydrogen peroxide, and finally rinsed with saline. The circumoral area is prepared in the usual fashion and isolated.

A modified Dingman self-retaining mouth retractor allows depression of the tongue and lateral retraction of the cheeks (Fig. 3). One-half percent lidocaine solu-

tion with 1/200,000 epinephrine is injected into the median raphe of the soft palate. A midline incision is made extending from the hard palate to the base of the uvula, deviating from the midline at its base. Stay sutures provide for lateral retraction and are held in place via the springs of the Dingman mouth retractor.

The operating microscope now provides magnification and illumination. Topical 5% cocaine is applied to the posterior pharyngeal mucosa and its midline is infiltrated with 0.5% lidocaine solution with 1/200,000 epinephrine. A midline incision is made into the posterior pharyngeal median raphe (Fig. 4A). This extends from the rosal clivus to the C2-C3 interspace. The posterior pharyngeal wall is now retracted laterally using stay sutures for self-retaining exposure. The prevertebral fascia and longus colli muscles are reflected free of their osseous ligamentous attachments to expose the caudal clivus and the atlas and axis vertebrae. The anterior longitudinal ligament and the occipital ligaments are dissected free of their bony attachments to expose further the caudal clivus, ante-

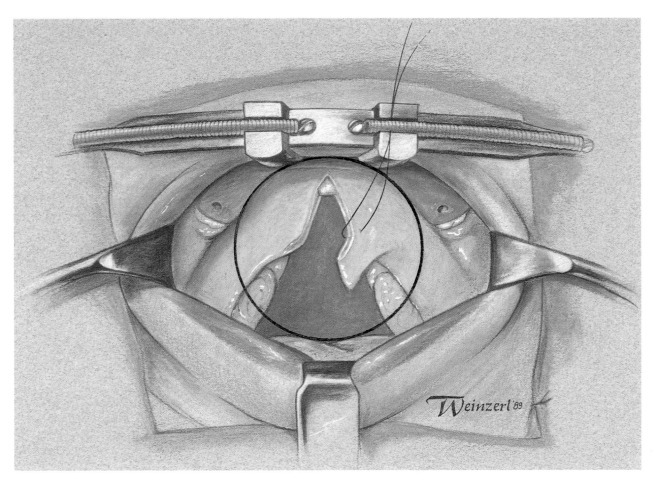

Figure 3. This drawing illustrates the exposure of the oral cavity and pharynx with the Dingman mouth retractors in place. The soft palate has been incised, exposing a portion of the hard palate at the apex of the incision. The view through the operative microscope is within the *circle*.

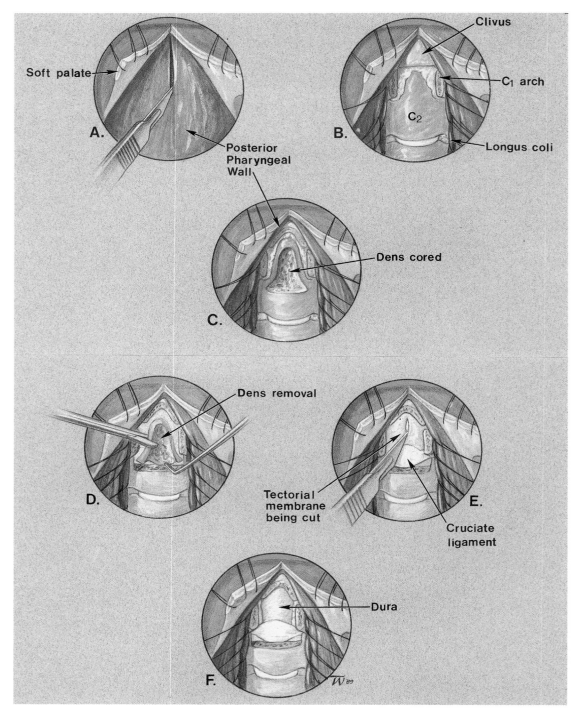

Figure 4. Drawing of views through the microscope. **A,** the soft palate is retracted laterally with stay sutures; the posterior pharyngeal wall is incised. **B,** the longus colli muscles as well as the posterior pharyngeal wall are retracted to expose the clivus, the anterior arch of C1, and the body of C2. The dens is revealed when the anterior arch of the atlas is resected. There is granulation tissue around the dens and behind the clivus. **C,** the caudal clivus is resected to expose the invaginated odontoid process which is now cored out. **D,** the shell of the odontoid process is removed along with a part of the body of the axis. **E,** the cruciate ligament is visible after removal of the odontoid process. The tectorial membrane is incised vertically. **F,** the dura bulges ventrally when decompression is complete.

rior arch of the atlas, and the anterior surface of the body of the axis (Fig. 4B). This exposure is between 3 and 3.5 cm in width (Fig. 5A). Further lateral exposure is inadvisable because of the risk of destruction of the eustachian tube orifices, entrance into the vertebral canal and damage to the vertebral arteries, and injury to the hypoglossal nerves.

The anterior arch of the atlas is now removed with a high-speed drill for a width of 3 cm. Resection of the caudal clivus is carried out in a similar fashion depending on the pathology (Fig. 4C). The soft tissue ventral to the odontoid process is cleared with rongeurs. The odontoid process is cored out in a rostrocaudal direction using a high-speed cutting burr initially and then a diamond burr. It is then separated from all of its ligamentous attachments using microsurgical technique (Fig. 4D). If there is chronic instability, pannus will be encountered. This should be carefully resected by cauterization and piecemeal removal. Division of the odontoid process at its base and downward traction is to be avoided because incomplete resection as well as a dural tear may result. The removal of the odontoid process is completed with up-biting Lee-Smith Kerrison rongeurs with a 1-mm footplate. Angled curettes and microbiopsy forceps also facilitate the removal (Fig. 5B).

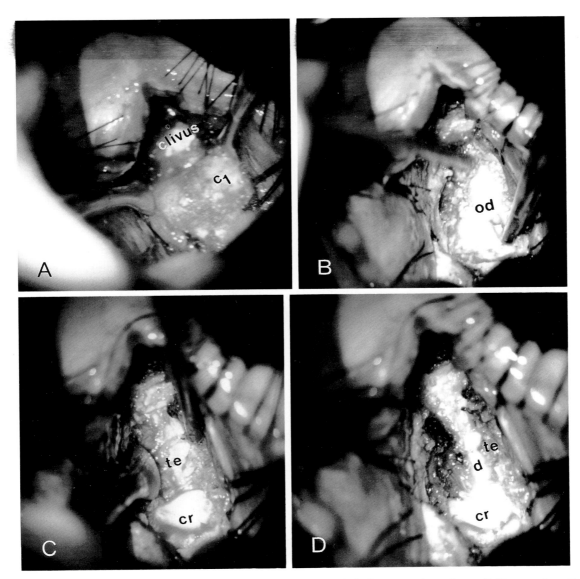

Figure 5. Microphotographs depicting the operative exposure and transoropharyngeal decompression of the craniovertebral junction of the patient depicted in Figure 1. **A,** exposure of the clivus, the arch of the atlas, and the body of the axis. **B,** the shell of the cored odontoid (od) being removed. **C,** the tectorial membrane (te) is seen above the cruciate ligament (cr) after the odontoid process is removed. **D,** the dura (d) bulges into the wound once the tectorial membrane (te) is incised.

Removal of pannus from behind the odontoid process and from the posterior fossa should be done piecemeal with angled and ring curettes.

Preoperative lateral pleuridirectional tomography, as well as axial magnetic resonance imaging, will guide the surgeon as to the extent of removal of the odontoid process or abnormal bony lesion (Fig. 4E). Extradural tumors, likewise, are now resected. The tectorial membrane must be incised carefully to allow adequate dural decompression (Fig. 4F). A blunt nerve hook inserted between the tectorial membrane and the dura prevents dural penetration (Fig. 5, C and D). Changes in brain stem latencies require gentle handling of tissues and minimal compression of the neural structures.

An intradural lesion at the upper cervical spine, craniocervical border, or behind the clivus necessitates a cruciate incision of the dura. The vertical component of this starts inferiorly proceeding up in a rostral direction with careful cauterization of the circular sinus at the foramen magnum. The dural turgidity may be reduced by draining spinal fluid through a previously placed lumbar subarachnoid drain. The dural leaves are reflected to the four quadrants to allow exposure of the lower pons, medulla, and cervicomedullary junction. Once the intradural operation is complete, it is essential to bring the dural leaves together with 4-0 polyglycolic acid sutures. Fascia harvested from the external oblique aponeurosis is now placed against the dural closure. This may be held in position by plasma glue if available. A fat pad reinforces the fascia.

Aerobic and anaerobic cultures are obtained from the depths of the wound prior to closure. Bacitracin powder and microfibrillar collagen are placed over the closure. The longus colli muscles are approximated in the midline with 3-0 polyglactin sutures. Anatomical approximation of the posterior pharyngeal musculature is obtained with similar sutures using an interrupted figure-of-eight technique. Then, horizontal mattress sutures approximate the posterior pharyngeal mucosa. There is no muscular layer over the clivus, and, hence, mucosal approximation must be done carefully at the rostral end of the incision. A blanket of Gelfoam is then placed over the mucosal closure of the nasopharynx.

The closure of the soft palate is done by bringing the nasal mucosa together with interrupted 3-0 polyglactin sutures. The muscularis as well as the oral mucosa of the soft palate are approximated with interrupted vertical mattress sutures of similar strength.

In situations where surgery is necessary through the clivus, or in patients with platybasia and a foreshortened clivus, the hard palate must be exposed and its posterior 8–10 mm resected using Kerrison rongeurs. During this step, it is essential to preserve the mucosa in the nasal as well as the oral aspects of the hard palate. This technique allows high nasopharyngeal exposure without splitting the mandible or doing a median glossotomy.

Postoperative Care

Following the operation, the patient's head is elevated to 10–15° and is maintained in 5–7 pounds of skeletal traction. This permits drainage of nasal and oral secretions without pooling at the operative site. Intravenous hyperalimentation is the rule for the first five to six days during which no oral intake is permitted. At the end of this time it is important to assess craniocervical stability with flexion-extension dynamic pleuridirectional tomography, visualizing the facets. Vertical instability is checked with and without cervical traction. Should instability be present, a dorsal fixation procedure is necessary. In the event that the craniocervical junction is stable, the tracheostomy is gradually allowed to close. The oral intake is advanced from a clear liquid diet at the end of the first week to a full liquid diet in a fortnight. Solid food is given at the end of the third week.

If the dura was opened and a fascial graft was used for repair, intravenous antibiotics and spinal drainage are continued for 10 days after surgery.

COMPLICATIONS

The most dreaded postoperative complication is cerebrospinal fluid leakage and meningitis. This may be immediate or delayed. An immediate cerebrospinal fluid leak is best handled via immediate reapproximation of the wound and closure in the manner described. A delayed cerebrospinal fluid leak implies retropharyngeal infection. This must be treated with intravenous antibiotics, spinal drainage, and elevation of the head. Intravenous hyperalimentation promotes wound healing by secondary intention. Should this not occur, a surgical closure becomes necessary.

Wound dehiscence can be avoided by delaying oral intake. Retropharyngeal infection may present itself with dehiscence within 7-10 days. Control of infection and possible lateral extrapharyngeal drainage of the site may be necessary. Mucosal coverage will occur if an adequate caloric intake is maintained.

Nasal speech and regurgitation of food are manifestations of dehiscence of the palate; closure of the separated edges may be done early or late. Inadequate and improper closure of the soft palate will lead to velopalatine incompetence.

Failure to recognize craniocervical instability can lead to disastrous vascular complications as well as cervicomedullary compression.

ANTEROLATERAL CERVICAL APPROACH TO THE CRANIOVERTEBRAL JUNCTION

DENNIS E. McDONNELL, M.D.

INTRODUCTION

Synonyms for this operation are the transcervical, anterolateral, parapharyngeal, or submandibular approach to the ventral craniovertebral junction (atlas, axis, and clivus). Surgical exposure of the ventral aspect of the craniovertebral junction has always been considered difficult and dangerous, and rightly so. Since 1956, when Smith and Robinson described gaining access to the anterior cervical spine by dissecting through fascial planes, surgeons have steadily become bolder in directly attacking pathologic processes involving the vertebral bodies or discs, and lesions in the ventral spinal canal. This approach is part of every spinal surgeon's armamentarium for dealing with the segments of C3 to T1. It has not gained popularity with treatment of conditions rostral to C2. The transoral route is presently the preferred ventral route to the atlas, axis, and clivus.

Surgeons have been hesitant to adopt this approach because of the complexity of anatomy, concentration of vital structures, and difficulty in exposure that is entailed in the approach to this region. However, there are some inherent advantages to this approach that might warrant consideration. This approach gives a sterile surgical field as opposed to the contaminated transoral field. It offers wider exposure of the lateral masses of C1 and C2 than is possible via the transoral route. Also, the lower cervical segments are available, if necessary, whereas they are not for the transoral route.

PATIENT SELECTION

Characteristically, a symptomatic lesion affecting the cervicomedullary junction of the central nervous system (CNS) is insidious, subtle, and relentless in its progression. The ultimate cause is mechanical compression of the CNS resulting in pain, myelopathy, and, ultimately, apnea and death, if the compression is not reversed in some way. The lesion may be congenital, developmental, or acquired and may involve the osseous elements, supportive ligaments, vascular structures, and/or the CNS. Craniovertebral instability may be superimposed, further compromising the patient.

It is essential that the anatomy of the lesion be imaged, misalignment be discerned, and instability be determined before a treatment plan can be decided for the patient. Plain x-ray films of the craniocervical junction should include anteroposterior, open-mouth, and lateral views. Dynamic flexion and extension in the lateral projection will help to assess instability. The magnetic resonance (MR) image will determine the position of the compressing lesion as well as the type and degree of CNS distortion present. The computed axial tomogram (CT) will give important information regarding the integrity of the bone of the body of C2, odontoid process, lateral mass articulations, arches of C1, and occipital structures. Positive contrast cisternography combined with CT and/or polytomography gives additional information regarding bone and soft tissue distortions.

A lesion within or distorting the ventral subarachnoid space extending from the pharyngeal tubercle of the basiocciput caudally to even the lower cervical segments is amenable to this approach. A lesion producing symptoms of pain, weakness, incoordination, dysphagia, nystagmus, deafness, other cranial nerve dysfunction, or urinary incontinence, and having an inherent tendency of progression, demands direct removal if the process is to be arrested. If the process is chronic, the patient may be debilitated and nutritionally compromised. The patient's respiratory reserve may be impaired which further increases the risk for any surgical procedure. A bedridden, debilitated, catheterized patient harboring a CNS compressive lesion presents a perplexing and difficult challenge to the surgeon. Anatomical, physiological, nutritional, psychological, and neurological factors must all be assessed before performing this pro-

147

cedure. Therefore, this cannot be rushed into; the risks must be assessed and an organized plan of action must be formed.

Retraction of the superior pharynx for exposure of this region results in swelling with relative compromise of the upper airway. Postoperative respiratory embarrassment should be expected and managed. Respiratory impairment will be aggravated by any preoperative myelopathy. Postoperative pharyngeal swelling will also impede oral alimentation. If there is generalized debility, then nutritional depletion will be compounded further by the stress of the surgery and impaired deglutition. Indwelling urinary catheter, vascular access lines, alimentation tube, endotracheal tube, and external subarachnoid drain may be in place for an extended time, raising the threat of systemic infection. A catabolic state will potentiate the risk of such infection. Therefore, nutritional support must be carefully planned preoperatively.

It is strongly recommended that a treatment plan algorithm, as described by Menezes, be followed in establishing a management plan for the patient with an upper cervical or craniovertebral lesion. By doing so, problems and complications can be reduced or avoided and chances for an optimal outcome improved. If craniovertebral instability is expected either pre- or postoperatively, then this must be specifically addressed preoperatively. Likewise, if the intradural compartment is purposefully entered (one of the advantages of this approach) then the cerebrospinal fluid (CSF) must be diverted, at least temporarily, to avoid a CSF collection under tension in the dissected cervical tissues or a CSF-cutaneous fistula.

Severe neurologic impairment is *not* a contraindication to this procedure. The statement, "the patient is too ill to tolerate surgery," just does not hold, if there is any neurologic function to preserve caudal to the lesion. Obviously, if there is coagulopathy, sepsis, systemic malignancy, or cardiac compromise, then such a patient is not a candidate for this surgery until these conditions are reversed.

The alternative procedure is the transoral approach. The best procedure most often is the procedure with which the surgeon has the most experience and is most comfortable. The transoral approach is most commonly used by surgeons approaching this region. Therefore, when dealing with extradural lesions localized to the C1 and C2 segments it may be preferred. However, such lesions are just as amenable via the transcervical route. If the lesion extends rostral to the pharyngeal tubercle of the basiocciput, then an alternative to the transcervical route should be considered. If the dura must be entered or the lesion extends caudal to C2, and not rostral to the pharyngeal tubercle, then the transcervical route is preferred.

PREOPERATIVE PREPARATION

The patient with a craniovertebral chronic compressive lesion is in serious jeopardy from compression and/or instability. The rationale for treatment is surgical correction of the pathological tension, distortion, and compression of the neuraxis in order to reestablish neural conductivity and to renew regional cervicomedullary blood flow. The treatment plan for these patients is often multistage and is outlined as follows:

1. Attempt reduction by cervical traction to establish realignment or to demonstrate irreducibility of any malalignment.
2. Tracheostomy/feeding gastrostomy or jejunostomy.
3. Anterior resection of the encroaching structures (bone, ligaments, pannus, exudate, or tumor).
4. Immobilization in skeletal traction between stages.
5. Occipito-C1–C2–C3 fusion by the posterior approach.
6. Halo brace immobilization, usually for six months.

These steps must be understood and accepted by the patient and family before commencing the anterior spinal operation.

Respiratory reserve will be a critical factor in the immediate postoperative management. Therefore, formal assessment of pulmonary function is crucial, particularly if there is a history of chronic lung disease. Tracheostomy and feeding gastrostomy should be done electively; the gastrostomy established one week preoperatively allows for it to mature so that it is immediately available for use. The tracheostomy is placed either at the time of gastrostomy or just prior to the transcervical procedure. Adequate nutrition is essential to avoid bacterial infections and to assist early mobilization. This is best ensured by preemptive and elective direct transabdominal enteric access.

Refrain from using preoperative antibiotics to avoid altering the patient's normal flora and establishing resistant nosocomial bacteria. A broad spectrum antibiotic (i.e., cefazolin) is given just prior to starting the procedure. A topical antibiotic is also placed in the irrigation (i.e., bacitracin).

If entry through the dura is planned, a lumbar subarachnoid drain should be placed before starting the procedure. It need not be draining during the procedure, but it is established for continuous drainage postoperatively. This reduces CSF hydrostatic pressure at the surgical site, thus avoiding a CSF fistula.

SURGICAL TECHNIQUE

Anesthesia

The patient is positioned supine while awake. If it is decided that a tracheostomy is not needed, then an awake intubation is done. The hypopharynx, larynx, and trachea are anesthetized locally with a topical anesthetic. The trachea is then intubated via the nasotracheal route. The fiberoptic bronchoscope is helpful and facilitates this maneuver. This avoids hyperextension, which may aggravate compression of the neuraxis. General anesthesia is maintained by an intravenous narcotic agent, and a combination of inhalation agents consisting of isoflurane, nitrous oxide, and oxygen. A low dose of sodium thiopental is given as well. If motor evoked potentials or the electromyogram is to be monitored, long-acting muscle relaxants should be avoided. Infiltration of the skin incision with 0.5% lidocaine with 1/200,000 epinephrine will aid hemostasis in the superficial tissues.

A lumbar subarachnoid drain is placed with the patient in the lateral decubitus position either under local anesthesia or after induction of general anesthesia. Great care must be used in positioning the patient for this, particularly if there is instability.

It is advantageous to monitor blood pressure through a direct arterial line, central venous pressure, end expiratory carbon dioxide tension, and neurophysiologic responses throughout the procedure. Monitoring of somatosensory cortical evoked responses from the stimulation of the median and common peroneal nerves is helpful. Motor evoked responses will probably also be measured as a routine in the future. An indwelling Foley catheter is often already in place for patients with advanced myelopathy. Hourly measurement of urine output is obtained as an additional guide to fluid balance. The intraoperative administration of diuretics is not ordinarily necessary for this procedure. Sequential compression pneumatic hose are placed on the lower extremities for prophylaxis against venous stasis and thromboembolism.

Operative Positioning

The operating table should be set up beforehand to accept the "C-arm" fluoroscope. Usually the C-arm is oriented in the transverse plane for lateral projection beneath the head of the table, so that it is out of the way of the anesthesiologist, surgeon, and assistant. Fluoroscopic control of the operative field is very helpful for maintaining orientation in the sagittal plane. For some tables it is necessary to place a padded radiolucent board on the table and to orient the head of the patient to overhang the foot of the table, to accommodate the C-arm coming in beneath the table and the patient's head, neck, and shoulders.

The patient's head is rotated 30° to the contralateral side and extended in order to raise the mandible up and away from the surgeon's line of sight to the field (Fig. 1). It is supported on a sponge doughnut or horseshoe headrest. Of course, if the patient's head is being maintained in a halo traction system, the sponge doughnut is not needed.

Skeletal traction is often necessary to maintain position in the face of spinal instability. If a halo ring is in place, an extra thick pad or short mattress can be used on the operating table to allow the patient's head to go into extension, by having the head overhang the end of the pad, supported by the halo ring and traction. Rope attached to the tongs or halo and 10 to 15 lbs of weight for traction can be hung over an ether screen support.

The anesthesiologist, anesthesia equipment, and monitoring devices are all at the head of the patient. The surgeon and assistant are opposite each other at the patient's side, and the scrub nurse is next to the surgeon toward the patient's feet.

The microscope is mounted with the assistant's observation port and laser. It will straddle the C-arm at the head of the table and be brought from the side opposite the surgeon. The laser console is positioned on the surgeon's side toward the patient's head. This allows the articulated arm to attach to the microscope opposite to the observer port and out of the way of the operating team. The high-speed drill can be kept sterile in a basin on a ring stand out of the way and brought into the field only when needed.

The neck and chin are shaved and scrubbed with detergent as is either the lateral thigh or lower abdomen, if a fascial graft is needed for subsequent dural closure. The neck incision is marked and injected with the local anesthetic/epinephrine combination.

Plastic adhesive towel drapes positioned around the marked incision sites will help isolate the operative areas which are then covered by an adhesive incise drape. This isolates the tracheostomy as well as other contaminated sites from the operative fields.

The operating microscope and laser articulated arm are draped with commercially available plastic drapes. The C-arm is also draped with transparent plastic drapes.

Skin Incision

The choice of incision is dependent on the surgeon's experience and the specific craniovertebral exposure required for the task at hand. Four choices are available: transverse, oblique-vertical, hockey-stick, and "T." The first description of this approach by Stevenson recommended the T incision. A vertical extension or direction of the incision is necessary only if exposure caudal to C4 is necessary. Otherwise, the transverse incision is quite adequate and cosmetically more appealing; it also serves to relatively protect the superior laryngeal nerve (SLN). Regardless of the incision, the secret to adequate exposure with this approach is wide dissection of the cervical fascial planes. The concept that the vertically oriented incision facilitates the exposure and obviates the necessity for wide fascial dissection is erroneous and misleading.

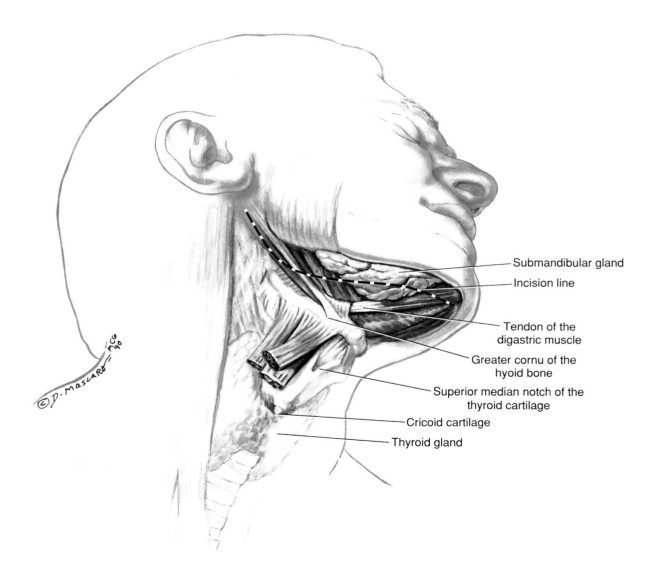

Submandibular gland

Incision line

Tendon of the
digastric muscle

Greater cornu of the
hyoid bone

Superior median notch of the
thyroid cartilage

Cricoid cartilage

Thyroid gland

Figure 1. The patient's position is oriented with the head extended and rotated contralateral to the side of approach. The curvilinear incision (*dotted line*) is 2 cm below and parallel to the edge of the mandible.

The transverse incision is my preference, and this will be the perspective presented here. The incision is 2 cm inferior and parallel to the lower edge of the mandible, and extends from the angle of the mandible posteriorly to the base of the mental protuberance *beyond the midline* anteriorly (Fig. 1). Care is taken to avoid the marginal mandibular branch of the facial nerve supplying the mental muscles of the lower lip.

The side of approach, right or left, depends on the lesion. If there is unilateral lower cranial nerve impairment, the approach should be made from the side of impairment to avoid possible injury to the intact contralateral cranial nerves. However, with this procedure the surgeon's perspective will be at approximately a 20° angle from the midsagittal plane and a 30° angle from the transverse/horizontal plane; this gives an easier view of deep structures contralateral to the side of approach. Therefore the side of approach is an important factor in preoperative planning, particularly with lesions eccentric from the midline. In dealing with midline lesions, the side of approach is usually that of the surgeon's preference.

Dissection and Exposure

The key to adequate exposure is wide sharp dissection of each layer or plane of the cervical fascia, beginning with development of a wide subcutaneous flap on each side of the incision superficial to the platysma muscle (Fig. 2). There will be anatomical landmarks that identify each plane and guide the surgeon's way. Each landmark is dissected free of its fascial investment and is preserved both anatomically and functionally. Fine-toothed forceps and delicate semisharp dissecting scissors are the instruments to use here. It is helpful, if not essential, for the surgeon's assistant to pick up the cervical fascia with fine-toothed forceps just opposite to the surgeon's forceps and follow along the surgeon's course, giving countertraction on the fascia as the dissection with scissors progresses. This maneuver helps to define the fascial plane being dissected. Likewise, the surgeon must move the forceps and lift the fascia close to the scissors, keeping the fascia taut with countertraction from the assistant's forceps at all times. The fascial planes are avascular with no major intervening structures. When lifted and opened, the areolar fibrous texture of the fascia is revealed. Its transparency allows a view of the structures it contains. Such perspective is gained only with countertraction on the fascia and sharp dissection. Wide opening of each fascial layer in a sequential, methodical manner will ensure adequate exposure of the deeper structures, while preserving the intervening structures. The dissection can be compared to that required on a cadaver in the anatomy laboratory for anatomical presentation. Therefore, this procedure requires a "cadaveric" dissection of the cervical

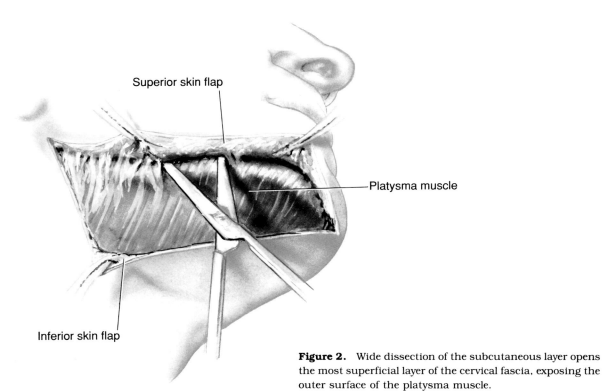

Superior skin flap

Platysma muscle

Inferior skin flap

Figure 2. Wide dissection of the subcutaneous layer opens the most superficial layer of the cervical fascia, exposing the outer surface of the platysma muscle.

fascia and its enclosed structures. Anatomical landmarks will lead the way.

The route will be through the platysma muscle to the submandibular trigone, beneath the submandibular gland, inferior to the digastric muscle, inferior to the hypoglossal nerve, superior to the greater cornu of the hyoid bone, past the lateral aspect of the superior pharyngeal constrictor muscle, to the retropharyngeal space and the precervical fascia. The previously dissected skin edges and subcutaneous flaps are retracted with a Weitlaner-type self-retaining retractor, thus exposing the superficial surface of the platysma muscle.

Platysma Muscle
The medial edge of the platysma is grasped in the midline. A hole is cut in the median fascial raphe to gain entrance to the next fascial layer. The dissecting scissors is used to undermine and develop the fascial layer in the midline vertically in a cephalocaudal direction. The fascial sheet thus formed is then cut vertically in the midline for a length of 6 cm from the mandibular symphysis to the median notch of the superior thyroid cartilage (Fig. 3). This defines the medial edge of the platysma muscle and initiates vertical access and will allow freer retraction. The medial edge of the platysma is grasped and elevated. The undersurface of the platysma is then dissected and freed. The platysma mus-

cle can then be transected across its fibers parallel to the direction of the primary incision for the full length of the exposure (Fig. 4). The edges of the platysma are further undermined to form muscle flaps along both the superior and inferior edges of the incision, which are then incorporated and spread apart by the Weitlaner retractor.

Submandibular Gland
The next fascial layer is identified by the submandibular gland which bulges forth beneath its transparent investment (Fig. 5). The inferior edge of the gland is grasped and elevated with the assistant giving countertraction. The fascia is then opened, undermined, and dissected parallel to the line of the incision. The facial artery and vein will be encountered crossing the field of dissection posterolateral to the submandibular gland. These vascular structures should be gently grasped and elevated by their adventitia. They are then dissected axially along their course. This maneuver further opens the submandibular fascial plane. The facial vein is clamped, transected, and ligated. The facial artery is preserved (Fig. 6). Dissection of the facial artery proximally in the lateral direction will lead to the carotid sheath, which is the lateral limit of the exposure. When the facial artery is dissected, it can be fully retracted and need not be sacrificed, as it serves as an orientation landmark. Elevating the inferior edge of

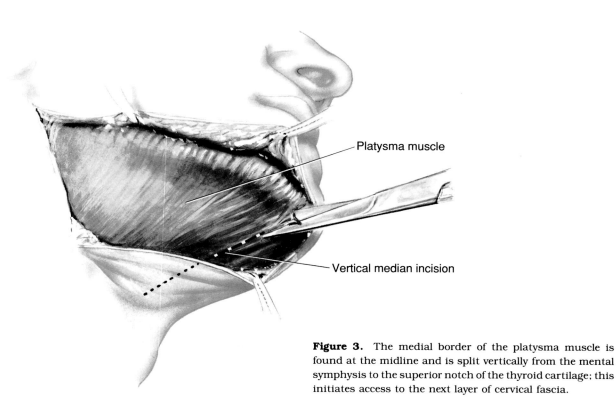

Platysma muscle

Vertical median incision

Figure 3. The medial border of the platysma muscle is found at the midline and is split vertically from the mental symphysis to the superior notch of the thyroid cartilage; this initiates access to the next layer of cervical fascia.

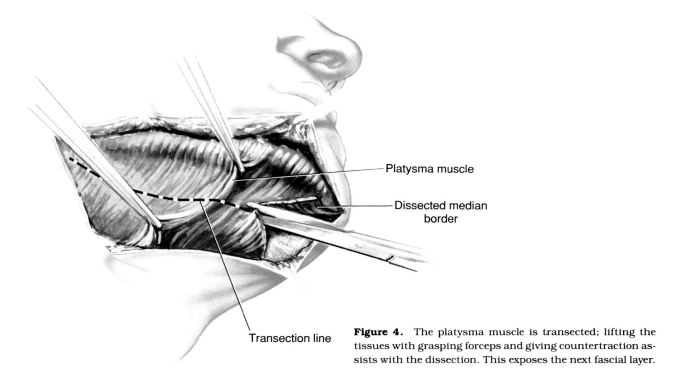

Platysma muscle

Dissected median
border

Transection line

Figure 4. The platysma muscle is transected; lifting the tissues with grasping forceps and giving countertraction assists with the dissection. This exposes the next fascial layer.

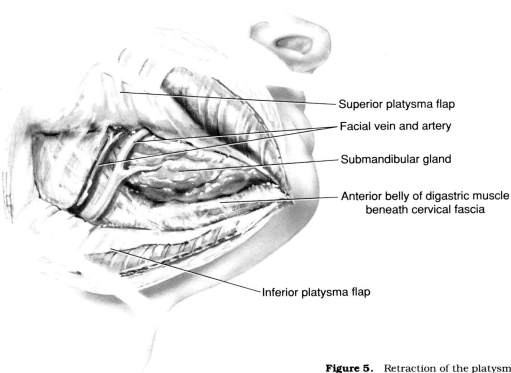

Superior platysma flap

Facial vein and artery

Submandibular gland

Anterior belly of digastric muscle
beneath cervical fascia

Inferior platysma flap

Figure 5. Retraction of the platysma exposes the submandibular gland and the facial artery and vein. Dissection of these structures opens the next layer of cervical fascia.

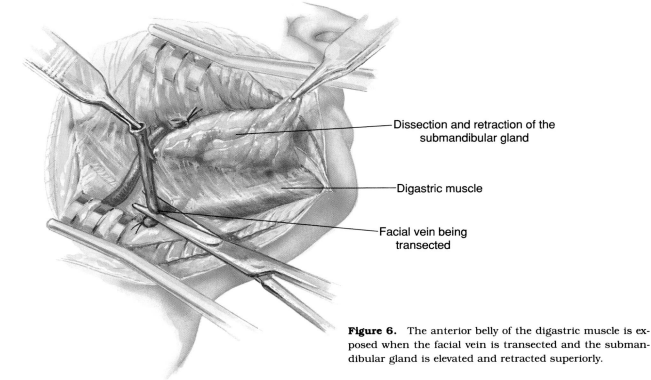

Dissection and retraction of the
submandibular gland

Digastric muscle

Facial vein being
transected

Figure 6. The anterior belly of the digastric muscle is exposed when the facial vein is transected and the submandibular gland is elevated and retracted superiorly.

the submandibular gland with the superior edge of the incision using the Weitlaner retractor exposes the next landmark, the tendon of the digastric muscle.

Digastric Muscle and Tendon
The next fascial layer is identified by the tendon of the digastric muscle, which is a substantial, glistening yellow-white cord running parallel to the course of the incision beneath the inferior edge of the submandibular gland (Fig. 7). The fascial sling around the digastric tendon attaching it to the greater wing of the hyoid bone is transected along the course of the tendon. This frees the tendon so that it can be retracted rostrally toward the mandible. This retraction is facilitated by dissecting the lower edge of the anterior and posterior bellies of the digastric muscle and freeing their undersurface. When the digastric tendon is retracted toward the mandible, the next fascial layer becomes evident. The hypoglossal nerve comes into view coursing just deep, slightly inferior, and parallel to the digastric tendon.

Hypoglossal Nerve
The hypoglossal nerve is gently dissected along its course and carefully preserved (Fig. 8). Posterolaterally the dissection is carried along the nerve trunk toward the descending hypoglossal ramus, which is another guide to the region of the carotid

artery. Again, it is not necessary to dissect along the medial border of the carotid sheath unless segments caudal to C4 are to be exposed. Thus freed, the hypoglossal nerve is retracted superiorly, exposing the hyoglossus muscle. The greater cornu of the hyoid bone now comes into view.

Hyoid Bone
The greater cornu of the hyoid bone can now be seen and palpated. The fascia overlying it is grasped and opened along the course of the hyoid bone to the carotid sheath (Fig. 9). The carotid artery is easily palpated and is the lateral-most limit of the dissection. It is retracted laterally by a right-angled, Army/Navy, or Sauerbruch retractor. This maneuver opens the retropharyngeal space. It is not necessary to cut any muscles, nerves, or vessels. At this point there is concern for compromise of the superior laryngeal nerve (SLN). The SLN courses deep to the internal carotid artery along the middle pharyngeal constrictor muscle toward the superior cornu of the thyroid cartilage. The SLN is therefore caudal and inferolateral to the route of the exposure described here. Entrance to the retropharyngeal space by this procedure is along the greater cornu of the hyoid bone and adjacent to the superior pharyngeal constrictor muscle. The SLN is not seen in the dissection of this approach. However, the SLN is vulnerable to stretch injury from retraction.

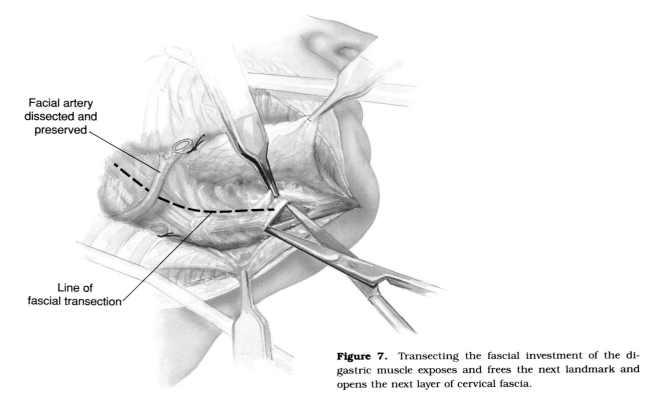

Facial artery
dissected and
preserved

Line of
fascial transection

Figure 7. Transecting the fascial investment of the digastric muscle exposes and frees the next landmark and opens the next layer of cervical fascia.

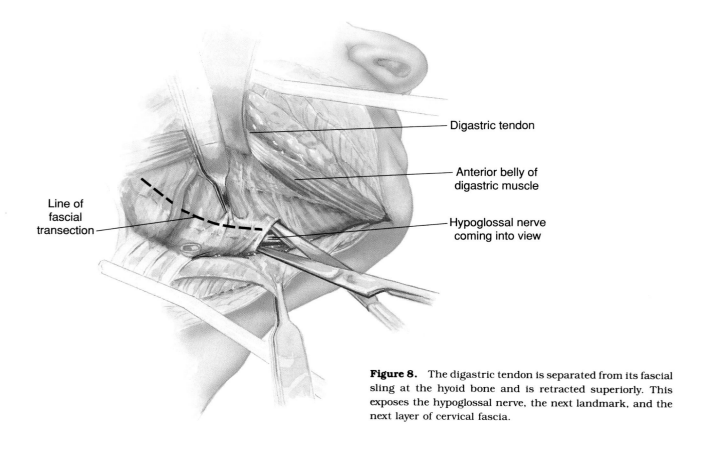

Line of
fascial
transection

Digastric tendon

Anterior belly of
digastric muscle

Hypoglossal nerve
coming into view

Figure 8. The digastric tendon is separated from its fascial sling at the hyoid bone and is retracted superiorly. This exposes the hypoglossal nerve, the next landmark, and the next layer of cervical fascia.

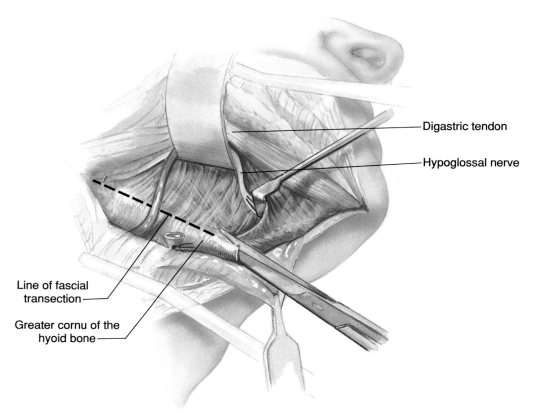

Digastric tendon

Hypoglossal nerve

Line of fascial transection

Greater cornu of the hyoid bone

Figure 9. Dissection of the hypoglossal nerve opens this layer of cervical fascia and allows retraction of the nerve to expose the next landmark, the greater cornu of the hyoid bone. Opening the fascia along the hyoid bone exposes the lateral wall of the superior pharyngeal constrictor muscle.

Wide dissection of the fascial planes as described here would tend to protect the SLN from retraction injury, as less force is required to separate the tissues that are freed by the fascial dissection. The SLN is not involved in the soft tissues retracted superiorly for this exposure; it would be vulnerable to transection if the deep cervical fascia was opened vertically in the lateral exposure here to gain access to C4 or lower cervical segments through this route. The SLN must be specifically identified and preserved if C4 or caudal segments are to be exposed by this route.

The superior constrictor muscle of the pharynx is retracted medially by a deep right-angled retractor. The retropharyngeal areolar tissue is opened with scissors. The fat pad in the retropharyngeal space confirms the location. The anterior surface of the cervical spine is easily palpated. The prominence of the anterior tubercle of C1 is noted and orients the surgeon by directing the palpating finger rostrally. The precervical fascia and muscles are now in view. The midline of the cervical spine orients the midsagittal plane and is identified between the longus colli and longus capitis muscles on either side, with the C1 anterior tubercle in the center (Fig. 10).

Longus Colli Muscles

The medial borders of the longus colli muscles are cauterized and elevated by sharp dissection from the anterolateral surfaces of C2 and C3. The muscles converge at the midline and cramp the surgeon's view of the midline. A tooth-bladed self-retaining retractor is now inserted with the blades engaged in the dissected medial walls of the longus colli muscles (the deep blades of the Cloward or Caspar retractor will do, but the Apfelbaum modified retractor system is more suited for this region).

This preliminary soft tissue retraction initiates access to deep structures. The microscope with CO_2 laser attached is now adjusted to the field. A quick glimpse with the fluoroscope in the lateral projection will assist the orientation. The laser is very advantageous in separating the longus colli and longus capitis muscles from their medial attachments (Fig. 11). Laser dissection facilitates the exposure of the anterior arch of C1 and the lateral mass articulation of the atlas and axis. It allows muscle separation up to the pharyngeal tubercle of the basiocciput. Visualizing these most rostral structures requires vertical retraction using a deep, narrow, right-angled retractor

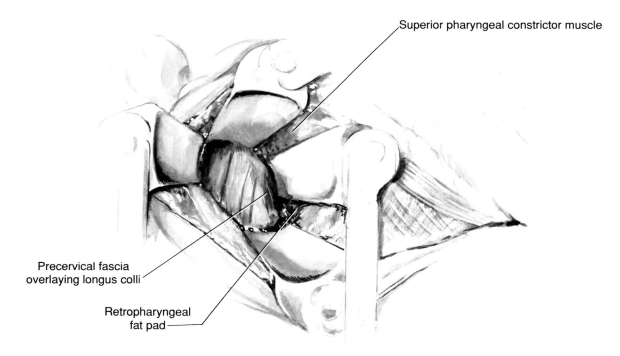

Superior pharyngeal constrictor muscle

Precervical fascia overlaying longus colli

Retropharyngeal fat pad

Figure 10.   Retraction of the superior pharyngeal constrictor opens the retropharyngeal space and exposes the precervical fascia and the longus colli muscles.

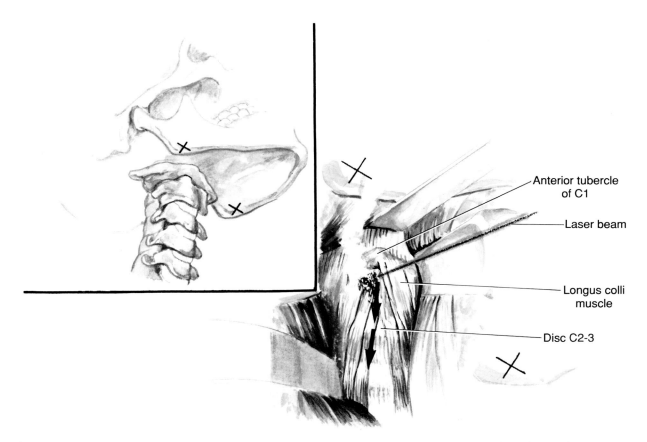

Anterior tubercle
of C1

Laser beam

Longus colli
muscle

Disc C2-3

Figure 11. The anterior tubercle of C1 identifies the midline. The longus colli muscles are dissected from the anterior arch of C1 and the anterior surface of C2 and C3. The laser controlled by the microscope attachment facilitates this.

blade. This retractor can be self-retaining or hand-held by an assistant. Here, again, the Apfelbaum retraction system offers an advantage in angulation of view. The medial one-half of the C1 and C2 lateral masses as well as the anterior rim of the foramen magnum and adjacent basiocciput (structures rostral to the anterior arch of C1) should be in view before proceeding further.

Median Tubercle of the C1 Anterior Arch

Aligning the surgeon's sight trajectory with the mid-sagittal plane and the conscious discernment of the angle of approach using the C1 anterior tubercle as a guide will help maintain proper orientation (Fig. 11). The perspective of view to the structures of interest is upward and angled at 45°. The inferior and anterior aspect of the arch of C1 and the base of the dens as well as the interval between the dens and lateral mass articulations are seen. Laser removal of overlying soft tissue clears the view. The dens, body of C2, and atlantotransverse ligament can be removed without removing the anterior arch of C1, if so desired. The transverse ligament is a tough, thick, well-defined, pale yellow ligamentous belt behind the dens. This ligament comes into view after the dens has been resected. It is a guide after the arch of C1 and the odontoid process are removed, but it may be obscured by some pathologic factors such as occur in rheumatoid arthritis.

Anterior Rim of the Foramen Magnum

The anterior rim of the foramen magnum is the next landmark just above the arch of C1. The basiocciput can be palpated and seen between the attachments of the longus colli and longus capitis muscles. This can be drilled away if entrance into the ventral aspect of the posterior fossa is required. The pharyngeal tubercle is the rostral-most landmark and limit to this approach.

Resection

A high-speed drill with a cutting burr is used to resect the bone (straight or angled handpiece). The drill should not encumber the surgeon's view. Usually the anterior arch of C1 can be removed to give a full view of the dens and adjacent articulations. The dens should be resected from the apex caudally, keeping its base intact (Fig. 12). It should be thinned out like an eggshell. The diamond burr is used at this point to avoid inadvertent tearing of the adjacent soft tissues. These lateral and posterior osseous cortical remnants are dissected with a Rosen-type microdissector from the periosteum and adjacent ligaments. They can be lifted away with either a 3-0 curette or a micro Kerrison rongeur. The medial wall of the lateral masses can be removed to widen the ventral exposure; this will be necessary if the lesion is intradural. The atlantotransverse ligament must now be identified to verify proper orientation (Fig. 13). This ligament along with the apical bursa and cruciform and tectorial ligaments must be removed. Separation from the underlying dura is accomplished by microdissection. The CO_2 laser slightly defocused at 5 to 10 watts allows removal of these structures without mechanical pulling. These ligaments and pannus can be thick, resilient, and difficult to remove when there has been long-standing instability at C1-C2. If the anterior rim of the foramen

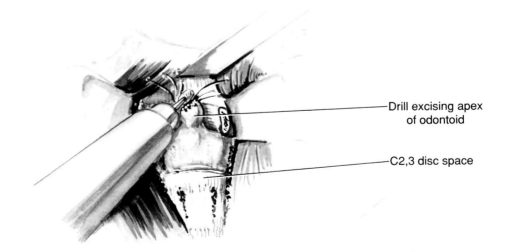

Drill excising apex of odontoid

C2,3 disc space

Figure 12.   The anterior arch of C1 has been removed, exposing the dens. The dens is best drilled away from its apex to its base.

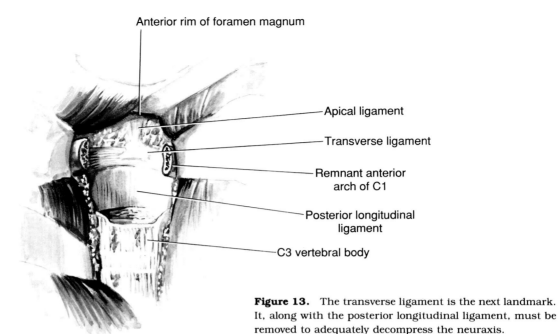

Anterior rim of foramen magnum

Apical ligament

Transverse ligament

Remnant anterior arch of C1

Posterior longitudinal ligament

C3 vertebral body

Figure 13. The transverse ligament is the next landmark. It, along with the posterior longitudinal ligament, must be removed to adequately decompress the neuraxis.

magnum is to be removed, it should be drilled away at this point using a diamond bit.

The ventral aspect of the dural sac must bulge and pulsate into the resection site (Fig. 14). Only then is adequate decompression of the neuraxis assured. The dura is recognized by its glistening pale gray color and longitudinal fibers. It may be transparent enough to reveal the pial vessels of the underlying spinal cord.

If the lesion is intradural, the dura can now be opened longitudinally. Traction sutures on the dural edge help to widen the exposure. The P-2 cutting needle on a 5-0 polydioxanone suture or the PR-1 needle on a 5-0 polyglycolic acid suture can be manipulated here for this purpose. If the lesion is a neoplasm, the laser is indispensable for atraumatic removal and compensates for the "long reach" required via this approach. Vascular lesions are dealt with as unique circumstances.

Control of the bleeding from venous sinuses and epidural veins can be challenging at times in this region. Microbipolar coagulation is the mainstay for hemostasis. Waxing bone edges will control bleeding from this source. I prefer microfibrillar collagen (Avitene) and gentle suction compression with a cottonoid pledget for control of bleeding around the dura and neuraxis.

Closure Techniques

Dural Closure

The dura cannot be closed primarily here. A dural graft will be needed, using either autograft or allograft

fascia. The graft is tacked on all four sides at several places using 5-0 suture on the P-2 needle; a running stitch can also be used. The milliwatt CO_2 laser can be used to "weld" the edges. The most effective dural closure supplement is fibrin glue. The commercial form of fibrin glue is not yet approved. I use cryoprecipitate instilled topically over the graft followed by spraying it with thrombin (Thrombostat). This results in a thick layer of coagulum which helps to seal the dural closure.

CSF Diversion

An external lumbar subarachnoid drain should be placed before commencing the procedure if an intradural procedure is planned. If the dura is inadvertently opened, the lumbar subarachnoid drain should be placed before the patient is transported from the operating room. The lumbar catheter should be tunneled subcutaneously for several centimeters before being brought out through the skin to the external reservoir. This will allow CSF drainage for several days and minimize infection at the CSF drain site. Drainage of about 300 ml of CSF per each 24-hour period will reduce hydrostatic pressure at the surgical site and avoid a CSF fistula.

Spinal Stabilization

Spinal stabilization is of critical importance and preoperative plans are implemented. Skull tongs are usually in place before starting, and light traction (5 to 10 lbs) is maintained throughout the procedure. Traction can be maintained as a temporizing measure

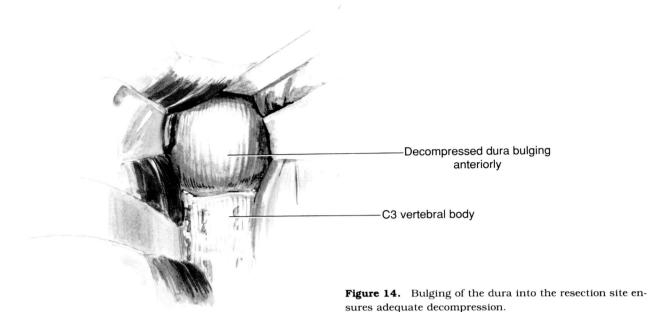

Decompressed dura bulging anteriorly

C3 vertebral body

Figure 14. Bulging of the dura into the resection site ensures adequate decompression.

postoperatively until final stabilization is accomplished. Osseous fusion in situ is an option. The C1–C2 lateral masses are available for interarticular arthrodesis via this approach. An intact C1 anterior arch can be used as a graft purchase. These alternatives imply a stable atlantooccipital articulation, which must be discerned.

An external orthosis (halo brace) is rarely adequate as the sole source for either temporary or long-term stability following this procedure. It is often essential as a supplement to surgical arthrodesis of the craniovertebral junction and is continued for several months.

Occipitocervical arthrodesis is required as a subsequent procedure in the face of craniovertebral instability. The patient is kept in skull traction until this is accomplished.

Drains

Subsequent buildup of serum or CSF in the dissection site is best evacuated via a closed suction silicone rubber catheter brought out from a separate stab wound. Usually this can be removed in 48 to 72 hours. This helps to relieve tissue pressure on the upper airway and reduce bacterial culture media in the wound.

Suture Closure

Absorbable rather than nonabsorbable suture material is preferred for wound closure. The platysma muscle is closed as a separate layer. Interrupted horizontal mattress stitches placed separately in the subcutaneous layer give strength to the closure. Skin edge

approximation with a continuous subcuticular stitch will provide a cosmetically pleasing scar, particularly if a transverse incision has been used.

Monitoring

Neurophysiologic Monitoring

Somatosensory and motor evoked responses are being used with increased frequency for these procedures. Their true efficacy and role are controversial and yet to be determined. Theoretically, they have merit in warning the surgeon of a potentially injurious maneuver and may be of benefit. Anesthesia methods must be modified to support such monitoring if it is used.

Radiographic Monitoring

The C-arm fluoroscope is a helpful, if not essential, adjunct for this procedure. It should be positioned for lateral projection at the outset and kept in place during the procedure. It offers the surgeon an ongoing means of orientation, monitors progress of the resection, and warns of any shift in alignment. In Figure 15, the intraoperative lateral fluoroscopic view shows the trajectory of view and the retractor position using this approach; the dissector is behind the dens and the anterior arch of C1 can be preserved if desired. The standard x-ray unit can be used as an alternative but is more inconvenient and time consuming.

SPECIALIZED INSTRUMENTS

Retractors

Adequate retraction is essential here because of the

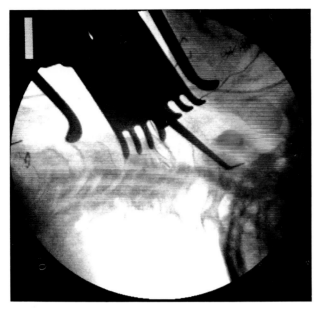

Figure 15. This lateral fluoroscopic view demonstrates the angle of access and the retractor position. The dissector is along the posterior wall of the dens.

deep access and angle of approach. Hand-held retractors are used during the cervical fascia and soft tissue dissection. A narrow pediatric Deaver retractor (modified by first straightening the bow and then bending the blade to a 90° angle so that blade tip measures 8 cm) can be used to lift soft tissues rostrally for initial precervical dissection of the superior corner at C1 and the clivus.

The deep blades of the Cloward or Caspar self-retaining retraction systems are adequate for ongoing retraction after dissection of the longus colli muscles. However, they are not designed for retraction in this region; therefore, their purchase on the tissues is not secure and they can migrate out of position. The surgeon must be aware of this as the procedure progresses. The Apfelbaum modification of the Caspar retractor is designed specifically for this region and may eliminate the retraction problem here. Additionally, some table-mounted retraction devices are being designed that may improve visualization. Regardless of the retraction system used, attention is directed to avoiding injury to the structures being retracted. There is no substitute for adequate soft tissue dissection to ease retraction strain and facilitate safe exposure using this approach.

Drills

A high-speed drill system controlled under microsurgical technique is required. The drill shaft must be long enough to avoid line of sight obstruction. The A

attachment for the Midas Rex drill or comparable handpiece works well; an angled handpiece for this drill is now available, which will facilitate its use. The long-angled handpiece of lower speed drills are applicable as well. Both cutting and diamond burrs are needed for safe bone resection.

Laser

The microsurgical CO_2 laser facilitates dissection of paraspinal muscles, resection of ligaments, and excision of pannus or tumor. Complete removal of offending lesions is possible even in hard-to-reach areas. Mechanical trauma is also avoided, thus improving the safety of the procedure. Use of safe microsurgical laser technique and appropriate energy densities is mandatory.

Ultrasonic Aspirator

The ultrasonic aspirator can be an advantage in the removal of selected soft tissue lesions, particularly if they are vascular neoplasms. The long-angled handpiece will be needed, because the short or straight pieces will not fit into the field and will obscure the line of sight.

Microinstruments

Microdissectors of various designs will be useful in the separation of soft tissue from bone, particularly around the dens. Micro Kerrison rongeurs, both 45° and 90°, and micro pituitary forceps will be needed for soft tissue removal. An angled or straight 2-0 or 3-0 curette will assist in delicate bone removal. Bayonetted instruments are needed to keep the line of sight free. Long, insulated bipolar forceps are indispensable for hemostasis.

Sutures

A small, strong, cutting, and semicircular needle is needed for suturing in this cramped space. The P-2 Ethicon needle works well here. The preferred suture is 5-0 polydioxanone which can be used as a dural traction suture, for dural patch repair, or for dural graft closure. An alternative needle and suture for this purpose is 5-0 Dexon Plus on a Davis & Geck PR-1 needle.

COMPLICATIONS

Neurological Complications

Increased motor paresis, respiratory paralysis, sensory loss, and systemic sympathectomy with loss of autonomic control are the devastating effects of neuraxis injury at the cervicomedullary junction. Aggravation of a preexisting myelopathy is always an inherent risk of operating in this region. This risk is even greater when instability is present. Often, instability is produced or increased with surgical resections in this region.

Tight compression of the neuraxis by misaligned bone, inflammatory granulation tissue, or neoplasm must be relieved to effect adequate decompression. Such manipulation always adds increased risk of aggravated insult to neural structures by direct trauma or damage to their vasculature. Microsurgical technique is critical to limiting these deleterious occurrences.

Peripheral and cranial nerves are at risk during dissection of the cervical fascia and retraction of the soft tissues of the submandibular triangle. The hypoglossal nerve is particularly vulnerable as it is directly dissected and retracted. Often there is transient tongue weakness lasting a few weeks. The marginal mandibular branch of the facial nerve can be severed or stretched as it courses around the angle of the mandible, thus causing a sagging of the lower lip. The vagus nerve can be stretched, usually by retraction; this is evidenced by hoarseness of the voice and is usually self-limited. These changes are most often due to dysfunction of the superior laryngeal nerve.

Vascular Complications

Injury to the carotid artery is a potential which is not likely to occur because the dissection is medial to it and the retraction is deep to it. Dissection and freeing of the medial rostral carotid sheath will reduce transmitted strain of retraction to the carotid artery. The vertebral artery is at risk of laceration particularly while drilling or curetting the lateral recesses of the C2 and C3 vertebral bodies and the intervening disk. The surgeon must keep these structures continuously in mind throughout the procedure.

Venous access may be a problem if the patient is debilitated. Peripheral veins may be thrombosed, and sepsis from indwelling peripheral and central venous lines is an ever-present burden. Central venous access is needed during the operative procedure to guide fluid balance and may be needed postoperatively for parenteral nutrition. Fastidious attention and sterile technique are required to reduce problems with venous access.

Peripheral venous thrombosis and pulmonary embolism is an ever-present threat to the patient who is bedridden or under prolonged anesthesia. Sequential compression pneumatic hose, mini-dose heparin, and a rotating bed may help reduce this risk.

Respiratory Complications

Upper airway obstruction from soft tissue swelling is a major postoperative problem with this procedure. This is particularly the case with myelopathic and debilitated patients. Even the patients who are neuro-logically intact may require a prophylactic tracheostomy to avoid this problem. At the very least, patients will require an endotracheal tube for several days to ensure an adequate airway. Pneumonitis either from aspiration or atelectasis must be combated continually in the immediate postoperative period. Positive end-expiratory pressure of 5 to 10 cm H_2O on the ventilator is prophylactic for atelectasis. A rotokinetic bed assists pulmonary drainage. A feeding jejunostomy may prevent aspiration.

Visceral Complications

Pharyngeal perforation will negate the advantage of the transcervical procedure over the transoral route. If undetected and not repaired it will lead to catastrophic septic fasciitis and/or a retropharyngeal abscess. Anatomic dissection of the fascial planes and cautious retraction are required to avoid this; with attention to detail, this problem is uncommon and can usually be avoided. It becomes a more imminent concern when scarring from previous operations in or radiation to this region obscures landmarks and tethers retraction. The use of smooth-tipped rather than tooth-tipped retractor blades may help avoid injury to the pharynx. I prefer the toothed retractor blades because they anchor more securely into the longus colli muscle edge. However, proper seating of the blades beneath the dissected medial edge of the longus colli muscle is mandatory.

A CSF fistula will occur if the subarachnoid space is opened and not specifically closed. A lumbar subarachnoid catheter will help prevent this from occurring and help close it when it does occur.

Structural Complications

Instability cannot be overemphasized. An aggravation of myelopathy occurs if this is not treated. Skull traction is required from the outset. A brace and/or surgical arthrodesis may be needed.

Nutritional Complications

Adequate nutrition is critical for recovery of any stressed patient. Nutritional insufficiency is compounded by a preoperative debilitated state, which is often the case with patients harboring lesions in this region. The pharyngeal and upper airway edema that occurs after this procedure will impede deglutition for several days. The resulting aggravation of a nutritional catabolic state can be averted by a preoperative gastrostomy or jejunostomy. Optimal nutritional support will also help to avoid sepsis and to facilitate early ambulation and rehabilitation of these patients.

Hemodynamic Complications

Hypovolemia and impaired sympathetic tone can combine, dangerously reducing cardiac output. Postural hypotension is regularly noted. This can further impair neurologic function. Attention to central venous pressure and fluid maintenance, and the administration of colloid/crystalloid parenteral fluid combinations for fluid balance support, will help avert this. Supplemental sympathomimetic agents may be used, either intermittently or continuously for an adequate response.

Avoiding Complications

Complications will occur even with the best laid plans, particularly with the involved surgical procedure described here. Patient selection and preparation will help reduce their incidence. Seven actions that will help obtain an optimal ultimate result, in my opinion, are:

1. Careful selection of a treatment plan based on an algorithm that considers reduction of malalignment and specific imaged anatomy of the neural compression;
2. Preemptive and elective
   a) Tracheostomy
   b) Feeding gastrostomy or jejunostomy;
3. Hydrodynamic control of CSF
   a) External lumbar subarachnoid drain (catheter tunneled under the skin)
   b) Permanent CSF-peritoneal shunt if required;
4. Wide anatomic dissection of fascial planes;
5. Microsurgical technique under fluoroscopic control;
6. Nursing on a rotokinetic bed with skull traction;
7. Intensive postoperative support.

CORRECTION OF MALPOSITION OF THE ORBITS

JOHN A. PERSING, M.D.

INTRODUCTION

Malposition of the orbits is a congenital deformity that is frequently seen in craniofacial anomaly centers. There are two commonly encountered forms of this abnormality involving the mediolateral axis of the orbits.

The first is telorbitism, which refers to a widened distance between the two orbits. This is to be distinguished from the second type, hypercanthorum, in which there is a widened distance between the medial canthi alone (the distance between the lateral canthi is normal). The widened distance between the canthi may be due to bone, soft tissue, or both being abnormally displaced laterally. In this chapter, only the condition of the bone displacement will be considered.

PATIENT SELECTION

The appropriate operative procedure for correction for the patient with hypercanthorum entails translocation of the medial portion of the orbits only, whereas in the patient with telorbitism both the medial *and* lateral orbital walls are translocated medially. Patients are chosen for the two different operative approaches based on the clinical measurement of a widened intercanthal distance (medial and lateral) and plain radiographic and computed tomography scan demonstration of widened bony intercanthal distance. Surgery is elected usually at approximately four years of age, unless a concurrent abnormality such as an encephalocele is present, providing the opportunity for one-stage treatment. Age four is chosen because this allows for correction of the abnormality when the bone is sufficiently strong to avoid inadvertent fracture, the orbit has reached relative maturity, and the child has not reached school age, so that major deformity can be corrected, or at least ameliorated, prior to critical peer interaction at school age.

PREOPERATIVE CONSIDERATIONS

The risks of the operative procedure include potential

injury to the brain and visual system, including enophthalmos, extraocular muscle entrapment, optic nerve damage, cerebrospinal fluid leakage, and recurrence of the intercanthal deformity postoperatively. It is unclear as to whether translocation of the orbits medially in early childhood negatively affects midfacial growth.

Preoperative preparation includes prophylactic use of intravenous antibiotics at the time of surgery to cover anaerobic flora in the frontal and paranasal sinuses, and prophylactic, short-term, anticonvulsants. No steroids are used.

A comprehensive anesthetic technique is advocated which includes orotracheal intubation, monitoring for blood loss with central venous catheters, arterial line, and Foley catheter, and monitoring for air embolus by Doppler, end-tidal CO_2, and nitrogen monitors. Hypotension is induced by increasing concentrations of the inhalation anesthetic agent at the time of craniotomy to minimize blood loss. Autologous or designated donor blood transfusion is preferred if blood transfusion is necessary. Spinal drains are placed in the lumbar cistern following the induction of anesthesia. The drains are not opened, however, until burr holes have been made and the craniotomy is about to be performed. The child's trunk and extremities are wrapped with a soft gauze to maintain body heat, and all irrigation fluids are warmed before use to prevent hypothermia.

SURGICAL TECHNIQUE

The initial preparation for the treatment of patients with hypercanthorum or telorbitism is the same. The patient is placed supine with the head on a well-padded headrest and the neck slightly extended. Draping of the patient includes full exposure of the scalp to the region of the midportion of the vertex of the skull and to the level of the mouth caudally. Hair removal in the scalp, if performed at all, is minimal, to a maximum of 1 cm wide, corresponding to the course of the bicoronal incision. Hair anterior to the skin incision line is braided to remain out of the way during the operative procedure and is covered with masking tape or heavy aluminum foil. A bicoronal incision is performed, extending down to the level of the tragus anteriorly, to allow for easy dissection periorbitally. The dissection of the anterior scalp flap is performed in a supraperiosteal plane to the level of the orbital rims, followed by elevation of the periosteal flap from the same bicoronal incision site to be used later as a covering flap for the anterior cranial fossa floor defect created by the orbit translocation procedure.

Bilateral pterion burr holes and one parasagittal burr hole posterior to the coronal suture are placed. A bifrontal craniotomy line is drawn on the skull leaving approximately 1 cm height of frontal bone superior to the apex of the superior orbital rim. A bifrontal craniotomy is performed. The outer table of the midline frontal bone in the glabellar region is removed with a side cutting burr, and the frontal bone is fractured forward. Alternatively, as frequently is the case in the region of excess bone in the glabellar region, a burr hole may be placed in the area of intended bone removal (Fig. 1A).

Hypercanthorum

In patients with hypercanthorum, the remaining bifrontal bone segment is bisected, leaving a supraorbital bar, approximately 5–6 mm in width, cephalad to the medial portion of the orbital rim. If the nasal profile is acceptable, a segment of midline bone may be left approximately 3 mm wide to simulate a new nasal bridge. Two additional approaches exist, however, if the nasal profile is unacceptable. The midline bone may be removed entirely, leaving a 5-mm bone seg-

ment laterally on each medial orbital rim (Fig. 1B). When the orbital rims are translocated medially, the medial border of the orbital rim defines a new, more acceptable nasal profile. The second and most often used alternative is to leave a 3-mm segment of nasal bone in the midline to serve as a base scaffolding for on-lay bone graft augmentation of the dorsum of the nose. With all these techniques, the medial orbital osteotomy is usually performed with a sagittal or oscillating saw to avoid unwanted fracture of the nasal and lacrimal bones.

The frontal lobes are allowed to reposition posteriorly by cerebrospinal fluid drainage for an osteotomy in the orbital roof extending posterior to the midpoint of the globe's anteroposterior axis (Fig. 1C). The medial limit of the osteotomy is the lateral cribriform plate, avoiding injury at this time to the olfactory nerve fibers. Characteristically, the cribriform area is excessively widened and will obstruct medial translocation of the orbital rim. Therefore, the anterior-most olfactory fibers are divided, and the proximal segments of these nerve fibers and surrounding dura are oversewn to prevent cerebrospinal fluid leakage postoperatively. The anterolateral portion of the ethmoid air cells are removed by rongeur, to allow subsequent unobstructed movement of the orbits medially.

If the medial canthi position relative to one another and to the anteroposterior axis of the nasal bone is acceptable, effort is made to preserve their attachment to the lacrimal bone. To avoid displacement of the canthi during dissection, a subcilliary, conjunctival or Caldwell-Luc incision is made infraorbitally to complete the caudal dissection and osteotomy paralleling the superior orbit osteotomy (Fig. 1, D–F).

Figure 1. **A,** a burr hole is placed in the glabellar region at the site of intended bone removal (*green*) to allow for safe dissection of the midline dura and sagittal sinus. Orbital osteotomies are located, as shown, to include provision for removal of the medial inferior portion of the nasal process of the maxilla so as not to impinge on the nasal airway following medial orbital translocation. A supporting frontal bone bar, approximately 5 mm tall, is left above the medial superior orbital rim. **B,** *1,* the midline nasal bone has satisfactory projection but the breadth is too great. The midline nasal bone is left in situ, and resection of excess bone occurs in the paramedian location (*green*). *2,* the midline projection is unacceptable. The midline bone is removed and the medial orbital walls, when translocated medially, form the new nasal profile. *3,* the existing nasal profile is deficient but, rather than excising the midline nasal bone, it is allowed to remain

in situ to serve as base scaffolding for dorsal augmentation by placement of a cantilevered bone graft. **C,** *1,* view of the anterior skull base from above. The orbital roof osteotomy extends from the midportion of the orbit laterally to the cribriform plate medially. *2,* the osteotomy extends posteriorly well behind the midpoint of the axis of the globe. Bone is removed medially (*green*) adjacent to the cribriform plate to allow for medial translocation of the orbital roof. **D,** in order to place osteotomies in the inferior orbital region, either a transconjunctival, Caldwell-Luc, or subciliary incision is made. **E,** in transconjunctival and subciliary approaches, a preseptal dissection is preferred to expose the inferior orbital rim. **F,** the inferior orbital osteotomy is placed at the level of the infraorbital foramen in children to avoid damage to developing tooth buds.

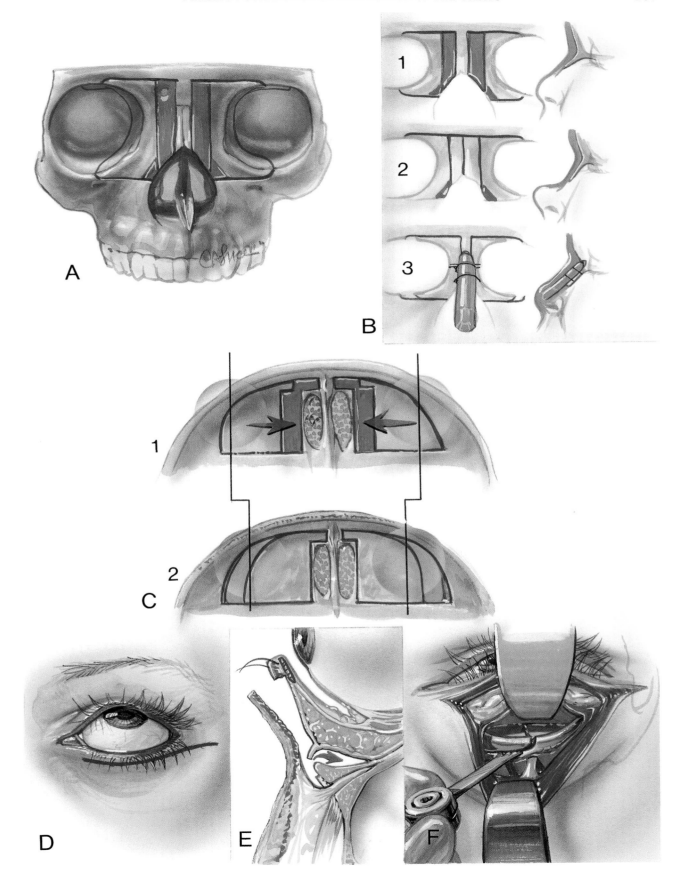

A transversely oriented osteotomy is placed in the paramedian frontal bone, leaving 5–6 mm width of frontal bone as the medial extension of the supraorbital bar.

If the midline nasal bone is to remain in situ, the osteotomy line does not extend into the plane of the medial nasal bones. The segment complex of frontal, ethmoid, and more laterally situated nasal bones is removed by osteotome bilaterally (Fig. 2A).

The medial rim with superior and inferior rim extensions, in the form of the letter "C," are mobilized. Ordinarily, the greatest resistance to movement is encountered in the deep nasomaxillary region. Prying of the rim with an osteotome usually frees the bony and soft tissue attachments. Care must be taken, however, to avoid injury to the naso-lacrimal duct during this maneuver. As the orbits are translocated medially, infolding of nasal cartilage (septal and upper lateral) and mucosa usually results, requiring trimming of the excess tissue. The openings in the mucosa are oversewn to prevent gross air and bacterial contamination into the epidural space postoperatively. The medial orbital walls and the nasal bones are trimmed with the air drill to approximately 3–4 mm wide so that the overall distance between dacryon and dacryon is approximately 10 mm or less (Fig. 2B). Trimming is done at this time rather than earlier, to avoid fracture of the medial orbit during the prying maneuvers. The nasal process of the maxilla is aggressively trimmed to avoid occlusion of the airway as the orbital rim is moved medially. The orbital rims are placed in position but are not yet secured.

If the medial canthi need to be repositioned, a transnasal medial canthapexy may be performed. It is easier to perform the initial stages of the canthapexy prior to stabilization of the orbital bones because of the greater visibility afforded by the mobile and widely separated bone segments. A drill is used to open the entry point into the posterior superior lacrimal bone (Figs. 2, C and D, and 3A) to avoid fracture of this fragile bone. If the medial orbital wall is exceedingly thin and does fracture, a split calvarial bone graft (Fig. 3B) from the parietal region may serve as a substitute for the medial orbital wall. It will provide stabilization of the medial canthus and avoid anterior as well as lateral migration of the canthus postoperatively. The medial orbital rims are then translocated medially and secured to each other and the frontal supraorbital bar.

If the midline nasal profile remains unacceptable after translocation of the medial orbits, a cantilevered costochondral bone graft may be secured to the existing nasal profile (Fig. 3, C and D). Costochondral rib grafts are the primary choice graft material because the cartilaginous tip, unlike even calvarial membranous bone, resists resorption extremely well. To lessen the likelihood of epidural infection postoperatively, the pericranial flap previously elevated at the time of anterior scalp flap dissection is tacked over the ethmoid air cells on the anterior cranial base. The scalp flap is then closed in two layers, galea and skin.

Figure 2. **A,** dissection is carried out posterior to the lacrimal crest medially. An oscillating saw is used to complete the superior and inferior orbital osteotomy. The posterior medial orbital wall osteotomy is completed by an osteotome. Particular attention is necessary to remove enough bone in the ethmoid air cell region to allow for unimpeded translocation of the medial portion of the orbital rim. **B,** following mobilization of the orbital rims, the midline bone and remaining medial orbital rims are trimmed (*green*) with a shaping burr to achieve the thinnest possible final nasal midline (ordinarily 8 to 10 mm encompassing the medial orbital walls and the midline bony strut). **C,** the medial canthi are elevated with an accompanying periosteal pennant from the dorsum of the nose. **D,** a drill hole (*green*) is placed in the posterior superior lacrimal bone for the periosteal pennant and the canthus to be passed transnasally.

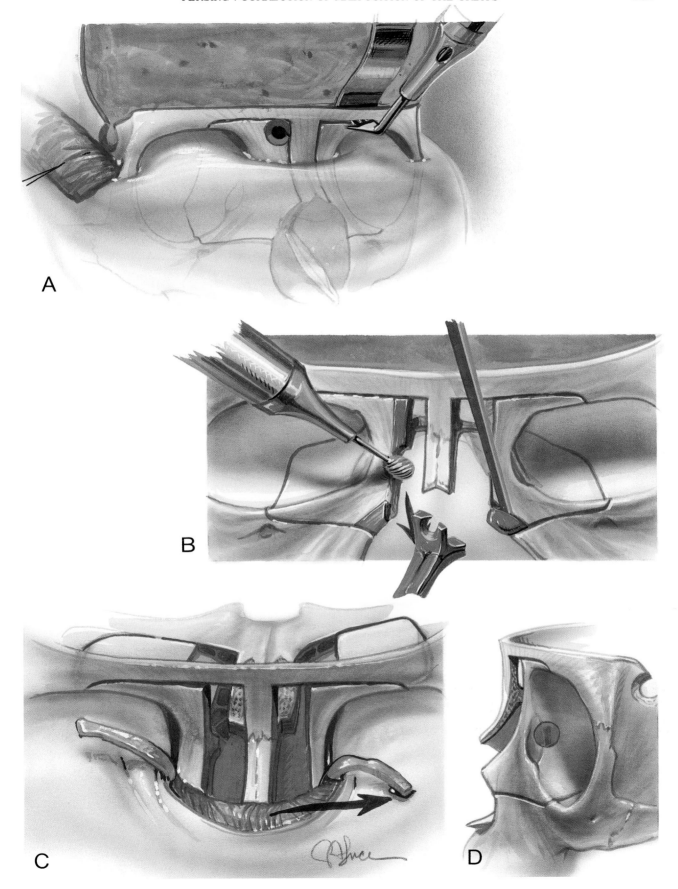

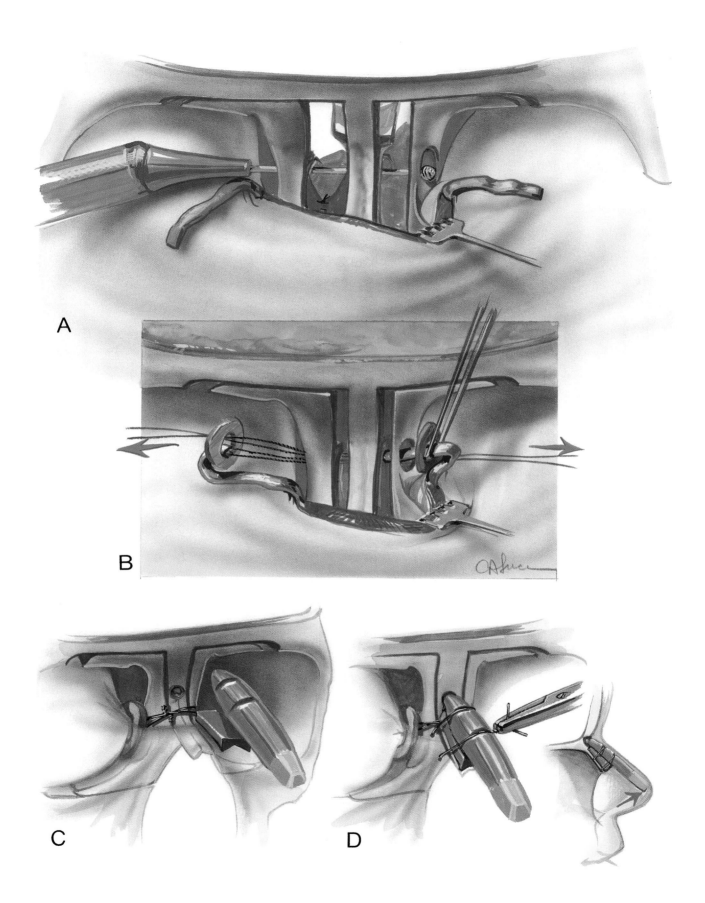

A

B

C

D

Figure 3. **A,** an air-driven burr is used to penetrate the lacrimal bone perpendicular plate of the ethmoid to allow threading of the canthal tendon. Any significant opening in the nasal mucosa is oversewn. **B,** if the lacrimal bone is too fragile or otherwise unusable, a split calvarial bone graft can be used to serve as a buttress substitute for the lacrimal bone. The canthal periosteal pennants are tightened following medial translocation and fixation of the orbital rims. **C,** augmentation of the nasal bridge is accomplished following translocation of the orbits by placing a wedge of bone beneath the cantilevered costochondral cartilage graft. **D,** the graft is secured to the underlying medial orbital rims by transosseous wiring.

Hypertelorism (Telorbitism)

For patients with hypertelorism (telorbitism), the operative approach is much the same as just described for hypercanthorum, but, in addition, the lateral orbit is moved with the medial, as a single unit.

The patient is positioned supine, following placement of a lumbar cerebrospinal fluid drain, and a bifrontal craniotomy including temporalis muscle elevation is performed. The supraorbital bar is left 1 cm wide at the level of the orbital rim apex (Fig. 4, A–C). The supraorbital bar will be transversely bisected when translocation of the orbit is performed, leaving a 5-mm-wide supraorbital bar for fixation, and a 5-mm-wide orbital rim at the rim's apex. The orbital roof and lateral orbital wall are cut posterior to the midpoint of the globe following careful posterior repositioning of the anterior tip of the temporal lobe. If correction of an accompanying orbital malrotation is not necessary, horizontally oriented osteotomies are placed on the anterior surface of the maxilla through or below the level of the infraorbital foramen (Fig. 4D). In young children, the more cephalad osteotomy is desirable to avoid injury to developing tooth roots. Olfactory fiber section and frontonasoethmoid resections are performed as described previously for the treatment of hypercanthorum.

In patients with hypertelorism, the medial canthi may require repositioning. This is performed by transnasal canthopexy as described earlier (hypercanthorum). Likewise, the need for repositioning of the lateral canthi approximately 2 mm above the medial canthi on the horizontal axis also may be evident. After the orbits have been translocated and secured, the attachment point for the lateral canthi in most cases, is placed just inside the orbital rim (Fig. 4, E–H). When severe exorbitism (globe protrusion beyond the eyelids secondary to a constricted orbit volume) coexists, the canthi are attached to orbital rim bone on the external surface of the zygomatic process of the frontal bone. This reduces the projection of the globe beyond the eyelid. The temporal fossa is filled with calvarial bone chip grafts and the temporalis muscle is advanced forward to be attached to the orbital rim, in order to prevent an "hourglass" deformity or hollowing postoperatively in the temporal region.

The incisions are closed in two layers, galeal and skin. The nose is packed with a petroleum-based gauze. No drain is inserted in the galeal region to avoid aspiration of nasopharyngeal bacteria into the subgaleal space.

Figure 4. **A,** a bifrontal craniotomy is performed with a 1-cm-tall supraorbital bar left above the apex of the orbital rim. It is bisected leaving a 5-mm-thick supraorbital rim which may be translocated medially, following removal of paramedian frontal and nasal bone (*green*), and a 5-mm supraorbital bar to which the orbital rim bone is affixed. **B,** note resection of the nasal process of the maxilla to avoid impingement on the nasal airway. **C,** the orbits are then translocated medially. **D,** bone grafts are inserted posterior to the lateral rim of the orbit and in the region of the zygoma to prevent a postoperative hourglass deformity. A drill is used to trim the lateral portion of the supraorbital bar. **E,** the normal position of the lateral canthus is approximately at or 2 mm above the level of the medial canthus. **F,** drill holes are placed in the frontal process of the zygoma. The lateral canthus is attached transosseously to the internal surface of the zygomatic process of the frontal bone, if the patient does not demonstrate globe proptosis. **G,** if the patient has accompanying significant proptosis, the canthus is placed on the *external* surface of the frontal process of the zygoma in an effort to reduce the malrelationship between the globe and the eyelids and restore normal lid/globe anatomic relationships (**H**).

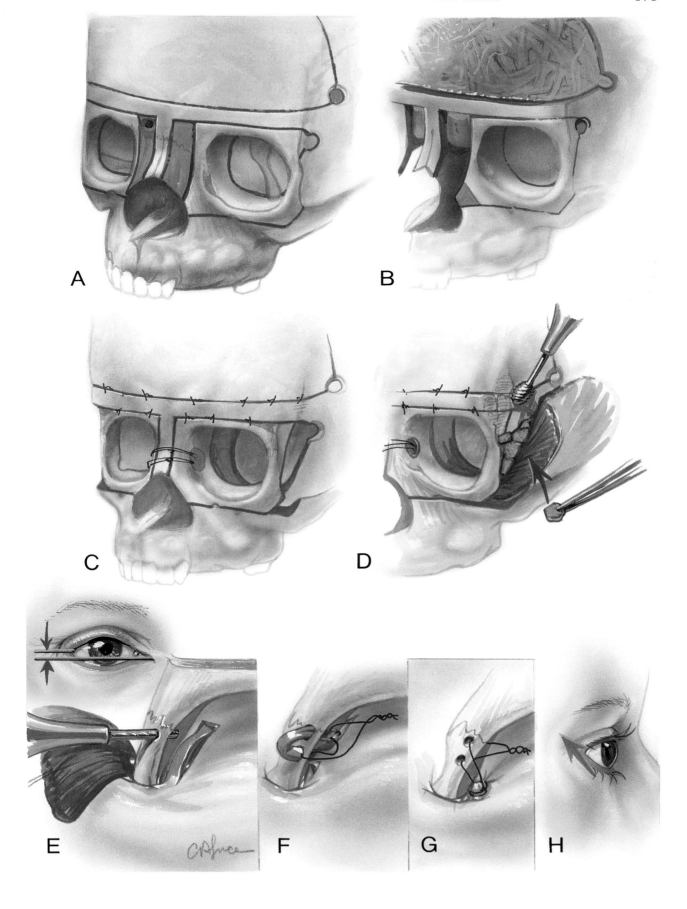

POSTOPERATIVE CARE

The patients are monitored postoperatively by clinical measures, and intracranial pressure (ICP) monitoring is not used routinely. This is because placement of a lumbar cistern drain allows for false low recordings of intracranial pressure despite clinical evidence of cerebral edema. This may lead to a tardy diagnosis of elevated ICP or intracranial hemorrhage. Because of this, pain control postoperatively should still allow for clinical assessment of neurologic status.

COMPLICATIONS

Complications from the operative procedure are relatively few. The major immediate concerns relate to cerebral edema and/or intracranial hemorrhage, and injury to the visual system, either to the globe or optic nerve by trauma or hematoma, or to the extraocular muscle system. Also, it is important to note that if sufficient bone is not removed from the medial portion of the cribriform plate as the orbit is translocated medially, there is the possibility of impingement of the medial rectus muscle on the corner of the remaining bone, which may require reoperation. Later concerns include cerebrospinal fluid leakage, subdural or epidural infection, and osteomyelitis. The possibility of cerebrospinal fluid leakage and meningitis should be significantly reduced by watertight dural closure supported by the use of fibrin glue at the suture line, with further support by the pericranial flap overlying the dural closure. Unresolved problems are soft tissue relaxation at the medial canthal region resulting in an apparent redevelopment of hypercanthorum, and the possibility of growth disturbance on the nasomaxillary and midface regions, with surgery performed in early childhood.

REMOVAL OF CERVICAL OSSIFIED POSTERIOR LONGITUDINAL LIGAMENT AT SINGLE AND MULTIPLE LEVELS

RALPH B. CLOWARD, M.D.

INTRODUCTION

Ossification of the posterior longitudinal ligament (OPLL) has been recognized as a cause for cervical spinal stenosis resulting in severe compressive myelopathy. This lesion was first described by Japanese authors in 1960 and numerous articles have since delineated its pathology and recommended techniques for its surgical treatment. Although it is quite prevalent in the Far East, OPLL is encountered less often in Caucasians. It is considered important in the differential diagnosis of cervical myelopathy. My experience with this lesion antedates the initial 1960 published report by almost 10 years. My first case was diagnosed in 1951 and has been followed for 38 years. The first operated patient, by laminectomy in 1956, did not improve.

Since 1958, all of my OPLL operations have been by the anterior surgical approach. Direct access to the lesion regardless of its size and extent was accomplished by removing the greater part of the vertebral bodies and the intervening discs. The resulting spinal defect was filled with a large, well-fitting cadaver bone graft obtained from the bone bank and sterilized with ethylene oxide gas.

TWO OPERATIVE TECHNIQUES

Multiple Level OPLL

If the ossified lesion extends longitudinally over two or more levels of the spine and occupies a minimum of 60% of the anteroposterior diameter (Fig. 1, A–E) a multiple level surgical technique is used. The surgical opening in the spinal canal must expose the length of the symptomatic lesion and be wide enough to expose the extremes of the lesion to facilitate its total removal. There must be extra room to insert a dural patch if necessary.

Operative Technique

The standard anterior surgical approach for treatment of cervical disc lesions described elsewhere in this Atlas is used. A generous stripping of the longus colli muscles is essential to obtain the wide transverse exposure. Two sets of self-retaining retractor blades with teeth will expose the number of disc spaces required for the vertical exposure. All discs are excised and the disc spaces are completely cleaned to the maximum depth of the disc space where the hard bony lesion is encountered.

The Cloward anterior cervical instruments are employed, using the guide, the guard, and the drill attached to a Hudson drill handle (Fig. 2A). The largest drill, 16 mm in diameter, is used. The depth to be drilled is determined by measuring the disc space with the depth gauge and then projecting the drill 1 or 2 mm longer. The drill, therefore, will encounter and remove a millimeter or so of the anterior surface of the OPLL.

Successive drill holes are made in the adjacent, cleaned out disc spaces at two, three, or four levels (Fig. 2B). If the patient has small vertebral bodies, the bone between the drill holes may be totally removed by the large drill. With large vertebral bodies, a narrow isthmus of bone will remain. This is nibbled away with a large bone rongeur (Fig. 2C). The remainder of the large opening in the spine is shaped with a high-speed drill using a "pineapple" burr (Fig. 3A). The upper and lower rounded ends of the exposure are squared off, and then the lateral walls are joined and finally bevelled slightly, wider at the top than the bottom. The lateral margins of the OPLL are carefully separated from the loose areolar attachments to the dura. Then, the lesion is shaved down with a high-speed diamond drill. Starting at its thickest area, it is gradually reduced to a thin shell (Fig. 3B). A small hole is made in the thinnest area to expose the dura. The thin angled osteophyte elevator is inserted and the underside of the lesion separated from the dura. The upbiting 3

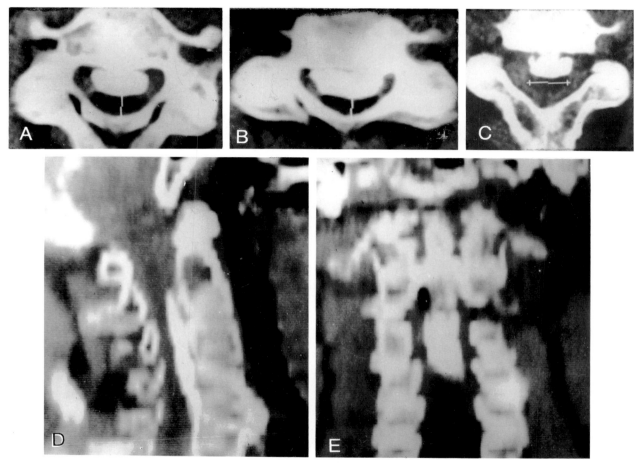

Figure 1. Multilevel OPLL. **A–C,** a computed tomogram, axial view, showing the thick ossified ligament occupying greater than 60% of the sagittal diameter of the spinal canal.

D and **E,** sagittal and coronal reconstructed views showing the longitudinal extent of the OPLL.

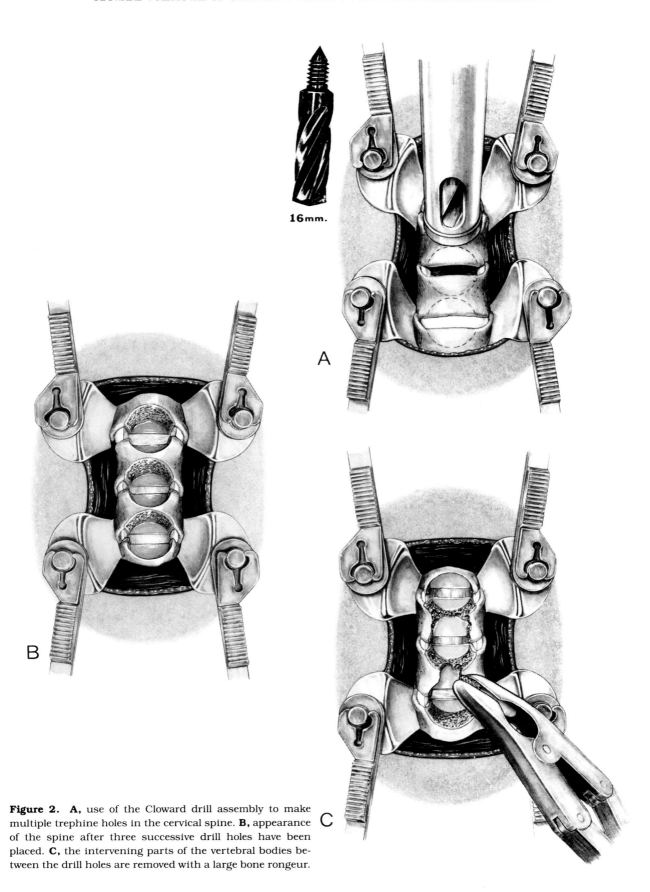

Figure 2. A, use of the Cloward drill assembly to make multiple trephine holes in the cervical spine. **B,** appearance of the spine after three successive drill holes have been placed. **C,** the intervening parts of the vertebral bodies between the drill holes are removed with a large bone rongeur.

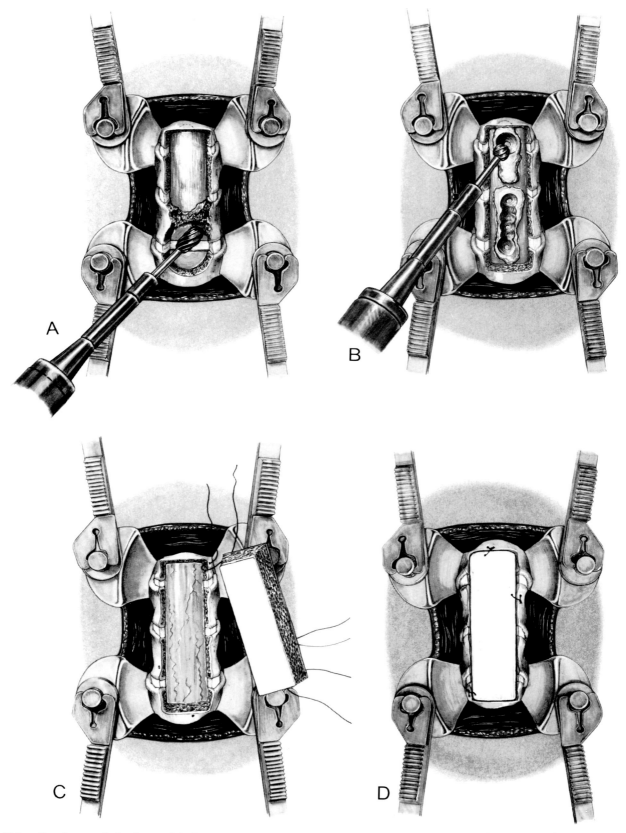

Figure 3. **A,** use of a high-speed drill to complete the bone removal and convert the bone defect into a smooth, bevelled, rectangular channel. **B,** drilling the ossified posterior longi-tudinal ligament. **C,** insertion of the bone graft. **D,** technique of securing the bone graft.

mm 40° cervical rongeur is inserted and the remaining shell of the bony lesion is nibbled off bit by tiny bit, until it is completely removed. Removal of the lesion may be done under the microscope, although this is not essential.

If the dura is accidentally torn, the tear is sutured watertight with fine sutures. If the lesion has invaded and destroyed an area of dura, the defect should be patched watertight with a dural substitute. This is only possible with a wide dural exposure.

In one case in Japan, the dura had been invaded and incorporated into the OPLL over the entire length of the lesion (three levels). There was insufficient dura lateral to the lesion to attach any kind of dural substitute. Therefore, a large piece of Gelfoam was placed over the spinal cord and the bone graft inserted. The complications of free-flowing spinal fluid and meningitis almost cost the patient her life. The cerebrospinal fluid drainage stopped after nine months and the patient finally made a complete recovery.

A large bone graft is shaped with an air drill to fit tightly into the spinal defect so that the cancellous bone of the iliac crest is in close proximity to the sides of the spinal defect as well as to the ends (Fig. 3C) These long grafts are secured to the spine at the end or the side with small loops of wire (Fig. 3D) In Figure 4, postoperative x-ray films (Fig. 4, D and E) and computed tomography scans (Fig. 4, A–C) show long bone grafts and a wide spinal canal.

Postoperative Care

The postoperative care is the same as that of the anterior cervical disc operation. The patient requires only a soft collar postoperatively, with a tight-fitting secured bone graft.

Single Level OPLL

OPLL responsible for a severe neurologic deficit (radiculomyelopathy or quadriparesis) can occur from a

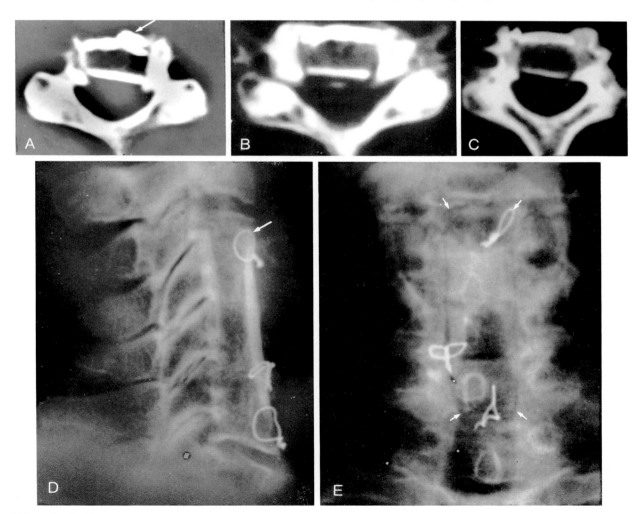

Figure 4. **A–C,** postoperative computed tomogram in axial view, showing a properly seated bone graft and evidence of completely excised OPLL. **D** and **E,** lateral and antero-posterior views of the cervical spine showing the bone graft secured to the cervical spine with wire loops (*arrows*).

lesion localized and confined to one level (Fig. 5) or result from trauma to the end of a longer OPLL. A conventional single level anterior discectomy is made with a large drill to make an opening sufficient to remove the intraspinal lesion. The hole in the disc space is made with a 14- or 16-mm drill and then enlarged with an air drill to a round or a rectangular contour. The opening into the spinal canal is sufficient to gain access to and totally remove the intraspinal lesion. The bone graft is fashioned to fit the spinal defect, which may be either round or rectangular (Fig. 6).

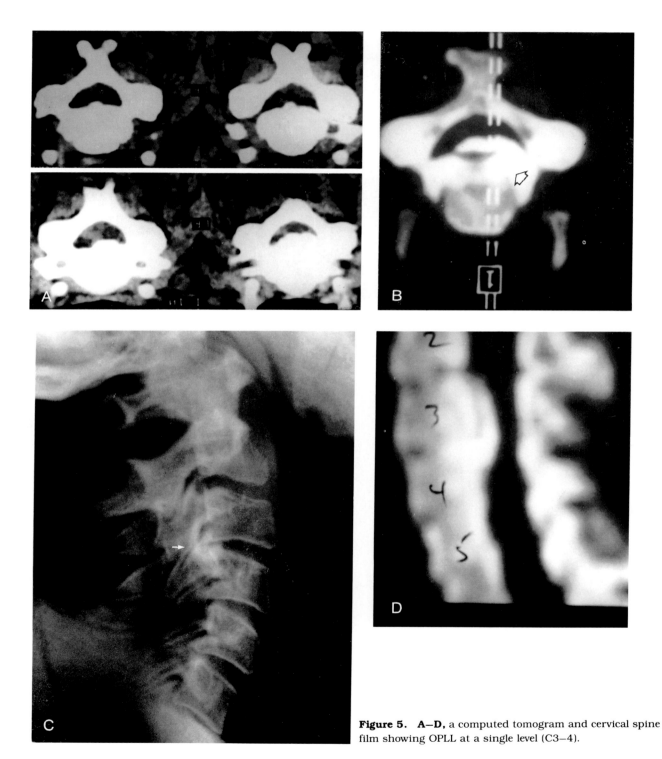

Figure 5. A–D, a computed tomogram and cervical spine film showing OPLL at a single level (C3–4).

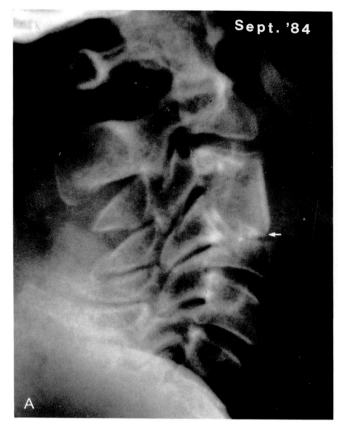

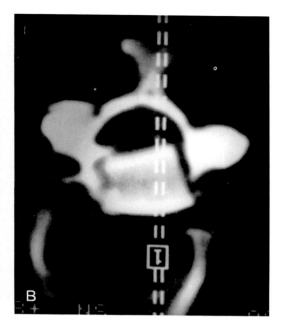

Figure 6. A postoperative film showing optimal placement of the bone graft and total removal of the OPLL.

CONCLUSIONS

Direct and total removal of ossified and hypertrophied posterior longitudinal ligaments of the cervical spine is extremely effective in relieving the symptoms and neurologic deficits of cervical myelopathy. Personal experience with this operation has demonstrated good to excellent results in 93—95% of patients. Over 75% of the patients operated upon have reversed their functional deficits and become neurologically normal.

TECHNIQUE OF VENTRICULOSTOMY

JOSEPH H. PIATT, JR., M.D.
KIM J. BURCHIEL, M.D.

INTRODUCTION

Ventriculostomy is a rudimentary neurosurgical skill. Because it requires no special manual dexterity, ventriculostomy is one of the first procedures mastered by the neurosurgical trainee, but even the experienced operator can encounter difficulties if basic aspects of technique are neglected. This chapter first describes cannulation of a normal ventricular system in general terms. The anatomic details of the frontal and the posterior approaches to ventriculostomy are then presented. Common errors are highlighted.

GENERAL CONSIDERATIONS

Ventriculostomy is a daily exercise on a busy neurosurgical service. The most frequent indication is the need for temporary decompression of the ventricular system in the setting of hydrocephalus. In the past, ventriculostomy has seen heavy use in the measurement of intracranial pressure (ICP), but several other techniques that entail less risk of ventriculitis are now available for use as a monitoring tool per se. If elevated ICP requires cerebrospinal fluid (CSF) drainage as a therapeutic measure, however, ventriculostomy is still indispensable. Ventriculostomy may also be a preliminary step in a variety of other neurosurgical operations, such as CSF shunt insertion, Ommaya reservoir insertion, excision of posterior fossa lesions that have caused hydrocephalus, and functional stereotactic procedures.

In theory, the ventricular system can be cannulated from any site on the surface of the skull, but in practice only two sites are in common use: one near the midline just anterior to the coronal suture and another just anterior to the lambdoid suture. Beginning at these sites and utilizing simple external landmarks, the surgeon can cannulate the ventricular system safely and easily. The precise location of the standard sites is discussed below. It is probably no more difficult to hit the ventricle from the one site than from the other, but it is our impression than the posterior site is more difficult. Selection of a site is usually determined by extraneous considerations such as the underlying disease process, the location of preexisting incisions and burr holes, and the surgeon's training and experience. In the absence of compelling reasons to the contrary, it is customary to perform ventriculostomy on the right side in order to minimize the risk of injury to the dominant hemisphere.

Whichever approach is selected, frontal or posterior, external landmarks guide ventricular catheter insertion, and these landmarks must not be obscured by surgical drapes. It is usually possible to feel the bridge of the nose through the drapes, but it is often impossible to locate the ear. One solution to this problem is to mark sites near the nasion and the tragus with plastic syringe container caps. These caps can be secured at the correct locations with the adhesive tapes used to affix precordial stethoscopes to the chest, and they are easy to feel through conventional draping. Alternately, the scalp, face, and ear can be draped all together in a single field with a large, transparent, adhesive plastic drape. The scalp is shaved widely in order to permit subgaleal tunneling of the Silastic ventricular catheter. The incision, the midline, and the course of the nearby sutures are marked before draping, not after.

Although a twist drill is adequate for most situations, a burr hole is advantageous because it allows hemostasis under direct visual control as well as flexibility in aiming the ventricular catheter. The dura is coagulated and opened widely, and the pia-arachnoid is opened as well. If an attempt is made to push a Silastic catheter with a wire stylet through a hole too small, the catheter will drag on the dural aperture, and the stylet will puncture the catheter tip and protrude into the brain parenchyma.

Once the site for the burr hole has been selected, the final position of the catheter is determined by three geometric variables: the alignment of the catheter in the sagittal plane, alignment in one other perpendicular plane, either the coronal or the axial, and the depth of catheter insertion. For infants and small children, the depth of catheter insertion can be estimated from the computed tomography (CT) scan, but in an adult with a nondisplaced ventricular system it is never necessary initially to insert the catheter more than 6 cm deep to the outer table of the skull. If it is properly directed, the catheter will encounter CSF at this depth. Strict control of the depth of insertion of the catheter and stylet minimizes the risk of neurological complications. Catheters are available with impregnated spots at the 5, 6, and 7 cm marks. Alternatively, the catheter may be marked with a loose ligature.

When the return of CSF is not immediate, the natural tendency to insert the catheter further must be resisted. If ICP is not greatly elevated, it is helpful for the anesthesiologist to normalize arterial pCO_2 so that the cranial cavity is sufficiently pressurized to force immediate venting of CSF out the catheter as soon as the ventricular system is punctured. An air lock in the lumen of the catheter may be eliminated by gentle irrigation with a small quantity of saline, and the distal end of the catheter may then be dropped in order to siphon ventricular CSF. If the catheter has been positioned in the frontal horn, body, or trigone of the lateral ventricle, the flow of CSF should be free. If it is not, the possibility that the catheter has been misplaced must be considered. Other less capacious CSF spaces that can be cannulated inadvertently include the temporal horn, the interhemispheric fissure, the third ventricle, the sylvian fissure, and even the basilar cisterns. An intraoperative plain skull radiograph or pneumoventriculogram will distinguish among these possibilities. If there is an open fontanel or a craniectomy defect, intraoperative ultrasonography may be useful as well.

When free flow of CSF has been achieved, the ventricular catheter can be advanced without the stylet to its final depth and tunneled under the galea to an exit site at least 5 cm distant.

The principal complications of ventriculostomy are central nervous system infection and intracranial hemorrhage, and they occur at low but not negligible rates. In the setting of ICP monitoring, positive CSF or catheter tip cultures are encountered at a rate of slightly less than 10%. In only about half of these instances is there CSF pleocytosis or other signs of established ventriculitis. The risk of infection for an individual patient rises with the duration of monitoring, the number of ventriculostomies performed, the requirement for other neurosurgical procedures, and the presence of intraventricular hemorrhage. To minimize the risk of infection, it is common practice to replace the ventriculostomy catheter after 5 days. Tunneling the catheter under the galea to an exit site at least 5 cm away from the site of insertion probably reduces the rate of infection as well. There is no consensus on the efficacy of prophylactic antibiotics. The risk of hemorrhage visible on CT along the course of the catheter may be as high as 2%, but, prior to the CT era, symptomatic hemorrhages requiring treatment were recognized at much lower rates. Failure to cannulate the ventricular system may be considered a complication, as well; in experienced hands the failure rate is as low as 1%.

Ventriculostomy is performed frequently for a wide variety of indications on the assumption that the risks of infection and injury to the brain are very low, but lapses in technique quickly vitiate the assumption of low risk. Adequate lighting, draping, positioning and immobilization of the patient, instrumentation, and anesthesia are all critical. Patient restlessness disrupts sterile technique and makes landmarks difficult to maintain. Insufficient anesthesia for incision of the scalp and for tunneling of the catheter allows surges in systemic arterial pressure and central venous pressure that can exacerbate intracranial hypertension. Hemorrhage from the cortical surface occasionally requires illumination, hemostatic agents, and the bipolar cautery for control. Although we recognize that accepted standards of practice vary from one medical center to another, we believe that requirements for anatomic control and surgical asepsis favor performance of ventriculostomy in the operating room with the assistance of an anesthesiologist whenever the patient's condition permits.

FRONTAL VENTRICULOSTOMY

The patient is positioned supine with the neck in a neutral position and the brow up.

Proper localization of the burr hole site is critical. A site 3 cm from the midline, at the midpupillary line, and 1 cm anterior to the coronal suture is recommended (Fig. 1). Sites closer to the midline risk encounters with the large bridging veins draining the frontal lobes into the sagittal sinus or, catastrophically, with the sagittal sinus itself; a distance of 3 cm makes adequate allowance for the usual uncertainty in determination of the midline. Sites further lateral invalidate the usual landmarks for directing ventricular catheter insertion. Sites further posterior begin to encroach on motor cortex, and anterior sites require incisions on the forehead. The coronal suture can almost always be palpated in the midline.

Once the site for a burr hole has been selected, it is necessary to align the catheter in the coronal plane and in the sagittal plane. In the coronal plane the catheter must be pointed at the glabella (Fig. 2A). In the sagittal plane the target is a point about 2 cm anterior to the tragus of the ipsilateral ear (Fig. 2B). If the landmarks have been successfully identified through the drapes, and if the catheter is properly aligned, CSF will be encountered at a depth of 6 cm. The terminal portion of the catheter will lie in the frontal horn of the lateral ventricle with its tip near the foramen of Monro (Fig. 2C).

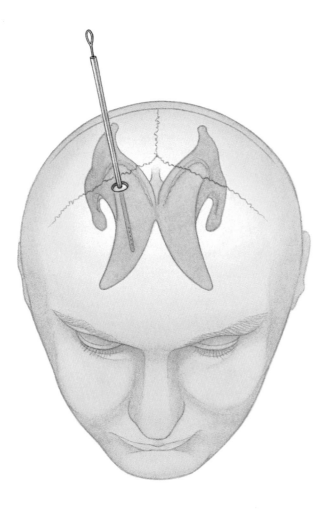

Figure 1. For frontal ventriculostomy a burr hole site is selected about 3 cm from the midline, at the midpupillary line, and 1 cm anterior to the coronal suture. In the coronal plane the catheter is directed toward the glabella.

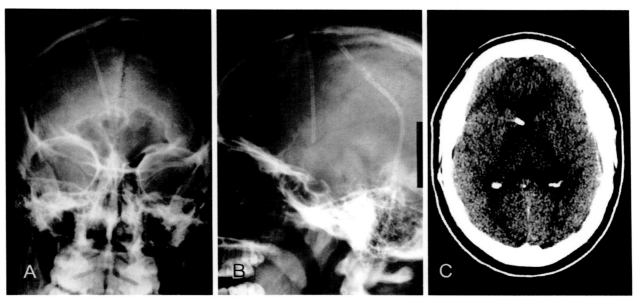

Figure 2. In the coronal plane the ventricular catheter is passed from an entry site 3 cm from the midline toward the glabella (**A**). In the sagittal plane the catheter is directed from an entry site just anterior to the coronal suture toward a point about 2 cm anterior to the external auditory meatus (**B**). The tip of the catheter comes to rest in the frontal horn close to the foramen of Monro (**C**).

POSTERIOR VENTRICULOSTOMY

The patient is positioned three-quarters supine with a roll under the ipsilateral shoulder and with the head turned fully toward the contralateral shoulder (Fig. 3). It is expedient for the head to rest with the brow at the horizontal plane or even slightly below.

Proper selection of the burr hole site is critical for posterior ventriculostomy as well. A burr hole near the midline allows insertion of a catheter down the length of the body of the lateral ventricle and also allows utilization of the medial canthus for orientation. A point 8 cm superior to the inion and 3 to 4 cm lateral to the midline is suitable (Fig. 4). These coordinates place the burr hole just above the lambdoid suture. For patients in whom the inion cannot be palpated, such as young infants, the lambdoid suture itself can be used for orientation: a site in the parietal bone just anterior to the suture 3 cm from the midline is satisfactory.

For posterior ventriculostomy a palpable marker at the glabella permits orientation through the drapes in both the sagittal and axial planes. From the posterior approach there is a natural tendency to wander across the midline, and the surgeon should take care to aim at the ipsilateral medial canthus in the axial plane. In the sagittal plane, the marker at the glabella is itself the target. If the catheter is properly directed, it will encounter CSF at a depth of 6 cm as it punctures the dorsolateral wall of the trigone of the lateral ventricle. From this point the catheter can be advanced into the body of the lateral ventricle without the stylet. For CSF shunts the depth of ventricular catheter insertion can be measured from the CT scan. It is customary to place the tip of the catheter at the most extreme end of the frontal horn in order prevent obstruction of the catheter perforations by choroid plexus (Fig. 5). For temporary ventricular drainage or for ICP monitoring, the depth of catheter insertion is less critical. As for frontal ventriculostomies, externalized catheters should be tunneled to an exit site several centimeters from the burr hole in order to minimize the risk of infection.

The most problematic aspect of posterior ventriculostomy is locating the site for the burr hole. The surgeon may be tempted to pick a more inferior site corresponding to the tip of the occipital horn, where the ventricular system is closest to the cortical surface. If, as in CSF shunt insertion, the goal is to place the tip of the catheter in the frontal horn, an inferior site is a mistake. From this approach the surgeon faces the difficult task of slipping the catheter up over the hump of the thalamus (Fig. 5). Instead, the catheter may fall into the temporal horn and, because the thalamus itself is the obstacle, it can be injured by the stylet. A more lateral site above and behind the pinna has been popular as well, perhaps because positioning the patient is simpler for this approach. The trigone of the lateral ventricle, viewed en face from this perspective, presents a large cross-sectional target area. It is, however, a shallow target, and from this lateral approach the surgeon must somehow persuade the catheter to turn frontally as soon as it encounters CSF. Furthermore, because the surgeon has no good landmark for orientation of the catheter in the axial plane, the thalamus and internal capsule are at risk for injury by a catheter directed slightly too far anteriorly.

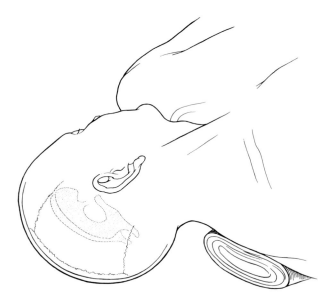

Figure 3. For posterior ventriculostomy it is necessary to place a roll under the ipsilateral shoulder in order to turn the head fully horizontal.

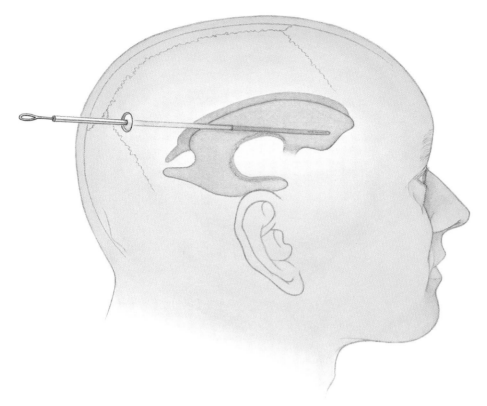

Figure 4. For posterior ventriculostomy a burr hole is placed 8 cm above the inion and 3 to 4 cm off the midline, just anterior to the lambdoid suture. The catheter is directed toward the medial canthus in the axial plane and toward the glabella in the sagittal plane.

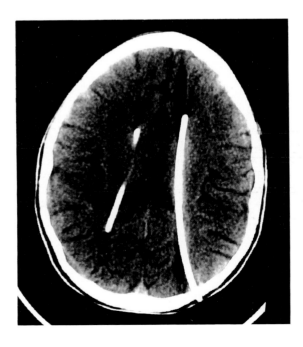

Figure 5. For posterior ventriculostomy the optimal length of the ventricular catheter can be estimated from the CT scan. In this patient the left ventricular catheter is slightly too long, but such an error has the advantage of placing the catheter tip perforations anterior to the choroid plexus and reducing the risk of catheter obstruction by ingrowth of tissue. The right ventricular catheter was inserted through a burr hole situated inferior to the recommended site; this catheter had to be guided up over the hump of the thalamus, as its passage in and out of the plane of the CT scan indicates.

CEREBELLAR MEDULLOBLASTOMA

ARTHUR E. MARLIN, M.D.
SARAH J. GASKILL, M.D.

INTRODUCTION

Medulloblastoma is a midline tumor occurring in the posterior fossa. While these tumors occur throughout life, they are far more common in children than in adults. They represent 15–20% of brain tumors in children with a peak incidence at 8 years of age and a 2:1 male/female ratio. The tumor was first described by Bailey and Cushing in 1925. They believed it originated from the pluripotential medulloblast—a primitive cell which has never been identified. More recently, the tumor has been thought to originate from cells of the subependymal region of the fetus and has thus been termed a primitive neuroectodermal tumor of the posterior fossa.

The classical presentation is usually that of increased intracranial pressure related to hydrocephalus. The average symptom duration is two months. The most common presentation is, therefore, morning headaches and vomiting, papilledema, and ataxia.

The diagnosis of a midline posterior fossa tumor is made by computed tomography (CT) or magnetic resonance imaging (MRI) (Fig. 1). Typically, on CT, the tumor has a slightly increased density and enhances with contrast. There tends to be a low signal intensity on T1 weighted MR images and enhancement with gadolinium. On T2 weighted images, the tumor has a high signal intensity. There are atypical features in about half the cases. In general, the tumor fills the fourth ventricle from the cisterna magna to the aqueduct of Sylvius, causing hydrocephalus.

With the diagnosis of a midline posterior fossa mass in a child, surgery is mandated because gross total removal provides the best outcome regardless of tumor pathology. Any alternative therapy produces a poorer outcome.

PREOPERATIVE CONSIDERATIONS

Timing of surgery will depend on the degree of hydrocephalus and state of the patient. Unless the child is in poor nutritional status and medical condition, the sooner the surgery, the better. If the patient is not medically stable, then increased intracranial pressure can be controlled with external ventricular drainage (EVD) until operative intervention is appropriate. With EVD, there is a definite but small risk of upward herniation. This risk can be further decreased by careful control of intracranial pressure with the avoidance of sudden cerebrospinal fluid (CSF) drainage and decompression. It is the senior author's preference to avoid EVD if possible and operate soon after the diagnosis is made. Pretreatment with steroids is thought to be beneficial and is always done, especially when there is some delay in surgery. If possible, steroids are not given until after the enhanced CT scan, as this may alter the enhancement. Anticonvulsants are not routinely used in posterior fossa surgery. Prophylactic antibiotics are given for placement of the external ventricular drain, if used, but are not routinely used for the surgery itself. There is no definitive study to suggest that they are effective in this circumstance.

We prefer to use the sitting position for medulloblastoma surgery (Fig. 2). Anesthesia technique therefore requires a central venous catheter and Doppler monitoring for venous air embolism. Arterial blood pressure, oxygen saturation, and end-tidal CO_2 are also monitored. Leg wraps are used to prevent hypotension. The patient is hyperventilated to decrease intracranial pressure. Mannitol or Lasix, however, are not routinely given. If, on exposure, the posterior fossa is tight, the lateral ventricle is cannulated and EVD is established.

POSITIONING AND DRAPING

The major debate of operative positioning centers on the sitting versus the prone or lateral decubitus (parkbench) type of position. The argument against the sitting position is the increased incidence of air embolism. The advantage of the sitting position is the excellent exposure and decreased intracranial pressure. Although air embolism is best known in the sitting position, it has been reported in the prone position and, in fact, occurs in any position where the head is higher than the heart. Because of the incidence of air embolism and the possible disastrous consequences,

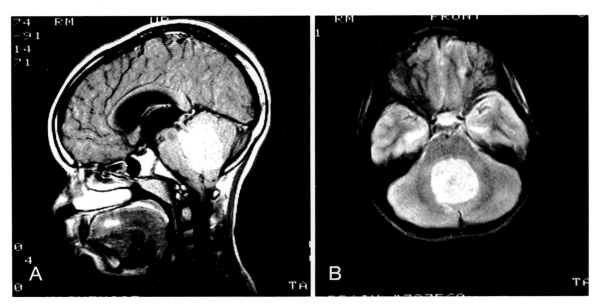

Figure 1. Sagittal (**A**) and axial (**B**) T1-weighted MRI scans with gadolinium enhancement of a midline medulloblas- toma. Note the relationship of the tumor to the floor of the fourth ventricle, aqueduct of Sylvius, and cisterna magna.

special precautions must be taken in the sitting position.

Pin sites should be wrapped with Vaseline gauze to eliminate these as a source of air embolism. Hemostasis must be meticulous. Air may enter the diploic spaces of the bone, so these must be carefully waxed. The Doppler monitor should always be loud enough so the surgeon can hear it to identify air at the same time as the anesthesiologist. The Doppler monitor should be tested several times with a rapid saline infusion during the operation. With changes in the Doppler sounds, the anesthesiologist should attempt to aspirate the air from the right atrium and the surgeon should attempt to eliminate the source. A wet lap sponge should always be available to cover the wound when air is identified. The wound is then gradually exposed to find the source. Jugular compression or Valsalva's maneuver may help.

Before surgery, all the members of the operative team should familiarize themselves with the head holder and stabilizing apparatus. If necessary, a drill should be done so that all involved know how to quickly and effectively change the patient's position to supine if needed. This is more readily accomplished in the sitting position than the prone, and the anesthesiologist has the best access to the patient in this position.

The patient's head is placed in the three-pin head holder. The foot board is used as a seat for a small child so the shoulders are at least three inches off the table when the head of the table is removed. The table is gradually placed in the sitting position with careful arterial pressure monitoring, first by flexing the table and then by elevating the back. The head is held straight by the surgeon while the fixation device is first secured proximal to the patient, and then tightening proceeds distally. The head should be flexed, taking care not to compromise venous drainage or the airway. A spiral, flexible endotracheal tube is used. The chin should be about a finger's breadth off the chest. Once secured in this fashion, the entire table and patient, now as a single unit, can be tilted slightly forward. During the procedure, upward and downward movement of the table will be required. Draping should allow for this movement. The arms are folded and supported on the patient's lap to prevent a traction brachial plexus palsy.

Once positioned and shaved, the incision is marked (Fig. 2). The inion is the major landmark. The occipital squama, C1, and C2 will need to be exposed. In general, an incision 4 cm above the inion and 8 cm below to about the spine of C5 will be adequate. A burr hole incision is also marked in case EVD is necessary. This is 4 cm lateral to the inion and 6 cm above it. The position of the inner canthus of the eye from this incision should be noted before draping so a ready pass can be made into the ventricle, if necessary. The incision is then infiltrated with saline in small infants, or Xylocaine with epinephrine, to allow for dissection of the skin edges and hemostasis. The initial drapes are held in place with skin staples, which most adequately and expeditiously secure them. Sheets and a craniotomy drape with an incorporated window and irrigation collection bag are used.

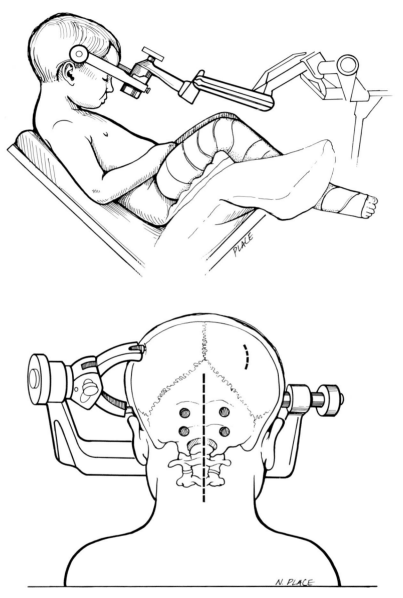

Figure 2. *Top*, the sitting position is demonstrated. *Bottom*, the incision is made with respect to the inion, 4 cm above and 8 cm below.

SURGICAL TECHNIQUE

The skin incision is made and Raney clips placed on the skin edges. To do this, each skin edge needs to be dissected with blunt dissection in the scalp and sharp dissection in the neck, taking care to leave the fascia intact. A gauze is used over the skin in infants and small children to prevent necrosis from the pressure of the Raney clips. The skin is then dissected laterally, using retraction with Weitlaner or cerebellar retractors, exposing the fascia. The fascia and muscles are opened in a Y fashion (Fig. 3) to decrease the likelihood of a postoperative pseudomeningocele. The intersection of the limbs of the Y should be low on the skull for easiest closure but still over the skull. The upper limbs of the Y are incised with the cutting current down to bone. Using periosteal elevators, the muscle is then stripped to the nuchal line. Care is taken not to go beyond this line as that would eliminate the advantage of the Y. As the muscle is stripped, emissary veins will be encountered on both sides. These need to be waxed. The V flap is retracted with a heavy suture. The surgeon then continues the midline incision, stripping the muscles from the arch of C1 and the spine and laminae of C2. The remaining muscles on the occipital squama must be stripped laterally on each side to the region of the mastoid process, which may be poorly developed in a child.

Two burr holes are now placed in the occipital squama on each side of the midline. After stripping the dura from the bone, a craniectomy with rongeurs or a craniotomy with an air drill, such as the Midas Rex, can be performed. The bone here need not be replaced because the angle of the skull and the heavy musculature provide protection. The bone is removed superiorly until the inferior portion of the transverse sinus is visualized, and laterally to the region of the mastoid. The sigmoid sinuses need not be exposed. Care should be taken in the midline. Here, the bone can have a "keel-like" projection intracranially, and the occipital sinus can be quite large. Also, care should be taken with the arch of C1, which may be cartilaginous in the young child. The craniectomy should be performed before the removal of the arch of C1 and the spine of C2; these provide protection in case an instrument slips. The inferior pole of the tumor should be exposed; the preoperative MRI will indicate the need to remove C1 and C2. Bone edges are carefully waxed to prevent air embolism.

Assessment of the intracranial pressure in the posterior fossa can now be made. It is surprising that even with large lesions, with the sitting position and hyperventilation, the dura will not be tight. If this is the case, it can be opened as described below.

If the dura is tight, then the burr hole incision is made. The calvarium is perforated. The dura is coagulated and incised. An external ventricular drain is placed. This is tunneled to exit at a distance from the incision. CSF is slowly allowed to escape until the dura can be opened without cerebellar herniation. Care must be taken not to decompress the ventricles too rapidly, as an extraaxial hematoma, subdural or epidural, may result. Intracerebral hemorrhage may even occur.

The dura is also opened in a Y fashion with the inferior limb slightly off the midline (Fig. 4). First, the dura is opened over each hemisphere to the region of the occipital sinus. At this point, either small hemostats or hemoclips are used to isolate the sinus before it is transected. The sinus is then tied off with a 4-0 silk suture and the clips or hemostats removed. The V dural flap is elevated and retracted superiorly with a suture. The dural opening is then extended inferiorly off the midline to the caudal portion of the foramen magnum or the inferior pole of the tumor. These dural flaps are retracted by suturing them to the paravertebral muscles. The table-patient unit is tilted further forward to provide better visualization.

The foramen magnum and usually the tumor are visualized. Using a 22-gauge needle, the arachnoid of the foramen magnum is penetrated. CSF can be taken for cytology; the significance of this cytology, however, is unclear. The arachnoid is then widely opened. This can be done with the needle or forceps.

If the inferior pole of the tumor is seen, it is gently elevated with a small retractor or Penfield dissector. The floor of the fourth ventricle is visualized and a cottonoid is placed on it (Fig. 5). If the tumor is not visualized, the cerebellar tonsils are elevated, the floor of the fourth ventricle is visualized, and a cottonoid is placed.

At this point, the Yasargil self-retaining retractor is brought into the operative field. The cerebellar hemispheres are slightly retracted, if necessary, to clearly expose the vermis. The arachnoid and pia over the midline vermis are coagulated with bipolar cautery, and a linear incision is made into the vermis. Using blunt dissection, this is extended until the tumor is encountered. Planes laterally are then developed using bipolar coagulation, gentle retraction, and cottonoids. At this point, biopsies are taken. Medulloblastomas are usually friable and quite readily suctioned.

As one extends deeper and superiorly, the plane between tumor and cerebellum may become indistinct, but the demarcation between normal and abnormal tissue is readily visible. The tumor should be manipulated very gently with careful concern regarding the anatomy involved. If the tumor is not readily suctioned, the Cavitron ultrasonic aspirator (CUSA) should be used. The table can be further tilted and elevated. Working at the exposed surface, the tumor

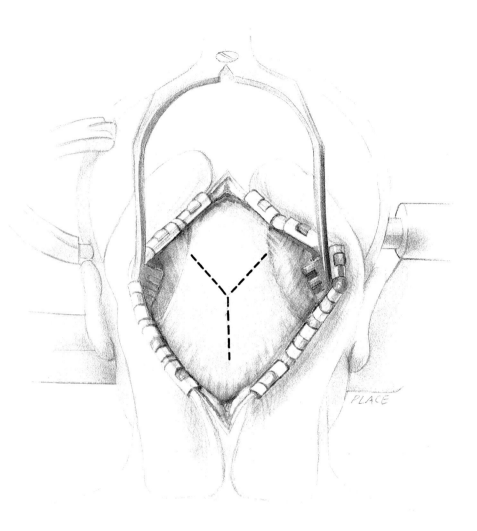

Figure 3. The Y-shaped fascial incision is shown.

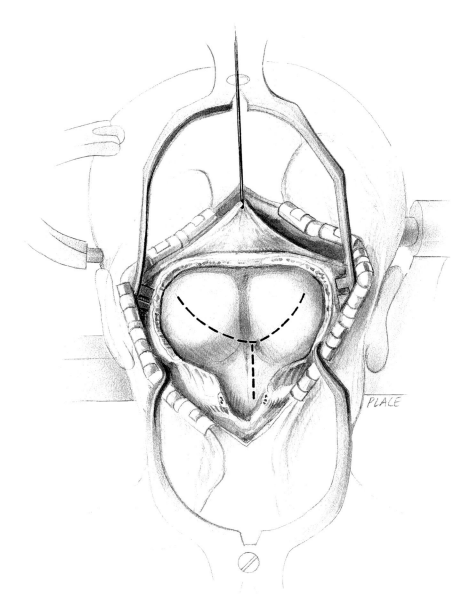

Figure 4. A Y-shaped incision is made in the dura, taking care to tie off the occipital sinus
superiorly, and making the inferior limb slightly off the midline.

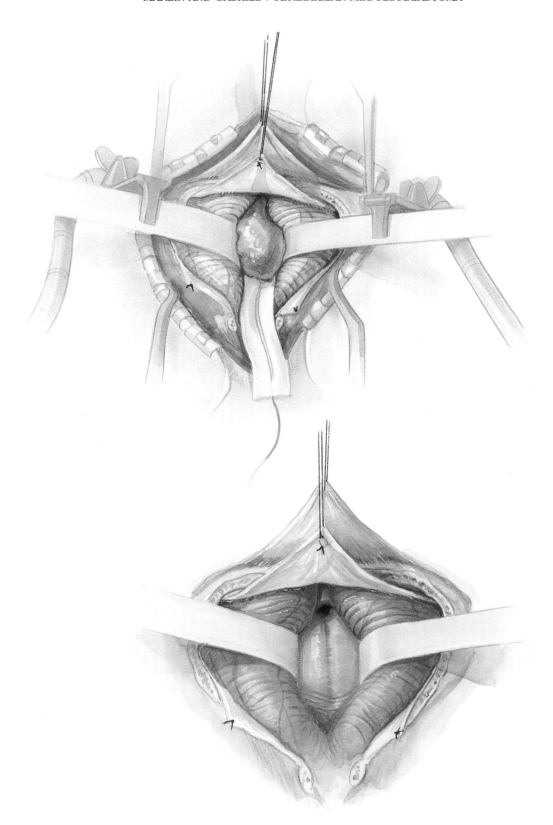

Figure 5. *Top,* tumor is seen after the dura is opened and the vermis is partially split. The vermis will be further split, and the tumor plane developed. A cottonoid is placed on the floor of the fourth ventricle. *Bottom,* after tumor resection, the enlarged aqueduct of Sylvius can be visualized.

will come inferiorly into the field. Working with gentle suction, the rostral portion of the fourth ventricle and aqueduct will come into view. Once seen, attention should be turned caudally to the cottonoid on the floor of the fourth ventricle. The tumor should now be gently lifted from the fourth ventricle and the cottonoid advanced rostrally. This portion of the tumor can now be removed with forceps and suction. The first goal of surgery, to unblock the aqueduct, has now been accomplished.

Using the CUSA, the remaining tumor is now removed. Up to this point, there is usually oozing from the tumor which is not easily controlled until the tumor is removed. Large bleeding vessels are controlled with bipolar coagulation. If the tumor does not readily come off the floor of the fourth ventricle or is invading the floor, it is "shaved" off with gentle suction here, and the brain stem is not violated. Most commonly, the tumor does not invade the floor of the fourth ventricle and is readily lifted from it. In this fashion, the second goal of surgery, gross total tumor removal, is accomplished.

Once hemostasis has been achieved, the tumor cavity is inspected for possible residual tumor (Fig. 5). Hemostasis can be assessed by Valsalva's maneuver or jugular venous compression. Questionable areas of tissue are sent for frozen section. No hemostatic agents are left behind.

Once satisfaction has been achieved, the dura is closed with 4-0 silk. If watertight dural closure cannot be obtained, a fascial patch is used. Gelfoam is used to cover the dural closure. The paravertebral muscles and fascia are now closed with 2-0 Vicryl sutures. A good fascial closure is very important to prevent a pseudomeningocele. The subcutaneous tissue is closed with 3-0 Vicryl. The skin is closed with 3-0 Vicryl in a subcuticular fashion followed by the application of Steristrips.

POSTOPERATIVE CONSIDERATIONS

The table is now tilted back to the original position, and the three-pin head holder is removed. A soft cervical collar may be used for comfort. The patient is extubated in the sitting position and is kept sitting for the first 48 hours.

Within 48 hours after surgery, a CT scan, without and with contrast, is done to assess the extent of tumor removal and the degree of hydrocephalus. This must be compared to the preoperative study. Significant pneumocephalus will be apparent, but some decrease in ventricular size should be obvious. A significant number of patients, perhaps 40%, will subsequently need a ventriculoperitoneal shunt.

One week postoperatively, CT myelography is done to rule out metastases and stage the patient for adjunctive therapy. With this, CSF is sent for cytology, and bone marrow aspiration is performed. Currently, CT myelography appears superior to MRI for evaluation of spinal metastases. This will probably change in the near future.

SHUNTING OF A POSTTRAUMATIC SYRINX

DAVID J. GOWER, M.D.

INTRODUCTION

Cavitation of the injured portion of the spinal cord following trauma is a common phenomenon. As a consequence of this posttraumatic cavitation, a syrinx may form within the substance of the cord from several months to many years following the injury. The presenting symptoms and signs of a syrinx are varied and may be as subtle as a slight change in sensory level or as dramatic as intractable pain. A constant awareness of the potential for syrinx formation in the patient with a spinal cord injury is the most effective way to ensure that these lesions are found.

DIAGNOSIS

Prior to the advent of magnetic resonance image (MRI) scanning, the diagnosis of posttraumatic syringomyelia was difficult. One technique used to search for a syrinx was postmyelographic computed tomography (CT) scanning, looking for an increase in the radiodensity of cysts within the spinal cord (Fig. 1). Another commonly used technique was air myelography. The "collapsing cord sign" was indicative of a positive test. Both of these tests had faults that produced both false negatives and false positives. MRI scanning has significantly improved the accuracy of syringomyelia diagnosis and follow-up (Fig. 2, A and B). The entire spinal cord may be visualized in a sagittal plane, and the extent of a posttraumatic syrinx may be seen. Unfortunately, a large percentage of patients with spinal trauma also have some form of internal fixation device in place to facilitate spinal stabilization. Such ferrous materials may disrupt the image of the spine obtained with the MRI and prevent visualization of some critical areas of the spinal cord. Sampling of information from the spinal cord above or below the metal artifact is still possible and treatment planning may be carried out using this information.

PREOPERATIVE PREPARATIONS

As with all types of surgical procedures, preoperative

discussions with the patient should include discussion of risks versus potential benefits of therapy. In addition to the standard risks associated with any surgical procedure, some authors have reported dramatic loss of neurologic function following decompression of the syrinx.

The position for placement of the syrinx to subarachnoid shunt is the major preoperative decision to be made. In general, the shunt catheter should go into the most dependent portion of the syrinx cavity but above the level of injury in a complete lesion. MRI images should be able to show the extent of the cyst, position of the cyst within the substance of the cord, and some of the intracystic anatomy. The best surgical

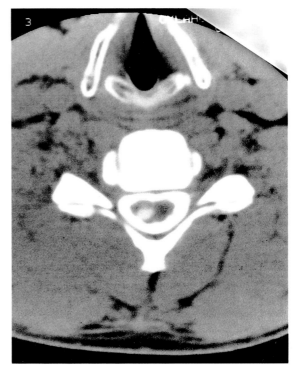

Figure 1. An example of a delayed contrast CT scan of a cervical posttraumatic syrinx. Note the area of contrast enhancement within the parenchyma of the spinal cord.

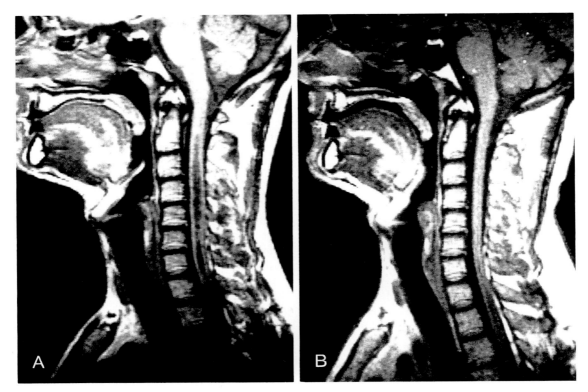

Figure 2. **A,** a 35-year-old patient four years after a lower thoracic compression fracture with an incomplete spinal cord injury. The patient presented with an ascending sensory level and midthoracic pain intractable to medical therapy. Note the large syrinx extending from C2 down into the thoracic spinal cord. **B,** one month following a thoracic syrinx to subarachnoid shunting procedure. The syrinx is now decompressed in the cervical region and the patient's pain is improved.

method for treatment of a syrinx is to shunt the collected spinal fluid back into the subarachnoid space or into the peritoneal cavity. The shunt tubing in the spinal cord should be placed in the most dependent area of the cyst but with consideration of the concentration of function (i.e., thoracic rather than cervical). The size of the cyst at each level is also important, and it is preferable to place the tubing in an area with the greatest amount of dilation to reduce the risk of injury to remaining function of the cord. In those patients with thoracic or conus lesions, placement of the shunt in the thoracic region is preferable to the cervical area. The drainage end of the shunt should be placed in the subarachnoid space but in some cases of trauma this may not be possible and the patient should be prepared for possible diversion of cerebrospinal fluid into the peritoneal cavity.

Anesthetic Considerations

General anesthesia is the anesthetic of choice. While some surgeons are capable of performing complex operations upon the spine under local anesthesia, the risk to the patient with small amounts of movement while placing the tubing may be great. Preoperative medications may include a course of dexamethasone and/or a cephalosporin prophylactic antibiotic. The patient should be mildly hyperventilated to reduce intracranial/intraspinal pressure and the potential for rapid dilation of the syrinx following the opening of the dural envelope. Pneumatic sequential compression stockings are usually used on the patient's lower extremities to reduce the risk of deep venous thrombosis and potential pulmonary embolism. Monitoring of somatosensory evoked potentials in conjunction with possible rectal sphincter electromyography may also be useful.

Operative Positioning

The patient should be positioned prone on the table in a manner appropriate for the area of the spinal cord that is to be approached. Chest rolls are helpful in decreasing venous congestion and reducing bleeding. Patients with a cervical lesion should be placed in tongs on a circular headrest with care being taken to protect the eyes or in a three-point fixation system. The arms should be placed at the side with appropriate padding. With a thoracolumbar approach, the patient should be positioned in a prone position with the arms up on armboards. Before the skin of the patient is prepared, an x-ray film of the area should be taken to locate the correct position for the shunt; a radiopaque marker may be placed upon the skin to identify the location. A mark should be made on the skin lateral to the site of the incision with a skin marker or with a needle, but the scratch should not cross the midline.

Draping

The wound should be draped out in the standard fashion so that the mark for proper location is easily seen in the operative field. The site of the incision should be marked with an appropriate skin marker and should be covered with an adhesive drape that may or may not be impregnated with iodine. The field should be wide enough to allow access to the abdomen should a syrinx to peritoneal shunt be required. Frequently during this period of time the circulating nurse in the room will pass the shunt tube onto the back table. The tubing should be in contact with the room air for the minimum amount of time to decrease the risk of dust attaching to the surface by electrostatic attraction. The tubing should be placed directly into a solution of Bacitracin (50,000 units in 250 ml of saline) and kept in the solution until ready to insert into the spinal cord.

SURGICAL TECHNIQUE

Skin Incision

The skin incision should be in the midline. Since the appropriate vertebral level was previously identified radiographically, the incision should be centered over this level. The length of the incision usually can be limited to 7–10 cm.

Operative Procedure

The paraspinous musculature should be retracted using an appropriate retractor, and the wound should be made meticulously free from bleeding sites. The lamina over the site that had been previously decided upon should be removed using a high-speed drill. In most cases only a single level needs to be removed with some of the bottom of the lamina above and the top of the lamina below also drilled away. Wide exposure on the side of the proposed shunt should be carried out. The bleeding from the bone edges may be controlled with bone wax or Gelfoam pressed into the diploë; the bleeding from epidural veins is controlled using bipolar electrocautery. The gutters between the dura and the bony edge are lined with Gelfoam moistened with thrombin in order to control bleeding, and the wound is lined with cotton sheets.

The dura is opened by a small nick with a sharp instrument, leaving the arachnoid intact (Fig. 3). One method of further opening the dura is to insert the tip of a blunt nerve hook and gently pull the instrument superiorly to split the dura along the natural lines of division. One should be careful to leave at least 2–3 mm of unopened dura at each end of the wound in order to facilitate later closure in a water-tight fashion.

The actual site for the myelotomy should be considered once the dura is open. Midline opening of the spinal cord will potentially damage the dorsal columns and decrease the patient's proprioceptive function from the lower extremities and should be avoided. The preferable area to enter the cord is in an area of obvious thinning or in the dorsal root entry zone. The

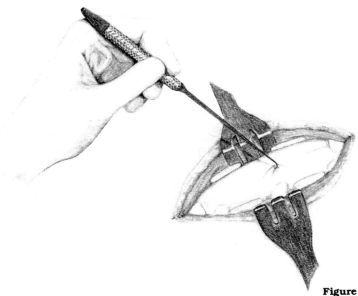

Figure 3. A sharp hook is used to elevate the dura so it may be opened with a scalpel.

side of the entry should be determined prior to the operation by careful examination of the MRI scan. Damage to the thoracic dorsal root entry zone will give at worst a dermatomal patch of numbness around the patient's thorax.

The arachnoid should be opened paramedian and spinal fluid released. The edges of the arachnoid can be gently picked up using a forceps and tacked to the edge of the dura using hemaclips. Usually two to three hemaclips are necessary to ensure that the arachnoid is tacked up out of the way. This portion of the procedure will allow an easy identification of the subarachnoid space to ensure that the placement of the subarachnoid portion of the syrinx to subarachnoid shunt is not in an extraarachnoid position. The subarachnoid space should be observed at this time. In most cases there should be minimal scarring and access to the subarachnoid space, but, where access is poor, a shunt of cerebrospinal fluid into the peritoneal cavity may be necessary.

Attention should be directed to the spinal cord where the pia mater is cauterized using the bipolar cautery on a low power setting. Care should be taken not to damage large vessels on the surface of the cord. In those patients whose spinal cord appears reason- ably normal without dilation or thinning, a 26-gauge needle should be passed into the cord to puncture the cyst and ensure that the syrinx extends into the operative site. The fluid within the posttraumatic syrinx should be clear and colorless. Yellow fluid or bloody fluid would imply a different pathologic process. A myelotomy approximately 1 cm in length is made by first incising the pia with a No. 11 blade and then using bipolar forceps and a microdissector to open the cord into the cyst longitudinally.

In patients with syringomyelia secondary to trauma, often the syrinx is asymmetrical (Fig. 4) with several blind pouches that do not allow the easy passage of the shunting catheter. The proximal arms of the shunt (Fig. 5) should be passed in each direction within the syrinx cavity (Fig. 6). The entire length of the shunt tube should be used, if possible.

In those cavities that are not large enough to accommodate the entire shunt tube, the tube should be trimmed so that it does not stretch or distort the spinal cord. Great care should be taken while inserting the tube into the spinal cord to ensure that the tubing is within the syrinx cavity and is not dissecting a separate plane outside the cavity through the parenchyma of the cord. After placement of one end of the small "K" or "T" tube, it is necessary to kink the tubing at its midpoint and have an assistant hold the middle connector while the other end of the tubing is passed into the syrinx cavity. The spinal cord should receive the minimal amount of manipulation possible while at the same time maintaining the smallest possible myelotomy so that the tubing does not slip out. Once the tube is in place, the distal end of the tube intended for the subarachnoid space needs to be placed.

The dentate ligaments can be identified on the lateral aspect of the spinal cord. The distal tube should be placed under the leaf of arachnoid that has been pre-

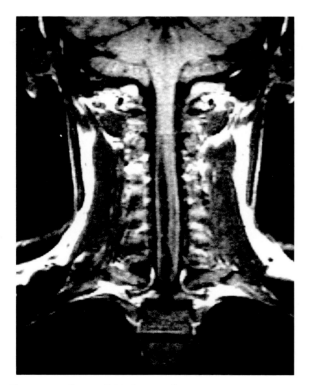

Figure 4. Cervical MRI scan demonstrating a posttraumatic syrinx. Note that the cavity is irregular and is paramedian. This information should be considered when planning placement of a syrinx to subarachnoid shunt tube.

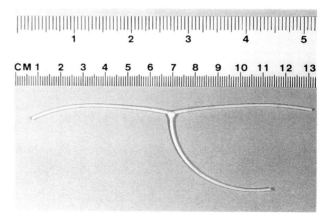

Figure 5. Photograph of the small silicone plastic tubing used to form the syrinx shunt. The tubing is very flexible and may be custom fit to the syrinx cavity.

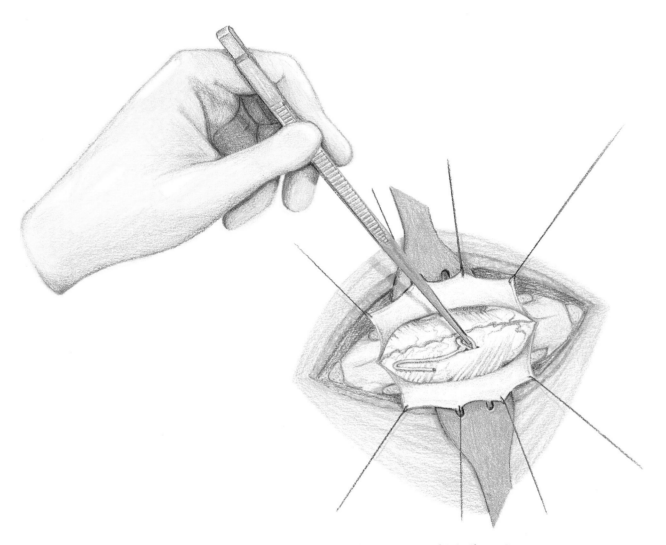

Figure 6. The proximal arms of the shunt are passed into the syrinx.

served along the dura, and passed ventral to the dentate ligament (Fig. 7). This will ensure that the tubing is subarachnoid. There should only be a minimum of bleeding during this procedure, and all bleeding must be stopped and the wound completely dry before closure is started. If ultrasonography is available, it can be used to examine the spinal cord at this time to look at the tubing within the syrinx cavity. Comparison of the spinal cord before and after placement of the shunt tube should ensure that the syrinx is adequately drained.

In those patients with poor access to the subarachnoid space, the distal aspect of the shunt should be connected to a standard peritoneal shunt catheter which is passed through a subcutaneous tunnel to a separate incision on the flank. The tubing is passed into the peritoneal cavity and the separate wound closed. The tubing should be carefully tacked to the paraspinous tissue in a manner that will not kink the tubing. This is sometimes best accomplished by bringing the tubing down in a loop around the next spinous process before bringing it out through the fascia. If at all possible, one would hope to see cerebrospinal fluid leaking from the distal end of the catheter before its placement into the peritoneal cavity.

Closure

Closure is started by removing from the wound the metal clips that were used to hold the arachnoid back. These are taken off the field and not left within the wound. The arachnoid is allowed to fall back into position. The dura is then closed using either an interrupted or running stitch. Stitches should be placed very close together to ensure the best chance of a watertight closure.

After closure of the dura, Valsalva's maneuver performed by the anesthetist increases the subarachnoid pressure; any leaks that are identified should be reinforced using sutures. In those patients in which dural closure is difficult, fibrin glue consisting of cryoprecipitate mixed in equal proportions with topical thrombin is helpful in producing a watertight closure. Several stitches can be placed to reapproximate the muscle bellies and then sutures placed for the tight closure of the fascia, again to reduce the chances of cerebrospinal fluid leakage. The skin is usually closed with a running nylon suture in a locking stitch to provide a firm barrier against cerebrospinal fluid leakage. Percutaneous drainage of the wound should be avoided if at all possible since this will leave a track to the surface. Skin sutures should be left in these wounds for longer than the usual period of time, sometimes up to two weeks, to ensure that the wound is well-healed.

SPECIALIZED INSTRUMENTATION

Removal of the lamina in these patients should be done with a high-speed drill. The Midas Rex drill is particularly well-suited because of the large number of bits available and the speed with which the drill turns.

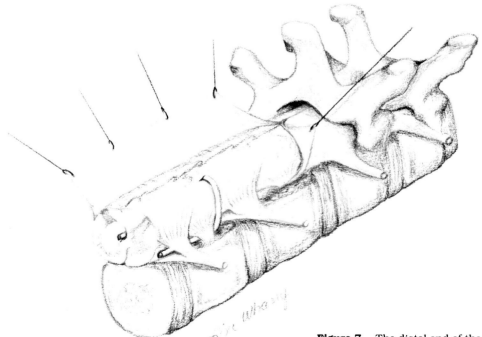

Figure 7. The distal end of the shunt is placed within the subarachnoid space ventral to the dentate ligament.

The M8 or AM8 bits are particularly good for this type of laminectomy. Microinstrumentation and an operating microscope are also of value while placing the shunt tubing into the syrinx cavity. Intraoperative ultrasonography is an interesting but not a necessary component of the procedure to ensure that the tube is in place and the syrinx adequately drained.

POSTOPERATIVE COMPLICATIONS

Neurological deterioration postoperatively should be evaluated in a method that is appropriate to the extent and rate of deterioration. Those patients who awaken with catastrophic neurologic deficit should be studied on an urgent basis with CT or MRI scanning or wound re-exploration if appropriate. In those patients who awaken with a mildly worsened neurologic deficit, conservative therapy and observation may be indicated since the manipulation of the spinal cord may have made the patient temporarily worse.

Cerebrospinal fluid leaks should be treated in an aggressive manner. Small leaks from the wound can be treated by reinforcing stitches of the wound edges. Major leaks of cerebrospinal fluid should probably be re-explored and the dura again closed at the site of leakage. In those patients in whom it is necessary to re-explore for cerebrospinal fluid leakage, use of fibrin glue or autologous blood patching is helpful in reducing the problems of continued leakage postoperatively.

A small superficial wound infection or stitch abscess can be treated by local wound care. Superficial wound infections should be treated by gentle cleansing of the wound with removal of debris. Deep infections should be treated in the operating room by opening the fascia and packing the incision. Like most shunting devices, infection of the tubing would necessitate removal of the prosthesis from the spinal cord. Most likely, this form of infection would present as meningitis, and it would be unlikely that this could be cured with antibiotics alone.

DIRECT SURGICAL TREATMENT OF VEIN OF GALEN MALFORMATIONS

HAROLD J. HOFFMAN, M.D.

INTRODUCTION

The clinical presentation of a patient with a vein of Galen malformation is entirely dependent on the severity of shunting through the fistula. Neonates with galenic malformations characteristically have multiple fistulae (Fig. 1) which shunt more than 25% of their cardiac output through the malformation, resulting in high output congestive heart failure. In addition, low diastolic blood pressure reduces coronary blood flow and results in myocardial ischemia which aggravates the heart failure. Preferential flow through the malformation bypasses the cerebral cortex, leading to cerebral ischemia (Fig. 2). These infants are gravely ill because of their associated cerebral and myocardial ischemia and cannot be managed medically. Direct surgical attack on these neonatal malformations of the vein of Galen can rarely be done with safety. Modern interventional neuroradiologic techniques can lead to obliteration of many of the fistulae feeding the galenic malformation. In doing so, the patient can be rescued from intractable heart failure and, if any residual malformation is left, surgery can be used to deal with this in a well patient who is no longer in heart failure and whose brain has been salvaged from ischemia. In using such interventional techniques one must be cognizant of the characteristic constriction in the draining straight sinus, which is probably a protective mechanism (Fig. 3).

The older infant and young child with a galenic malformation typically has very few fistulous connections to the vein of Galen (Figs. 4 and 5). Although these children may show evidence of heart failure, they characteristically present with a greatly dilated vein of Galen which occludes the aqueduct and posterior third ventricle and produces hydrocephalus. These patients are candidates for surgical obliteration of the fistula.

Older children and adults with galenic malformations frequently have a relatively low flow angiomatous network supplying the vein of Galen. These patients are rarely candidates for surgical attack on the lesion.

PREOPERATIVE PREPARATION

The patient who has heart failure should be treated medically and by interventional neuroradiologic techniques. Because these patients can suffer cerebral ischemia, they are prone to seizures and anticonvulsant medication should be used. If significant hydrocephalus is present, this should be treated with a cerebrospinal fluid diversionary shunt.

OPERATIVE PROCEDURE

Anesthesia

Neonates and infants have a small blood volume which can be severely compromised during surgery for a galenic malformation. Central venous and arterial lines are mandatory for monitoring purposes. A warming blanket must be used to reduce heat loss during the operation. Mannitol, steroids, and hyperventilation can aid in producing a relaxed operative field. The neonates and infants cannot be placed in a pin fixation headrest because of fear of penetrating the skull. An infant horseshoe headrest is sufficient.

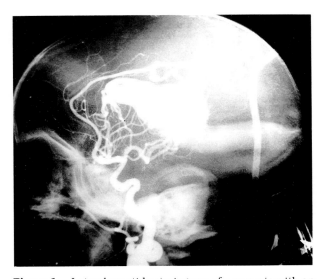

Figure 1. Lateral carotid arteriogram of a neonate with an aneurysm of the vein of Galen showing multiple fistulous feeders entering the aneurysm.

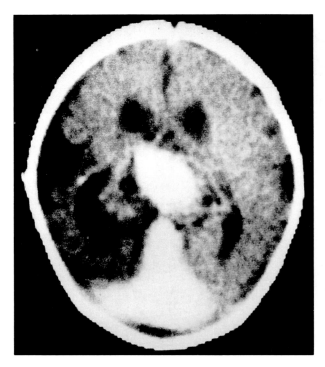

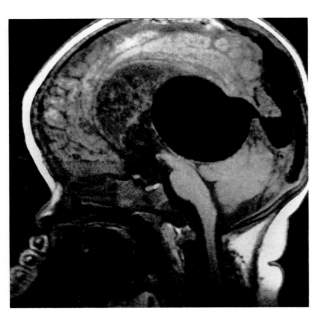

Figure 3. Magnetic resonance imaging scan of an infant with an aneurysm of the vein of Galen showing characteristic constriction in the straight sinus.

Figure 2. Computed tomography scan of a neonate with an aneurysm of the vein of Galen and ischemic damage to the right cerebral hemisphere.

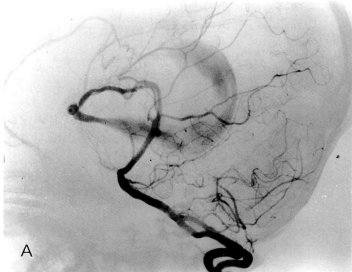

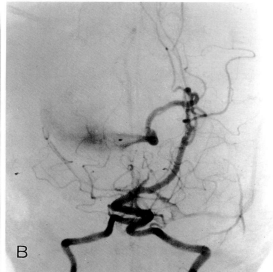

Figure 4. Lateral (**A**) and anteroposterior (**B**) views from a vertebral arteriogram of an infant with an aneurysm of the vein of Galen showing a large fistulous branch of the posterior cerebral artery which enters the aneurysm at its anterosuperior border.

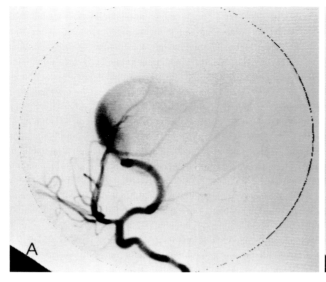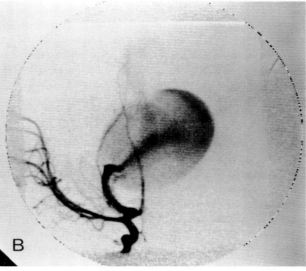

Figure 5. Lateral (**A**) and anteroposterior (**B**) views from a carotid angiogram showing a large fistulous branch of the posterior cerebral artery which enters the aneurysm at its inferolateral border.

Operative Routes

A variety of routes have been used to deal with a galenic malformation. These include transcallosal, subtemporal, and transtentorial routes.

The transcallosal route is the approach of choice for those galenic malformations in which the feeding vessels enter the lesion over the dome of the sac, particularly at its anterosuperior aspect. In those patients with multiple feeders entering from both sides it may be necessary to stage the transcallosal route—going in from one side initially and then approaching from the other side at a subsequent occasion.

The subtemporal approach is the best route to those malformations that are fed by one or occasionally by a union of both posterior cerebral arteries. The fistula can be clearly visualized by this route and successfully clipped or ligated.

The transtentorial route should be used only for those malformations in which there is a single feeding vessel entering at the level of the tentorial notch. By opening the tentorium the surgeon can obtain a clear view of this vessel which is usually a branch of the posterior cerebral artery that can directly enter the vein of Galen. However, in neonates with a massive dilated venous drainage system the tentorium is extremely vascular; opening into it risks massive hemorrhage and so the transtentorial route is not used in such patients.

Transcallosal Route

The patient is positioned supine with the head ele-vated 30° above the body and placed on a horseshoe headrest in anatomical position so that the nose faces directly forward (Fig. 6A). The vertex is then prepared and draped. The skin incision is square, with the anterior limb of the incision just behind the coronal suture and the medial portion of the incision just across the midline on the far side, extending back to just in front of the lambda from which the posterior transverse limb of the incision runs parallel to the anterior transverse limb. A free bone flap is turned and the dura opened. Care should be taken to preserve parasagittal draining veins. The dural opening is made in such a fashion as to preserve as many of the draining veins as possible.

Utilizing self-retaining brain retractors, the hemisphere is retracted away from the falx and the corpus callosum exposed (Fig. 6B). The corpus callosum is frequently thinned out by the underlying aneurysmal vein of Galen. In neonates there may be very large anterior cerebral arteries lying on the corpus callosum and penetrating through it into the aneurysm. Using suction or the ultrasonic aspirator, an opening is made through the corpus callosum which brings one on to the dome of the aneurysm. The aneurysmal sac is not adherent to brain and its wall is sufficiently thick that it can be mobilized so as to visualize the feeding arteries. As many feeding arteries as one can safely occlude should be clipped utilizing titanium clips (Fig. 6C). If one is successful, the sac will collapse or become less tense and the color of blood will change from red arterial blood to blue venous blood.

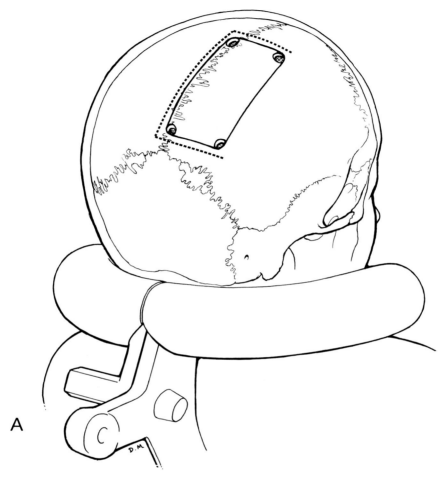

A

Figure 6. A, a line drawing showing the skin incision (*dashed line*) and bone flap for the transcallosal approach. **B,** retractors are on the falx and the right cerebral hemisphere. One draining vein has been divided in the course of elevating the dural flap. A distended feeding anterior cerebral artery branch can be seen beneath the arachnoid on the corpus callosum. **C,** the anterior cerebral feeder has been clipped. Retractors are separating the divided edges of the corpus callosum incision. The anterior cerebral artery feeder is entering the aneurysm at its anterosuperior border. A posterior cerebral artery feeder can be seen entering posteriorly and laterally on the aneurysm.

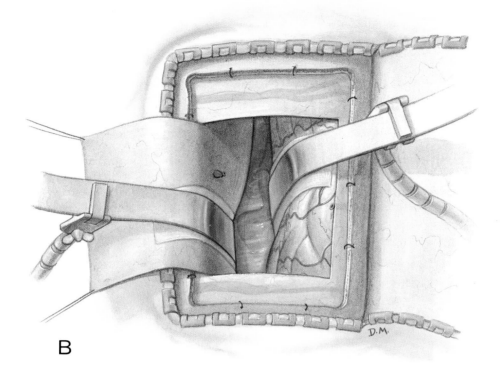

B

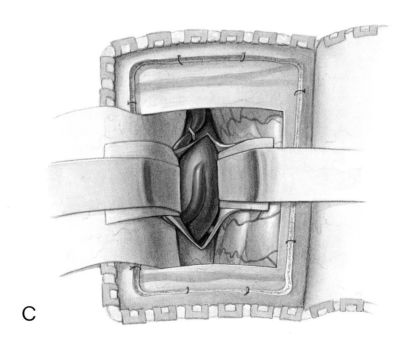

C

Figure 6. (*Continued*)

Subtemporal Route

In patients with a single branch of the posterior cerebral artery creating a fistulous tract into the vein of Galen or occasionally into the vein of Rosenthal and from there into the vein of Galen, a subtemporal route can be used to visualize the feeding vessel and directly ligate or clip it. This route is particularly useful in infants with a single posterior cerebral artery branch feeding directly into a greatly dilated vein of Galen.

The patient is positioned prone with the head turned to expose the side of the subtemporal approach (Fig. 7A). The skin incision extends from in front of the ear to above the squamosal temporal suture and goes back to the mastoid. An osteoplastic flap is turned and the dura opened. If the brain has been properly relaxed by treatment of the hydrocephalus and utilization of mannitol and hyperventilation, the temporal lobe can be easily retracted (Fig. 7B), the tentorial edge visualized, and the feeding posterior cerebral artery branch going into the aneurysm ligated or clipped (Figs. 7C and 8).

Transtentorial Route

If the feeding vessel comes in more posteriorly, it is useful to open the tentorium and retract upward on the temporal and occipital lobes and downward on the cerebellum in order to expose the aneurysm and find the feeding vessel which can enter the vein of Rosenthal, thus distending it as well as the vein of Galen.

The patient is positioned in much the same fashion as for the subtemporal route (Fig. 9A). However, the flap is more posteriorly placed so that one elevates the brain behind the vein of Labbé (Fig. 9B). The tentorium can be cut using a blunt hook and utilizing the monopolar cautery to coagulate and cut this structure. Once the fistulous vessel is exposed as it enters the vein of Rosenthal or vein of Galen, it can be clipped (Figs. 9C and 10).

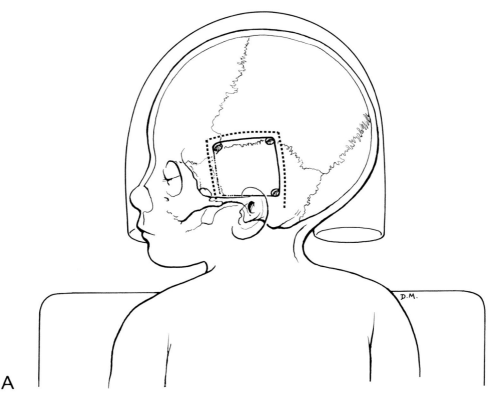

A

Figure 7. A, a line drawing showing the skin incision (*dashed line*) and bone flap for the subtemporal approach. **B,** a retractor has elevated the temporal lobe. The vein of Labbé is preserved. **C,** the temporal lobe has been further elevated, fully exposing the tentorial edge, the feeding posterior cerebral artery branch, and the aneurysm. A clip has been placed on this feeder.

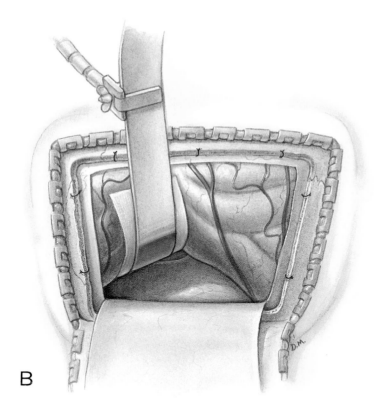

B

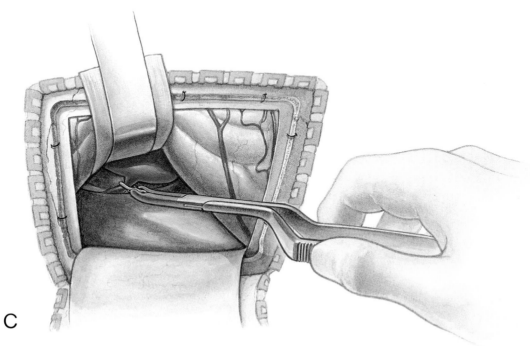

C

Figure 7. *(Continued)*

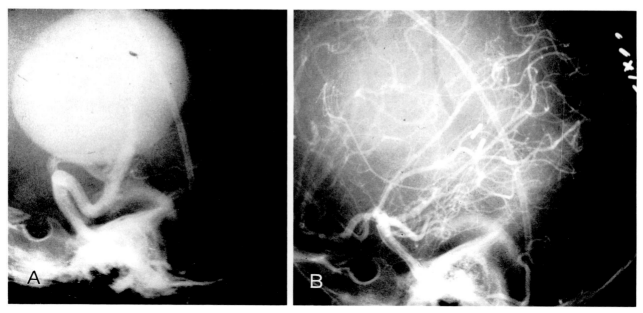

Figure 8. A, a lateral vertebral arteriogram showing a fistulous posterior cerebral branch entering the base of the aneurysm. **B,** a postoperative lateral vertebral arteriogram of the same patient showing the ligated fistulous branch and no filling of the aneurysm.

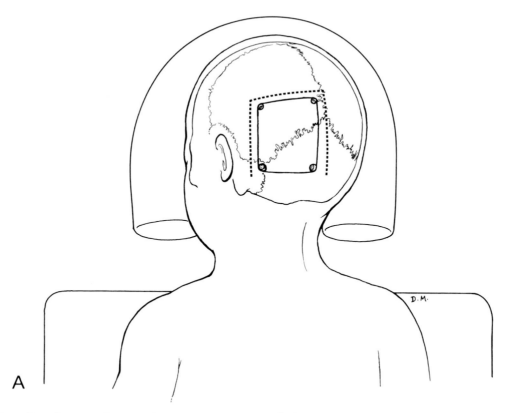

Figure 9. A, a line drawing showing the skin incision (*dashed line*) and bone flap for the transtentorial approach. **B,** a retractor is elevating the occipital lobe, exposing the tentorium. **C,** with further elevation of the occipital lobe and with the tentorium divided, a large feeding posterior cerebral artery branch is seen entering a distended vein of Rosenthal which is continuous with the vein of Galen.

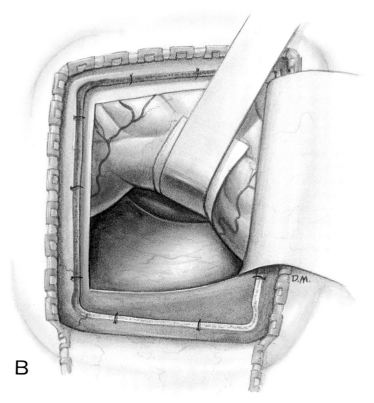

B

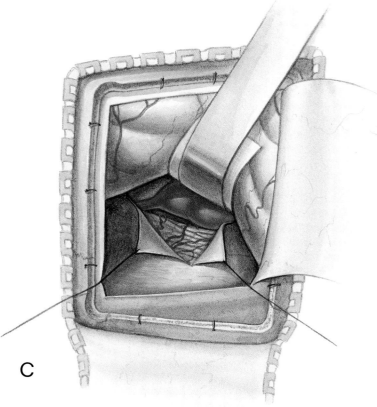

C

Figure 9. *(Continued)*

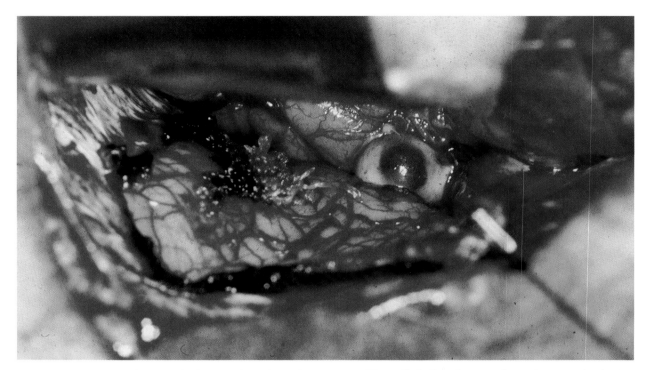

Figure 10. Operative photograph showing the split in the tentorium and the appearance of an aneurysmally dilated vein of Rosenthal after clipping of a posterior cerebral artery feeder.

Closure Techniques

The dura is tacked up to the bone flap and an epidural drain is left in place for 12 hours. The bone flap is reattached using nonabsorbable sutures. The scalp is closed in two layers using absorbable sutures in the galea and staples in the skin.

Monitoring

Normal perfusion pressure breakthrough has been reported in patients following direct surgery on an aneurysm of the vein of Galen. In most of these patients, the surgery has involved interfering with the venous drainage from the aneurysm. I believe that if the surgery is restricted to cutting off the arterial supply to the aneurysm and leaving the venous drainage intact, no problems should occur with normal perfusion pressure breakthrough. However, cortical blood flow can be measured using a thermal diffusion flow probe which will allow any postoperative hyperemic edema to be anticipated. It is important during the operation to not let the patient become hypovolemic and to maintain an adequate central venous pressure and a normal systolic blood pressure.

COMPLICATIONS

The wall of an aneurysm of a vein of Galen can on occasion be relatively thin and so the aneurysmal sac must be treated with care to avoid disastrous hemorrhage. As mentioned, normal perfusion pressure breakthrough has been reported, complicating surgery for vein of Galen aneurysms. If the surgery is restricted to occluding the feeding arteries entering the vein of Galen, normal perfusion pressure breakthrough should not occur. Such a maneuver is effective with these lesions in that, unlike the usual arteriovenous malformation, these feeding arteries are large fistulous tracts going directly into the vein of Galen, which has a normal but enlarged venous drainage.

SPINAL NERVE SCHWANNOMA

PHYO KIM, M.D.
BURTON M. ONOFRIO, M.D.

SELECTION OF PATIENTS

Intraspinal schwannomas may be subdivided as those purely intraspinal, abutting on, but not extending beyond, the lateral limits of the mid-pedicle, or those dumbbell-shaped, extending lateral to the pedicle. Dumbbell tumors may be primarily within the spinal canal with a minimal extent lateral to the pedicle, or primarily extraspinal into the posterior triangle of the neck, or into the thoracic, abdominal, or pelvic cavities with a minimal intraspinal component.

Most patients present with pain of long duration in the involved dermatomes; however, they may present with a mass in the posterior cervical triangle or may have an "incidental tumor" found on routine chest x-ray (Fig. 1). Various forms of long tract deficits may cause hand and/or leg numbness and weakness if spinal cord or cauda equina compression is the early sign of the presence of tumor. When a sacral tumor is present, sacral pain, saddle hypalgesia, or a urinary or anal sphincter disorder may be the first noted abnormality.

In a patient with von Recklinghausen's disease, multiple tumors are present. Determining the one or ones that are symptomatic may pose a difficult problem, as well as choosing which ones may be safely and appropriately removed while not upsetting the homeostasis the other nonsymptomatic lesions have at that time with other brain and/or spinal cord segments.

The definitive diagnosis of spinal nerve schwannoma is made on the basis of radiographic studies. Plain x-ray films of the spine (especially the appropriate oblique view) may show enlargement of the intervertebral foramen (Fig. 2) or erosion of the adjacent vertebral bodies, pedicles, or transverse processes (Fig. 3). The cortical margins of the bone are usually well-maintained, denoting the slow growth pattern of these benign lesions. The tumor mass may be visualized by plain and enhanced computed tomography (CT) scans. Magnetic resonance imaging scans using T1 weighted imaging with gadolinium enhancement and T2 weighted imaging, either of the entire spine or tailored to the appropriate segments, best defines the mass and the soft tissue interphase with the spinal cord or cauda equina. Water-soluble contrast myelography and postmyelogram CT scanning show the relationship of the mass with the subarachnoid space. Myelography is particularly useful to rule out dural and arachnoid diverticulae which may be confused with solid or cystic tumors, especially in the posterior mediastinum. These spinal fluid diverticulae may not require surgery since they are usually innocuous incidental lesions. Postmyelogram CT scanning may indicate, especially in dumbbell tumors, those which are

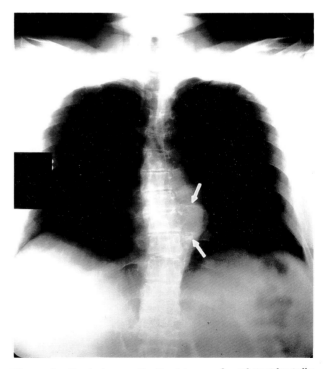

Figure 1. Posterior mediastinal tumor found incidentally on a routine chest x-ray film (*arrows*). Note left T9-T10 rib erosion with intact bony cortical margins indicative of an indolent tumor growth pattern.

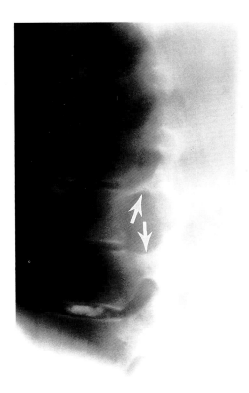

Figure 2. An oblique thoracic spine film shows marked foraminal enlargement with intact pedicle and facet cortical margins (*arrows*).

amenable to total removal solely by the anterior approach (Fig. 4).

If the segment is functionally critical, namely, spinal roots at the levels of C5-T1 and L3-S1, many surgeons have attempted partial root preservation, fearing significant functional loss to a limb. Recent studies at the Mayo Clinic showed that detectable neurologic deficit occurs only infrequently after division of the root (C5-T1, L3-S1) together with the tumor. The trend was consistent throughout the cases irrespective of tumor size and extension (intradural, extradural, and intra-extradural mass). The postoperative deficits, which appeared in a small group, were partial, and good functional recovery was always achieved after physical therapy. Therefore, if the tumor is infiltrating diffusely into the host nerve root(lets), our current practice is to remove the entire involved root to achieve complete tumor removal.

To plan an appropriate skin incision, especially in cases of a thoracic region tumor, a skin marker is placed at the level of the lesion either during myelography or using fluoroscopy the night before the operation. When the sitting position is to be used for laminectomy for tumors in the cervical region, patients should undergo a thorough cardiac examination to rule out atrial septal defects. Intraoperatively, the anesthesiologist takes measures to prevent air embolism, such as placing a central venous catheter in the atrium and attaching a Doppler monitor probe on the

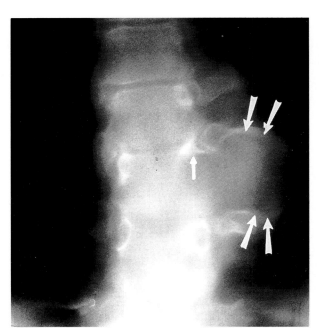

Figure 3. Anteroposterior tomogram shows left vertebral body, pedicle (*single arrow*), and proximal rib (*double arrows*) erosion.

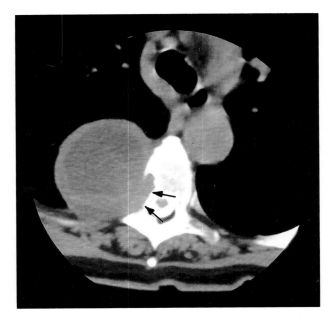

Figure 4. Although vertebral body erosion has occurred, as shown on this postmyelogram CT scan, this multidensity posterior mediastinal tumor causes no significant deformation of the subarachnoid space (*arrows*) and was removed entirely from the anterior, transthoracic approach.

anterior wall of the chest. Intraesophageal echocardiography may be useful in detecting and visualizing the presence of air in the atrium during the surgery. Maintenance of a normal blood pressure range intraoperatively is critical to prevent neurologic complications secondary to defective spinal cord autoregulation. Prophylactic antibiotics (we use vancomycin, 1 g, intravenously) are given during the induction of anesthesia. Somatosensory evoked potential monitoring is used to minimize the risks of injury in tumors causing significant compression of the spinal cord or cauda equina.

SURGICAL PROCEDURE

Concerning solely extradural tumors, when the extradural segment of the parent nerve root proximal to the tumor is long enough, an anterior approach with piecemeal removal and intraforaminal debulking will deliver the root safely into view and permit a silver clip application proximally, thus precluding a spinal fluid leak. If the tumor is fibrous, not lending itself to debulking into the foramen or if the origin of the tumor from the root is too close to the common dural sac, a combined anterior and posterior approach will be needed (Fig. 5).

If the dumbbell tumor is in the cervical segments and has a significant intraspinal segment, we prefer a posterior approach with a total facetectomy at the appropriate level. In the vast majority of cases, even when large, the extraspinal tumor may be delivered piecemeal. The surgeon, staying within the tumor capsule posteriorly, gently pulls on the tumor capsule while placing countertraction on the structures abutting

the capsule. Using bipolar coagulation, meticulous hemostasis may be achieved and clear visibility reduces the chance of injury to the carotid sheath and vertebral artery (Fig. 6).

For thoracic dumbbell tumors extending 1 cm beyond the lateral aspect of the facet on the anteroposterior imaging studies, the patient is placed in the lateral position and the chest, abdomen, and back are

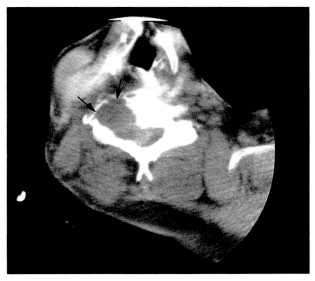

Figure 6. This tumor has not extended beyond the confines of an eroded and expanded cervical spine segment (*arrows*) and may be removed totally using the posterior laminectomy approach. Water-soluble myelography with postmyelogram CT scanning should be used to define the possibility of an intradural component prior to surgery.

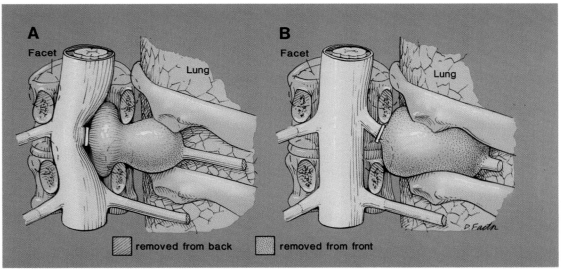

Figure 5. **A** and **B,** the parent root foramen, harboring a tumor, has been enlarged in both examples. The tumor in *A* demands a posterior and anterior approach. The tumor in *B* may be removed totally with an anterior approach.

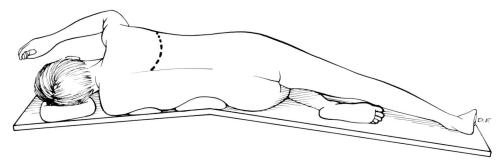

Figure 7. The lateral position used for the thoracotomy when employing the anterior approach may be modified intraoperatively to allow a posterior laminectomy approach, in the non-obese patient, by rotating the patient forward, exposing the thoracic spines posteriorly.

prepared and draped. A thoracic surgeon performs an intercostal incision between the ribs corresponding to the vertebral segment involved (Fig. 7). The team approach maintains safety in reflecting the aorta on the left or the vena cava on the right. The head of the rib caudal to the foramen is removed. If the tumor is on the T8 nerve root, the head of the T9 rib is removed to visualize the foramen involved. The intercostal artery and veins may be safely controlled both proximal and distal to the tumor and clipped. The tumor is debulked, maintaining the tumor capsule integrity if possible. As the debulking is carried medially through the foramen, visualization of the parent nerve proximal to the tumor may be possible if the tumor is soft or partially cystic. If a clip can safely be applied to the root proximal to the tumor, a posterior approach is not needed. If the tumor is fibrous or there is not a suitable proximal uninvolved segment of nerve long enough to clip, the procedure is terminated, silver clips applied to the tumor margins, the chest incision closed, a drain inserted into the pleural cavity and attached to underwater suction, and the patient turned to the prone position. The back is prepared and draped and the spinous processes of the adjacent vertebral segments along with laminae and facet joint are exposed widely. A total hemilaminectomy of the cephalad and caudal segments is done on the appropriate side. The total facetectomy is performed at the involved foraminal level, the ligamentum flavum is removed, and a plane is achieved medial to the tumor. The parent root is found and doubly clipped or ligated to prevent a spinal fluid leak, and the remaining tumor is removed. An orthopedist evaluates the need for a fusion at this juncture.

In aesthenic patients, the anterior intercostal approach in the lateral position may be extended to include the posterior vertebral elements for facet and lamina removal without closing the chest. By rotating the patient 45° anteriorly, the posterior vertebral elements may be explored with the chest still open.

Extending the safety limits of either the anterior or posterior approach is to be avoided. If needed, the two approaches using the same anesthetic are well-tolerated in the thoracic, lumbar, or sacral segments. Working in the depth of one approach to avoid a second incision risks spinal cord, major vessel, or visceral damage and that philosophy is to be avoided (Fig. 8). For dumbbell sacral tumors, an anterior transdural approach plus a second phase, same anesthetic, prone posterior approach, is usually needed (Fig. 9).

Solely intradural tumors demand adequate visualization to delineate the proximal and distal parent nerve root, to prevent avulsion from the ventral spinal cord with disastrous subpial hemorrhage. Removing the lamina and performing a facetectomy, flush with the pedicle, on the side of the tumor, ensure an adequate field for safe tumor removal.

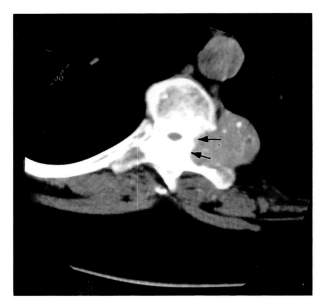

Figure 8. The foramen is massively eroded by tumor. However, because of a tight irregular tumor common dural interface (*arrows*), intracapsular subtotal tumor removal anteriorly will likely need to be followed by a posterior partial hemilaminectomy and total foraminotomy to allow safe and total tumor removal.

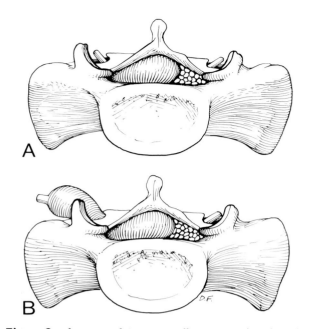

Figure 9. **A,** a sacral tumor totally contained within the sacral canal needs only a posterior approach. **B,** any extension anterior to the sacral foramen will need an anterior and posterior approach.

When an intradural tumor extends through the foramen anteriorly in the cervical segments, the tumor and nerve root are removed piecemeal. A fascia lata or homologous dural graft is used to close the dura laterally after the tumor removal has been accomplished (Fig. 10, A and B). Rarely is there a need for a second stage procedure anteriorly to remove "unreachable" tumor extending anteriorly. If there is residual tumor, the second stage anteriorly is done several weeks later after the dural graft has been well-incorporated, to prevent a cerebrospinal fluid collection in the anterior neck after the second stage procedure.

Dumbbell intradural thoracic tumors with significant anterior extension should also be staged to avoid a spinal fluid leak communicating with a negative pressure intrapleural space, possibly precipitating low pressure headaches and postoperative subdural intracranial hematomata caused by the persistent cerebrospinal fluid pleural fistula. For dumbbell intradural tumors affecting the spine below the diaphragm, the posterior and anterior approach may be done the same day, with the surgeon attempting a watertight dural closure. The lack of a significant negative pressure system intraabdominally makes a persistent extraspinal cerebrospinal fluid collection unlikely.

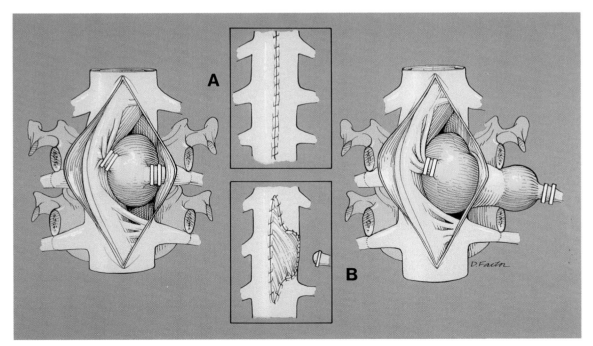

Figure 10. **A,** totally intradural tumor, **B,** an intra-extradural extraspinal dumbbell tumor.

Our preference in case of a laminectomy for a cervical region tumor is the sitting position, since this allows excellent exposure with gravity drainage of blood and cerebrospinal fluid, maintaining a relatively bloodless field. A Gardner headholder with three pins is placed on the head, with the pins on the frontal or parietal area avoiding the temporal squama. The upper half of the table is raised about 60°, and the lower half is raised to elevate the legs. The headholder is secured to a frame connected to the siderail of the table, and the neck is positioned in moderate flexion to make the alignment of the vertebrae approximately vertical. The flexion of the neck should not be excessive to prevent occlusion of the jugular vein or anterior cord compression in patients harboring moderate spondylosis. To minimize the risk of air embolization pertinent to the position, meticulous precautions should be made, such as waxing all exposed bone edges and remaining subperiosteal as much as possible when reflecting the muscles prior to performing the laminectomy.

COMBINED CRANIOFACIAL RESECTION FOR ANTERIOR SKULL BASE TUMORS

EHUD ARBIT, M.D.

JATIN SHAH, M.D.

INTRODUCTION

The rationale for combined craniofacial resection of a skull base tumor is that this procedure can achieve a complete monoblock excision of the tumor with adequate margins. Our experience suggests that this is the most effective approach to local control of disease, and, in combination with radiation therapy and chemotherapy, it may also improve long-term survival.

A wide variety of tumors may involve the anterior skull base. They may be grouped into three main categories according to their site of origin: 1) tumors that originate in the nasal cavity or paranasal sinuses and extend to the skull base; 2) tumors arising from the orbital contents or lacrimal gland, which may ultimately erode the orbit and skull base; and 3) tumors of intracranial origin that transcend the skull base to involve the orbit, nasal cavity, paranasal sinuses, or infratemporal fossa. The last group are usually either meningiomas or metastases.

The most common tumors in these areas are malignant and arise in the paranasal sinuses. Most are of epithelial origin and include, in order of frequency, epidermoid carcinoma, undifferentiated carcinoma, and adenocarcinoma. Fewer than one-third of these tumors are of salivary gland origin. Approximately 10% are esthesioneuroblastomas arising from the olfactory epithelium. There are also rare cases of various sarcomas, lymphomas, metastases, and ectopic meningiomas. Tumors of paranasal sinus origin most often occur in the fifth and sixth decades of life, with the exception of the esthesioneuroblastoma, which is more common in the third and fourth decades of life.

PRESENTING SYMPTOMS

Presenting symptoms and signs are seldom characteristic and are often confused with those of sinusitis or allergic rhinitis. The most common complaints are nasal stuffiness, obstruction, nonspecific sinus dis-

charge, and occasionally local pain. Less frequent symptoms include periorbital edema, pain over the cheek and forehead, and excessive lacrimation. Rare symptoms include epistaxis and cerebrospinal fluid (CSF) rhinorrhea.

Neurologic symptoms indicate that the disease is more advanced, with extension of the tumor beyond the sinuses or into the cranial cavity. Anosmia indicates involvement of the olfactory nerves and is commonly associated with esthesioneuroblastoma and olfactory groove meningioma. However, essentially all tumors that erode the cribriform plate or infiltrate the nasal cavity can cause anosmia. Hypesthesia or pain in the cheek may indicate extracranial involvement of the maxillary nerve or erosion of the skull base in the foramen rotundum area. Ocular motor signs and diplopia may result either from nerve involvement or displacement of the globe, due either to intraorbital extension of the tumor or to intracranial invasion through the foramen lacerum into the middle fossa, cavernous sinus, and/or superior orbital fissure. Trismus usually indicates involvement of the pterygoid fossa.

RADIOGRAPHIC EVALUATION

Invaluable clinical information may be gained by the radiographic evaluation of the paranasal sinuses, skull base, and adjacent brain. Visualization of soft tissue detail relative to osseous walls and air spaces in the sinuses, as well as delineation of disease processes beyond the boundaries of the sinuses, are indispensable in determining operability and in planning radiotherapy. Radiographically, it is important to assess the extent of the soft tissue mass in the infratemporal fossa, in the parapharyngeal space, and in the frontal and temporal fossae. Critical to determining operability are the pterygoid region, nasopharynx, sphenoid sinus, cavernous sinus, orbital apex, and cerebrum. Edema in the frontal lobes, in the absence of an enhancing tumor, suggests that the dura is involved and in some instances bridged by microscopic foci of tumor.

Before the decision is made as to operability, in cases where the tumor originated in the paranasal sinuses, patients routinely undergo biopsy to determine the histology of the tumor. Treatment planning and discussion with the patient are facilitated by this information, as the prognosis depends largely on the type of tumor present.

The indications for combined craniofacial resection are still somewhat subjective. Cases that should be considered include those in which the tumor originates in the nasal cavity, maxillary antrum, or orbit, extends to the frontal ethmoid or sphenoid sinus complex, and may or may not involve the base of the skull and dura. The objective is to achieve a gross monoblock resection of the tumor with clear surrounding margins. When this goal is impossible—e.g., because of invasion of the cavernous sinus or cerebrum beyond the frontal lobes—craniofacial resection is contraindicated.

SURGICAL TECHNIQUES

Before surgery, nasal cultures are obtained. Patients are also evaluated by a prosthodontist so that prostheses to replace parts of the palate, maxilla, or orbit can be made if necessary. Antibiotics and glucocorticosteroids are started preoperatively.

The operation is performed under general anesthesia with endotracheal intubation. The tube is placed in the mouth on the side contralateral to the procedure, and the oral cavity is packed with gauze to avoid the subsequent postoperative aspiration or swallowing of pooled blood. Arterial and venous lines are placed, as is a central venous pressure line. The patient is turned on his side, and two spinal needles (18-gauge) are introduced for continuous intraoperative drainage of CSF. After these preparations, the patient is returned to the supine position. The needles are secured through the gap in the operating room table and mattress, and connected to an intravenous extension line, which in turn is connected to a large glass syringe. The entire drainage system is sealed in sterile plastic bags. This closed system allows for continuous drainage, while saving CSF, which can be used at the end of the procedure for reexpansion of the brain.

Following initial preparation, the head is fixed in a three-pin Mayfield headrest in a straight supine position, with a mild elevation and a 15–20° extension. This fixed position permits visualization of the anterior fossa as far back as the anterior clinoid processes, while providing adequate working exposure of the cribriform plate and planum sphenoidale with minimal brain retraction. The eyes are protected with corneal shields and the head is shaved and prepared with Betadine. While the head is being prepared, a split thickness skin graft is obtained from the thigh and preserved in antibiotic and saline solution, for later use in covering the mucosal defect.

The scalp incision—usually a bicoronal scalp incision—is outlined with a marking pen (Fig. 1A). After infiltration with an epinephrine/Xylocaine solution, the skin is incised as deep as the galea, carefully preserving the integrity of the underlying pericranium. After incision of the galea, a subgaleal plane is developed, the posterior scalp flap is retracted as far as possible, and the pericranium under this posterior part of the flap is incised and elevated with a periosteal elevator (Fig. 1B). The anterior scalp flap, with attached pericranium, and the temporal muscle on one or both sides, are elevated from the skull and from the superior temporal lines. This subperiosteal dissection proceeds to the supraorbital ridges and glabella (Fig. 1C).

At this point, a free cranial bone flap is raised (Fig. 2). Usually this is a bifrontal flap; however, for smaller lateral lesions, we have used a one-sided flap that scarcely crosses the midline. In raising the bone flap, we try to avoid burr holes in the low frontal area. The Midas Rex high-speed drill/knife is effective in sawing through the anterior wall of the frontal sinus (Fig. 2). To provide visualization and maneuverability in the posterior frontal region with minimal cerebral retraction, it is important to raise a low flap, the inferior margins of which are the superior orbital ridges, regardless of the location of the frontal sinus. After being elevated, the flap is removed from the operating field. The frontal sinus mucosa is exenterated with pituitary rongeurs, and the sinuses packed with Gelfoam and antibiotic solution. The posterior wall of the frontal sinus can be sawed with a high-speed drill or removed piecemeal with rongeurs. While the bone flap is elevated, it is important to preserve the integrity of the dura, and all dural tears should be repaired immediately.

Because most craniofacial operations are performed for extradural tumors, dissection in these instances is strictly extradural. The dura is gently elevated off the orbital roofs and the anterior fossa. It may be helpful during this maneuver to vent CSF, thereby shrinking the intradural volume, and to use a self-retaining retractor (e.g., Greenberg or Leyla retractor). Dural dissection of the orbital roof is fairly simple. However, separation of the dura from the multifidous crista galli at the midline can be more difficult. We often elect to free the crista from its base with sharp instruments or narrow-tipped rongeurs, and to elevate the dura with part of the crista. The olfactory

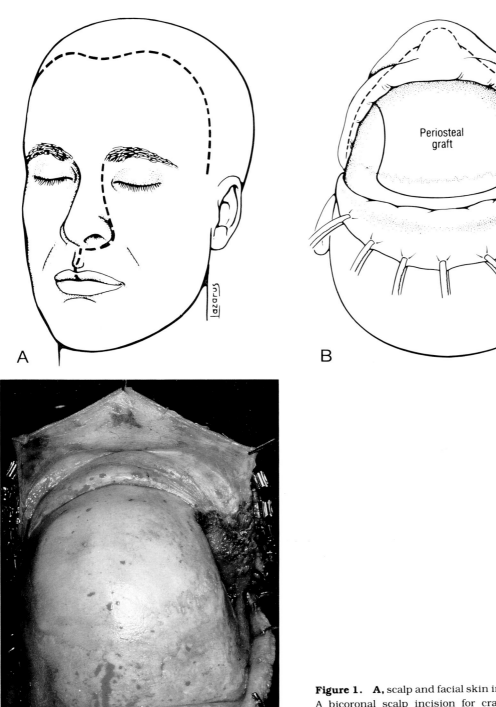

Figure 1. **A,** scalp and facial skin incisions (*dashed lines*). A bicoronal scalp incision for craniotomy and a Weber-Fergusson incision for the facial exposure are shown. **B,** the scalp flap is reflected posteriorly to permit elevation of the pericranial (periosteal) graft. **C,** the pericranial flap is reflected anteriorly as far as the supraorbital ridges.

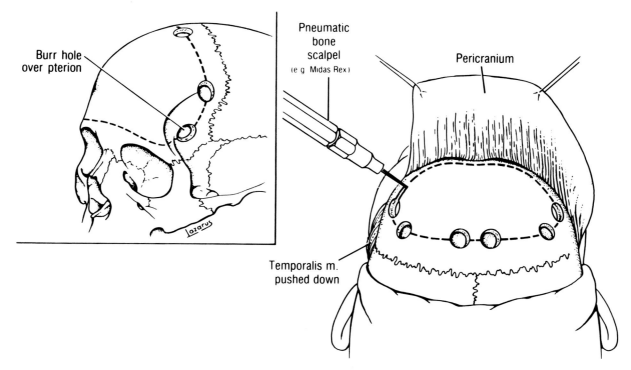

Figure 2. Burr holes are made and the frontal bone overlying the sinuses is cut with a pneumatic bone scalpel.

rootlets are cut sharply from the cribriform plate (Fig. 3). If any holes were created during dissection in the dura overlying the crista galli and cribriform plate, these are now sutured meticulously.

In cases where the tumor bridges the dura and extends intracranially, no attempt is made initially to separate the basal dura from the skull base. Instead, the dura is opened along the floor of the anterior fossa. The falx cerebri is transected, and frontal lobes are elevated and inspected. By careful dissection, the tumor usually can be separated from the brain parenchyma and then removed. Ideally, the tumor is separated first from the brain parenchyma, and then the entire circumference of the dura is incised, in order to include all of the involved dura in the specimen. The intracranial tumor and the dura are then separated from the skull base and removed from the operating field. Afterward, the remaining basal dura is elevated from the base of skull, using the same steps as for tumors that do not invade the intracranial compartment. When the dura has been elevated and exposed, the dural defect is sutured either primarily, if there is enough dural tissue, or using a pericranial graft or temporalis fascia graft. Meticulous closing of the dura is crucial in preventing a CSF leak and potential infection.

The next phase of the operation is to prepare for extirpation of the remaining specimen. This is accomplished by an osteotomy through the planum sphenoidale and the roof of the ethmoids on either or both sides (Fig. 4). If the bone is thin, a fine osteotome is used. On the other hand, for thicker bone, the Hall microdrill or Midas Rex knife is appropriate. After mobilization of the superior surface of the specimen, the bone flap is temporarily replaced and secured loosely to the skull in order to protect the brain during the facial resection.

The facial component of the operation begins with a Weber-Fergusson incision using either a Dieffenbach or Lynch extension, depending on whether a medial, partial, or total maxillectomy, with or without orbital exenteration, is indicated (Fig. 1A). In cases where tumor extends into the antrum, a medial maxillectomy with exenteration of the nasal cavity and palatal fenestration, or partial maxillectomy removing only the hard palate on that side, is performed. The skin incision is deepened from the facial soft tissues to the periosteum, and the cheek flap is elevated and retracted laterally with skin hooks (Fig. 5A). At the upper end of the incision, the medial canthal ligament is identified, detached, and marked for reapproximation at the end of the procedure. The infraorbital nerve is sectioned inferiorly, and the anterior wall of the maxilla is exposed (Fig. 5, *B* and *C*). The hard palate is preserved whenever possible, in order to spare the

patient impairment in swallowing and speech. The nasal septum, however, is frequently removed to provide access to the ethmoid sinuses.

For tumors requiring palatal resection, a dissection is made through the hard palate either at or just off the midline, in order to spare as many teeth as possible for fixation of a dental prosthesis. The incision is carried through the midline of the hard palate and the ipsilateral soft palate. Laterally, the osteotomy proceeds through the zygomatic arch. If the orbit is preserved, the medial orbital walls are carefully freed from the periorbita. By reflecting the nose and the nasal septum laterally, it is possible to remove the entire specimen with the ethmoid sinuses of the opposite side.

After the facial specimen has been freed, the neurosurgeon rejoins the operation and removes the specimen en bloc from the facial and cranial sides. The resected specimen usually includes the tumor, the entire cribriform plate, the superior and middle turbinates on one or both sides, and occasionally the orbit. During the separation of the specimen, difficulty arises at the point where the maxilla is attached to the pterygoid plates. Here the specimen must be freed by blunt, and often blind, dissection from the sphenopalatine fossa. In cases where an orbital exenteration is indicated, the optic nerve and the ophthalmic artery are exposed at the orbital apex, the ophthalmic artery is ligated and cut, and the optic nerve is sharply transected at the optic foramen.

After the specimen has been removed, hemostasis is established. Irregular bone edges are rongeured or smoothed for reconstruction. All redundant mucosa is carefully trimmed and removed to prevent formation of postoperative polyps.

Reconstruction of the skull base takes place in three stages. The first stage is the closure of the dura, either primarily or using a free graft, either of temporalis fascia or of pericranium. In the second stage, the pedicled periosteal flap is rotated, laid over the bony defect on the floor of the anterior cranial fossa, and secured both to the basal dura and the bony skull base (Fig. 6). In cases where the orbit has been exenterated, it is simpler to secure the pedicled flap to the basal dura and bone through the orbital defect. The last stage of reconstruction includes the application of a split thickness skin graft to the exterior of the periosteal flap. The skin graft is applied from the facial aspect and meticulously positioned into the bony crevices and over the soft tissue surfaces. It is important to achieve a good approximation of the graft against the pericranial flap. The graft is sutured peripherally to the undersurface of the skin flaps and held in position with a snug packing of Xeroform gauze.

The craniotomy and facial incisions are closed using standard techniques. However, before the bone

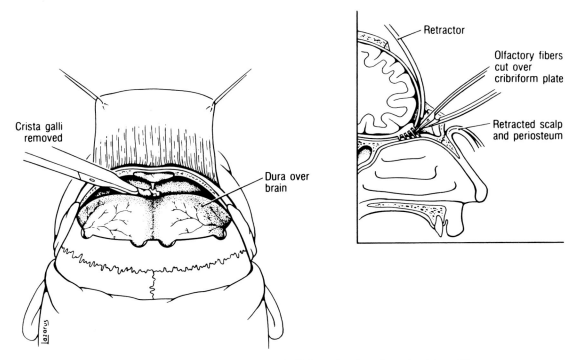

Figure 3. The dura is dissected off the orbital roofs and crista galli.

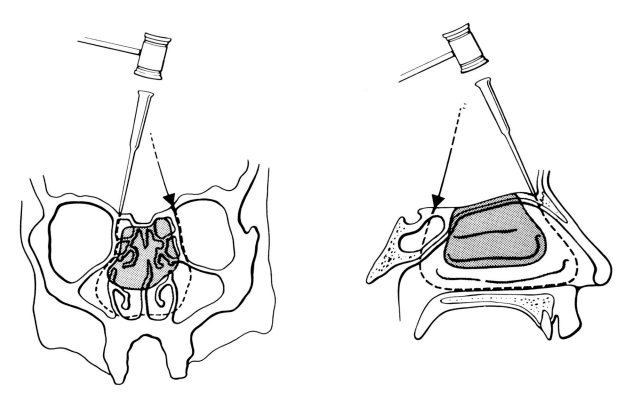

Figure 4. The frontal floor is separated along the planum sphenoidale and the roof of the ethmoid air cells; the use of an osteotome or microdrill is appropriate.

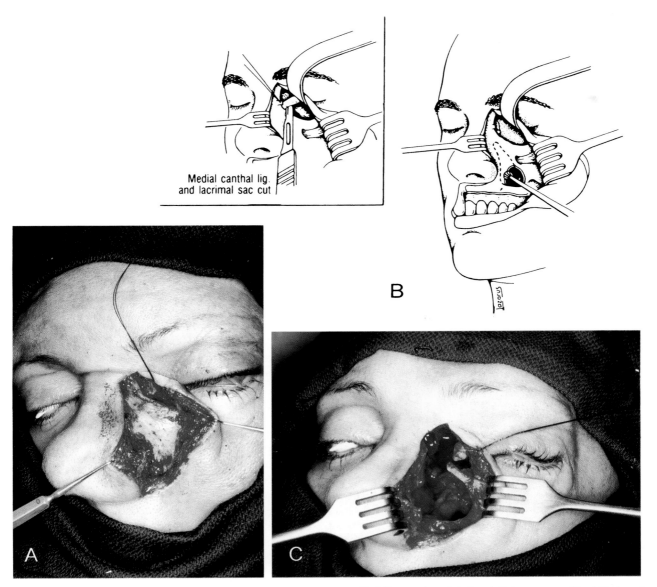

Figure 5. **A,** the facial skin is incised and the cheek flap is elevated and retracted with skin hooks. **B** and **C,** the medial canthal ligament and infraorbital nerve are identified and transected. A maxillectomy is performed.

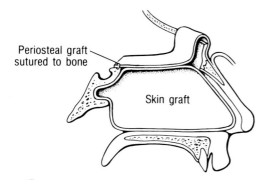

Figure 6. Reconstruction of the anterior skull base. After closure of the dura, the pedicled periosteal flap is applied and secured to the bony margins of the skull defect and to the basal dura. A split thickness skin graft is applied from the facial aspect to the maxillectomy defect and the undersurface of the periosteal flap.

flap is replaced, CSF is reintroduced through the lumbar drains to expand the brain and fill the subarachnoid spaces. Bone grafting may be necessary for cosmetic reasons, especially to fill defects in the glabellar region (Fig. 7, A–C). After the bone flap is replaced, the epidural space is minimized with tenting dural sutures. An epidural suction drain such as a Jackson-Pratt drain is routinely used and the scalp is closed in two conventional layers.

The spinal needles are removed. The patient is transferred to an intensive care unit, where vital signs and neurologic status are monitored for 24 hours. Intravenous broad-spectrum antibiotics, anticonvulsants, and steroids are routinely prescribed in the postoperative period. The drains are kept in place for 2–3 days, and the antral packing is kept in place for 5–10 days, during which time the patient remains on antibiotics. When the packing is removed, the defect is either repacked loosely or covered with an interim dental prosthesis. The skin grafted area is irrigated on a daily basis after the packing is removed, and, if necessary, necrotic shreds of the skin graft are debrided to expedite epithelialization of the exposed surfaces.

For the first three days after surgery, the patient is kept in the recumbent position, in order to avoid the egress of CSF or ingress of air, which would cause tension pneumocephalus. Fluids should be restricted to prevent brain edema.

COMPLICATIONS

Combined craniofacial resection is a fairly extensive procedure, in which two distinct compartments, the intradural-subarachnoid space and the paranasal sinuses, are entered into and made contiguous. Given these circumstances, the rate of complications associated with the procedure itself is quite low, and may reasonably be considered acceptable. Careful patient selection, preoperative planning, and meticulous adherence to basic surgical and neurosurgical techniques all reduce the associated risks. The reported mortality, including that observed in our patients, ranges from 3 to 5%. Morbidity, including minor and major complications, ranges from 15 to 20%.

Complications regarded as minor include local seromas, sloughing of the skin graft, and pneumocephalus. Major complications include cerebral edema, contusion, or hemorrhage, infection, meningitis, tension pneumocephalus, and CSF fistula. Although little can be done to prevent minor complications, these usually resolve spontaneously.

To prevent the more serious complications, several important measures can be taken. Prevention of brain edema and contusion is of the utmost importance. Working lumbar drains to vent CSF, and comprehensive use of hyperventilation and diuretics (mannitol and Lasix) throughout the long procedure are paramount. CSF fistulae can be prevented by achieving watertight dural closure and skull base repair. It is recommended that dural openings be addressed as they occur, and closed either primarily with 4-0 Nurolon sutures or by tissue grafting. If a CSF fistula does occur, we recommend placing the patient in the supine position with one or two indwelling lumbar drains, and reducing the intracranial pressure for a few days. In most cases, the CSF fistula will resolve spontaneously. However, CSF leaks lasting a few days are not uncommon. If a leak persists, the insertion of an indwelling lumbar drain for continuous CSF venting is indicated. The need to reexplore the wound to repair a CSF leak is exceedingly rare.

Tension pneumocephalus may be a life-threatening condition unless it is promptly addressed. Usually it is due to enlargement of a trapped pocket of intracranial air from the time of surgery, compounded by a CSF leak. Meticulous dural repair, reexpansion of the brain at the end of the operation, placement of subdural and/or epidural drains intraoperatively, and maintenance of the recumbent position for at least two days postoperatively all reduce the risk of tension pneumocephalus. If it does occur, however, drainage must be promptly begun, to vent air and decrease the intracranial pressure. After verification by computed tomography scan or skull films that there is no underlying brain parenchyma, a polyethylene venous catheter placed through one of the burr holes provides effective drainage.

Infection may become a life-threatening situation, whether in the form of meningitis, infection of the bone flap, or empyema. Preventive measures are essential. Prior to surgery, nasal cultures should be taken and antibiotics begun; antibiotics should be given continu-

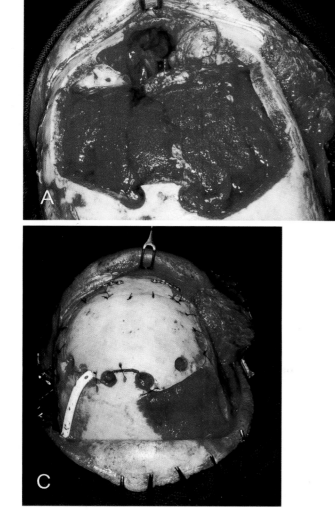

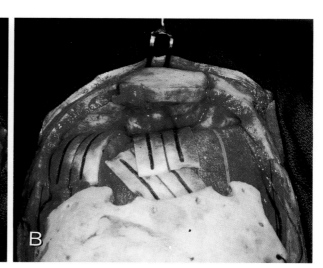

Figure 7.   A, in this case, tumor involved the frontal sinus, frontal bone, and medial aspect of the orbit. The involved bone has been removed to expose the nasal cavity and the orbital adipose tissue. **B,** to reconstruct the skull defect in the glabellar region, a split thickness bone graft has been harvested from the right posterior frontoparietal area and has been carved to provide for a cosmetically acceptable repair. **C,** the view of the cranium prior to closure. The bone graft harvested from the right posterior frontoparietal area is in position at the glabellar region and has been fixed in place with Synthes miniplates and screws. A Jackson-Pratt drain has been left in the epidural space.

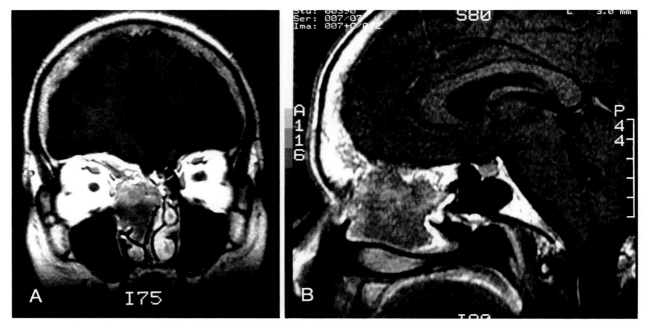

Figure 8.   **A** and **B,** a typical case for craniofacial resection. Coronal and sagittal magnetic resonance images demon- strate a paranasal sinus tumor eroding the anterior skull base; note the absence of intracranial tumor and edema.

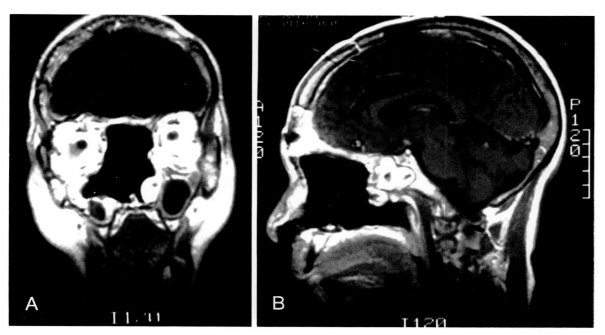

Figure 9.   **A** and **B,** coronal and sagittal magnetic resonance images after resection. Note the extent of the resection and the reconstruction.

ously until the nasal packing is removed. Any rise in the patient's temperature should be regarded as serious. If pyrexia develops, meningitis should be considered immediately and ruled out by lumbar puncture.

RESULTS

The prognosis for patients who undergo combined craniofacial resections is generally favorable (Figs. 8 and 9). The overall median survival in our series is five years. Survival time depends largely on the histological type and grade of the tumor, and on the presence or absence of intracranial involvement. Excellent local control can be achieved in well-differentiated adenocarcinoma and squamous cell carcinoma. However, successful control is less likely with anaplastic epithelial tumors and sarcomas. Although intracranial extension adversely affects prognosis, limited intracranial invasion is not necessarily a surgical contraindication. In patients with neurologic dysfunction for whom the prospect of local control by chemotherapy or radiation therapy is poor, palliation may be sufficient reason for surgery, since the morbidity of the procedure itself is fairly low.

Radiation therapy and chemotherapy are important adjuncts to surgery. Even for patients with well-differentiated tumors that have been removed with clear margins, we advocate postoperative radiation and perhaps chemotherapy. At this stage, control of potential microscopic residual disease may depend on these treatments. In tumors that are of higher grade, have less clearly defined margins, or invade the intracranial space, we often use preoperative radiation and chemotherapy to shrink the tumor first to make surgical resection possible.

SUMMARY

Tumors involving the base of the skull can be resected successfully using a combined craniofacial approach, with minimum morbidity and acceptable mortality. Unfavorable prognostic factors include intracranial extension, high-grade histology of the tumor, and previous treatment failure. With the sophisticated diagnostic techniques now available, particularly brain imaging methods, tumor margins can be defined preoperatively with increasing clarity. As methods of adjuvant therapy become more effective, craniofacial procedures will be appropriate in a wider variety of cases, and their benefits will increase accordingly.

DIAGNOSTIC OPEN BRAIN AND MENINGEAL BIOPSY

RICHARD P. ANDERSON, M.D.
HOWARD H. KAUFMAN, M.D.
SYDNEY S. SCHOCHET, M.D.

INTRODUCTION

There are circumstances in which patients with obvious brain disease may require specific diagnosis, and this can only be accomplished through the evaluation of brain tissue. This occurs in two circumstances:

1. Chronic bilateral cerebral symptoms and signs associated with progressive dementia and/or profound behavioral change; or
2. Unilateral, often localizable findings which are frequently associated with other signs of meningoencephalitis.

In addition, biopsies should be performed only when the results of these studies have the potential for modifying therapy or are useful in genetic counseling. A list is provided below to give a clearer understanding of those disease categories in which biopsy is useful and/or necessary in arriving at a final diagnosis.

Infections
  Bacterial cerebritis (*Whipple's disease, nocardiosis, mycobacterial infection*)
  Fungal cerebritis (*aspergillosis, mucormycosis*)
  Parasitic disease (*toxoplasmosis*)
  Viral encephalitis
  Chronic leptomeningitis

Collagen Vascular Disorders
  Sarcoidosis
  Granulomatous angiitis
  Various vasculitides
  Various connective tissue diseases

Dementias of Childhood
  Alexander's disease
  Canavan's disease
  Lafora's disease
  Neuroaxonal dystrophy
  Ceroid lipofuscinosis—rarely indicated

Dementias of Adulthood
  Pick's disease
  Creutzfeldt-Jakob disease
  Alzheimer's disease—rarely indicated

Neoplasms
  Primary and metastatic

Acute problems requiring brain biopsy would include certain cases of encephalitis and suspected vasculitis. Opinions vary as to the need for biopsy in the diagnosis of herpes simplex encephalitis now that relatively less toxic drugs such as acyclovir are available. Nevertheless, occasional biopsy specimens from patients clinically diagnosed as having herpes simplex encephalitis have disclosed other disease processes such as fungal infections that required different therapy. Granulomatous or isolated angiitis can be diagnosed only from cerebral biopsy specimens. The prognoses for these disorders have been improved markedly by the use of immunosuppressive therapy.

Biopsy may be appropriate in certain subacute and chronic diseases. These include patients suspected of having chronic bacterial encephalitis (Whipple's disease and possibly Lyme disease), or chronic meningitis, in whom the diagnosis cannot be established from the cerebrospinal fluid. In rare instances, biopsies may be appropriate in chronically ill patients if the results are of importance in providing accurate genetic counseling. Very rarely, biopsies may be justifiable as a source of tissue for research on diseases of unknown etiology and pathogenesis.

Another category of brain biopsy that has received less attention is the sampling of additional tissue at the time of a therapeutic procedure. This would include removal of brain tissue or meninges at the time of ventriculostomy, cerebrospinal fluid shunting, or evacuation of a hematoma. These tissues should be handled with the same care as other diagnostic biopsy specimens because much valuable information may be obtained from these specimens. For example, cortex obtained when a hematoma is evacuated should be examined by techniques appropriate for the detection of amyloid angiopathy, arteriovenous malformation, or neoplasm.

The initial step in the performance of brain biopsy is discussion among the individuals requesting the biopsy, performing the biopsy, and examining the biopsy specimens. This discussion will help in selecting the most appropriate biopsy site and utilizing these tissues optimally.

The timing of biopsy should also be considered. When possible, the biopsy should be performed during a working day to ensure that the technical staffs in the various laboratories are available and are thoroughly familiar with the specialized diagnostic procedures that may be needed for optimal utilization of the tissue. Even in the case of patients suspected of having herpes simplex encephalitis, antiviral therapy can be initiated and the biopsy performed the next day when proper laboratory support has been mobilized, as this will not impair the test results. Flexibility tailored to the individual case with communication among all is the most important factor.

SURGICAL TECHNIQUE

Anesthesia and Medication

General endotracheal anesthesia is used most commonly, but if the patient is cooperative, biopsies may be done with light sedation and local anesthesia. If increased intracranial pressure is a factor, mannitol and hyperventilation may be utilized. Prophylactic anticonvulsants to avoid a known risk of seizures should be given preoperatively, but despite this, seizures are a potential complication. Prophylactic antibiotics are used, but if an infectious process is suspected, should

not be given until after the specimen is taken. As previously mentioned, in cases of herpes simplex encephalitis, pretreatment with acyclovir will not alter the findings significantly for several days to weeks.

Operative Technique

For a temporal lobe biopsy, the patient is positioned supine on the operating table, and, when it is to be used, general endotracheal anesthesia is induced. With a doughnut pad under the head, the head is turned to the side at a level above the heart, and a towel roll is placed under the shoulder. We flex the patient slightly at the hips and knees (Fig. 1). A small area of scalp is shaved, and the operative site is prepared. A 5-cm curvilinear incision is drawn 1 cm anterior to the external auditory meatus which extends up from the zygoma and turns posterior above the ear to approximately 1 cm above the pinna (Fig. 2). The region is draped with paper drapes and a Betadine-impregnated adhesive plastic sheet.

The proposed incision is infiltrated locally with 0.5 to 1.0% lidocaine with 1/100,000 epinephrine. It takes from 5 to 15 minutes to achieve maximum vasoconstriction with epinephrine. The incision is then made with a No. 10 blade through skin, fascia, and muscle down to periosteum. The bone is cleared with a periosteal elevator. Retraction is maintained with a Weitlaner retractor. A Hudson brace and McKenzie perforator are employed to create a burr hole. (In an awake patient, power drills are unnecessarily loud, potentially frightening, and rather expensive.)

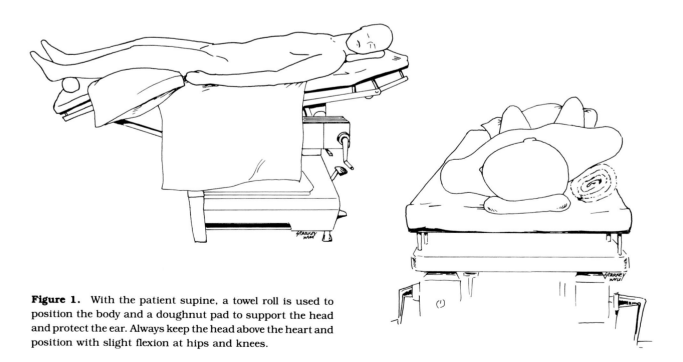

Figure 1. With the patient supine, a towel roll is used to position the body and a doughnut pad to support the head and protect the ear. Always keep the head above the heart and position with slight flexion at hips and knees.

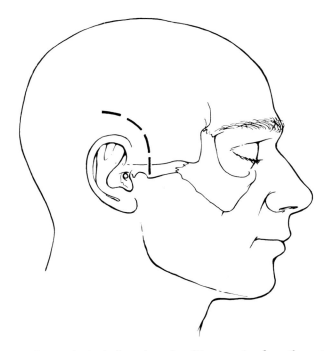

Figure 2. The incision is 1 cm anterior to the external auditory meatus from the zygoma to 1 cm above the pinna and about 5 cm long.

Using rongeurs, the craniectomy can be enlarged to a 2–2.5 cm diameter (Fig. 3). Cautery is subsequently avoided until the tissue has been removed. A dural hook is used to lift the dura and a No. 11 blade to make either a cruciate or a curvilinear incision. A sample of meninges may be removed if needed. Sufficient brain tissue should be obtained so that the appropriate studies can be undertaken. Generally, this can be done from a cube measuring 1.0–1.5 cm in each dimension. Specimens should include cortex and white matter, and, whenever possible, a sulcus. Using a No. 11 blade, a four-sided incision is made 1.0–1.5 cm on a side, and at least 1.5 cm deep (Fig. 3, *inset*). This is undermined with a Penfield No. 3 dissector and lifted out with a cupped forceps.

The tissue for histopathologic studies and electron microscopy must be handled as gently as possible. Even when manipulated with great care, neurons at the pial surface and near the margins of resection will be shrunken and angular (Fig. 4). Conversely, neurons deep in the interior of a large specimen will often become abnormally swollen. When they are mild, handling artifacts complicate but do not preclude accurate diagnosis. Vacuolar artifacts from improper handling (and suboptimal tissue processing) are especially troublesome when Creutzfeldt-Jakob disease is being considered. The morphologic diagnosis of this condition is based in part on the recognition of subtle intracytoplasmic vacuoles that must be distinguished from artifactual changes.

When viral and other cultures are indicated, tissue for these studies should be placed immediately in sterile containers and sent directly to the appropriate laboratories from the operating room so as to avoid the risk of contamination. Although isolation of the etiologic agent remains as the most definitive procedure for infectious disease, the use of immunofluorescent and immunoperoxidase techniques, as well as in situ hybridization has extended the role of the morphologist in the diagnosis of these conditions. Some hint of the diagnosis should be derived from the clinical data or from gross morphologic features so that only necessary and appropriate stains are used.

After the specimen is removed, electrocautery and Gelfoam are used to achieve hemostasis. It may be difficult to close the dura; indeed, if a dural specimen is taken, this may be impossible. The wound is then irrigated and the layers above the dura and bone are closed tightly. A running locked skin suture extending just beyond the ends of the incision will ensure a watertight closure.

Specimens from other sites may be desirable, depending on such things as disease process, imaging characteristics, and electroencephalographic localization. Biopsy of silent areas should be carried out using appropriate skin and bone flaps. In small peripheral lesions, computed tomography localization and intraoperative ultrasonography are very useful to minimize the size of the incision and the craniectomy and the amount of brain manipulation.

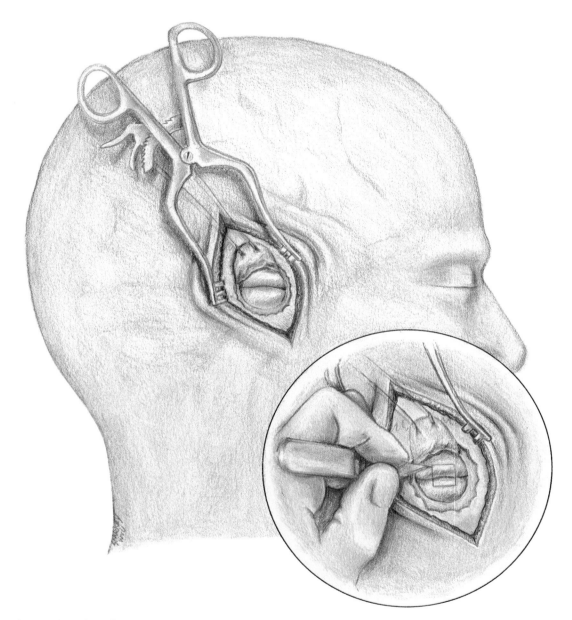

Figure 3.   A 2.0–2.5-cm diameter craniectomy is performed and the dura opened to expose the lower aspect of the temporal lobe. *Inset*, remove a cube 1.0–1.5 cm on a side and 1.0– 1.5 cm deep. If possible, include a sulcus. Undermine with a No. 3 Penfield dissector and remove with cupped forceps.

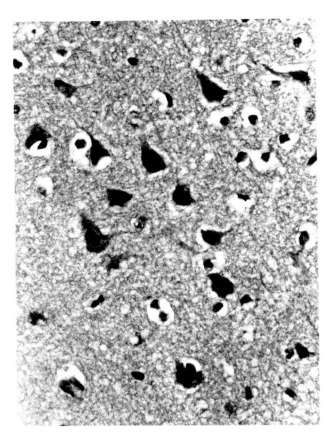

Figure 4. Artifactual changes include shrunken angular neurons with pyknotic nuclei seen at the margin of a biopsy specimen. H & E × 650.

Lastly, highly infectious agents carry risks to the surgical team and those who come in contact with the equipment. Extreme caution with complete body coverage of team members and care to protect all team members from "sharps" should be followed. Since every operative case is potentially infectious, universal blood precautions are employed as standard practice. In patients suspected of having a highly contagious disease such as AIDS or Creutzfeldt-Jakob disease, additional precautions may be taken. All unnecessary equipment is removed from the room. Disposables are used if possible, cabinet and room entry are limited, and an outside circulator should be present to allow persons in the room to remain within the room. For slow viruses, special cleaning of nondisposables with steam autoclaving at 132°C for one hour or soaking in 1 N sodium hydroxide for one hour is recommended.

Contributors

A. LELAND ALBRIGHT, M.D.
Associate Professor
Department of Neurosurgery
University of Pittsburgh School of Medicine
Pittsburgh, Pennsylvania

ISSAM A. AWAD, M.D.
Vice Chairman
Department of Neurological Surgery
The Cleveland Clinic Foundation
Cleveland, Ohio

DANIEL L. BARROW, M.D.
Associate Professor
Department of Neurosurgery
Emory University School of Medicine
Atlanta, Georgia

DERALD E. BRACKMANN, M.D.
Clinical Professor of Otolaryngology
University of Southern California School of
    Medicine
Los Angeles, California

PAUL J. CAMARATA, M.D.
Resident
Department of Neurosurgery
University of Minnesota
Minneapolis, Minnesota

CHRISTOPHER E. CLARE, M.D.
Chief Resident
Department of Neurosurgery
Emory University School of Medicine
Atlanta, Georgia

DONALD F. DOHN, M.D.
Chairman
Department of Neurological Surgery
The Cleveland Clinic Florida
Fort Lauderdale, Florida

STEPHEN J. HAINES, M.D.
Associate Professor
Division of Pediatric Neurosurgery
Department of Neurosurgery
University of Minnesota
Minneapolis, Minnesota

PATRICK J. KELLY, M.D.
Professor
Department of Neurological Surgery
Mayo Medical School
Rochester, Minnesota

DAVID C. McCULLOUGH, M.D.
Chairman
Department of Neurological Surgery
Children's Hospital
Washington, D.C.

PREM K. PILLAY, M.D.
Fellow
Department of Neurological Surgery
The Cleveland Clinic Foundation
Cleveland, Ohio

GEORGE T. TINDALL, M.D.
Professor and Chairman
Department of Neurosurgery
Emory University School of Medicine
Atlanta, Georgia

ERIC J. WOODARD, M.D.
Assistant Professor
Department of Neurosurgery
Emory University School of Medicine
Atlanta, Georgia

Contents

VENTRICULOPERITONEAL SHUNTING

DAVID C. McCULLOUGH, M.D.

INTRODUCTION

Ventriculoperitoneal shunting is the preferred method for cerebrospinal fluid (CSF) diversion in hydrocephalus of children and adults. The technique was conceived and first attempted early in the 20th century and was revived in the 1950s, with indifferent results. Introduction of silicone conduits with elastic properties eventually contributed to clinical success. After 1970, ventriculoperitoneal shunting supplanted various other diversionary methods including ventriculoatrial shunting.

SELECTION OF PATIENTS

Because the majority of cases of hydrocephalus are not relieved by direct surgical intervention, CSF diversion with implantable devices has become the conventional therapy for this condition. The common use of ultrasound, computed tomography (CT), and magnetic resonance imaging (MRI) has disclosed increasing numbers of potential candidates for shunt procedures. Some surgeons recommend that any patient with large ventricles should be treated, but most conservatively advocate shunting only when there is a potentially reversible deficit or a progressive condition. Infantile congenital hydrocephalus is almost always progressive. Patients with acquired noncommunicating hydrocephalus and symptomatic acquired communicating hydrocephalus will usually require intervention.

The determination of progressive hydrocephalus may be difficult in other circumstances. Serial developmental and neurological examination in infants, neuropsychological studies in older children and adults, or radiographic evidence of progressive ventriculomegaly can affirm the need for CSF shunting. If a block is correctable by definitive surgery, or, if there is uncertainty as to the progressive nature of hydrocephalus, shunt treatment should be deferred.

Active ventriculitis, fresh ventricular hemorrhage, or peritoneal or systemic infection present specific contraindications to early shunting. Spontaneous compensation of the hydrocephalic condition may fol-low the removal of obstructive neoplasms and certain posterior fossa cysts. Posthemorrhagic hydrocephalus following intraventricular hemorrhage in neonates is often evanescent. Temporizing measures such as serial lumbar punctures or the administration of osmotic diuretics may suffice for communicating hydrocephalus in premature infants.

Occasionally, radionuclide or contrast medium ventriculography and cisternography assist in the detection of progressive hydrocephalus. Abnormal pressure waves during continuous intracranial pressure monitoring support the diagnosis of a progressive condition in older children and adults.

Permanent CSF bypass is seldom an emergency procedure. However, in the cases of acute acquired hydrocephalus or a rapidly decompensating congenital condition with increased intracranial pressure, delay may be detrimental. When neurological and radiographic data raise questions of fresh hemorrhage, active infection, or the possibility of direct surgical cure (e.g., posterior fossa tumor or cyst), temporary ventriculostomy may stabilize the situation and permit careful preoperative investigation and planning.

PREOPERATIVE PREPARATION

A single ventricular tap is recommended before surgery to exclude active infection and examine CSF contents in posthemorrhagic or postinfectious hydrocephalus of infancy. Although shunts may function satisfactorily in the face of extremely high CSF protein levels, it is prudent to delay until the protein concentration is below 200 mg %.

Selection of Components

Simplicity should prevail in the selection of devices for implantation in humans. I favor a specific system that eliminates some potential complications and makes others easier to manage. The flanged ventricular catheter allows for a certain margin of error in placement of the proximal tip of the device. Furthermore, it seldom becomes entangled with choroid plexus and, therefore, produces a lower incidence of bleeding when extraction is necessary. Spring-wire reinforcement of the ventricular catheter wall eliminates the need for insertion of a flange to ensure patency as the catheter angles sharply downward from its dural insertion site. The reservoir valve device permits percutaneous needle access to CSF. The diaphragm valve incorporated in the distal part of the reservoir is quite predictable in its performance. It provides unidirectional flow for functional evaluation on rare occasions when this is needed. A single proximal valve is used so that the surgeon can expose the system, survey flow from all components, and, if necessary, change the resistance with one incision. A flat-bottom device secured to the periosteum inferior to the burr hole eliminates the annoying possibility of disconnection between the reservoir and the (then inaccessible) ventricular catheter upon extraction of a burr hole reservoir during a revision. The open-ended peritoneal catheter with three series of side slits avoids an additional resistance in the system while allowing CSF egress from proximal apertures if the distal end of the catheter becomes occluded.

SURGICAL TECHNIQUE

The procedure is performed under general endotracheal anesthesia after intravenous thiopental induction. Special warming lights and airway humidification with warming counteract hypothermia in small infants. Prophylactic vancomycin (10 mg/kg) is administered as soon as the intravenous line is inserted in the operating room.

Correct patient positioning is critical to the smooth implantation of the shunt. The patient is placed at the top edge of the operating table to the operator's side and the head is turned sharply to the side opposite the insertion. The head is elevated for occipital access and the neck and trunk are extended with supporting cushions under the shoulders to facilitate subcutaneous tunneling (Fig. 1A). A meticulous 10-minute sequential skin preparation with povidone-iodine scrub and paint solution is then performed. Proposed incisions are outlined with a surgical marking pen. After palpating to exclude hepatomegaly, an abdominal incision is marked over the right upper quadrant. Surgical drapes include an adherent plastic that is impregnated with povidone-iodine over incision and tunneling sites (Fig. 1B), excluding the anterior fontanelle if ultrasound is to be used to guide the insertion of the ventricular catheter.

When inserting the shunt from the occipital site (Fig. 1), judgment of the appropriate distance from the skull surface to a point in the anterior horn just in front of the foramen of Monro is guided by measurement from preoperative CT scans. In older children and adults who tend to have smaller occipital horns, a frontal burr hole is preferred. Then the length of the ventricular catheter is determined by measurement of the distance from the proposed burr hole at the skull surface in a straight line to a point just superior to the midpoint of the bregma-interaural line (locus of the foramen of Monro).

The shunt is inserted from the right side unless the left lateral ventricle is significantly larger (Fig. 2). A curved incision with its long arm vertical is made 2.5–4 cm superior to the inion and 2.5–3.5 cm lateral to the occipital midline. If a frontal burr hole is used, the incision site is slightly anterior to the coronal suture and 2.5–3.0 cm lateral to the midline. A small scalp flap is turned. Clips or hemostats are used at the wound edges and care is taken to avoid violation of the periosteum during the initial incision. The scalp flap may be secured with a self-retaining retractor. A small cruciate periosteal incision is performed just inferior to the scalp incision line and a burr hole is drilled. The dura is coagulated with bipolar forceps and a 2-mm round dural opening is produced using a hook and a No. 11 knife blade. The arachnoid layer is lightly coagulated and knicked.

Shunt components are removed from sterile packages only immediately prior to placement. Skin incision contact with shunt parts is avoided and the gloves of the surgical team are changed and washed prior to handling the shunt components. The ventricular catheter is introduced with a wire stylet toward the inner canthus on a line directly between the horizontal planes of the supraorbital ridge and the bregma (Fig. 2). I prefer a flanged catheter which is situated with its tip in the anterior horn to avoid choroidal attachment. Intraoperative ultrasound (using the anterior fontanelle as an ultrasonic window) is useful for direct guidance in infants. Alternatively the tip is advanced to the premeasured point 1 cm anterior to the foramen of Monro (or 1 cm above the foramen on frontal placement) as determined from the CT scan. After insertion to the appropriate length, CSF flow is checked and the distal end of the catheter is immediately clamped to the drapes.

A 4–5-mm abdominal incision is made in the right upper quadrant passing through the subcuticular tissue. A peritoneal trocar is passed posteriorly and medially in the direction of the umbilicus as the anesthesiologist induces a Valsalva effect to tighten the abdominal muscles (Fig. 3). After the stylet is removed 30–60 cm of an open-ended peritoneal catheter (with three sets of side slits) is introduced through the trocar sleeve (Fig. 4) and the sleeve is removed.

A semisharp stainless steel tunneling device may be passed through the abdominal incision from the scalp incision subcutaneously (Fig. 5). In older patients a tiny cervical incision is often performed. Then, the tunneling device is passed from that level taking care to tunnel anterior to the clavicle. The proximal end of the peritoneal catheter is backed through the sub-

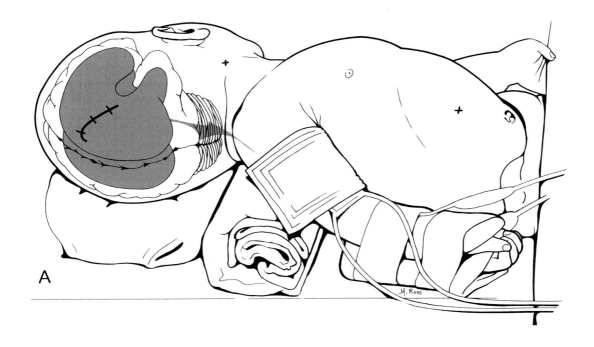

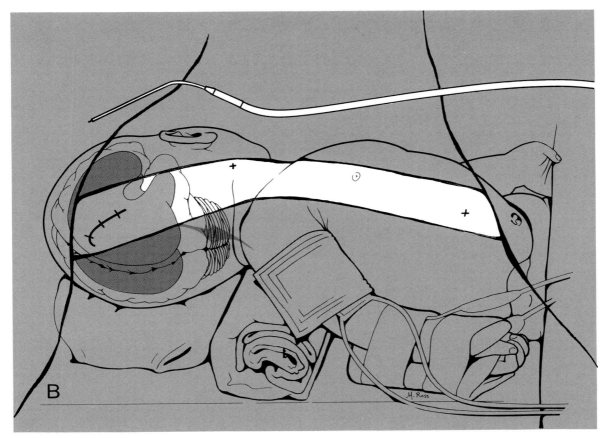

Figure 1. **A,** positioning of an infant for ventriculoperitoneal shunting. **B,** the prepared and draped surgical field with marks at incision sites.

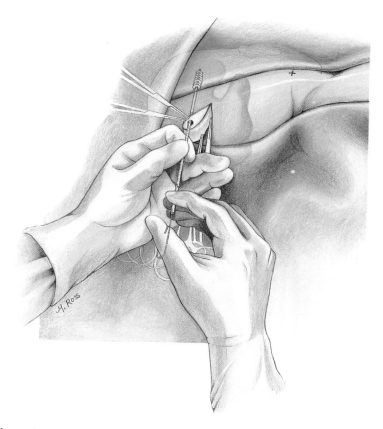

Figure 2. Insertion of a ventricular catheter from a right posterior entry site.

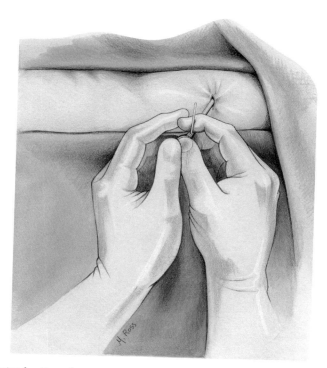

Figure 3. Introduction of a peritoneal trocar at a right upper quadrant incision site.

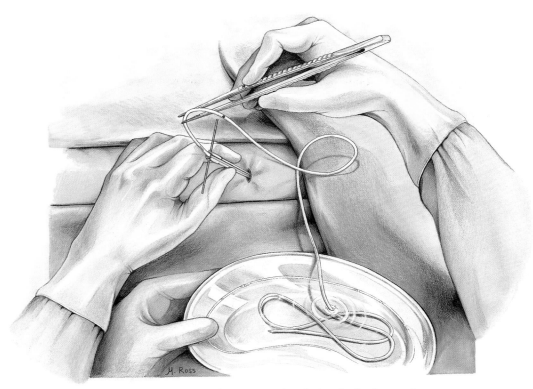

Figure 4. Introduction of a peritoneal catheter via the trocar sleeve.

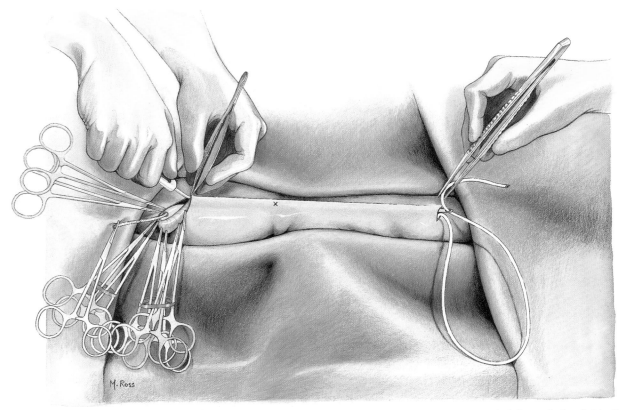

Figure 5. A tunneling device introduced from the scalp incision site to the abdominal incision site. The proximal end of the peritoneal catheter is threaded through the slot in the tunneler tip.

cutaneous tunnel. After the subgaleal space under the scalp flap is dissected to accommodate a proximal reservoir, the tunneling device is used to bring the proximal end of the peritoneal catheter from the cervical incision to the scalp (Fig. 5). Excess tubing is trimmed from the proximal end of the catheter. The catheter is then attached to a proximal flow control reservoir valve (Fig. 8). Low resistance reservoirs with diaphragm valves are used for infants less than one year of age. Larger or standard size medium pressure flow control reservoir valves are used for older infants, children, and adults. The reservoir and distal catheter are injected with a bacitracin irrigating solution (50,000 units in 200 ml of injection saline). Then, the distal end of the ventricular catheter is trimmed to its appropriate length and attached to the proximal end of the reservoir valve. Silk ties (2-0) are firmly teased into the connector grooves and tied tightly. The reservoir base is sutured to the periosteum with 4-0 silk. Occasional leakage around the exit point at the dura may require the application of Gelfoam which is secured by suturing the periosteum over the burr hole. After the reservoir is secured to the periosteum any excess loop of tubing at the peritoneal incision site is "stuffed" in (Fig. 6), making certain there is no subcutaneous coil (Fig. 7). Synthetic absorbable sutures are used to close the periosteum at the burr hole as well as the galea. Nonreactive synthetic sutures are used to close the skin and a compression scalp dressing is applied to discourage leaking until ventriculoperitoneal flow is well established. The cervical and abdominal incisions are closed in a similar fashion.

POSTOPERATIVE CARE
Postoperatively the patient is maintained in a horizontal position for 12 to 24 hours. Vancomycin prophylaxis (10 mg/kg, every 6 hours) is continued for 36 hours. Gradually, the head is elevated depending on the condition of the anterior fontanelle or the tolerance of the older patient. Alimentation is usually initiated within 12 hours unless there is abdominal distension and hypoperistalsis. Patients may be discharged from the hospital on the second postoperative day.

COMPLICATIONS AND PROGNOSIS
In spite of potentially frequent and varied complications, mortality and morbidity can be surprisingly low if a meticulous follow-up system is provided. This includes regularly scheduled office visits, periodic CT scanning, and convenient access to a neurosurgical service for symptomatic patients. Ventriculoperitoneal shunts are not electively lengthened for axial growth when parents are observant and a responsive care system is available.

Early postoperative complications include obstruction due to malposition of the device or inaccurate selection of components with excessive resistance in the system. Older, taller patients often require very gradual mobilization because of postural head pains related to intracranial hypotension.

Immediate infection is rare, but most septic incidents occur within the first two months of insertion or revision of a shunt. They usually manifest with obstructive symptoms, fever, cellulitis, and leukocytosis. Blood cultures are often positive. Most organisms can be cultured from percutaneous reservoir taps. Staphylococcal organisms predominate. In centers where shunts are frequently inserted in children, procedural infections rates approach 2%. The most reliable therapy is complete shunt removal with temporary external drainage and appropriate systemic antibiotics. A new device can be inserted after obtaining at least two consecutive negative cultures 48 hours apart.

Injury to an abdominal organ occurs in 0.4% of patients. This often presents as an infectious-obstructive episode, but extrusion of the catheter via the intestinal tract has been observed.

Although older patients with very large ventricles are at risk for overdrainage leading to subdural effusions and hematomas, less than 5% of pediatric patients develop this complication. An asymptomatic subdural effusion should be monitored clinically and with serial imaging. Most will resolve spontaneously.

Obstructive complications will inevitably occur. The majority involve the distal portion of the device. Patients with high CSF protein values at the initiation of therapy may require several shunt revisions during the first postoperative year. After about the sixth year, patients treated in infancy may present with obstruction due to axial somatic growth and relative shortening of the peritoneal catheter. Obstruction may also result from rarely encountered peritoneal pseudocysts, ascites due to peritoneal absorptive failure, peritoneal adhesions, internal debris, or breakage and disconnection of shunt components. The use of modern kink-resistant silicone tubing with avoidance of older, delicate, spring-reinforced peritoneal catheters has virtually ended the occurrence of disconnection and catheter migration.

A small cohort of pediatric and adolescent patients with CSF diversion receives considerable attention because of frequent bouts of vomiting, headache, and lapses of consciousness. The patients tend to have small ventricles, diminished extraventricular CSF spaces, and a thick skull. In my experience less than 4% of treated patients were suspected of having this "syndrome." The majority of these actually had true proximal shunt obstruction solved by appropriate catheter replacement in the frontal horn. In the re-

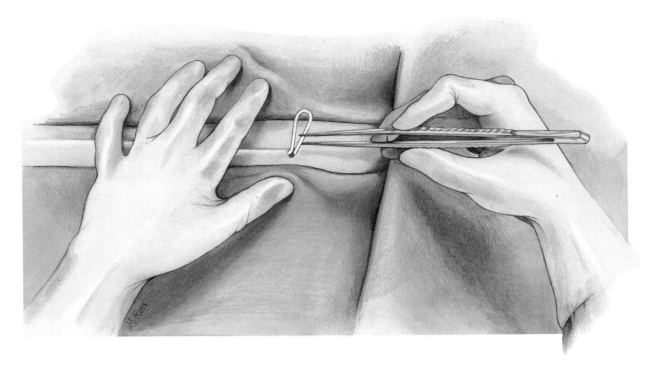

Figure 6.   Stuffing the excess peritoneal catheter via a small abdominal incision.

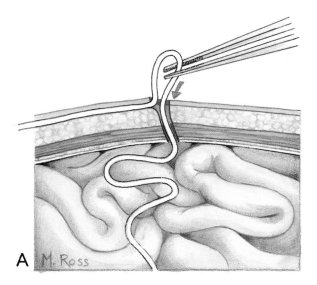
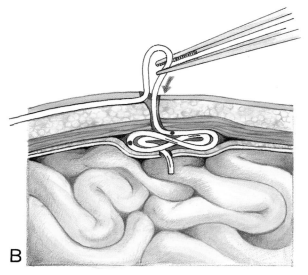

Figure 7.   **A,** the correct positioning of the peritoneal catheter after stuffing. **B,** an incorrect position of the peritoneal catheter which is coiled in an extraperitoneal location after attempted stuffing.

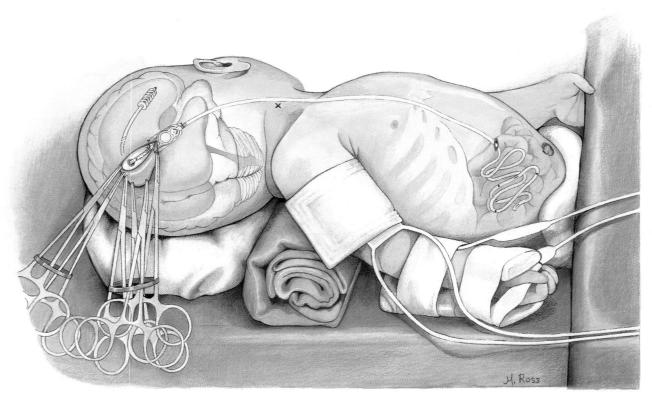

Figure 8. A properly inserted ventriculoperitoneal shunt in an infant. Note the anterior position of the proximal tip of the ventricular catheter, the location of the proximal reservoir valve under the skin flap, and the generous coil of open-end peritoneal catheter within the abdomen.

mainder, corrective procedures such as augmenting valve resistance and subtemporal craniectomy may be required to manage symptoms and prevent decompensation.

Current mortality and morbidity data reveal that 95% of children with nontumoral hydrocephalus survive for over 10 years and about 65% are intellectually normal. For infants with overt hydrocephalus at birth, the outcome is less favorable with about half demonstrating normal intelligence. Shunt-independent arrest is seldom observed. In patients followed an average of 15 years, 75% have required at least one revision and several have required as many as eight repeat operations. The mean number of revisions has been two procedures per patient.

VENTRICULOATRIAL SHUNTING

PAUL J. CAMARATA, M.D.
STEPHEN J. HAINES, M.D.

INTRODUCTION

The ventriculoatrial (VA) shunt was introduced as a method of treatment for hydrocephalus in the 1950s and was the first predictably successful valve-regulated cerebrospinal fluid (CSF) shunt. Technical developments have since made ventriculoperitoneal shunts reliable and, because they are easier and quicker to insert and revise, and have less propensity to systemic bacteremia if infected, they are the initial treatment of choice for hydrocephalus for most patients. There are some patients in whom a VA shunt is the procedure of first choice, such as those patients with fibrosis or inflammation in the peritoneum from remote or recent infections or multiple previous abdominal operations. The peritoneal cavity of some patients, particularly small infants, may occasionally not have sufficient absorptive capacity to handle the necessary amount of cerebrospinal fluid.

INDICATIONS

Ventriculoatrial shunts are indicated for the treatment of hydrocephalus, either obstructive or communicating, which is not transient in nature. Other indications for shunting, which may occasionally require VA shunting, include the treatment of pseudotumor cerebri and drainage of arachnoid cysts and subdural hygromas unresponsive to other therapeutic measures.

CONTRAINDICATIONS

Bacteremia or infection of the CSF or proposed shunt tract are absolute contraindications to the placement of a VA shunt. In the presence of infection elsewhere in the body, a shunt should be inserted only in very unusual circumstances. Congestive heart failure and pulmonary hypertension may both interfere with shunt function and be aggravated by the additional fluid load delivered to the heart; these are relative contraindications to the procedure, especially in infants. Abnormal venous anatomy and previous jugular or subclavian vein thrombosis are relative contra-

indications. Where both VP and VA shunting are contraindicated, shunts to the pleural space, the gall bladder, the ureter, the bone marrow, the subarachnoid space, and other areas have been reported to be successful.

PREOPERATIVE PREPARATION

Preoperatively the patient or his or her parents are informed that the major risks of the procedure are those of infection and shunt malfunction, either of which would necessitate revision or replacement of the shunt. When a VA shunt is placed in an infant, malfunction due to growth-related migration of the atrial catheter into the superior vena cava is so predictable that elective revision at about two years of age has been recommended by some. There is a slight risk of intracranial hemorrhage (which may be increased in patients with marked hydrocephalus). Remote risks of air embolism, cardiac rupture and tamponade, and thromboembolism are mentioned, as are the attendant risks of general anesthesia.

Where possible, an antiseptic bath or shower is administered preoperatively. The hair should be shaved immediately preoperatively. An appropriate dose of an anti-staphylococcal antibiotic is administered upon anesthetic induction.

Anesthetic Considerations

Most patients with hydrocephalus can be presumed to have some degree of increased intracranial pressure (ICP). Because of this a gentle anesthetic induction is preferred, being careful to avoid any manipulations that would increase ICP, i.e., Valsalva maneuvers, coughing, prolonged hypoventilation. Appropriate inhalational or intravenous anesthetics that decrease ICP and preserve cerebral autoregulation are used, combined with hyperventilation if deemed necessary. Succinylcholine is avoided because of its propensity to increase ICP.

Special Equipment

A C-arm fluoroscopic unit is extremely helpful in verifying correct catheter placement. Operating room personnel must remember to don lead aprons prior to scrubbing. It is also useful to have intravenous contrast material available. Heparinized saline is necessary to flush the atrial catheter, as well as an antibiotic saline solution with which to irrigate the shunt system and wounds. The appropriate shunt system is chosen preoperatively, and a central venous pressure monitoring device must be available to monitor pressure waves as the atrial catheter is advanced.

Positioning

The basic principle of positioning the patient is to provide clear access to the head for ventricular puncture and to the neck for cannulation of the venous system. Therefore, following induction of satisfactory general endotracheal anesthesia, with the patient in the supine position the head is turned to the appropriate side. In the preferred setting, the head is turned to the left to provide access to the right neck. Because of the vascular anatomy, right-sided cannulations are

often easier than left-sided ones. The ear may be taped forward and thereby easily draped out of the field. Soft padding is placed beneath the shoulders to expose the anterior triangle of the neck (Fig. 1, A and C). The skin in the operative field and surrounding area is then prepared with an appropriate antiseptic soap. Prior to draping, the landmarks for ventricular access and access to the venous system are drawn on the skin (Fig. 1 B). A mark is placed approximately 2.5–3 cm from the midline and 11–12 cm posterior to the nasion in the adult (or approximately one-seventh of the distance from the coronal suture to the nasion in the child). A line is then drawn from this mark toward the inner canthus of the ipsilateral eye. Another line is drawn that passes through this point and a spot 1 cm anterior to the tragus of the ipsilateral ear. If these lines are taken to represent imaginary planes in partial sagittal and coronal directions, their intersection forms a line that should pass through the foramen of Monro (Fig. 2).

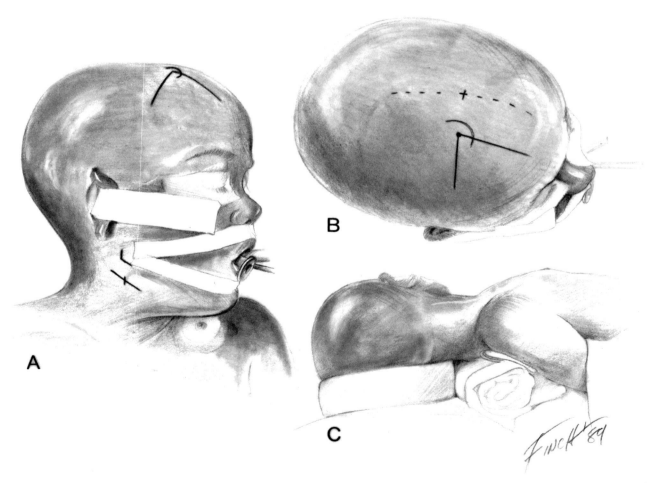

Figure 1. Lateral (**A**) and vertex (**B**) views of incision landmarks. Note the intersecting lines drawn to represent two planes. The ventricular catheter should be passed along the line that is the intersection of these two planes. **C,** side view of padding placed under the head and shoulders for optimal positioning.

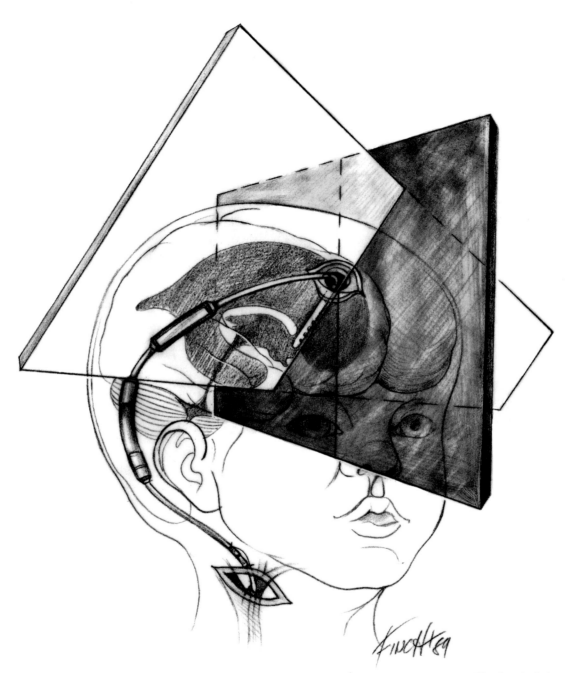

Figure 2. A ventricular catheter traveling along the intersection of the two drawn planes will be directed at the foramen of Monro.

Sterile drapes are then applied in such a manner as to allow for access to head and neck sites. In draping the head, it is helpful to place a sterile towel with one border on the midline to use as a landmark in placing the burr hole. If intraoperative ultrasound is to be used in the case of an infant, the anterior fontanelle should be draped into the operative field.

The shunt hardware, including ventricular and atrial catheters, valve system, reservoir, and connectors, should be chosen before the procedure, opened, and placed in an antibiotic-saline solution on the instrument table before the incision is made. We avoid the use of bacitracin because its foaming action may interfere with the function of some valves. It is prudent to have several valves with different pressures readily available. The valve system to be used should be tested according to the manufacturer's recommendations to ensure its appropriate function. It should be filled with saline solution, all air bubbles removed, and clamped on one end with a rubber shod mosquito clamp to keep it full of fluid. To the greatest extent possible, one should avoid touching the skin and shunt system with the gloved hand to minimize the risk of postoperative infection.

SURGICAL TECHNIQUE

The operation is carried out in a logical, stepwise fashion. We prefer to place the ventricular and vascular catheters as the last part of the operation because of the risk of dislodging either catheter before it is secured in final position.

Step One—Isolation of the Common Facial Vein

A 2-cm transverse neck incision is made one finger breadth below and parallel to the ramus of the mandible in an adult, and a proportionally smaller distance below the jaw in children. This should be centered just medial to the medial border of the sternocleidomastoid muscle (Fig. 3). The platysma is split in the direction of its fibers, and using a combination of blunt and sharp dissection along the avascular plane medial to the sternocleidomastoid muscle, the common facial vein is identified. The vein is isolated for about 1 cm of its length, and two ligatures of a size appropriate to the size of the vessel are placed around it. The vein is then ligated using the most cephalad tie.

Recently, we prefer to use a percutaneous technique similar to that used for placing central venous catheters. Usually the internal jugular vein is used for access, though the subclavian may be used, and the procedure is identical to cannulation for standard central venous catheters. For the internal jugular vein, a thin-walled, 18- or 20-gauge needle which is contained in most central venous access kits is used. The skin is punctured approximately 4–6 cm (2–3 finger breadths) above the clavicle along the posterior border of the sternocleidomastoid muscle or a proportionate distance in a child. The tip of the needle should be aimed at the sternal notch (Fig. 4). Alternatively, the carotid artery can be palpated and the needle aimed lateral to it. For the subclavian vein, the needle is inserted just below the junction of the middle and inner thirds of the clavicle and aimed at the sternal notch.

Once the vein is punctured, the syringe is removed and a flexible J-wire (0.021 inch in diameter for older children and adults) is inserted through the needle; its position can be checked with fluoroscopy. The needle is removed when the wire is verified to be in the superior vena cava. A small 1-cm incision is made at the point of entry to facilitate passage of the introducer and to connect the shunt system with the atrial catheter and bury it. A standard, tear-away introducer sheath over a vessel dilator is then passed over the wire through the subcutaneous tissue and into the vein. The wire and dilator are removed and a finger is placed over the sheath to prevent the introduction of air. The atrial catheter can now be threaded through the sheath to its proper position described in Step 4 below.

Step Two—Placement of a Cranial Burr Hole

The ventricular catheter may be placed into the frontal or occipital horn of the lateral ventricle depending on the preference of the surgeon and the individual patient's ventricular anatomy. We prefer the frontal approach because our experience indicates that such shunts function better than parieto-occipitally placed ones. The patient's nondominant hemisphere is selected because of the remote risk of parenchymal damage caused by hemorrhage at the site of insertion. A curved incision is made with its base directed inferiorly so that no portion of the incision will be overlying the shunt apparatus. The burr hole is then made using a standard hand or power drill at the predetermined site, bone wax is applied, and the exposed dura is covered with a saline-soaked sponge or cottonoid patty until later in the procedure.

Step Three—Placement of the Valve System

At this point the valve system is passed subcutaneously from the cranial incision to the neck incision, passing in front of the parietal boss and behind the ear. Care must be taken to avoid the very thin skin just behind the ear and not to have the bulky portion of the valve or reservoir over a bony prominence where they may cause pressure erosion of the skin. Depending on the size of the patient, a small transverse incision may be necessary behind the ear so that the distal tubing may be passed the remainder of the distance to

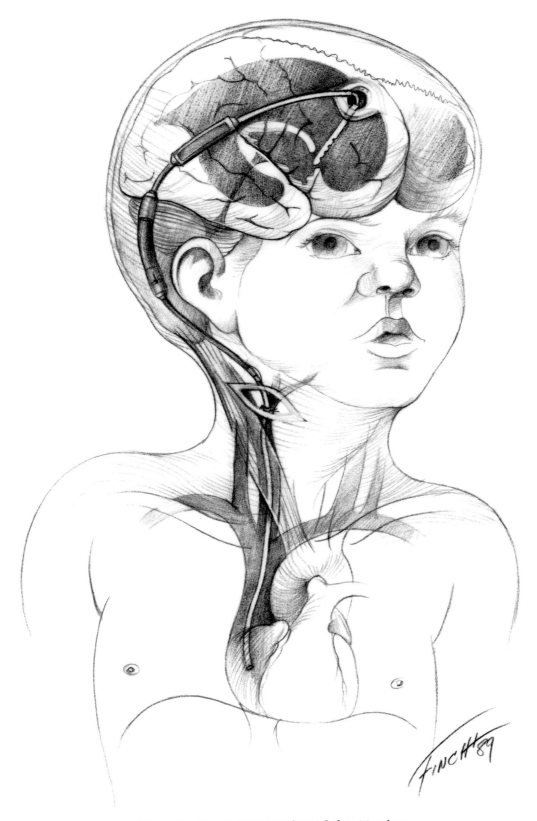

Figure 3. Complete ventriculoatrial shunt in place.

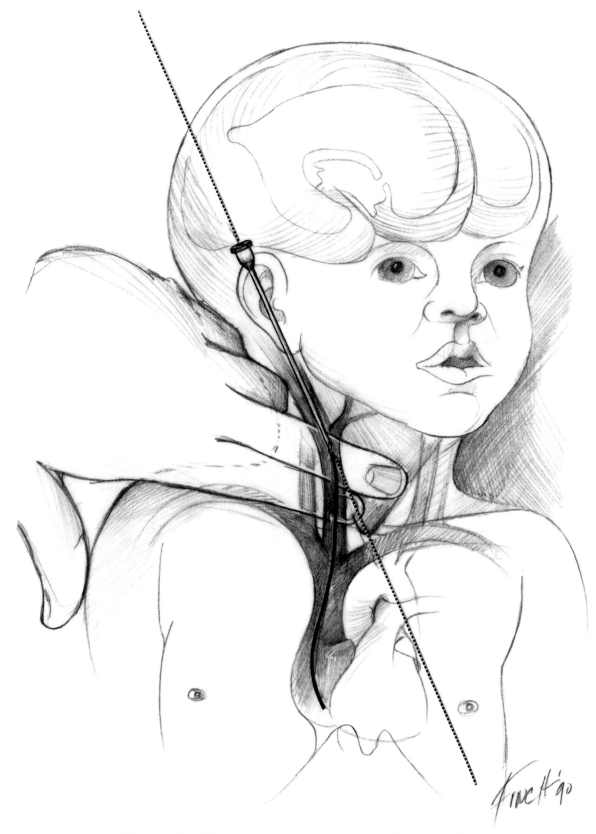

Figure 4. Guidelines for percutaneous placement of the atrial catheter.

the neck incision. We prefer using the Cordis-Hakim shunt system, which is easily passed in this manner using a curved passing device included with the system. Other shunt systems may require minor technical variations. The proximal shunt system tubing is then cut to the appropriate length and a right-angled connector is attached using a permanent suture. Both ends of the system are clamped with rubber shod clamps in order to maintain the system fluid-filled and free of air bubbles, and to avoid inadvertently pulling the tubing out of the incision, and are covered with sponges moistened in an antibiotic solution. The purpose of placing the valve-reservoir system first is to minimize the number of manipulations once the vein and the ventricle have been catheterized. When the venous or ventricular catheter is placed early in the procedure, it may be dislodged inadvertently. Because of this possibility, we then place the atrial catheter, and the ventricular catheter last.

Step Four—Placement of the Atrial Catheter

The goal in placement of the atrial catheter is, to position the catheter midway between the superior vena cava (SVC)-right atrium junction and the tricuspid valve. A variety of techniques are available to confirm this placement, the least reliable of which is the chest x-ray, upon which we do not rely. A more accurate, yet simple, way of correctly placing the catheter utilizes continuous pressure wave recordings as the catheter is advanced.

A small venotomy is made in the common facial vein, and the atrial catheter is introduced through it into the jugular vein. Alternatively, the catheter may be introduced directly into the internal jugular vein. In this case a purse string suture should be placed prior to making the venotomy. The catheter has been filled with an isotonic heparinized saline solution with the proximal end connected to a pressure transducer for continuous monitoring in a closed system, to prevent air aspiration. The ligature is cinched around the catheter just enough to prevent back bleeding yet allow the catheter to advance easily. A characteristic change is noted as the catheter is advanced first from the superior vena cava into the right atrium and then into the right ventricle (Fig. 5). The catheter is then withdrawn until the atrial pressure tracing is again identified. Fluoroscopy is often used during advancement of the catheter. If necessary, the catheter may be made visible by the injection of an appropriate quantity of contrast material. When the proper position has been identified, the remaining ligature is tied around the catheter so that it cannot move, but still will permit free flow of CSF. This should be ensured by aspirating to remove air bubbles and then flushing the distal catheter with heparinized saline. A rubber shod clamp is placed proximally, and a straight metal connector is tied to the catheter which is then covered with an antibiotic moistened sponge.

Step Five—Placement of the Ventricular Catheter

The goal in placement of the ventricular catheter is to place the tip in the frontal horn just anterior to the foramen of Monro. In an infant, ultrasound through the anterior fontanelle can often be used to direct the catheter placement in this fashion.

The center of the exposed dura is coagulated with a needle-point monopolar cautery to create an opening with a diameter equal to that of the catheter. The catheter should be marked in some fashion so that it is not advanced excessively (beyond 7 cm in the adult). A standard Silastic ventricular catheter with multiple side holes at its tip and an internal stylet in place is then advanced through the dural opening utilizing the guidance lines and planes described above until CSF return is evident. (We do not use flanged ventricular catheters because of the tendency of the choroid plexus to grow into the interstices of the catheter. This can lead to intraventricular hemorrhage when the catheter is removed during a revision.) Usually the resistance encountered when the catheter pops through the ventricular ependymal surface is easily felt. The stylet is then removed and the catheter advanced approximately 1 cm. A depth of 5–6 cm is usual in the adult and is proportionally less in children. A manometer may be connected to the catheter, and the ventricular pressure may be measured and recorded. The catheter is then clamped with a rubber shod clamp, cut, and connected to the valve system with the right-angled connector. The connector should then be secured to the periosteum with a single stitch.

The system is now inspected to ensure spontaneous flow of CSF from the valve, and the atrial catheter is again aspirated and flushed and connected to the valve system with a straight connector. The sutures are tied across the connector, to further protect against disconnection.

The position of the atrial catheter is again checked fluoroscopically. The tip of the catheter should be seen overlying the seventh thoracic vertebra. All wounds are inspected and irrigated with antibiotic saline solution and then closed in the standard fashion. The galea is first closed with interrupted 3-0 or 4-0 absorbable sutures, and the skin is closed according to the surgeon's preference. The posterior auricular and cervical incisions are closed in two layers, and sterile dressings are applied.

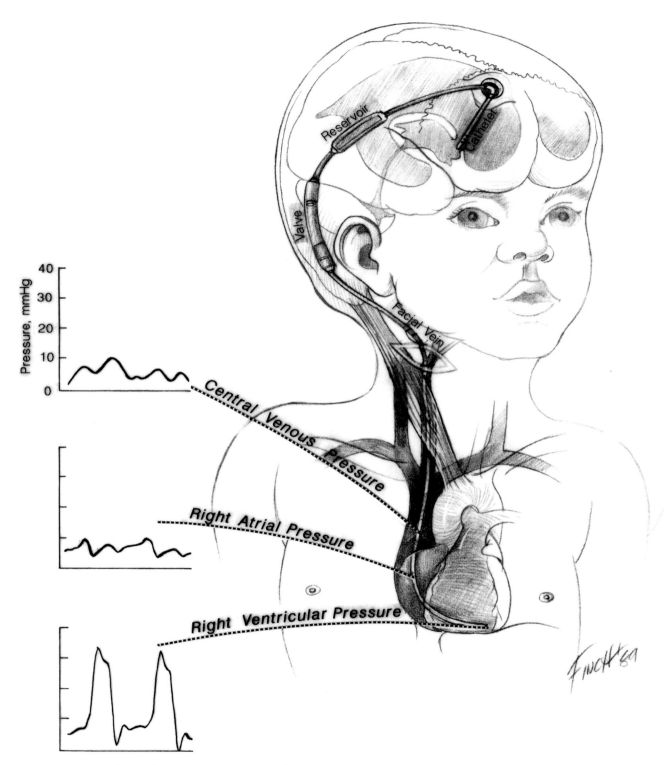

Figure 5. Typical pressure wave form readings seen with advancing catheter positions.

INTRAOPERATIVE PROBLEMS

Difficulty in Locating the Ventricles

We find the above method of passing the catheter most successful in cannulating the anterior part of the frontal horn of the lateral ventricle. If unsuccessful, three passes are made at slightly different angles, at no time passing the catheter to a depth greater than 7 cm in an adult. Passing the catheter perpendicular to a plane tangent to the skull at the point of entry is often helpful. As mentioned, ultrasound can be used in a child with an open anterior fontanelle.

Difficulty Passing the Atrial Catheter in a Patient with Normal Vascular Anatomy

Once the catheter enters the vein, it usually passes straight into the superior vena cava and right atrium. If any difficulty is encountered, a standard J-wire commonly used for central vascular access can be passed into the vein and almost always easily directed into the atrium under fluoroscopy. The catheter can then be threaded over the wire.

Difficulty Passing the Atrial Catheter in a Patient with Abnormal Vascular Anatomy

If a problem with venous access is anticipated, such as a patient who has had multiple VA shunts, previous SVC or jugular thrombosis, or multiple previous central venous access lines, it is advisable to obtain preoperative venography to define the anatomy. Where the internal jugular has been previously sacrificed or thrombosed, the external jugular may be of use. It is also possible with the aid of an interventional radiologist to catheterize a vein in a retrograde fashion from the groin using an angiographic catheter. One may then cut down directly on the wire, and this may be used to pull the catheter into the atrium.

Difficulty Positioning the Atrial Catheter

We find the method of using continuous pressure recordings the easiest and most accurate way of placing the tip of the catheter correctly in the atrium. The use of contrast material under intraoperative fluoroscopy is another method. Or, using the saline-filled atrial catheter as an ECG lead, the characteristic biphasic P-wave changes seen in the atrium may be identified. Two-dimensional intraoperative echocardiography has also been used successfully for this purpose.

POSTOPERATIVE CARE

Anteroposterior and lateral x-ray films of the skull and thorax should be obtained within the first two postoperative days to verify catheter positions and continuity of the system. A computed tomographic scan should be done within the first few weeks after surgery in the case of a first-time shunt placement to document ventricular size at a time when the shunt is known to be functional. This can be invaluable in assessing shunt function in the future.

We monitor the electrocardiogram (ECG) for the first 24 hours postoperatively because of the possibility of arrhythmia. One may wish to nurse the patient in the supine position for the first day if the intracranial pressure was particularly high to protect against collapse of the cerebral mantle.

COMPLICATIONS

Malfunction of the shunt system and infection are the two most common complications of the procedure and may occur at any time after operation, including in the recovery room. The former may be a consequence of an indolent CSF infection, obstruction of any part of the valve or tubing by proteinaceous debris or fibrosis, or disconnection. We believe the technique of securing all connections with a nonabsorbable suture tied across the connector can help prevent disconnection.

Infection can be minimized by the use of perioperative antibiotics, and by keeping the handling of the shunt system to a minimum. When at all possible, the system should be manipulated with instruments rather than the gloved hand. When tapping the shunt reservoir the skin should always be adequately prepared with the appropriate shave and antiseptic wash. Patients with a ventriculoatrial shunt should be advised to follow standard bacterial endocarditis antibiotic prophylaxis before any surgical or dental procedure.

CONCLUSIONS

Ventricular shunting procedures are commonly thought of as "minor" neurosurgical procedures. Given short shrift in training and low priority in practice, the operation may give suboptimal results. However, with meticulous technique and skillful execution, the ventriculoatrial shunt can be a safe and effective tool in the neurosurgeon's armamentarium for the treatment of hydrocephalus.

EXCISION OF ACOUSTIC NEUROMAS BY THE MIDDLE FOSSA APPROACH

DERALD E. BRACKMANN, M.D.

INTRODUCTION

The middle fossa approach for the removal of acoustic tumors was developed by Dr. William F. House in the early 1960s. It has been shown to be a safe approach with a minimum of mortality and morbidity. In this chapter, the approach for removal of an acoustic tumor will be described.

INDICATIONS AND PATIENT SELECTION

The middle fossa approach offers several advantages for the removal of small, laterally placed acoustic tumors. First, the majority of the dissection is extradural, thereby lowering morbidity. Second, the lateral end of the internal auditory canal is exposed which ensures removal of all of the tumor. With the retrosigmoid approach, the most lateral end of the internal auditory canal cannot be exposed safely without entering the labyrinth. Third, positive identification of the facial nerve is possible at the lateral end of the internal auditory canal. This facilitates tumor dissection from the facial nerve in this area.

For middle fossa acoustic tumor removal, we select patients who have a tumor that extends no further than 1 cm into the cerebellopontine angle. If the tumor is medially placed and does not extend to the fundus of the internal auditory canal, the retrosigmoid approach is preferred. A tumor that involves the distal end of the internal auditory canal is better approached via the middle fossa.

Candidates for hearing preservation surgery are those who have serviceable hearing, i.e., usually no greater than a 40-dB pure tone loss with residual speech discrimination of at least 80%. Preservation of wave form with only a slight increase of latencies on the auditory brain stem response is a favorable prognostic sign. Loss of function of the superior vestibular nerve as indicated by a reduced vestibular response on electronystagmography is also a favorable sign indicating a tumor in the superior compartment of the internal auditory canal. Tumors in the superior compartment are less likely to intimately involve the cochlear nerve and are also more likely to displace the facial nerve anteriorly rather than be located beneath the facial nerve.

There are also disadvantages to the middle fossa approach. The first is that with this approach, the surgeon must work past the facial nerve to remove the tumor. This subjects the facial nerve to more manipulation than does the translabyrinthine approach. A second problem sometimes encountered is postoperative unsteadiness resulting from partial preservation of vestibular function. This problem also occurs with the retrosigmoid approach, but it rarely occurs with total vestibular denervation with the translabyrinthine approach. Careful section of the remaining vestibular nerve fibers reduces the incidence of postoperative unsteadiness but also increases the risk of hearing loss.

The final potential problem with the middle fossa approach is limited access to the posterior fossa in the event of bleeding either at surgery or postoperatively. Although this has not occurred in our series, a problem could arise if significant bleeding occurred from the anterior inferior cerebellar artery.

OPERATIVE MANAGEMENT

Anesthesia

This operation is performed under general endotracheal anesthesia using inhalation agents. Facial nerve monitoring is routinely used so that muscle paralysis is not used except for the initial induction of anesthesia. Diuretics and mannitol are usually used to promote diuresis.

Positioning and Preparation

The patient is placed supine on the operating table with the head turned so that the operated ear is facing up. No external fixation is utilized. The surgeon is seated at the head of the table. The remainder of the operating room setup is shown in Figure 1.

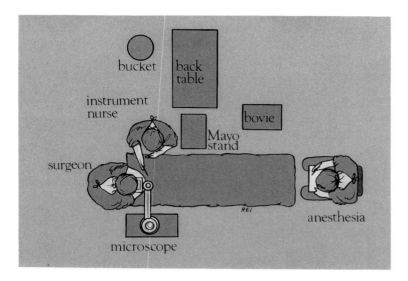

Figure 1. The operating room arrangement. The surgeon is seated at the head of the table.

A large area of hair removal is required because the incision extends far superiorly. The area of preparation extends nearly to the top of the head and far anteriorly and posteriorly. The skin is prepared with Betadine scrub and self-adhering plastic drapes are applied.

Incision

The middle fossa incision begins within the natural hairline just anterior to the base of the helix and extends superiorly approximately 7 to 8 cm, curving first anteriorly and then posteriorly (Fig. 2). Curving the incision allows the surgeon to spread soft tissue widely to gain more access anteriorly. Bleeding vessels are controlled with cautery. The surgeon often encounters a branch of the superficial temporal artery which is ligated with nonabsorbable sutures to avoid late postoperative bleeding and hematoma formation.

The initial incision extends to the level of the temporalis fascia. Finger dissection develops the plane of the temporalis fascia along the temporal line. An incision is then made posterosuperiorly along the insertion of the temporalis muscle onto the squamous portion of the temporal bone. The temporalis muscle is freed from the temporal bone and retracted anteroinferiorly. Elevation of the temporalis muscle in this fashion preserves its nerve and blood supply so that it could be utilized later for a temporalis muscle transfer to the lower face in case of persistent facial paralysis. The temporalis muscle is elevated to the temporal line and held in place with self-retaining retractors.

Elevation of the Bone Flap

A craniotomy opening is made in the squamous portion of the temporal bone (Fig. 3). The opening is approximately 4 cm square and is located two-thirds anterior and one-third posterior to the external auditory canal. It is important to place the craniotomy opening as near as possible to the floor of the middle fossa. This usually requires hand retraction of soft tissue by an assistant.

A medium cutting burr and continuous suction-irrigation are used. The bone flap is thicker superiorly as the squamoparietal suture is approached. It is important not to lacerate the dura during the bone removal for this could allow herniation of the temporal lobe. Herniation can best be avoided by leaving a thin plate of bone over the dura. The bone can then easily be fractured and removed. We prefer to make a bone flap rather than a burr hole and rongeur enlargement so that the temporal bone flap can be replaced at the end of the procedure. This results in less tissue retraction in the area of the incision, thus improving the cosmetic appearance. Replacement of the bone flap also reduces the possibility of transmission of brain pulsations to the skin, which is cosmetically undesirable.

Bone bleeders are commonly encountered and are controlled with bone wax. It is important to keep the edges of the bone flap parallel. This facilitates placement of the middle fossa retractor.

Once the surgeon has drilled nearly through the temporal bone flap, a joker elevator is used to separate the underlying dura and the bone flap is removed. Sharp edges are trimmed from the bone and it is placed in normal saline solution during the operation.

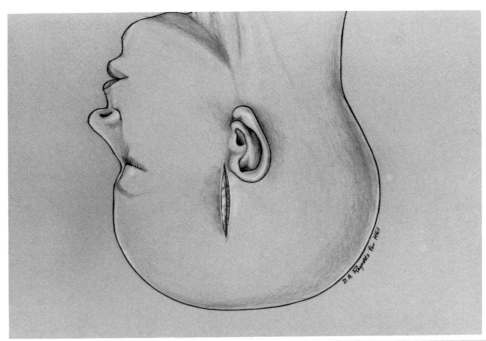

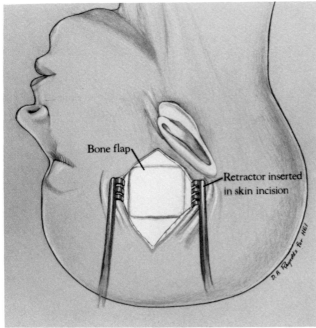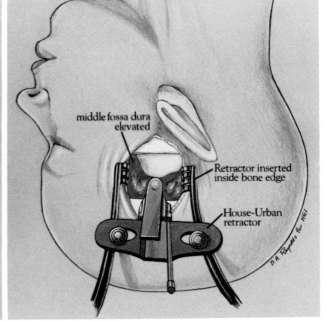

Figure 2 (_Top_). The incision extends 7–8 cm superiorly from the natural hairline and is 0.5 cm anterior to the helix.

Figure 3 (_Lower left_). The bone flap is made two-thirds anterior and one-third posterior to the external auditory canal.

Figure 4 (_Lower right_). A middle fossa retractor is firmly locked in place, and dural elevation is begun.

Elevation of the Dura

The dura is separated from the margin of the craniotomy defect with the joker elevator. Any sharp bone edges are removed with the rongeur. Occasionally, the inferior bone cut is above the floor of the middle fossa. This excess bone is removed with the rongeur. At times, there will be bleeding from the branches of the middle meningeal artery on the surface of the dura. This is best controlled with bipolar cautery with care being taken not to burn a hole in the middle fossa dura. The level of cautery must be reduced to the minimum necessary to coagulate the vessel. It is important to maintain the integrity of the dura since any defect may allow herniation of the temporal lobe. If a small tear is produced, it should be closed with dural silk suture to prevent extension and herniation. After separation of the dura from the edges of the craniotomy defect, the House-Urban retractor is put in place and firmly locked. The blade of the retractor is then set in place and gentle elevation of the dura from the floor of the middle cranial fossa is begun (Fig. 4).

The House-Urban retractor contains three adjustments, allowing for the desired placement of the retractor. The first adjustment affords movement of the entire blade mechanism in an inferior-superior direction. Once the blade is properly centered at the depth of the middle fossa dissection, this adjustment is secured at a position that gives maximum exposure but does not impinge on the superior edge of the craniotomy opening.

Dural elevation is carefully begun from posterior to anterior. As the dura is elevated, the tip of the blade is advanced. The two other adjustments are arranged appropriately. One adjustment allows for anterior-pos-terior movement of the tip of the retractor blade. The other adjusts the placement of the tip of the blade in a superior-inferior direction.

The structures within the temporal bone as viewed from above are shown diagrammatically in Figure 5. The first landmark to be identified is the cranial entrance of the middle meningeal artery at the foramen spinosum. This marks the anterior limit of the dural elevation. Frequently, venous bleeding is encountered in this area. It may be necessary to control this bleeding by placing a firm pack of Surgicel into the foramen spinosum.

The surgeon's attention is then directed posteriorly and the medial elevation of the dura is accomplished from posterior to anterior. First the petrous ridge is identified posteriorly. Care is taken in this area because the petrous ridge is grooved by the superior petrosal sinus which the surgeon must avoid entering. If the sinus is inadvertently entered, bleeding can usually be controlled by extraluminal packing with Surgicel. However, small pieces of Surgicel must not be placed in the lumen of the sinus because they can produce a pulmonary embolus.

The dura is then elevated from the floor of the middle fossa medially from posterior to anterior. In approximately 5% of cases, the geniculate ganglion of the facial nerve will not be covered by bone. Blind or rough elevation of the dura in such cases can result in damage to the facial nerve. It is best to gently elevate the dura from the temporal bone rather than to scrape the elevator along the bone of the middle fossa.

The posterior to anterior elevation avoids raising the greater superficial petrosal nerve. If this nerve were elevated and the dissection carried posteriorly,

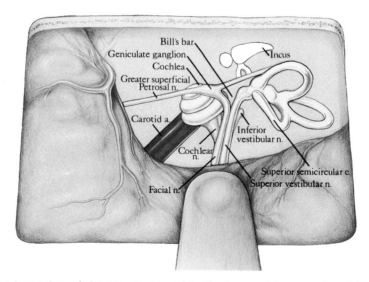

Figure 5. The relationship of the structures within the temporal bone as viewed from the middle fossa.

the geniculate ganglion and facial nerve would again be subject to injury. In the literature on the middle fossa approach to the gasserian ganglion an up to 5% incidence of facial paralysis has been reported. With careful dural elevation performed with the aid of the surgical microscope, this complication can be avoided in all cases.

As dural elevation proceeds, the arcuate eminence is encountered. At times, this is an obvious landmark but sometimes it is indistinct. The positive landmark is the greater superficial petrosal nerve which passes parallel to the petrous ridge, anteriorly from the geniculate ganglion. This nerve lies medial to the middle meningeal artery. Once the greater superficial petrosal nerve has been identified, it is carefully followed to the hiatus of the facial nerve and the blade of the middle fossa retractor is readjusted (Fig. 6).

A word of caution is necessary regarding pressure on the bone of the floor of the middle fossa. Both in the area of the tegmen and over the internal carotid artery the bone may be very thin and rarely even dehiscent. Although injury to the internal carotid artery has not occurred in our cases, care must be taken to avoid this complication. At this point the major landmarks of the middle fossa approach have been identified. These are the middle meningeal artery, the arcuate eminence, the greater superficial petrosal nerve, and the facial hiatus. Therefore, the surgeon is ready to begin bone removal over the internal auditory canal. There is often considerable bleeding from small vessels on the surface of the dura and the floor of the middle fossa. This bleeding is particularly troublesome since it pools into the most dependent portion of the wound where the bone removal is to begin. Considerable bleeding from any one vessel must be controlled. It is usual, however, for oozing to occur from multiple sites. We have found that such bleeding will stop spontaneously and it is best to proceed with the operation at this point.

Exposure of the Internal Auditory Canal

A large diamond burr and continuous suction-irrigation are brought in and careful removal of bone to identify landmarks of the temporal bone is begun. It is important to use the largest burr early in the bone removal since it offers the most protection against accidental injury to the geniculate ganglion, facial nerve, or superior semicircular canal. Attention is directed to the greater superficial petrosal nerve and bone is gently removed from the area of the hiatus until the geniculate ganglion is identified. A thin shell of bone is usually left over the geniculate ganglion but the ganglion itself is readily apparent through the bone (Fig. 7). By this time, bleeding has usually sub-

sided. If not, it is advisable to spend the time necessary to control the bleeding before proceeding.

The labyrinthine portion of the facial nerve is then followed from the geniculate ganglion to the internal auditory canal (Fig. 8). The labyrinthine portion of the facial nerve courses parallel to the plane of the superior semicircular canal. A smaller diamond burr is necessary for this bone removal since the ampullated end of the superior semicircular canal lies only a few millimeters posterior to the facial nerve at this point and the cochlea lies only a few millimeters anteriorly.

Some surgeons prefer to proceed with removal of bone over the internal auditory canal following the identification of the superior semicircular canal. The internal auditory canal makes an angle of 45 to 60° with the superior semicircular canal. We have found it easier to positively identify the internal auditory canal by following the facial nerve. We have not experienced problems with facial nerve paralysis by using this technique. Continuous monitoring of the facial nerve alerts the surgeon when the facial nerve is exposed.

Once the internal auditory canal has been identified, bone removal is continued medially until the entire superior surface of the internal auditory canal is exposed. As the surgeon proceeds medially it is possible to enlarge the exposure because the superior semicircular canal courses posteriorly and the dissection is medial to the cochlea (Fig. 9). Bone removal is continued until the porus acusticus is removed. The superior petrosal sinus grooves the petrous ridge and care is taken not to enter the superior petrosal sinus.

Great care must be taken to remove the bone without entering the dura because the facial nerve lies directly against the dura. It is best to leave an eggshell thickness of bone over the entire surface of the internal auditory canal until all of the bone removal has been completed.

Bone removal must be extensive for middle fossa acoustic tumor surgery. Medially, bone removal is carried far anterior and posterior to the internal auditory canal. The superior petrosal sinus will be lying free in the dura following removal of the petrous ridge. Care must be taken to avoid bleeding but should it occur it may be controlled with extraluminal packing of Surgicel or with clips.

The dissection is limited posteriorly by the superior semicircular canal. Bone is carefully removed from the entire extent of the internal auditory canal which allows exposure of approximately three-quarters of the circumference of the canal at the porus. It is not possible to achieve this degree of exposure in the lateral portion of the internal auditory canal because of the restricting position of the ampulla of the superior semicircular canal and the cochlea. When bone removal has been completed medially, the lateral end of

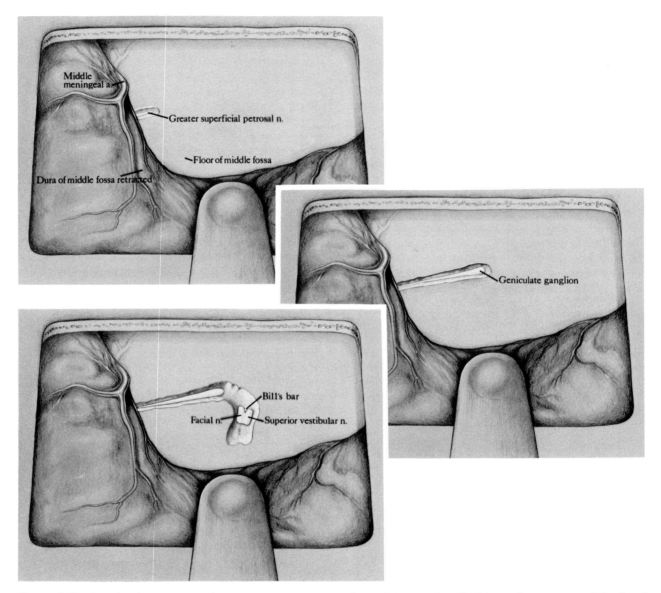

Figure 6 (Top). The dura is elevated and the greater superficial petrosal nerve is identified medial to the middle meningeal artery.

Figure 7 (Middle). Bone is removed from the greater superficial petrosal nerve until the geniculate ganglion is identified.

Figure 8 (Bottom). The labyrinthine portion of the facial nerve is uncovered from the geniculate ganglion to the internal auditory canal.

the internal auditory canal is dissected and the vertical crest of bone separating the facial nerve from the superior vestibular nerve (Bill's bar) is identified.

This completes the bone removal. The fine eggshell layer of bone is then removed and the dura is opened along the posterior aspects of the internal auditory canal (Fig. 10). The facial nerve lies anteriorly and the first exposure of the internal auditory canal should be away from the facial nerve. The dural flap is carefully elevated from the underlying tumor and the facial nerve is identified at the lateral end of the internal auditory canal where the vertical crest of bone (Bill's bar) allows positive identification. The superior vestibular nerve lies posteriorly at this point and a fine hook is used to begin the separation of the superior vestibular nerve and tumor from the facial nerve.

Tumor Removal

The vestibulofacial anastomotic fibers are cut and the superior vestibular nerve is cut at the end of the internal auditory canal. Separation of the tumor from the

end of the internal auditory canal and the facial nerve is begun next (Fig. 11). The principle of the tumor removal is that the tumor is freed from the facial nerve and the internal auditory canal and is delivered posteriorly out from under the facial nerve. For this reason, it is most important to remove all of the bone from the posterior aspect of the internal auditory canal.

Freeing of the lateral end of the tumor, particularly in the inferior compartment of the internal auditory canal, is one of the most difficult parts of the dissection. This difficulty is attributable to the poor view of the most lateral aspect of the inferior compartment of the internal auditory canal. The removal is accomplished with a long hook that is used to palpate the end of the internal auditory canal. It is best to totally section both the superior and inferior vestibular nerves to prevent postoperative unsteadiness (Fig. 12). A partial vestibular denervation is more likely to result in unsteadiness than is total removal of both vestibular nerves.

The tumor is gently teased out of the lateral end of

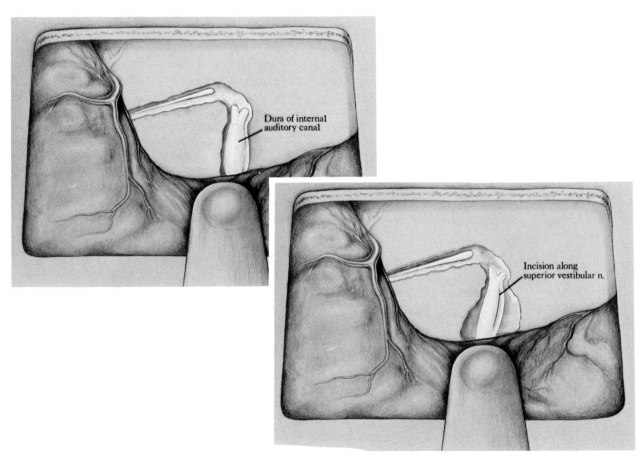

Figure 9 (Upper left). Bone is removed from the entire length of the internal auditory canal, including the porus acusticus.

Figure 10 (Lower right). The lateral end of the internal auditory canal has been dissected and the vertical crest (Bill's bar) identified. The dura is then incised at the posterior margin of the internal auditory canal.

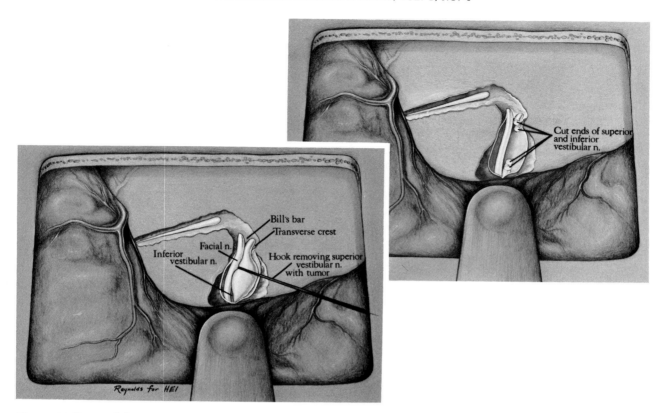

Reynolds for HEI

Figure 11 (*Lower left*). The tumor is separated from the facial nerve at the end of the internal auditory canal. It is carefully freed from the facial and cochlear nerves and delivered posteriorly.

Figure 12 (*Upper right*). The tumor has been removed. It is best to section the inferior vestibular nerve to minimize the risk of postoperative unsteadiness.

the internal auditory canal. The blood supply to the cochlea usually runs between the facial and cochlear nerves and in most cases is preserved with those nerves. At times, however, the arterial supply to the cochlea is interrupted, resulting in hearing impairment even though preservation of the cochlear nerve was achieved.

Once the lateral end of the tumor has been freed, the plane between the cochlear and facial nerves and tumor becomes apparent. This plane is then carefully developed through the use of fine hooks and the Rosen separator. Tumor dissection is continued medially and a search for the anterior inferior cerebellar artery is begun. The artery may loop up into the internal auditory canal inferior to the cochlear nerve or the tumor may displace it into the cerebellopontine angle. Great care must be taken to identify and not injure this most important artery.

After the anterior inferior cerebellar artery has been identified, it is freed from the surface of the tumor by careful blunt dissection with the Rosen elevator. The final problem is freeing the most medial aspect of the tumor. Before this, it is often necessary to partially remove the tumor with small cup forceps. This pre-

vents stretching of the facial nerve. During the course of the dissection, the surgeon must be careful not to injure the facial nerve with suction. This possibility is reduced by the use of the fenestrated neurotologic suction tip. Freeing of the medial end of the tumor with small hooks allows its removal (Fig. 12). Continuous intraoperative monitoring of facial nerve activity greatly facilitates dissection of the tumor from the facial nerve and is utilized routinely.

After total tumor removal, the tumor bed is irrigated profusely. Bleeding from small vessels usually subsides during the irrigation. At times, larger vessels will require bipolar cautery for control of bleeding.

Inadvertent injury to the anterior inferior cerebellar artery is always a possibility during removal of the medial aspect of the tumor. Control of bleeding would be extremely difficult in this situation because of limited access. Fortunately, this has not occurred in our experience; if it should, it might be necessary to remove more bone in the area of the superior semicircular canal to expose more of the posterior fossa dura in order to gain access for the application of a clip. If bleeding should still not be controlled, it might be necessary to perform a postauricular approach and translabyrinthine exposure of the cerebellopontine angle to achieve this control.

Wound Closure

Closure of the defect in the internal auditory canal is accomplished with a free graft of temporalis muscle. The temporal bone flap is then replaced and the temporalis muscle resutured to its insertion. The subcutaneous tissue and skin are closed in layers and a sterile dressing is applied. If there is excessive oozing, a Penrose drain is utilized.

COMPLICATIONS AND MANAGEMENT

An epidural hematoma is an uncommon early postoperative complication. The incidence of this may be reduced by the use of a drain where there is excessive oozing. Meticulous attention to hemostasis is a necessity. Patients with this complication will exhibit signs of increasing intracranial pressure. Treatment is immediate evacuation of the hematoma on the intensive care unit. The patient is then taken to the operating room where more definitive control of the bleeding is accomplished.

Other complications are those that are common to any intracranial procedure, such as meningitis. Temporal lobe injury from retraction on the temporal lobe was an early concern but has not been a problem in our series. We have had no patients who have had signs of cortical injury such as hemiparesis or aphasia. Hearing loss and facial paralysis are expected complications in some of these patients as with any acoustic tumor removal.

DISCUSSION OF SERIES

As of June 1989, over 2500 acoustic neuromas had been removed at the Otologic Medical Group (Los Angeles, CA). The middle fossa approach had been used to remove 106 of these tumors as of December 1986. The size of these tumors varied from 0.4 to 2 cm. Hearing was preserved in 63 patients (59%). In 37 patients (35%), hearing was the same as before surgery. There was a partial loss of hearing in 26 patients (25%). In the remainder, a total sensorineural hearing loss occurred despite preservation of the cochlear nerve in 89% of patients. Hearing roughly correlated with tumor size: hearing preservation is better for smaller tumors.

Eighty percent of patients had normal facial nerve function one year after middle fossa surgery for removal of an acoustic tumor. Another 9% had Grade II function and the remainder a greater degree of weakness. No patient had a total facial nerve paralysis. These statistics demonstrate the increased risk to the facial nerve in the middle fossa approach. In the translabyrinthine approach, with tumors of this size, 88% have normal facial function. The attempt at hearing preservation offered by the middle fossa approach does increase the risk to the facial nerve.

Other than hearing loss and facial weakness, there were no other serious complications in this series. There were no deaths.

CONCLUSION

The middle fossa approach is the preferred method for removal of small, laterally placed acoustic neuromas.

UPPER THORACIC SYMPATHECTOMY BY A POSTERIOR MIDLINE APPROACH

PREM K. PILLAY, M.D.
ISSAM A. AWAD, M.D.
DONALD F. DOHN, M.D.

INTRODUCTION

Current indications for upper thoracic sympathectomy include intractable palmar hyperhidrosis and, to a lesser extent, Raynaud's disease, reflex sympathetic dystrophy, and other sympathetic mediated pain syndromes. A variety of approaches for upper thoracic sympathectomy have been employed. These include anterior transthoracic, preaxillary transthoracic, supraclavicular, posterior thoracic, thoracic endoscopic, and percutaneous/stereotaxic approaches. The posterior approach is the most advantageous to neurosurgeons because it incorporates an exposure similar to that of thoracic laminectomy, and it allows bilateral exposure of the sympathetic chains and ganglia at a single sitting and via a single incision. The standard approach developed at our institution is a posterior midline approach, with bilateral 3rd rib costotransversectomy allowing a one-stage bilateral excision of the 2nd thoracic sympathetic ganglia. This is a modification of the technique described by Cloward and is based on the observation that the 2nd thoracic sympathetic ganglion provides exclusive innervation of sweat glands of the palm. If axillary sweating is also a prominent complaint, both the T2 and T3 ganglia are removed.

POSITIONING

Our preference is to perform this procedure in the sitting position because we believe that it affords a better exposure, with easier instrument handling than in the prone position. The possibility of air embolism is less of a concern because the operative wound is nearly at the level of the heart. The use of a central venous line is usually not necessary. After endotracheal general anesthesia, the patient is placed in the sitting position on a Gardner chair (Fig. 1) or by appropriately flexing the operating table. The head is held by elastic straps to a padded horseshoe rest applied to the face and is held erect by means of a metal frame slotted into the sides of the chair. The use of head-pins is avoided as these may be a source of air embolism.

Localization of the T2 spinous process is done by placing a radiopaque marker on the skin and obtaining a lateral cervical/upper thoracic x-ray film. The skin is scratched over the T2 spinous process, which is approximately at the level of the T3 costotransverse junction (Fig. 1). The patient's back is then shaved, cleaned, prepared, and draped.

OPERATIVE PROCEDURE

Exposure

A midline linear skin incision is made centered over the T2 spinous process approximately 10–15 cm in length. This will allow exposure of the T1–T3 spinous processes and laminae. The subcutaneous fat is cleanly divided to expose the underlying deep fascia (Fig. 2). A monopolar electrocautery knife is then used with a periosteal retractor to expose the spinous processes in the midline, followed by subperiosteal dissection of the paraspinal muscles off the laminae and costotransverse junctions from medial to lateral. The wound is held open with angled D'Errico retractors. Confirmation of the correct level is done by placing metal clips on either side of the transverse process and obtaining an intraoperative posteroanterior chest roentgenogram (Fig. 3). Compulsion about correct localization will avoid the undesirable complications of inadvertent stellate (T1) ganglionectomy with associated Horner syndrome, or a more caudal (below T2) ganglionectomy without adequate palmar sympathectomy.

Using a Leksell rongeur, the costotransverse junction bone is thinned out. Bone removal is then completed with Kerrison rongeurs after stripping the underlying pleura away with a Penfield instrument. In this manner a 3-cm section of the costotransverse

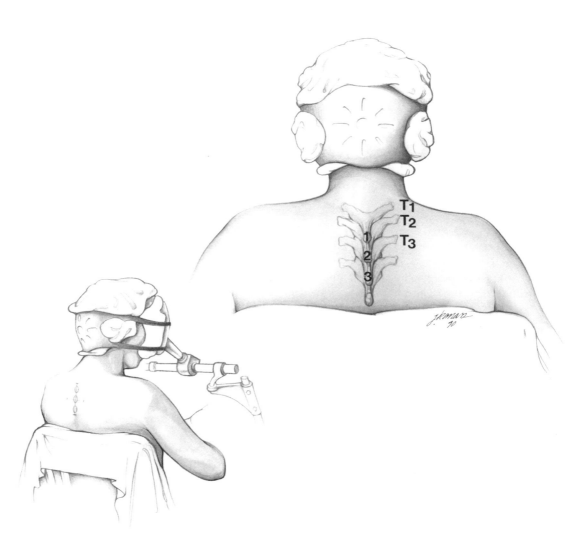

Figure 1. Operative positioning. The T2 spinous process is marked using lateral cervicothoracic radiographic guidance. The incision extends from T1 to T3 and is centered on the spinous process of T2. Because of downward slanting of the spinous processes, the center of the incision is at the level of the 3rd costotransverse junction. Because the incision is approximately at the level of the heart, no central venous line is placed for air embolism monitoring. To further minimize this risk, skull pins are not used, and the head is fixed instead to a padded horseshoe cerebellar rest using elastic bands.

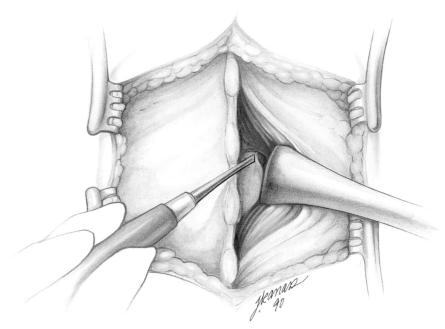

Figure 2. Paraspinal muscle dissection. The midline incision is extended to the spinous processes. Using electrocautery, the paraspinal musculature is stripped in a subperiosteal fashion.

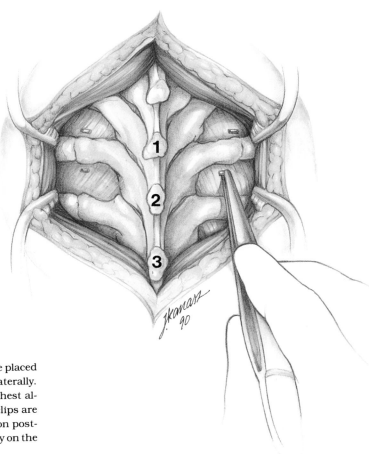

Figure 3. Intraoperative localization. Metal clips are placed above and below the 3rd costotransverse junction bilaterally. An intraoperative posteroanterior x-ray film of the chest allows verification of the correct level (3rd rib). These clips are subsequently removed so they will not be confused on postoperative films with other metallic clips placed directly on the sympathetic chain.

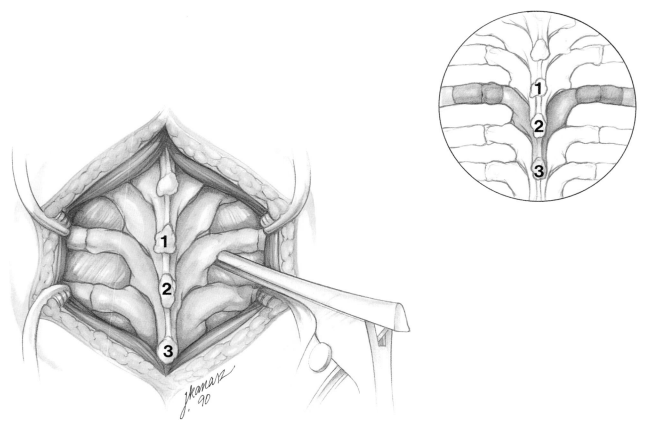

Figure 4. Bone removal. Using Kerrison rongeurs, bilateral T3 costotransversectomies are performed. The area of resection should extend to the pedicle medially and should include approximately 3 cm of the head of the rib (*inset*). The spinal canal is not entered by this bony removal.

junction is resected (Fig. 4). Care is taken to avoid too medial a bony exposure as inadvertent damage to the nerve roots and dura may occur with entry into the spinal canal. This procedure is carried out bilaterally. The bone edges are waxed and hemostasis carefully secured before the next step of identification of the sympathetic chain and ganglia.

Identification of the Sympathetic Chain and Ganglionectomy

A pair of Smithwick sympathectomy dissectors are used in the next step of this procedure. The spatula end of the instrument is used to depress and sweep the pleura in a medial to lateral fashion, while the hook end is used to probe for the chain. This is usually visualized as a fine gray glistening strand under loupe (× 2.5) magnification. This strand is usually followed superiorly to the T2 costotransverse joint level. The T2 ganglion can be identified as a prominent ovoid bulb along the sympathetic chain, with rami communicans tethering it to the adjacent intercostal nerve (Fig. 5).

A tonsillar hemostat is used to retract the ganglion downward (caudally), while sharply isolating the ganglion from the adjacent intercostal nerve. The neuroganglionic segment is then resected en bloc between two clips applied to the sympathetic chain cephalad and caudad. The clips provide a permanent radiographic marker of the sympathectomy and may help prevent regeneration of sympathetic innervation. The T3 ganglion may be included in the caudal end of the neuroganglionic segment if axillary sweating is a prominent complaint (Fig. 6). Prior to closure, the wound is irrigated with saline solution and Valsalva's maneuver initiated by the anesthetist to identify any pleural air leak which would predispose to a pneumothorax.

Wound Closure

Closure is carried out in a standard fashion. A few deep muscle stitches are placed using 1-0 Nurolon or silk sutures, followed by a watertight fascial closure with 2-0 Nurolon or silk sutures. The subcutaneous

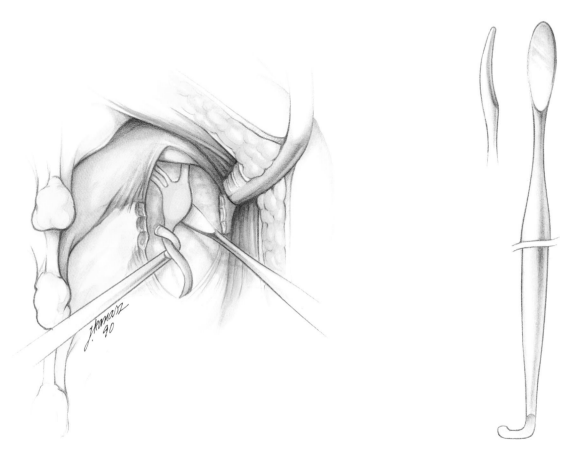

Figure 5.   Dissection of the sympathetic chain. The Smithwick dissector is used (the hook end in one hand, and the spatula end in the other hand) to free up the epipleural adhesions and retract the visceral pleura away from the spinal column. The hook end is then used to find and deliver the sympathetic chain. Further dissection with the Smithwick instrument cephalad allows the identification of the T2 ganglion. Its communications with the intercostal nerve are sharply divided. The ganglion is further delivered downward to visualize the sympathetic chain above it.

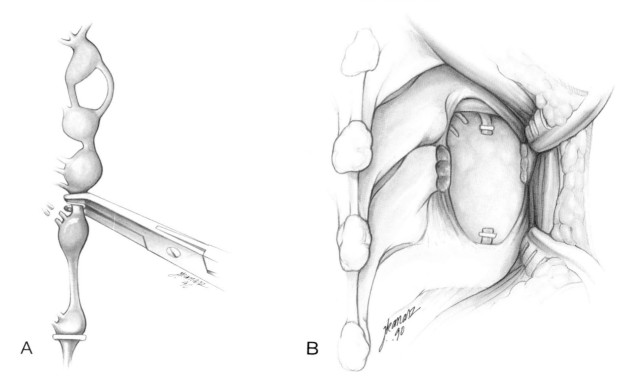

A   B

Figure 6. A, metal clips are placed above the T2 spinous process cephalad (making sure not to include the next higher ganglion which is the stellate ganglion), and another clip caudad at or below the 3rd sympathetic ganglion. **B,** the specimen is sent for rapid frozen pathologic confirmation of sympathetic ganglion, while the epipleural space is explored using irrigation and Valsalva's maneuver to ensure the absence of a tear in the visceral pleura which would predispose to postoperative pneumothorax. The management of a visceral pleural tear is discussed in the text.

layer is apposed with 3-0 Dexon or Vicryl and the skin closed with interrupted 3-0 Nurolon or nylon sutures. In the presence of an air leak from a pleural tear, this is located and a small red rubber catheter (No. 8 French) is placed within the pleural space. The wound is then closed in layers around the red rubber catheter until just prior to the last fascial stitch. The other end of the catheter is then placed in a basin of saline solution and positive intrapleural pressure is used by the anesthetist to drive air out through this underwater seal. The catheter is withdrawn during Valsalva's maneuver and wound closure is completed.

After application of the wound dressing, the head straps are removed, the patient transferred to the supine position, and anesthesia is reversed and the patient extubated. The palms of the hands should be warm and completely dry *immediately* following surgery.

POSTOPERATIVE CARE

An x-ray film of the chest (upright expiration view) is obtained in the recovery room and again the next day to exclude a pneumothorax. Vigorous incentive spirometry is encouraged in the postoperative period.

Parenteral narcotics and muscle relaxants are typically required for 1 or 2 days, followed by oral analgesics as needed. The patient is ambulated 24 hours after surgery and is usually sent home by the 3rd or 4th postoperative day. The skin sutures are left in for 14 days and the patient is restricted from lifting and strenuous activities for 4–6 weeks. A transient period of palmar moisture can be noted a few days after surgery (after initial palmar dryness); this has been attributed to *denervation hypersensitivity* of the sweat glands. This is never of the same intensity as preoperatively and only lasts 1 to 2 days; it warrants patient reassurance. Occasional neuritic discomfort is encountered in the axillae and interscapular region, especially following excessive manipulation of the intercostal nerve. This typically resolves spontaneously.

From 1960 to 1988, 440 patients with severe hyperhidrosis were selected for upper thoracic sympathectomy at the Cleveland Clinic. There was no operative mortality. The main complications were wound infection (2.9%), and pneumothorax requiring chest tube insertion (<1% of patients). Air embolism has not been a problem in any patient despite the use of the sitting position. All patients operated upon for hyperhidrosis had immediate relief of palmar sweating. Ninety-two percent of patients had long-term satisfaction with surgical results after a mean follow-up period of 7.2 years. A major cause of dissatisfaction was the occurrence of *compensatory sweating.* This occurred in other body areas in up to 35% of patients in the postoperative period, but was felt to be a persistent troublesome complaint in less than 5% of patients on longer follow-up. Frank recurrent palmar hyperhidrosis occurred in only three patients, 3, 5, and 6 weeks post-surgery, respectively. One of these patients with persistent unilateral hyperhidrosis had reexploration and ganglionectomy (missed at the first procedure) and was left with dry hands.

The results of this operation for Raynaud's disease and sympathetic mediated pain have been less gratifying, with less than half the cases deriving significant lasting benefit.

In conclusion, the upper thoracic (T2) ganglionectomy performed via the posterior approach is a safe, effective, and durable operation for the treatment of intractable essential palmar hyperhidrosis. It has allowed patients of all walks of life to improve social and occupational interactions without the hindrance, stigma, and embarrassment of excessive palmar sweating. The operation has also had limited application in other pathophysiologic situations mediated by sympathetic hyperactivity.

CAROTID ENDARTERECTOMY

DANIEL L. BARROW, M.D.
CHRISTOPHER E. CLARE, M.D.

INTRODUCTION

Atherosclerotic lesions of the cervical carotid artery usually occur at or near the common carotid bifurcation. These lesions may result in cerebral ischemia or infarction due to hemodynamic impairment of carotid blood flow or distal embolization. Although both of these mechanisms are important, embolization appears to play the dominant role in carotid system ischemia. Carotid endarterectomy is the surgical procedure for removing these atherosclerotic lesions from the region of the carotid bifurcation. Although the operation has significant intuitive appeal, the appropriate indications for carotid endarterectomy are the subject of ongoing debate. Several studies have demonstrated that patients with ischemic neurologic symptoms referable to the distribution of a significantly stenosed and/or ulcerated carotid artery experience a decreased risk of stroke following a successful carotid endarterectomy.

INDICATIONS AND ASSESSMENT OF RISK

The decision to perform a carotid endarterectomy should be based on a number of factors other than the mere presence of an atherosclerotic lesion of the carotid bifurcation. Important factors in the decision-making process include the patient's symptoms, physiologic state, collateral circulation, and underlying health. Carotid endarterectomy is primarily indicated for patients with clear ischemic neurologic symptoms ipsilateral to a significant carotid stenosis and/or ulceration. In certain situations, after consideration of all variables, a patient will be treated with systemic anticoagulation or antiplatelet agents rather than surgery. Patients with amaurosis fugax, central retinal artery occlusion, venous stasis retinopathy, transient ischemic attacks (TIAs) in the carotid distribution, prolonged reversible ischemic neurologic deficits, and mild-to-moderate fixed ischemic neurologic deficits are at risk for ischemic hemispheric damage.

The indications for carotid endarterectomy in a large group of patients with asymptomatic neck bruits, asymptomatic carotid stenosis, and vertebrobasilar symptoms associated with carotid artery stenosis are quite controversial. We do not recommend further work-up of patients with asymptomatic bruits. Because the natural history of asymptomatic carotid lesions is not well defined, we reserve endarterectomy for only those asymptomatic patients with severe stenosis (<2 mm residual lumen) or deep ulcerations. We have not performed a carotid endarterectomy for vertebrobasilar symptoms. However, after a critical analysis of the competence of the circle of Willis and collateral blood flow, some surgeons have thought that blood flow to an insufficient vertebrobasilar circulation can be augmented by removing a hemodynamically significant carotid lesion.

In all patients, the decision must be individualized after considering the patient's age, risk factors, and surgical risks for the particular institution and surgeon. The grading system developed by Sundt and associates groups patients according to predetermined risk factors and is useful in predicting the risks of surgical intervention:

Group 1. Neurologically stable with no major medical or angiographically defined risks, with unilateral or bilateral ulcerative-stenotic carotid disease;
Group 2. Neurologically stable with no major medical risks but with significant angiographically defined risks;
Group 3. Neurologically stable with major medical risks, with or without significant angiographically defined risks;
Group 4. Neurologically unstable, with or without associated major medical or angiographically defined risks.
Patients in groups 3 and 4 are at greatest risk for non-neurologic and permanent neurologic complications, respectively.

PREOPERATIVE ASSESSMENT

All patients with cerebrovascular symptoms should be evaluated to determine the cause of the symptoms and to assess the risk of stroke. Those patients with frequent TIAs, stroke-in-evolution, or acute onset of a mild deficit are at greatest risk and should be evaluated urgently.

We do not rely heavily on noninvasive tests of the carotid artery in clinical decision making. Good quality angiography is essential in the evaluation of patients being considered for carotid endarterectomy. Visualization of the origins of the cranial vessels in the thorax and of their extracranial and intracranial distributions are all important. In the symptomatic patient, angiography is usually performed after the patient has had appropriate medical evaluation and computed tomography (CT) or magnetic resonance imaging (MRI) of the head. The CT or MRI will usually rule out the presence of a mass lesion, such as a tumor, that may cause symptoms mimicking cerebral ischemia. These studies will also reveal old or new infarcts that may alter the timing of surgical intervention or show a "silent" lesion in the distribution of an otherwise asymptomatic carotid lesion.

Prior to surgery, the patient's cardiopulmonary status is carefully evaluated. Carotid atherosclerosis is an important indicator of systemic atherosclerosis. In patients with significant cardiac disease, a Swan-Ganz catheter may assist in fluid management in the perioperative period.

Patients with a recent transient ischemic attack or progressing focal cerebral ischemic event will frequently be placed on heparin while awaiting surgery. If symptoms continue despite adequate anticoagulation, these patients are considered surgical emergencies. Other patients selected for endarterectomy are scheduled for surgery as soon as possible unless they have had a recent major stroke or recent myocardial infarction which necessitates a delay. Patients awaiting an elective endarterectomy are placed on 325 mg of aspirin per day before surgery; this is continued postoperatively.

SURGICAL TECHNIQUE

Anesthesia

General endotracheal anesthesia is induced with thiopental sodium (3–5 mg/kg) and paralysis is obtained with pancuronium or vecuronium bromide (0.1 mg/kg). Lidocaine (1.0 mg/kg) or fentanyl (0.05–0.1 mg) is used to diminish a cardiovascular response to intubation. Anesthesia is maintained with a nitrous oxide/oxygen mixture and isoflurane (0.5–1.5%). Respirations are controlled to maintain an end-tidal CO_2 between 35 and 38 mm Hg. The patient is given glucose-free fluids during and after the operation. Anesthesia monitoring includes urine output, arterial blood pressure measurements, arterial blood gas analysis, end-tidal CO_2 determinations, and electrocardiographic monitoring. Monitoring of cerebroelectrical function is carried out with conventional 16-channel electroencephalography (EEG).

Operative Positioning

The patient is placed in the supine position with the head on a foam rubber "doughnut." The head is extended and turned slightly away from the side of the operation (Fig. 1). One or two rolled sheets are placed under the shoulder blades to facilitate extension of the

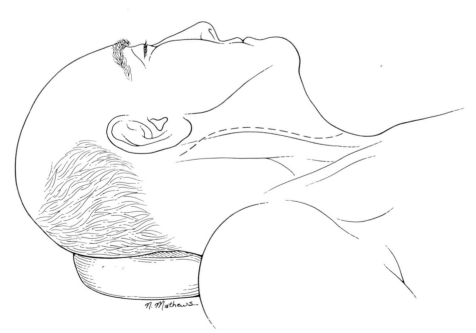

Figure 1. The patient is placed supine with the head on a foam rubber doughnut and turned slightly away from the side of the operation. The skin incision (*dashed line*) is made along the anterior border of the sternocleidomastoid muscle. It is curved superiorly to facilitate distal exposure without injuring the marginal mandibular branch of the facial nerve.

head. Rotation of the head will bring the internal carotid artery to a more accessible position laterally than its normal position behind the external carotid in an anteroposterior plane. The amount of head turning needed for optimal exposure can be determined from the preoperative anteroposterior angiogram. To diminish the risk of dislodging embolic material from the atherosclerotic plaque, the neck is not scrubbed but is prepared with povidone-iodine solution. If there is any suggestion from the preoperative angiogram that a venous patch graft will be needed or if the operation is a repeat procedure, a distal lower extremity is shaved, prepared, and draped for exposure of the saphenous vein for obtaining the graft.

Skin Incision

The skin incision is placed along the anterior border of the sternocleidomastoid muscle (Fig. 1). This may be curved medially at the lower end to a point just above the sternal notch. The superior limb is curved posteriorly from a point about 1 cm below the angle of the mandible toward the mastoid process. This superior curve is designed to avoid injury to the marginal mandibular branch of the facial nerve. The exact length of the incision is dictated by the position of the carotid bifurcation and the morphology of the plaque as demonstrated on the angiogram. The skin incision is carried down to the platysma muscle, dividing the transverse cervical nerve, which results in unavoidable numbness anterior to the skin incision.

Operative Procedure

The platysma is divided sharply, and meticulous hemostasis is maintained. A self-retaining retractor is placed into the wound with the medial side more superficial to avoid injury to the laryngeal nerves (Fig. 2). Dissection is carried out along the anterior border of the sternocleidomastoid through the loose areolar tissue that lies between this muscle and the strap muscles overlying the trachea. The plane of dissection is followed down to the internal jugular vein, which, as a key landmark for the exposure, lies lateral, parallel, and slightly anterior to the internal and common carotid arteries. Extreme care is taken to avoid manipulation of the carotid bifurcation and proximal internal carotid artery to minimize the risk of dislodging embolic material from the plaque. If the artery is palpated, as in a patient with a thick neck, it should be performed only on the common carotid artery and far away from the bifurcation.

Once the jugular vein is identified, dissection is along the medial border of the vein (Fig. 3). The common facial vein, which crosses the carotid at the level of the bifurcation, is doubly ligated and divided. It is usually necessary to section the omohyoid muscle to obtain adequate proximal exposure. The carotid sheath is incised over the common carotid artery. Tacking the sheath to the external cervical fascia helps elevate the carotid in the wound. Two self-retaining retractors are placed into the external fascia, further elevating the carotid from the wound.

As dissection is carried superiorly, the descendens hypoglossi nerve may be divided as it joins the hypoglossal nerve proper to prevent undue traction on the latter structure and to mobilize it for distal dissection of the internal carotid artery (Fig. 3). The superior thyroid artery is identified and dissected circumferentially. It is mandatory to gain access to the distal internal carotid artery. To do so, it may be necessary to divide the digastric muscle and mobilize the hypoglossal nerve. Injection of a local anesthetic into the carotid body and sinus is not routinely performed. However, if the anesthesiologist notes any change in vital signs during dissection of the bifurcation, 2–3 ml of 1% lidocaine is used to temporarily block the effects of carotid sinus stimulation.

The common and external carotid arteries are dissected free from their underlying beds only in those areas where umbilical tapes or clamps are placed around them. The umbilical tapes placed around the internal and common carotid arteries are threaded through rubber tubing to fashion a Rummell tourniquet. These should be placed well above and below the plaque as determined by the angiogram, observation of thickness in the vessel wall, or gentle palpation.

A No. 9 French malleable multiperforated suction tube is placed adjacent to the common and internal carotid arteries and fixed into position by stapling it to the surgical drapes.

Prior to carotid artery clamping, 100 units/kg heparin is given intravenously. Bolus doses of thiopental sodium (150–250 mg) are given until 15- to 30-second burst suppression is seen on the EEG recording. The barbiturate is continued by bolus injections or constant infusion to maintain burst suppression until internal carotid artery flow is reestablished. A phenylephrine infusion is occasionally required to maintain systemic blood pressure in the normal range. Hypotension must be avoided.

Once the heparin and barbiturates have circulated, the internal carotid artery is occluded first with an aneurysm clip. The common carotid artery is immediately occluded with a Fogarty vascular clamp, and temporary aneurysm clips are placed on the external carotid and superior thyroid arteries (Fig. 4).

The arteriotomy is begun in the common carotid artery with a No. 11 scalpel. Potts arterial scissors are used to extend the arteriotomy distally beyond the termination of the plaque in the internal carotid artery (Fig. 5). The true lumen of the vessel is entered,

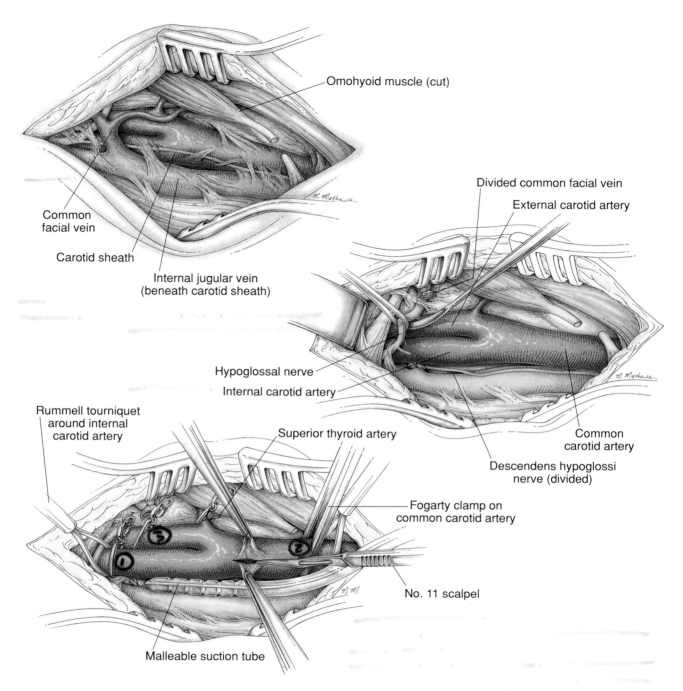

Figure 2 (Top). The loose areolar tissue anterior to the sternocleidomastoid is separated and a self-retaining retractor placed no deeper than the platysma muscle. The omohyoid muscle has been divided to improve proximal exposure.

Figure 3 (Middle). The common facial vein has been doubly ligated and divided, and the carotid sheath has been opened. Division of the descendens hypoglossi allows greater mobilization of the hypoglossal nerve and reduces the risk of traction injury to the latter.

Figure 4 (Bottom). The common and external carotid arteries have been dissected free from their underlying beds where clamps are placed around them. Rummell tourniquets have been fashioned for the common and internal carotid arteries in the event a shunt is necessary. Once heparin and barbiturates have circulated, the internal carotid artery is occluded first with an aneurysm clip. Next, the common carotid artery is occluded with a Fogarty clamp and aneurysm clips are placed on the external carotid and superior thyroid arteries. The arteriotomy is initiated with a No. 11 scalpel.

and no attempt is made to perform an extraluminal dissection of the plaque from the artery. Great care must be taken to ensure that the back wall of the carotid is not damaged. The arteriotomy incision should extend up the midline of the vessel to facilitate later closure of the arteriotomy. The arteriotomy into the common carotid artery is continued until the plaque ceases to be ulcerated and the wall of the vessel becomes more normal in texture. The atherosclerotic plaque is carefully dissected from the internal carotid artery with a microdissector or small spatula (Fig. 6). The plaque is removed by following the pathological cleavage plane created by the atherosclerosis between the intima and the fine layer of media. During the dissection, a vascular pickup is used to hold the wall of the artery as the assistant holds the edge of the

plaque. The spatula is moved from side to side, developing the plane described above, which is usually readily separated. Dissection proceeds halfway around the wall before repeating the separation from the other side. A clean feathering away of the plaque is usually possible in the distal internal carotid artery but not in the common carotid artery. The plaque is transected sharply in the common carotid artery and elevated to visualize the orifice of the external carotid.

In removal from the external carotid artery, the plaque is elevated from the wall through the orifice of the vessel (Fig. 7). As it thins, the vessel is everted, and the plaque is grasped with a hemostat and pulled inferiorly. Although this is a blind procedure, it usually breaks cleanly from the wall of the external carotid artery. Patency of this artery may be determined by

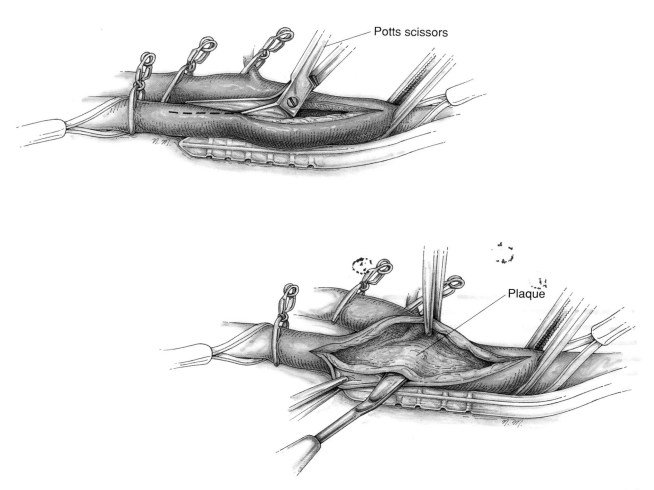

Figure 5 (Top). The arteriotomy is extended distally with Potts arterial scissors. The opening should extend up the midline of the vessel and within the true lumen of the artery. The arteriotomy is extended distally until the limit of the plaque on the posterior wall of the internal carotid artery is identified. The arteriotomy into the common carotid is con-

tinued until the plaque ceases to be ulcerated and the wall of the vessel becomes more normal in texture.

Figure 6 (Bottom). The plaque is removed by developing and following the pathological cleavage plane created by the atherosclerosis between the intima and media.

intraoperative angiography or by palpation of the superficial temporal artery pulse following restoration of blood flow.

The cut edges of the proximal end of the common carotid artery are everted, and the plaque is cut circumferentially 1–2 cm below the end of the arteriotomy (Fig. 8). This allows plaque removal below the end of the arteriotomy incision, making closure of the vessel easier and avoiding proximal stenosis. Once the plaque has been removed, the operating microscope is positioned to allow both the surgeon and assistant to have clear binocular vision. Loose fragments of atherosclerotic material and abnormal intima are meticulously removed under continuous heparinized saline irrigation. The irrigation fluid and blood are cleared from the wound by the Microvac suction tube. With the operating microscope, the distal internal carotid artery is carefully inspected, and any elevation of the intima beyond the end of the plaque is carefully trimmed with microscissors. If there is an abrupt step off or if the intima is loosely adherent to the media, double-armed sutures of 7-0 Prolene are placed vertically from the inside of the vessel outward so they traverse the intimal edge and are tied outside the adventitial layer. The arteriotomy is closed using a running 6-0 Prolene suture, starting at the distal end of the incision (Fig. 9). The use of the operating microscope to place small, closely spaced stitches results in a tight, nonleaking suture line without compromising the lumen of the vessel.

Prior to final closure, back bleeding from all the vessels is allowed to expel air and debris from the lumen of the repaired segment. The superior thyroid artery is not reclipped, allowing continuous back bleeding during placement of the final sutures to avoid air being trapped in the vessel. Following final closure of the arteriotomy, the arteries are reopened in a specific order. The external carotid artery is opened initially, followed by the common carotid artery. The common carotid artery is briefly reclosed just before the internal carotid artery is opened to allow any embolic material to be washed into the external carotid artery. The common carotid artery is then unclamped.

Placement of a Shunt

A shunt is used when there are changes in the EEG that do not immediately respond to a trial of induced hypertension. We prefer the Sundt internal shunt. The plaque is removed from the distal internal carotid artery prior to shunt placement (Fig. 10). The distal end of the shunt is first placed into the internal carotid artery. Back bleeding from the internal carotid artery will fill the shunt with blood. Then the proximal end is placed into the common carotid artery and

secured with the Rummell tourniquet. Plaque removal is completed by working around the shunt.

An alternate method of shunt placement is first to insert the shunt into the common carotid artery and secure it with the Rummell tourniquet. The shunt is held closed at its midportion with vascular forceps, briefly opened to confirm blood flow and evacuate any debris in the shunt tubing, and then placed into the lumen of the internal carotid artery.

Regardless of the technique, the shunt should easily thread up the internal carotid artery, and no force should be used to advance the shunt or intimal damage and dissection may result.

In its removal, a suture is placed loosely around the shunt to facilitate extraction. Prior to completely closing the arteriotomy, the shunt is withdrawn through a small open segment of the arteriotomy. The arteriotomy closure is then completed in a routine fashion.

Wound Closure

The retractors are removed and sufficient time is spent to obtain excellent hemostasis because the heparin is not reversed. The platysma and subcutaneous tissue are reapproximated and the skin closed with a 4-0 Vicryl subcuticular suture and Steristrips.

POSTOPERATIVE CARE

With the use of barbiturates, many patients are obtunded for a short period of time following recovery from anesthesia and may require continued intubation until they are alert. However, these patients may be examined, as brain stem function is readily tested and the patients will move their extremities in response to noxious stimulation.

Blood pressure is carefully monitored both in the recovery room and in the intensive care unit. Patients generally spend 24–48 hours in the intensive care unit following surgery. Once the patient tolerates liquids, aspirin is restarted and is continued indefinitely.

ALTERNATIVES IN SURGICAL TECHNIQUE

There are a number of technical variations in performing a carotid endarterectomy that are quite acceptable. Excellent surgical teams have advocated the routine use of venous patch grafts, routine shunting, local anesthesia, and many other personal preferences. It is important that the surgical team becomes comfortable with its method and frequently assesses its results.

Closure with a Venous Patch Graft

It is our custom to make liberal use of a venous patch graft in the closure of an endarterectomy, although it

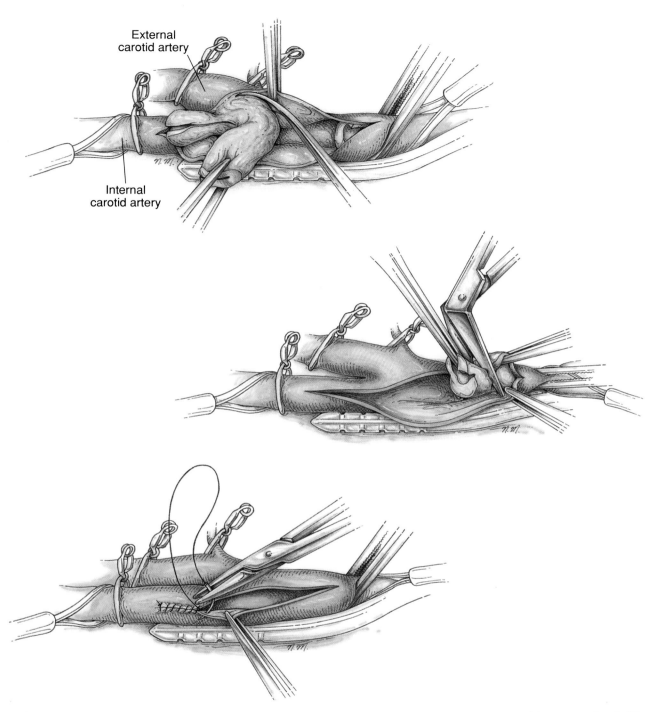

External carotid artery

Internal carotid artery

Figure 7 (Top). The plaque has been removed from the internal carotid artery initially so that a shunt may be placed more safely if necessary. The plaque has been sharply excised from the wall of the common carotid artery with Potts scissors. Next, the plaque is elevated and dissected from the external carotid artery by working through its orifice with a spatula. Once the plaque becomes thin, it is grasped with a hemostat and pulled inferiorly.

Figure 8 (Middle). The cut edges of the proximal end of the common carotid artery are everted and the plaque cut circumferentially 1−2 cm below the end of the arteriotomy. This maneuver makes closure of the proximal arteriotomy easier and avoids stenosis below the end of the arteriotomy incision.

Figure 9 (Bottom). The arteriotomy is closed under the operating microscope with running 6-0 Prolene sutures.

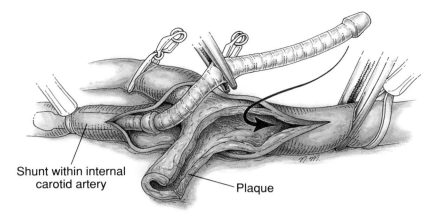

Shunt within internal
carotid artery

Plaque

Figure 10. In the event that a shunt is required, the plaque is initially removed from the distal internal carotid artery. The shunt is grasped in the center with hemostats and placed into the internal carotid artery. The hemostats are temporarily opened to allow back bleeding to fill the shunt with blood. The proximal end is then placed into the common carotid artery and secured with the Rummell tourniquet.

is not employed routinely. A venous patch graft is used in all cases of reoperation or if there is a suggestion from the arteriogram that the internal carotid artery is small. We believe that use of the operating microscope allows for closure of the arteriotomy with small suture bites and little compromise of the vessel lumen, thus reducing the need for a patch graft.

The venous graft is harvested from the saphenous vein just anterior to the medial malleolus at the ankle. A segment of vein 6–8 cm in length is removed, and the direction of flow is maintained. The vein is opened along a longitudinal seam by initially creating a small incision with the Potts scissors and advancing the partially opened scissors along the vein (Fig. 11). The distal end of the patch graft is preshaped and the vein stored in heparinized saline until ready for use.

The saphenous vein patch graft is sewn into place under the operating microscope with a 6-0 running double-armed Prolene suture (Fig. 12). The initial suture is critical and is placed through the apex of the graft and most distal point of the arteriotomy. This suture should be placed from the exterior of the graft to the interior and from the intimal surface of the internal carotid artery to the adventitial surface. Once the distal half of the graft has been sewn into place on both sides, the proximal end of the graft is shaped to conform to the proximal portion of the arteriotomy.

Shunting

Attitudes toward the use of shunts during endarterectomy range from those surgeons who routinely place shunts in all patients to those who do not monitor and never use a shunt. Our preference is to monitor patients with EEG, use barbiturates to increase the brain's tolerance for ischemia, and selectively employ shunts in those patients with asymmmetry in the EEG. Sundt and associates have had outstanding results using intraoperative cerebral blood flow measurements and EEG to determine the need for a shunt without the addition of barbiturates.

Barbiturate Anesthesia

Many surgeons perform carotid endarterectomies under local or general anesthesia without the use of barbiturates. The advantage of local anesthesia is the ability to neurologically monitor the patient during surgery. Barbiturates reduce the metabolic requirements of neural tissue and have been shown to modify or prevent cerebral injury from focal, reversible ischemia. They are most effective if given prior to the period of temporary focal ischemia and at a dosage that achieves burst suppression of the EEG. For these reasons, we routinely administer thiopental sodium prior to carotid cross-clamping and maintain burst suppression of the EEG with thiopental until the flow is reestablished. Spetzler and associates have advocated the routine use of barbiturates for carotid endarterectomy and reported a 1.5% morbidity and mortality in a series of 200 consecutive endarterectomies.

Despite the barbiturate-induced burst suppression of the EEG, asymmetry of the recordings between the two hemispheres can be readily appreciated. This allows for the placement of a shunt if a trial of induced hypertension does not correct the asymmetry.

In our opinion, the added cerebral protection of barbiturates will provide the time necessary for a meticulous, unhurried endarterectomy. The often-reported barbiturate hypotension has not been a prob-

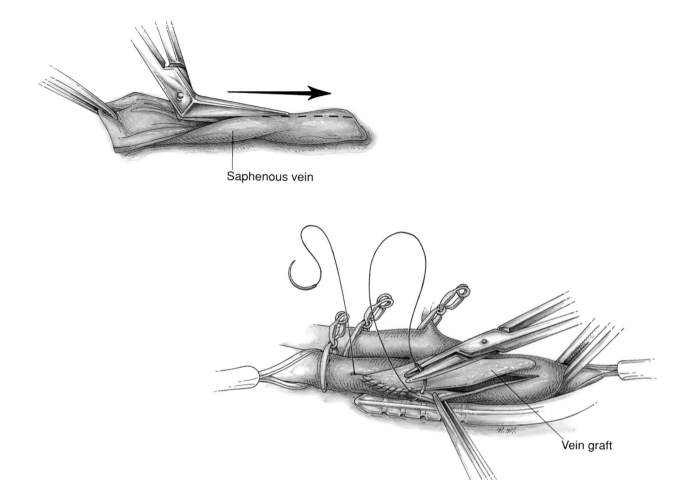

Saphenous vein

Vein graft

Figure 11 (*Top*). To prepare a saphenous vein graft, the vein is opened with Potts scissors. The inferior margin of the vein is grasped with forceps and the partially opened Potts scissors are advanced to produce a truly linear incision (*dashed line*).

Figure 12 (*Bottom*). In closure of the arteriotomy with a saphenous vein patch graft, the distal end of the graft has been preshaped and is sewn into place under the operating microscope with a 6-0 running double-armed Prolene suture. Sutures should be placed from the exterior of the graft to the interior and from the intimal surface of the internal carotid artery to the adventitial surface.

lem in our patients. Although barbiturates may delay a detailed postoperative neurologic evaluation, we think that the benefits far outweigh the risks.

Operating Microscope

Many excellent surgical teams perform carotid endarterectomies using only loupe magnification and headlight illumination. We have found that the superior illumination and magnification afforded by a microscope provides exceptional visualization of the operative field, especially the distal internal carotid artery. After removing the atherosclerotic plaque, the surgeon brings the microscope into the field to complete a meticulous endarterectomy by removing small fragments of plaque and diseased intima. With the microscope one can inspect the critical region of the distal internal carotid to be certain there is a smooth internal surface. Arteriotomy closure performed under the microscope is unequaled in our opinion. The sutures are placed with small close bites of a precise thickness of the vessel wall. Such a closure avoids stenosis of the internal carotid, reduces the need for a patch graft, and invariably results in a completely dry arteriotomy closure.

Intraoperative Angiography

Technical complications of carotid endarterectomy include residual plaque, intimal flaps, stenosis, and thrombosis. Such defects may cause a perioperative stroke through occlusion of the carotid artery, distal embolization, or delayed recurrent stenosis. Some surgeons elect to perform postoperative digital or conventional angiography to detect such defects. Others use noninvasive carotid testing to determine the presence of technical deficiencies.

With the availability of compact, portable, digital intraoperative angiography equipment, we have found intraoperative angiography to be simple and quite helpful. Technical errors are identified during the operation and can be corrected immediately. Once the arteriotomy is closed and flow reestablished, a 19-gauge butterfly needle is placed into the common carotid artery proximal to the endarterectomy site. After the fluoroscope is put into place, about 10 ml of 60% meglumine iothalamate is manually injected as rapidly as possible. If intraoperative angiography equipment is not available, a standard, single-shot conventional x-ray film exposed during contrast injection will provide adequate detail. If a large x-ray plate is positioned under the neck and head, an adequate film of the cervical and intracranial vessels can be obtained.

COMPLICATIONS OF CAROTID ENDARTERECTOMY

Any therapeutic advantage of a carotid endarterectomy is easily negated if the morbidity and mortality are excessive. A low perioperative morbidity and mortality rate in the range of <4% is mandatory for any potential benefit of the operation to be realized. Unfortunately, these rates range from 1.5% to more than 20% in the literature.

Complications may result from technical errors in performing the operation or as a consequence of the underlying systemic atherosclerosis these patients frequently have. Unfortunate consequences of carotid endarterectomy may be divided into non-neurological and neurological complications.

Non-neurologic Complications

Cardiac Ischemia

The atherosclerosis necessitating carotid endarterectomy generally reflects systemic vascular disease, including that of the coronary arteries. Myocardial infarction is the most serious systemic complication following carotid endarterectomy and accounts for the majority of postoperative deaths. In the study by Fode and associates of 1234 carotid endarterectomies, the incidence of myocardial infarction was 4.9% in those patients who had a significant cardiac history, although it was much lower in those who had no such history. Thus, close perioperative monitoring of cardiac function, including pulmonary artery catheterization as well as strict avoidance of severe hyper- or hypotension, is necessary in those with a significant cardiac history.

Wound Infection

Wound infection following endarterectomy is uncommon. Staphylococcal organisms are usually the offending agents. This complication is best managed by reexploration of the wound with irrigation and debridement. If the infection appears to involve deeper fascial layers, an arteriogram should be performed to exclude the possibility of a false aneurysm.

False Aneurysm

This rare complication should be considered whenever there is a persistent hematoma or infection. The diagnosis is made by arteriography, and treatment consists of excision of the aneurysm wall with repair of the artery, using a saphenous vein patch graft. This complication is more common when synthetic patch grafts are used to close the arteriotomy, especially if a deep wound infection occurs.

Wound Hematoma

Postoperative swelling of the wound may be due to hematoma or lymphatic fluid. This is usually a self-limiting process that will resolve in a few weeks. However, if airway compromise (usually due to hematoma) is present, the wound should be reexplored, the fluid collection evacuated, and the source of bleeding controlled.

Neurologic Complications

Embolization or Thrombosis

Distal embolization may occur at any time during or after the operative procedure. The highest risk for this complication is during dissection and manipulation of the artery and placement of a shunt. Minimizing manipulation and dissection in the region of the plaque will reduce the risks of embolization. Placing the clip on the internal carotid artery prior to occluding the common and external carotid arteries also reduces the chance of distal embolization, as does appropriate back bleeding prior to completion of the arteriotomy closure.

Another potential source of intraoperative or postoperative emboli or thrombosis is the newly exposed media of the artery, which is quite thrombogenic. Avoiding reversal of the heparinization may allow the formation of a platelet "pseudoendothelium" and may decrease the incidence of this problem. Perioperative treatment with aspirin may also reduce the incidence of embolic and thrombolic complications.

Ischemia during Carotid Occlusion

Most patients are able to tolerate the temporary carotid occlusion necessary for performing an endarterectomy. In the Mayo clinic series, where cerebral blood flow was measured during carotid endarterectomy, 8% of patients had levels below 10 ml/100 g/min. This level of cerebral blood flow is below the threshold necessary for maintenance of cellular integrity and will result in cerebral infarction.

We use barbiturates during the period of time the carotid is occluded to protect the brain from ischemia. If there is EEG evidence of ischemia, a shunt is placed to provide collateral blood flow during the operation.

Postoperative Hemorrhage

This rare complication may result from poorly controlled postoperative hypertension, especially in the setting of a high-grade carotid stenosis that has been opened. Sundt and associates have suggested that a normal perfusion pressure breakthrough phenomenon, similar to that observed in some patients undergoing resection of an arteriovenous malformation of the brain, may be a mechanism of postoperative hemorrhage. It is postulated that patients with a high-grade carotid stenosis are chronically hypoperfused; the intracranial vessels become dilated to maintain perfusion and lose the ability to autoregulate. These chronically dilated vessels are then unable to handle the restored perfusion pressure after endarterectomy.

Reperfusion of a recent stroke with hemorrhage into the infarct is another potential mechanism for this complication. Solomon and associates reported that 0.41% of patients undergoing carotid endarterectomy experienced a postoperative hemorrhage.

Seizures

This rare complication of carotid endarterectomy is usually seen within 1–2 weeks of surgery. It is postulated that this is due to edema secondary to relative hyperperfusion of the hemisphere. This complication is more common in patients who have had a preoperative stroke.

Cranial Nerve Injuries

A variety of cranial nerves are exposed to potential injury during a carotid endarterectomy, including the greater auricular, the marginal mandibular branch of the facial, the hypoglossal, and the superior and recurrent laryngeal nerves. Most cranial nerve injuries are due to traction and, unless inadvertently severed, will usually recover. If bilateral endarterectomies are planned, it is advisable to assess the function of the vocal cords prior to the second operation, as bilateral vocal cord paralysis due to bilateral recurrent laryngeal nerve injury is a serious complication that necessitates a tracheostomy.

TRANSSPHENOIDAL EXCISION OF MACROADENOMAS OF THE PITUITARY GLAND

GEORGE T. TINDALL, M.D.
ERIC J. WOODARD, M.D.
DANIEL L. BARROW, M.D.

INDICATIONS

Transsphenoidal surgery is the preferred approach for the surgical management of the majority of pituitary tumors, including macroadenomas. Indications for transsphenoidal surgery over transcranial approaches in large pituitary tumors include extension into the sphenoid sinus, associated cerebrospinal fluid (CSF) rhinorrhea, and invasion and/or destruction of the sphenoid bone with multidirectional intracranial extensions. This approach is also indicated when an intracranial operation would carry excessive risk for a patient (e.g., an elderly person in poor health or a patient with severely compromised vision). Occasionally, pituitary apoplexy warranting rapid decompression of the optic chiasm is another indication for a transsphenoidal approach.

CONTRAINDICATIONS

Transsphenoidal surgery is contraindicated when the patient has an infectious process involving the sphenoid sinus, a suprasellar mass associated with a normal sella turcica, or a "bottleneck" constriction between an intrasellar tumor and the suprasellar extension. A transcranial approach may also be considered in patients with significant intracranial tumor extension to the subfrontal, retrochiasmatic, or middle fossa regions.

A conchal sphenoid sinus is not a contraindication to the transsphenoidal operative approach as the use of a high-speed, angled drill allows the pituitary to be exposed safely.

PREOPERATIVE PREPARATION

As with any operation, preoperative assessment of patients undergoing transsphenoidal surgery is of paramount importance. To determine general health and tolerance of anesthesia, the patient's cardiovascular, respiratory, renal, hepatic, and endocrine systems should be evaluated, and a history of allergies, present medications, and prior anesthetic complications should be taken.

In patients with normal pituitary-adrenal function, 100 mg of hydrocortisone is routinely administered just before surgery; 50 mg is added to each liter of intravenous fluid during surgery, and 50 mg is given by mouth or intramuscularly in the recovery room and continued every 8 hours through the second postoperative day. Thereafter, the steroid dosage is tapered and subsequently discontinued or maintained at the level necessary for the patient's individual needs.

To reduce the risk of infection, a second-generation cephalosporin (e.g., cefuroxime) is also given just prior to surgery and continued for 24 hours postoperatively,

After the patient is anesthetized, an indwelling lumbar subarachnoid catheter or lumbar puncture needle is inserted and connected to a closed sterile drainage system. Pituitary tumors with suprasellar extension usually require withdrawal of CSF or the infusion of sterile saline to aid in removing the portion of the tumor above the sella. In the case of an intraoperative tear of the diaphragma sellae, the drain will aid in keeping the operative field dry during closure.

POSITIONING

In transsphenoidal operations, the endotracheal tube, esophageal stethoscope, and temperature probe are taped together and brought out the left side of the mouth. The endotracheal tube must be taped securely to the face. No oral airway is used.

Figure 1 provides an orientation for subsequent illustrations of the transsphenoidal approach. In the usual case, the skull clamp is placed with the pins in the temporal bones above the squama just below the parietal bossing (Fig. 2). If intraoperative x-ray examination or fluoroscopy of the sella is anticipated, e.g., with a presellar or conchal type of sphenoid sinus, a single pin is placed frontally, and two rear pins are placed in the occipital area. This allows free access to

intraoperative x-ray examination should the surgeon want to verify intraoperative location and monitor position of instruments in the sella and the suprasellar area (Fig. 3).

The head is tilted to the patient's left and elevated about 10° from the operating table with the surgeon standing on the patient's right side.

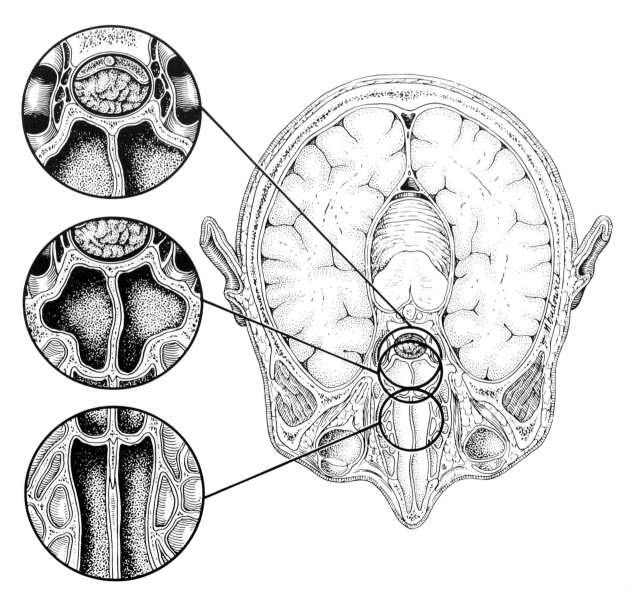

Figure 1. Orientation for illustrations of transsphenoidal approach for macroadenoma resection. The view is axial, with some of the subsequent *insets* depicting the procedure in a coronal plane.

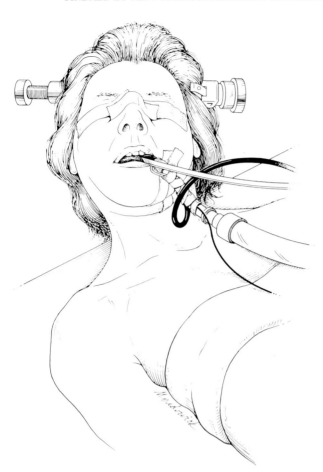

Figure 2. The patient is positioned with the head tilted to the left and elevated slightly. The skull clamp is placed just below the parietal bossing.

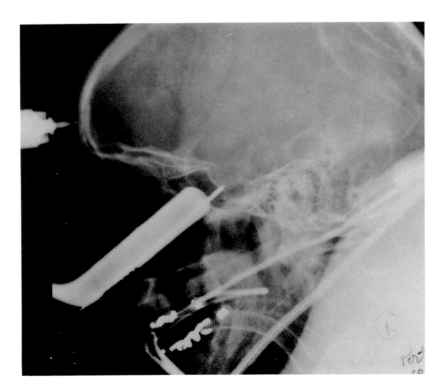

Figure 3. Lateral intraoperative skull film showing the position of a metal marker identifying the floor of the sella.

TRANSSPHENOIDAL SURGICAL PROCEDURE

Antiseptic solution (e.g., povidone) is applied to the nose and mouth, and the area is draped with sterile towels. The left lower quadrant of the abdomen is prepared and draped to obtain adipose tissue for later insertion into the sella turcica and sphenoid sinus. A separate set of sterile instruments is used to obtain the adipose tissue graft.

A small transverse incision is made in the upper gingival mucosa with a cutting cautery (Fig. 4). A cuff of mucosa on the inferior gingival edge should be left to be used for later closure. The incision is carried down to the maxilla, and a Freer dissector is used to separate the soft tissue in an upward direction to expose the piriform aperture, the floor of the nares, and the nasal mucosa.

With the cutting cautery in contact with the dissector, the tissue over the superior cartilaginous nasal septum is incised vertically (Fig. 5). Extending the incision slightly into the cartilage facilitates a subchondral separation of the mucosa from the nasal septum on one side.

Once the mucoperichondral plane between the septum and nasal mucosa is identified, it is developed inferiorly to the nasal spine using a small suction tip in the left hand and a dissector in the right hand (Fig. 6). At that level, the mucosa often adheres to the spine and considerable care should be taken to avoid a tear. The piriform aperture may have to be enlarged inferiorly and laterally with a small Kerrison punch.

Next, the nasal septum is fractured at its base anteriorly with a small osteotome, allowing it to be displaced to the opposite side. One of the palatine arteries, which is located anteromedially, may require coagulation at this point. Continued separation of mucosa from the nasal septum in a posterior direction is accomplished using a small sucker held in the right hand and a nasal speculum with long, thin blades held in the left hand. The blades are advanced and opened just enough to admit the tip of the sucker, which performs the actual separation of the mucosa from the nasal septum. At the posterior limit of the cartilaginous septum, a thin bony septum comprised of the superior portion of the vomer and inferior parts of the perpendicular plate of the ethmoid comes into view.

When the bony septum is in view, a speculum is introduced between the septum and mucosa and

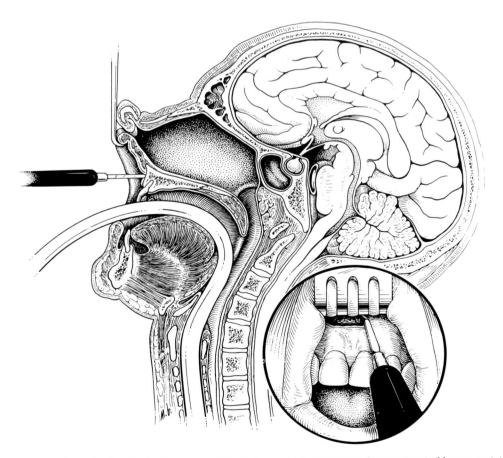

Figure 4. Incision in the gingival mucosa with electrocautery. The upper lip is retracted by an assistant.

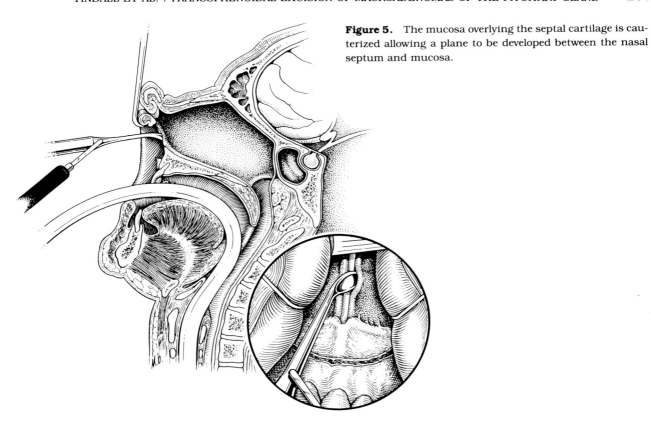

Figure 5. The mucosa overlying the septal cartilage is cauterized allowing a plane to be developed between the nasal septum and mucosa.

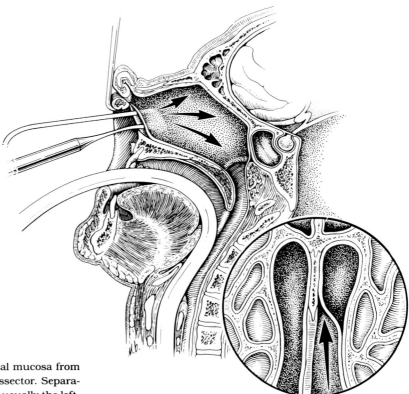

Figure 6. Method of separation of the nasal mucosa from the septum using a sucker tip and Freer dissector. Separation is made only on one side of the septum, usually the left.

opened (Fig. 7). This opening will fracture the thin perpendicular plate of the ethmoid near or at its junction with the sphenoid crest allowing one blade of the speculum to swing across the midline, thus exposing both sides of the anterior wall of the sphenoid sinus. The anterior wall of the sphenoid sinus with its characteristic "boat keel" appearance is a distinctive structure and is easily recognized. Although the speculum is inserted unilaterally, displacement of the nasal septum to the patient's right side makes the orientation midline (if the surgeon is using the left side). From this point on, the operating microscope is used with a 300-mm objective lens and ×12.5 oculars. The anterior wall of the sphenoid sinus is usually thin and can be opened with either Jansen-Middleton rongeurs, osteotomes, or Kerrison punches. The opening into the sinus can be started through the ostia of the sphenoid, located laterally at the 2 and 10 o'clock positions.

The size of the opening in the sinus is made slightly larger than the width of the speculum blades. The lateral extensions of the sphenoid opening are carried just far enough to visualize the most lateral aspect of the sella. The sphenoid sinus mucosa can be cauterized and shrunk using an insulated suction cau-tery. The speculum tip is advanced into the sinus and gently opened by hand only. This maneuver brings the surgeon closer to the sella and brings the long axis of the speculum directly in line with the center of the sella turcica (Fig. 8). It should be emphasized that although advancing the tips of the speculum into the sinus offers technical advantage, there is also potential danger of fracturing the sphenoid bone if force is used to open the speculum. Thus, one should not use excessive force (and certainly not a speculum-spreading instrument) when the tips of the speculum are positioned within the sphenoid sinus.

When the interior of the sphenoid sinus is visualized, recognition of the position of the sellar floor as it bulges into the sinus is straightforward. However, should any doubt exist, a lateral x-ray film of the skull can be obtained with a metallic marker such as a Kirchner wire lightly impacted into the anticipated position of the sellar floor (Fig. 3).

An opening is made in the anterior wall of the sella with a small osteotome placed on the sellar floor. Light mallet taps will fracture the floor and initiate the opening. Slight twisting of the impacted osteotome facilitates this maneuver. The opening is enlarged with a

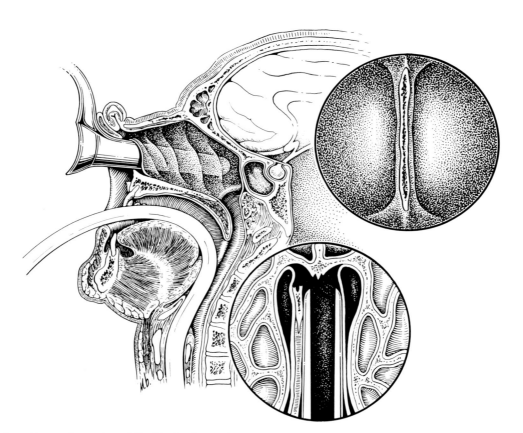

Figure 7. Insertion and opening of the bivalved speculum posteriorly fractures the thin, bony septum near or at the sphenoid crest and exposes the anterior wall of the sphenoid sinus on both sides of the midline.

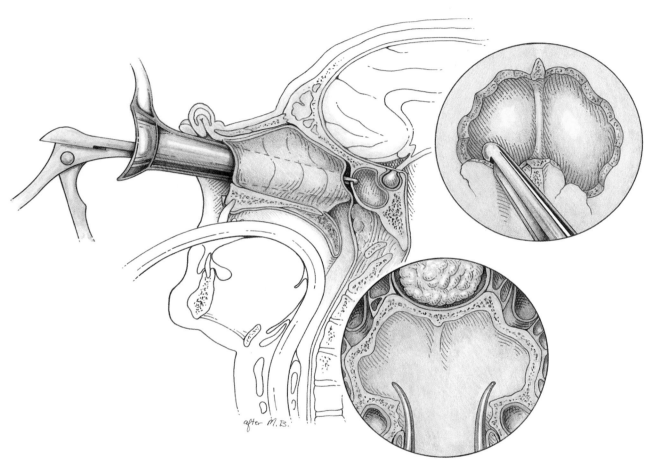

Figure 8. The anterior wall of the sphenoid sinus is opened and the flanged tips of a Cushing-Landolt speculum are gently placed within the sinus.

small punch laterally to the cavernous sinus and carotid bulge, inferiorly to the sella floor, and superiorly
to the intercavernous sinus (Fig. 9). Care must be
taken not to tear redundant dura with the rongeur
when opening the sella. A vertical incision is made in
the dura with a bayonet-handled scalpel having a No.
11 blade (Fig. 10), and a portion is excised in an elliptic
manner using angled microscissors (Fig. 11). If possible, a blunt hook is used to establish a plane between
the dura and pituitary gland or tumor. The dural
opening must not be extended too far superiorly or
laterally as entry into the suprasellar recess or cavernous sinuses can occur.

Macroadenomas frequently erode the floor of the
sella, appearing in the sphenoid sinus or extruding
into the sinus upon opening the dura. Usually the
tumor is readily visible and is removed easily with
blunt ring curettes, enucleators, and/or suction (Fig.
12). With large tumors, a thin, flattened pituitary
gland can be identified and spared. It is generally displaced posteriorly and superiorly.

In cases of suprasellar extension, the tumor can be
removed after evacuation of the intrasellar portion.
Preserving a cuff of tumor in the anterior and superior
aspect of the sella provides a handle to manipulate the
remaining suprasellar portion of the lesion. After the
bulk of the resection has been completed, the diaphragma sellae and tumor capsule can be inverted
into the sella by carefully raising the intracranial pressure with a slow infusion of Ringer's solution through
the lumbar subarachnoid catheter. The tumor is then
carefully peeled off the diaphragm with gentle suction.

The tumor bed generally stops bleeding once all
neoplasm is removed. In the absence of any CSF leak,
absolute alcohol can be applied to the resection bed for
about 5 minutes. This is an optional maneuver designed to destroy remaining tumor cells. This should
not be done, however, if there has been a tear in the
diaphragma sellae. The tumor bed and sphenoid sinus are then loosely packed with an adipose graft,
which may be held in place with fibrin glue. The speculum is withdrawn, and one or two absorbable catgut

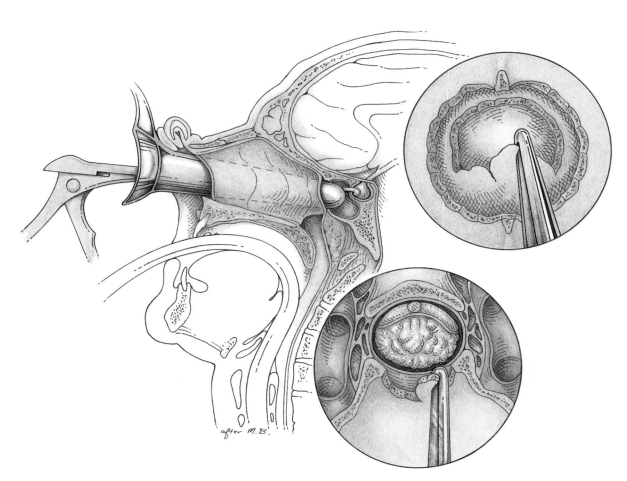

Figure 9. Removal of the sella floor with a small Kerrison rongeur.

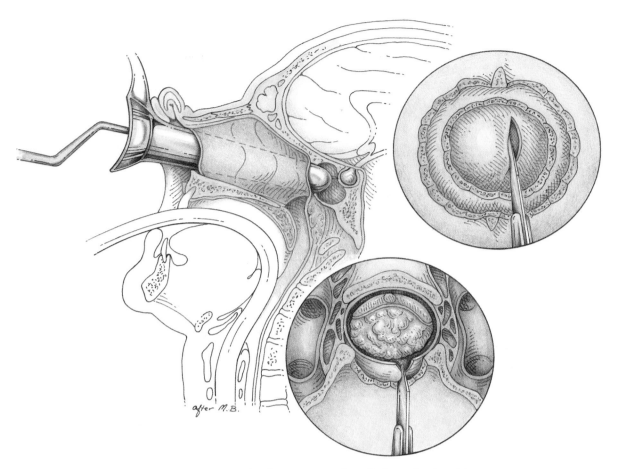

Figure 10   Incision in the dura covering the pituitary gland and tumor.

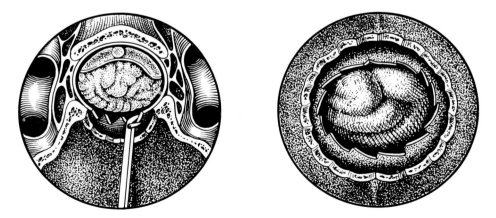

Figure 11.   Removal of an ellipse of dura using microscissors.

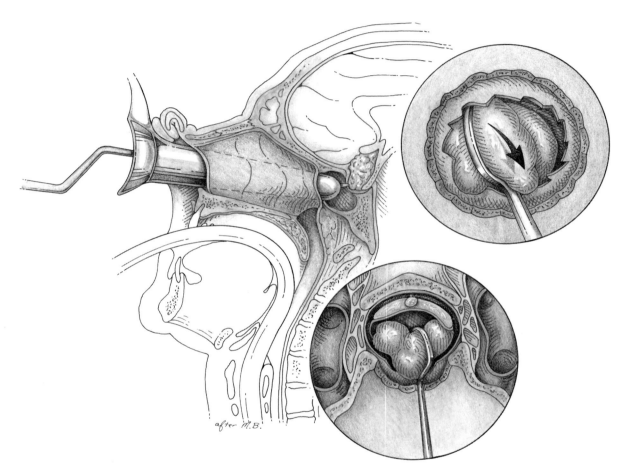

Figure 12. Resection of the tumor using a ring curette.

sutures are used to close the gingival mucosa. Soft rubber nasal airway tubes are placed in each nostril to reapproximate the nasal mucosa and are left in place for 24 hours. The nasopharynx and mouth are suctioned well, and the lumbar subarachnoid catheter is removed before the patient is awakened.

OPERATIVE MORBIDITY AND MORTALITY

Serious complications in patients undergoing transsphenoidal procedures are fortunately uncommon. In several large series, the incidence of operative death has been reported as 0.5%. Most fatal cases are associated with additional extenuating circumstances. Likewise, the incidence of nonfatal complications ranges from 1.1 to 13%, with an average of 3.6%.

Complications of transsphenoidal surgery may be classified anatomically as parasellar, intracranial, and sphenoid/nasofacial:

PARASELLAR
  CSF leakage
  Hypopituitarism
  Diabetes insipidus
  Cavernous sinus damage
  Intracavernous cranial nerve damage
  Intracavernous internal carotid artery
    damage
  Hemorrhage
  False aneurysm
  Carotid-cavernous sinus fistula
INTRACRANIAL
  Hydrocephalus
  Intracranial hemorrhage
  Hypothalamic damage
  Meningitis
  Optic chiasm or nerve damage
  Cerebral vasospasm
  Embolization
SPHENOID AND NASOFACIAL
  Sinusitis
  Mucocele
  Fracture of hard palate
  Fracture of cribriform plate
  Nasoseptal perforation
  External nasal deformity
  Devascularization or denervation of teeth

Because these have been described previously in standard texts, only a few of the more serious and/or frequent complications will be discussed.

CSF Rhinorrhea

The incidence of postoperative CSF leakage following transsphenoidal surgery depends primarily on the experience of the surgeon and the intrasellar pathologic findings. CSF leakage is common if the diaphragma sellae is disrupted during tumor removal, or in the case of an extensive macroadenoma directly eroding

this structure. Some delayed CSF rhinorrhea possibly occurs as a result of postoperative rupture of the diaphragma sellae where it herniates into the space left by removal of the tumor.

To prevent rhinorrhea, the intrasellar cavity and sphenoid sinus are filled with fat held in place with fibrin glue. The sellar floor may also be reconstructed with septal bone or cartilage, which helps to maintain the position of the fat graft and thus reduce the incidence of CSF leakage. Fat must be packed loosely to avoid producing a mass in itself. If the diaphragma sellae is torn or is intentionally opened during surgery, hyperventilation and/or lumbar drainage will diminish the CSF leakage during closure and permit a watertight seal.

Significant leakage of CSF usually manifests as a steady dripping of clear fluid, especially when the patient's head is placed in a dependent position. If only a few drops of clear to yellowish fluid are present, this likely represents nasal secretions or breakdown of the fat graft. If an adequate amount of fluid can be collected for quantitative analysis of glucose, a value greater than 30 mg/dl is diagnostic for CSF.

The initial approach to a persistent postoperative CSF leak should be conservative. One or more lumbar punctures are performed and CSF is removed slowly to as low a pressure as the patient's headache will tolerate. If the CSF leak persists, an indwelling spinal subarachnoid catheter is inserted percutaneously and left in place for 3 days, while the patient remains in bed with the head slightly elevated. The catheter is connected to a sterile reservoir, which is placed no higher than the lumbar puncture site. Should the fluid continue to leak following removal of the catheter, the transsphenoidal wound is reopened, and the sella and sphenoid sinus are repacked with adipose tissue.

Diabetes Insipidus

This may occur transiently or permanently following transsphenoidal surgery. Severe dehydration and electrolyte imbalance may result if the disorder is not promptly recognized. Treatment is with parenteral vasopressin (Pitressin) or intranasal desmopressin acetate (DDAVP).

Visual Complications

Damage to the optic nerves and/or chiasm may occur during removal of tumor from the suprasellar region. Attempts to remove adherent tumor or the tumor capsule from the optic apparatus may devascularize these structures and produce an irreversible visual deficit following infarction. This may be more common in patients who have been previously treated by craniotomy or radiation or who have poor vision preoperatively. Direct damage to the optic nerves may result from a fracture of the optic foramen and orbit produced by over-enthusiastic spreading of the bivalved speculum in the sphenoid sinus. Overpacking the sella with fat may cause pressure on the optic nerves and result in visual reduction; yet failure to leave a prop in the sella following removal of a large tumor leaves a cavity that possibly would allow prolapse of the optic nerves and chiasm. Pressure from a hematoma may damage the optic nerves and/or chiasm and may be reversible following prompt removal of the mass.

If vision appears to worsen postoperatively, an immediate computed tomography scan should be performed to identify a possible remediable cause, such as a hematoma or overpacked sella.

COMPUTER-DIRECTED STEREOTACTIC RESECTION OF BRAIN TUMORS

PATRICK J. KELLY, M.D.

INTRODUCTION

In order to resect an intra-axial tumor, a surgeon must visualize the tumor as a three-dimensional volume in space and know where surgical instruments are located with respect to that volume. However, there are several problems in the resection of deep-seated tumors which increase the risk and decrease the efficacy of surgery on these lesions. A deep-seated subcortical tumor may be difficult to find at nonstereotactic craniotomy. In addition, a glial neoplasm may have an irregular geometric configuration and it is difficult to stay oriented within these irregular extensions. Moreover, the histologic boundaries between a glial neoplasm and the normal or edematous gray and white matter may not always be clear at an open surgical procedure. Since deep-seated tumors are usually located in nonexpendible brain tissue, a surgical resection which strays out of tumor into brain parenchyma can result in severe neurologic complications. Computer-assisted volumetric stereotactic methods can be employed to help a surgeon localize the tumor and stay oriented within it. The following discussion concerns the instrumentation and methods presently used for computer-assisted volumetric resection.

INSTRUMENTATION

Stereotactic Frame

The COMPASS stereotactic system (Stereotactic Medical Systems, New Hartford, NY) was specifically designed for volumetric tumor stereotaxis. It evolved from a standard Todd-Wells stereotactic frame. The system consists of a fixed arc-quadrant, three-dimensional slide, and removable headholder (Fig. 1). It can be fixed onto a semipermanent base unit as shown in Fig. 2A, or mounted onto the lateral support rails of a standard operating table (Fig. 2B). In addition, data acquisition hardware (localization systems for computed tomography (CT), magnetic resonance imaging (MRI), and digital angiography (DA)) and computer

support hardware and software are also considered part of the system.

Headholder

The headholder consists of a base ring, four vertical supports, and skull fixation system. The headholder is fixed to the patient's skull by means of flanged carbon fiber pins.

Detachable micrometers are used to measure the distance between the end of the carbon fiber pins and the outer face of the vertical supports (Fig. 3). This provides a mechanism for accurate replacement of the frame if the data acquisition and surgery are not performed on the same day or if further stereotactic procedures are contemplated.

Arc-Quadrant

The 160-mm radius arc-quadrant attaches to horizontal arms which extend from the baseplate of the three-dimensional slide. Probes and retractors are directed by an attachment on the upper face of the arc. The arc-quadrant provides two angular degrees of freedom for approach trajectories (Fig. 4): a collar angle (from the horizontal plane) and an arc angle (from the vertical plane).

Three-Dimensional Positioning Slide

The headholder fits into a support yoke of a three-dimensional slide which moves the patient's head within the fixed arc-quadrant. Each axis of the three-dimensional slide is moved by a computer-controlled stepper motor or by hand crank if desired.

Stereotactic coordinates on the slide are detected by optical encoders on the x, y, and z axes which transmit the coordinates to digital readout scales and to the computer. In addition, Vernier scales on each axis for direct reading of stereotactic coordinates are provided as a backup to the optical encoders.

Computer System

Data acquisition, treatment planning, and stereotactic tumor resections are possible utilizing manual

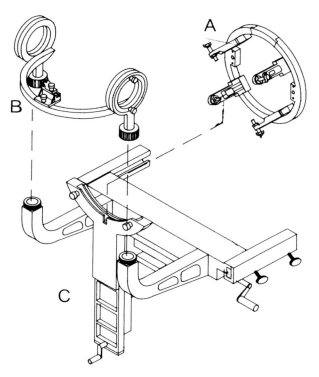

Figure 1. Components of the COMPASS stereotactic system which include a CT/MRI-compatible stereotactic headholder (**A**), a stereotactic arc-quadrant (**B**), and a three-dimensional positioning slide system, (**C**).

methods for calculation of stereotactic coordinates and cross-correlation of target points between the different imaging modalities. The computer is therefore not absolutely necessary. However, the computer saves a surgeon a great deal of time in calculating target points, interpolating imaging-defined tumor volumes, cross-registering points and volumes between CT, MRI, and DA, and in real-time interactive image displays during the surgical procedure. The computer makes volumetric stereotactic procedures practical and time efficient. At present, the COMPASS stereotactic frame is supported by a Vicom image processing system and Sun host computer. A Data General MV 7800 is used for backup and data storage.

Laser

The carbon dioxide laser is very useful in deep tumor stereotaxis and provides several advantages. First, the laser is convenient for removing tissue from a deep cavity and is relatively hemostatic. Second, the laser removes tissue by a narrow beam of light and thus there is one less instrument which must be inserted into a narrow surgical field. Finally, the laser beam can be computer-monitored and computer-controlled if desired.

Stereotactic Retractors

The stereotactic retractor system comprises cylindrical retractors, dilators, and an arc-quadrant adaptor. The retractor is a thin wall hollow cylinder 140 mm in length and 2 cm in diameter. Indexing marks on the retractor shaft are provided for measurement of insertional depth with respect to the stereotactic arc-quad-

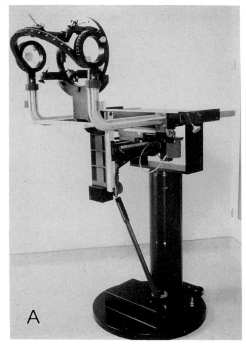

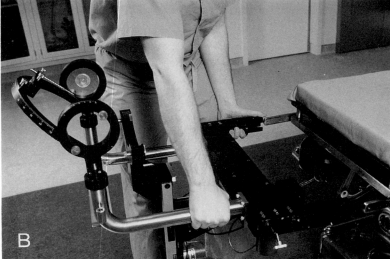

Figure 2. The stereotactic system can be mounted on a semipermanent base (**A**) or fixed onto the side rails of a standard operating table (**B**).

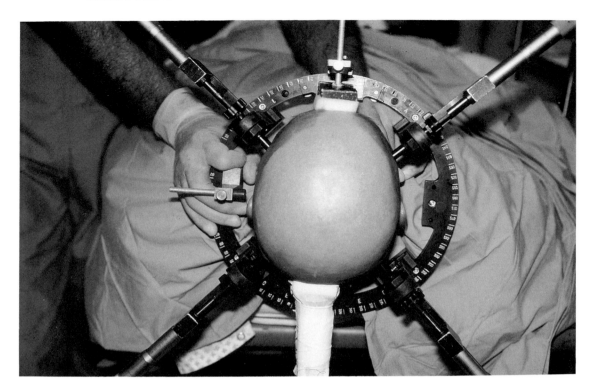

Figure 3. The stereotactic headholder is mounted to the patient's head by means of flanged carbon fiber pins which are inserted into holes drilled through the outer table of the skull into the diploë. Note the circular base ring of the stereotactic headholder with indexing marks at 5° intervals. Micrometer attachments are used to measure the distance between the outer face of the vertical support and the carbon fiber pin. This provides a mechanism for reproducibly replacing the frame for subsequent stereotactic procedures.

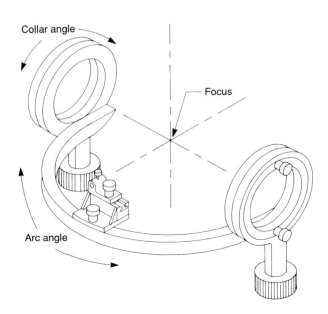

Figure 4. The stereotactic arc-quadrant provides two angular degrees of freedom. These are a collar angle or angle from the horizontal plane, and an arc angle which is an angle from the vertical plane. The attachment on the face of the arc directs a probe or a retractor perpendicular to the tangent of the arc-quadrant. Thus, these instruments will always arrive at the focal point of the arc-quadrant irrespective of the arc or collar angle. In the COMPASS system the patient's head is moved in x, y, and z axes to place an intracranial target point at the focal point of the stereotactic arc-quadrant.

rant. The retractor cylinder is directed perpendicular to the tangent and toward the focal point of the stereotactic arc-quadrant. Dilators which fit inside the retractor cylinder are 1 cm longer than the retractor. The distal end of the dilator is wedge-shaped and spreads an incision to the diameter of the retractor so that the retractor cylinder can be advanced. The retractor is used to maintain exposure by creating a shaft from the surface of the brain to the superficial aspect of a deep-seated tumor. In addition, the retractor itself provides a fixed stereotactic reference structure in stereotactic space to which computer-generated slice reconstructions of the CT/MRI-defined tumor volume are related.

Accessory Instruments

Extra long bipolar forceps with a shaft length of 150 mm are required to control bleeding in the surgical field when working through the stereotactic retractor. In addition, 150–160-mm-long suction tips, dissectors, and alligator scissors are also used.

Heads-Up Display
for the Operating Microscope

We developed a system by which the image output of a small video monitor mounted on the operating microscope is optically superimposed on the surgical field viewed through the microscope (Fig. 5). The com-

puter-generated image displayed on the video monitor is scaled by a system of lenses to the desired size. Thus, the surgeon sees the actual surgical field with the computer-generated rendition of that field based on CT and MRI superimposed.

PROCEDURAL ASPECTS

Data Base Acquisition

The CT/MRI-compatible COMPASS stereotactic headholder is applied under neuroleptic sedation and local anesthesia. Micrometer measurements are recorded at the application procedure. The headholder can then be removed following the data base acquisition and replaced in exactly the same position for the stereotactic surgical procedure at a later date.

The patient then undergoes stereotactic computed tomography, magnetic resonance imaging, and digital angiography. Separate localization systems for CT, MRI, and DA attach to the base ring of the COMPASS stereotactic headholder (Figs. 6 and 7). These create reference marks on CT, MR, and DA images from which stereotactic coordinates can be developed.

Stereotactic CT Scanning

The stereotactic headholder secures to a CT table adaptation plate on a General Electric 9800 CT scanner. The CT localization system consists of nine carbon

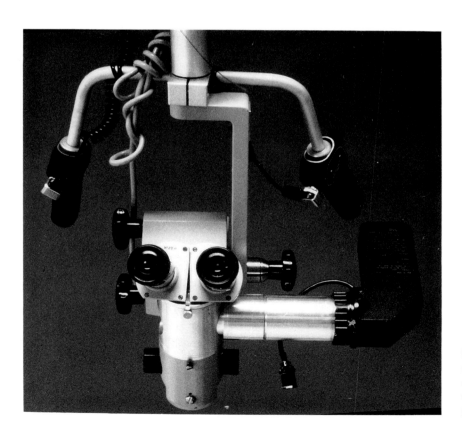

Figure 5. A "heads-up" display system for the operating microscope. The computer display is transmitted to the video monitor and then optically superimposed on the surgical field.

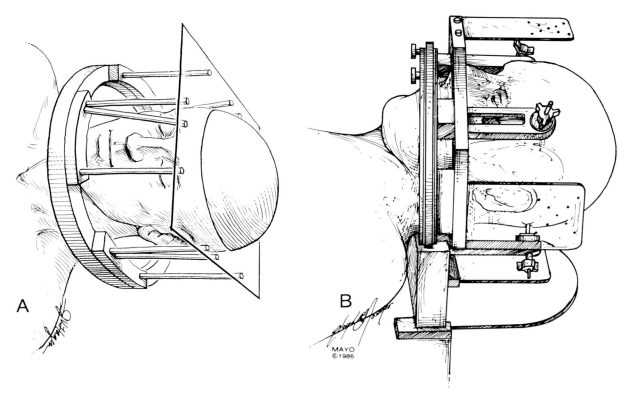

Figure 6. Principle of stereotactic localization systems for planar data such as computed tomography and magnetic resonance imaging and for projection images such as digital angiography. The CT (**A**) and MRI localization systems consist of "N"-shaped localization devices which create nine reference marks on each CT or MRI slice from which stereotactic coordinates can be calculated. The DA localization system (**B**) produces 18 reference marks on anteroposterior and lateral images which allow calculation of magnification, cross-correlation between DA and CT and MRI, and calculation of stereotactic coordinates from DA.

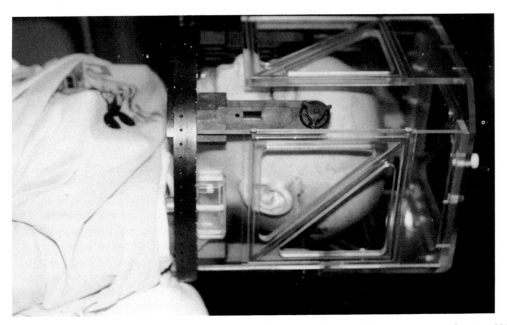

Figure 7. The MRI localization system which creates reference marks on axial, transverse, and sagittal MR images.

fiber rods arranged in the shape of the letter "N" located on either side of the head and anteriorly which create nine reference marks on each CT slice (Fig. 6A). Intravenous iothalamate meglumine is administered for contrast enhancement. Five-millimeter slices are gathered through the lesion, utilizing a medium body format.

Stereotactic Magnetic Resonance Imaging

Stereotactic MRI examinations are performed on a General Electric 1.5-tesla Signa unit. The MRI localization system consists of plates containing capillary tubes filled with copper sulfate solution arranged in the shape of the letter "N." Plates are arranged bilaterally, superiorly, anteriorly, and posteriorly (Fig. 7). This allows sagittal, coronal, and transverse image data acquisition. Nine reference marks are created on each sagittal, coronal, and axial MR image. Recently, MRI studies have been performed utilizing gadolinium diethylenetriamine pentaacetic acid contrast. In general, axial slices are useful for interpolation of tumor volumes. Sagittal and coronal images are useful in surgical approach planning.

Stereotactic Digital Angiography

The stereotactic head holder fits into a DF table adaptation plate on the General Electric DF 3000 or 5000 digital angiographic unit. Lucite plates which contain nine radioopaque reference marks located on either side of the head, anteriorly, and posteriorly create 18 reference marks on each anteroposterior and lateral DA image (Fig. 6B). The mathematical relationships between the fiducial marks and their locations on the DA images are the basis from which stereotactic coordinates for intracranial vessels can be calculated, and stereotactic target points derived from CT and MRI can be displayed on angiographic images. Digital angiography is performed utilizing a standard femoral catheterization technique. Orthogonal and 6° oblique arterial and venous phases are obtained in orthogonal and 6° rotated stereoscopic pairs.

Tumor Volume Interpolation

The archived data tapes from the CT, MRI, and DA examinations are transferred to the operating room computer system. Beginning with the lowest CT slice, the surgeon traces around the boundary of the tumor on each contiguous CT and MRI slice using the computer's cursor subsystem, and deposits multiple points around the boundary using the deposit key on the mouse. In addition, a single point located in the approximate geographical center of the lesion on one of the CT or MRI slices is digitized and retained as the reference target point. The digitized CT and MRI defined tumor contours are suspended in the computer's image matrix. Interpolated slices are then created at 1-mm intervals. The computer then fills in each of the digitized and interpolated slices with 1-mm cubic voxels. This creates a volume in space. Separate volumes for the CT- and MRI-defined contours are created. The interpolated CT- and MRI-defined volumes are constructed about the reference target point and calculations output which will center this point in the focal point of the stereotactic arc-quadrant frame.

The tumor volume can be reformatted for any desired rotation of the patient in the stereotactic frame (0 = supine; 90° = right shoulder down, lateral decubitus; 180° = prone; etc.). This facility allows a patient to undergo data acquisition in the most comfortable position, (i.e., supine) and to be operated upon in a position which will be comfortable and convenient for the surgeon. The actual numbers for patient rotation and arc and collar angles are determined during surgical planning.

Surgical Planning

Surgical planning is done at the computer console after the CT, DA, and MRI data tapes have been loaded on the operating room computer system. In the most ideal situation, data base acquisition and surgery take place on two separate days; the stereotactic head-holder is removed from the patient following data base acquisition and is reapplied at the time of surgery. Surgical planning can thus take place in a relaxed environment.

All solid intracranial tumors are resectible. The solid portion of glial tumors is defined by the volume of contrast enhancement on CT or MRI. However, brain tissue is always damaged in open surgical approaches to any tumor which is not directly on the surface of the brain. The object of surgical planning is to select the approach to a tumor which traverses the most expendable brain tissue. The actual direction of this approach is the surgical viewline. The surgical viewline is defined by and expressed in terms of patient orientation, and arc and collar trajectory settings on the stereotactic instrument. The computer can illustrate this approach by means of a shaded graphics display. The CT and MRI tumor volume displays can also be presented as slices cut perpendicular to this viewline.

Figure 8 summarizes the various approaches used in the resection of subcortical intra-axial tumors. These include transcortical, transsulcal, transsylvian, and interhemispheric approaches. Tumors located near the brain surface should be approached from the closest cranial entry point possible. Subcortical approach trajectories to deep tumors should traverse nonessential brain tissue in a direction parallel to major white matter projections.

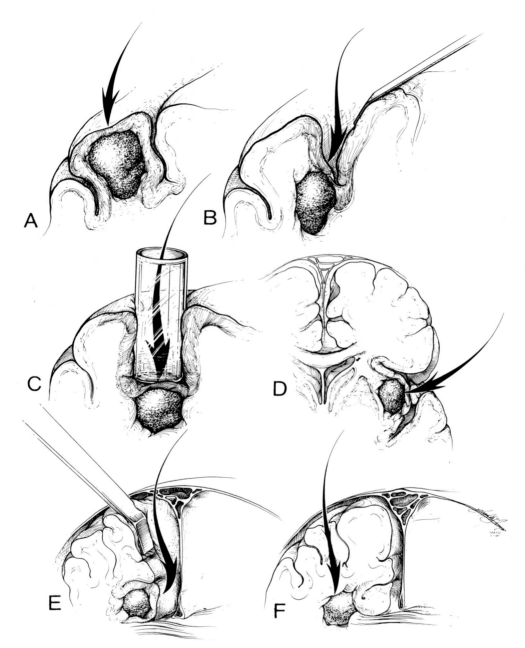

Figure 8. Summary of the various surgical approaches utilized in the exposure of subcortical tumors. These include transcortical (**A**), transsulcal (**B**), transsulcal (**C**), transsylvian (**D**), interhemispheric transcingulate (**E**), and transcortical (**F**) which would utilize a deep white matter incision as well.

The brain surface anatomy must be established in order to plan a safe approach to centrally located and deep-seated lesions. In some instances, deep sulci may also be used as a route to expose some deep lesions. Sagittal MR images are useful for the localization of specific fissures and sulci. Stereotactic stereoscopic cerebral angiography is also useful for finding the position of major sulci. The sulci are localized by identifying the deep vessel segments (apparent on the stereoscopic view) on the orthogonal arterial and venous phases of the stereotactic angiogram.

In particular, the position of the central sulcus, precentral sulcus, and precentral convolution must be established with respect to the tumor volume. The precentral sulcus can be split microsurgically to approach laterally lying precentral lesions. More medially located lesions under the precentral convolution are approached from an anterior direction, transcortically through the superior or middle frontal convolution or through the superior frontal sulcus. Posterior approaches through the superior parietal lobule are selected for the resection of lesions located behind the central sulcus. This approach is particularly useful for exposure of lesions near the atrium of the lateral ventricle. In this latter situation, the patient is rotated to 180° (prone position).

Trajectories for deep-seated lesions located in the basal ganglia or thalamus will depend in part on where

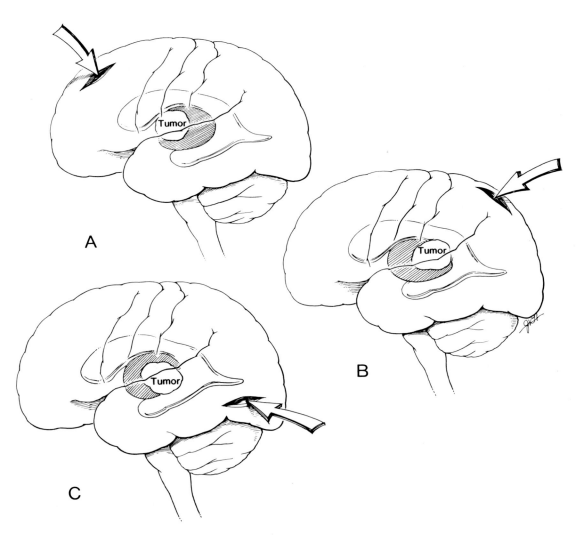

Figure 9. Three approaches are used for the exposure and resection of thalamic tumors. The route chosen will depend on the location of the tumor with respect to the normal thalamic anatomy. **A,** anterior thalamic tumors are approached utilizing a coronal trephination just behind the hairline in a trajectory which progresses posteriorly and me- dially through the anterior limb of the internal capsule. **B,** posterior dorsal thalamic tumors are exposed through the superior parietal lobule and lateral ventricle (patient rotation = 180°). **C,** posterior ventral lesions are exposed through a cortical and white matter incision at the temporo-occipital juncture.

the lesion is located with respect to the noninvolved portions of these nuclear groups. The approach to various thalamic lesions is illustrated in Figure 9. Anterior thalamic lesions are exposed by a retracted incision through the anterior limb of the internal capsule. Posterior dorsal lesions are resected utilizing an approach through the superior parietal lobule and atrium of the lateral ventricle with the patient prone (180° rotation). Posterior ventral thalamic lesions are approached through a cortical and white matter incision at the temporal-occipital junction (patient rotation of 135° is used for left-sided and 225° rotation for right-sided lesions).

Lesions in the anterior basal ganglia are approached from anteriorly and superiorly. Lesions in the posterior putamen are approached posterolaterally through the posterior temporal lobe.

Lesions in the posterior fossa are operated upon with the stereotactic frame placed in an inverted fashion (Fig. 10). Data acquisition is also performed with the head frame inverted. Midline lesions in the cerebellum or brain stem are exposed through the inferior vermis. However, midline approaches are uncomfortable for the surgeon if the patient is prone and the surgical approach is direct on the midline (arc angle 0). It is therefore best to rotate the patient 30°. This rotates the midline toward the surgeon so that he or she can stand to the patient's side and operate more comfortably (Fig. 11). Employing an arc angle of 30° returns the surgical approach to the midline. Com-

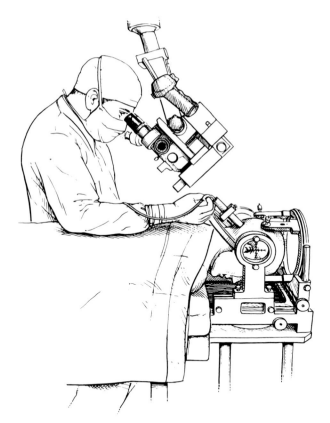

Figure 11. Setup for stereotactic resection of posterior fossa lesions. Note the inverted position of the head frame and the position of the surgeon.

puter software recalculates the target point for patient rotation, so that the frame adjustments continue to place the target point in the focal point of the arc-quadrant.

Lesions of the cerebellar hemisphere or lateral pons are approached in a lateral oblique trajectory from posterolateral to anteromedial. In this situation the patient is placed prone (rotation 180°) in the stereotactic frame. An arc angle of about 30–40° off the midline toward the side of the lesion is used.

The surgical approach should be comfortable for the surgeon. Patients can be rotated in the stereotactic headholder in order to provide the most comfortable working situation for the surgeon. Figure 12 illustrates the various patient rotations of the stereotactic headholder in the receiving yoke of the COMPASS three-dimensional positioning slide. The patient rotation selected will depend on the direction by which the surgeon intends to approach the tumor.

At the end of the planning session, the computer calculates and outputs target stereotactic coordinates and arc and collar angles, and reformats tumor volumes which account for patient rotation.

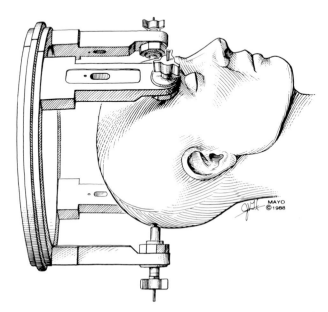

Figure 10. Inverted head frame position for resection of posterior fossa neoplasms. This position is utilized for data acquisition and surgery. It allows unencumbered access to the suboccipital area.

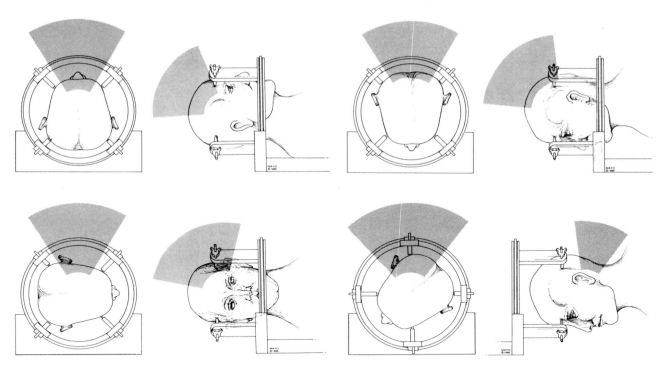

Figure 12. In the COMPASS stereotactic system the patient's head can be rotated to any position which will provide a comfortable working position for the surgeon. Only a few of these are illustrated here. *Top left,* the supine or 0° rotation is used for anterior approaches (*shaded area*). *Top right,* 180° rotation is used for posterior approaches. *Bottom left,* laterally lying lesions are approached employing a 90° head frame rotation for left-sided lesions and a 270° rotation for right-sided lesions. *Bottom right,* any rotation angle can be selected. A 225° rotation is used for approaches to the posterior medial temporal area as well as the posterior ventral thalamus. Rotations are also possible with the inverted frame position in the inverted head frame placement. The degree of rotation is aligned with an indexing mark on the yoke of the three-dimensional positioning system to confirm the rotation. The computer rotates all target, volumetric, and trajectory calculations to account for the rotation used.

Surgical Procedures

General endotracheal anesthesia is used. The stereotactic headholder is replaced utilizing the same pin placements and micrometer settings used during the data acquisition phase. The actual position of the patient's head depends on the headholder rotation selected, and this will be fixed in the stereotactic frame by placing the base ring of the headholder into the receiving yoke of the stereotactic frame. The index marks on the receiving yoke should line up with the degree index marks on the headholder at the desired rotation which was determined in surgical planning.

Four body positions are used to avoid compression of the jugular veins by the angle of the mandible on the transverse processes of the cervical vertebrae when the head is turned to the desired rotation position.

Supine: The supine position is used for head frame ("patient rotations") between 60° and 300°.

Lateral Decubitus: This position is used for head frame rotations between 60° and 120° (right side down) and between 240° and 300° (left side down). The down-side arm is extended forward. To maintain the position the bottom leg is bent at the knee, the top leg is straight. A pillow is placed between the legs.

Park Bench: The "park bench" or three-quarter prone position is employed for all head frame rotations between 180° and 240° (left side down) and between 120° and 180° (right side down). Here the patient lies on one side of the chest with the dependent arm behind to the side and down. The knee closest to the operating table is bent and the other leg straight with a pillow separating the legs.

Prone: This is rarely used for head frame rotations of between 150° and 210°. The patient's chest is supported by bilateral laminectomy-type chest rolls. The patient's body must be elevated by means of these rolls high enough so that the neck is not hyperflexed. In most situations, however, the park bench position is used instead of the full prone position for posterior approaches.

Following positioning of the body and securing the head frame in the receiving yoke of the stereotactic frame, the head of the operating table may be raised in order to place the patient's head above the heart to reduce the chance of a "tight brain."

The patient's scalp is prepared and draped as for a routine craniotomy. The sterile arc-quadrant is then secured to the support arms of the stereotactic frame. The tumor volume is positioned in the focal point of the stereotactic arc-quadrant. Entry and approach trajectory angles are set on the arc-quadrant.

Intracranial shifts in the position of deep cystic tumors and tumors near the ventricular system may occur after after skull and dura are opened, and cyst or ventricular fluid drained. The following step is therefore recommended. The guide tube on the stereotactic arc-quadrant is advanced to mark the scalp; it is withdrawn and a stab wound is made in the scalp. The guide tube is advanced to rest on the outer table of the skull. The skull is then opened with a stereotactically directed $1/8$-inch drill and the tumor is traversed with an open-ended biopsy cannula. A series of (0.5 mm diameter) stainless steel balls are deposited at 5-mm intervals along the viewline. The position of these markers is documented on anteroposterior and lateral stereotactic teleradiographs and will provide reference points for any subsequent intracranial shifts that may occur. The position of the tumor volume is translated accordingly within the computer image matrix to take this intracranial shift into account for subsequent image displays and stereotactic coordinate calculations.

The scalp is then opened with a linear incision which includes the stab wound. The incision follows parallel to the hairline in frontal approaches, is vertical in temporal, parietal, and posterior fossa approaches, and is usually transverse across the midline in parasagittal approaches. The skull is then opened using a 1.5–2-inch cranial trephine centered on the twist drill hole used to deposit the reference balls.

After removing the bone plug, the dura should be palpated. If it is tight and nonpulsating, the anesthesiologist should ensure that the $PaCO_2$ is 25 or less. Mannitol and/or barbiturates may be necessary to reduce intracranial pressure. The dura is then opened in a cruciate fashion. At this point, the procedure varies for superficial and for deep lesions.

Superficial Lesions

The location of the circular trephine opening in space is known. The edges of the cranial defect are used as a reference to which the computer-generated slices of the CT- and MRI-defined tumor volume can be referred.

A section of cortex having the same size and configuration of the most superficial tumor slice is removed with bipolar cautery and scissors. We have found that brain tissue is nonviable when tumor extends to within 5–7 mm of the cortical surface. Resection of this overlying brain tissue will result in no new neurologic deficit. A plane is then created around the tumor with bipolar cautery and suction. The computer displays the configuration of the trephine opening in relationship to the reformatted tumor outlines. The depth of the surgical instruments below the trephine opening is measured and related to the "slice distance" of the image displayed on the screen. Specifically, the "slice distance" is the distance of the image plane which is perpendicular to the surgical viewline from the zero point of the stereotactic arc-quadrant. The depth may be determined in the surgical field by measuring the distance between the outer face of the probe holder on the arc-quadrant and the external edges of the trephine opening.

The "heads-up" display on the operating microscope is very helpful in the stereotactic resection of superficial tumors (Fig. 13). The microscope field of view is moved until the image of the trephine opening projected into the microscope by the "heads-up" display unit is superimposed over the actual trephine opening in the surgical field. The tumor outline images are used as a template so that a plane between tumor and surrounding brain can be created. The positions of surgical instruments in the surgical field viewed through the microscope are also positioned in reference to the computer-generated image aligned to the surgical field.

In this way, high grade gliomas, some low grade gliomas, metastatic tumors, and vascular malformations can be removed as intact specimens with minimal bleeding.

Deep Lesions

As with the procedure for superficial tumors, the stereotactic coordinates which position the tumor in the focal point of the stereotactic frame, arc, and collar trajectory angles are set. A linear scalp incision is made, a 1.5-inch circular cranial trephination is performed, and the dura is tacked up and opened in a cruciate fashion. At this stage a cortical incision at least 2 cm long must be made. This can be made in the crown of a gyrus or in the depths of a sulcus. The incision is deepened into the subcortical white matter.

The retractor cylinder is mounted in the arc adaptor between the gently retracted gyral banks. The dilator is inserted and advanced until the dilator rests in the depths of the incision. The retractor cylinder is

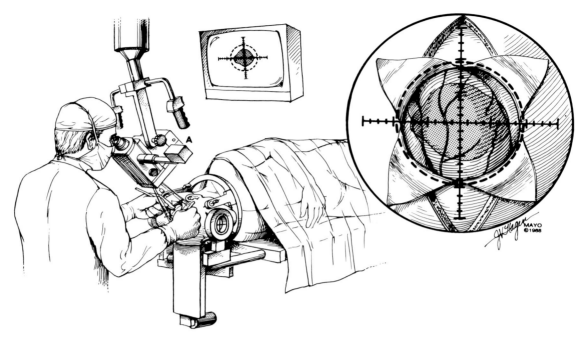

Figure 13. Method for stereotactic resection of a superficial tumor. The trephine opening has been placed stereotactically. The computer displays the position of a tumor volume slice at a specified distance along the viewline on a display monitor and into the "heads-up" display unit of the operating microscope (A). The image is scaled until the configuration of the trephine opening in the image display is exactly the same size and aligns to the actual trephine opening. The surgeon then uses the tumor slice image as a template which will aid in the isolation of the tumor from surrounding brain tissue.

advanced 5 mm over the dilator. Then the dilator is removed. The operating microscope is used to view the depths of the incision through the retractor. The subcortical linear incision is extended 5 to 10 mm deeper utilizing a focused CO_2 laser beam. The dilator is then reinserted and the cylindrical retractor advanced 5 mm further. The dilator is removed and the incision deepened further (Fig. 14, A–F).

Using this method a long subcortical incision from the surface of the brain to the tumor is made in small steps which consist of deepening the incision with the CO_2 laser and spreading the incision with the dilator over which the retractor is advanced and secured. At the outer border of the tumor, the incision is undercut medially and laterally, reflecting the laser beam off a stainless steel instrument inserted to the base of the retractor (Fig. 14, G and H). The dilator is then inserted, rotated 90°, and the retractor is advanced and secured. Thus a shaft is created from the stereotactic arc-quadrant to the superficial border of the intracranial lesion (Fig. 14I).

The retractor maintains the surgical exposure and provides a convenient reference for the depth of the stereotactic procedure since the radius of the arc-quadrant and the length of the retractor are known.

In addition, the operating room computer system displays the configuration of the cylindrical retractor as viewed by the surgeon (circle) in reference to reformatted CT/MRI-defined tumor slice outlines at a specified depth which usually corresponds to the insertional depth of the retractor. A calibrated millimeter reference grid is also displayed (Fig. 15).

The computer calculates a range along the viewline which indicates where tumor should first be encountered and where it should end along that given trajectory. Slices beyond the target point (at the focal point of the arc-quadrant) are given positive numbers (e.g., slice distance = +5).

The stereotactic removal of the tumor is performed differently than in conventional tumor surgery. In conventional surgery the center of the lesion is decompressed and then the walls of the cavity are resected. However, in stereotactic resection a plane of dissection between tumor and surrounding brain is established *before* decompressing the interior of the lesion. This prevents the walls of the cavity produced from closing in, rendering subsequent stereotactic computer images inaccurate.

Small deep tumors having the same size in cross-sectional area as the retractor are easily resected with good postoperative results. A plane of dissection around the tumor is developed using a slightly defocused laser beam (power about 25 to 30 watts, spot size 1 mm). The dissection proceeds circumferentially

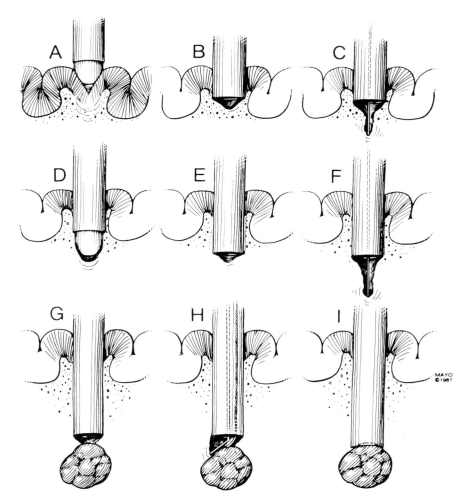

Figure 14. Use of the stereotactic cylindrical retractor. The sulcus is opened microsurgically. **A,** the sulcus is dilated utilizing gentle pressure on the dilator which is inserted through the retractor cylinder. **B,** the retractor is advanced to the depths of the sulcus and a cortical and subcortical incision is made with bipolar cautery and microscissors. **C,** the incision is deepened using a carbon dioxide laser. **D,** this incision is spread with the dilator. **E,** the retractor is advanced over the dilator. The dilator is removed. **F,** the incision is deepened with the laser. **G,** the superficial incision extends to the superficial border of the tumor. **H,** the brain tissue is dissected off the tumor with laser or bipolar forceps. **I,** the retractor is advanced to the superficial aspect of the tumor.

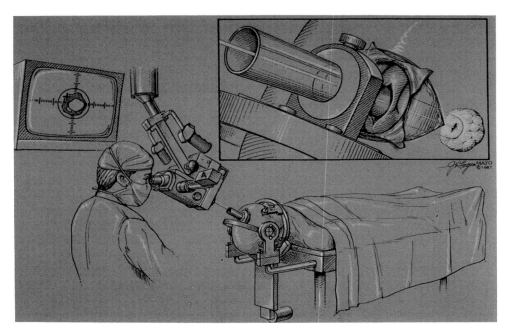

Figure 15. Stereotactic resection of a deep tumor requires a stereotactically directed cylindrical retractor, operating microscope, and surgical laser. The computer displays the configuration of the retractor with respect to its end and slices through the tumor volume cut perpendicular to the surgical viewline. This is displayed on the computer monitor as well as in the "heads-up" display of the operating microscope (A).

around each tumor level, progressing from the most superficial levels of the tumor to the deepest. The retractor is advanced as each level of 2 or 3 mm is dissected free of surrounding brain tissue until the widest cross-sectional diameter of the tumor is encountered. Then laser power is increased to 50–80 watts, the beam is defocused (spot size 2–3 mm), and the tumor is vaporized down to the level corresponding to the deepest insertional point of the retractor. Then, using the computer-generated slice image as a guide, the deeper portions of tumor are separated from surrounding brain using the laser beam at a lower power and on a smaller spot size as described above.

Tumors much larger than the retractor opening can also be removed with good postoperative results. The retractor is first advanced to the most superficial aspect of the tumor and using the slice image as a guide, a plane is established between tumor and brain tissue. The retractor position with respect to the tumor boundary is then set so that a plane of dissection between tumor and surrounding brain can be established on one side of the tumor. This is accomplished by first translating the image of the retractor on the computer image display of the tumor in order to have one side of the tumor within the retractor. The computer then calculates new stereotactic coordinates which will provide this situation with respect to the retractor. These new coordinates are executed automatically by the computer which activates the stepper

motors on the three-dimensional slide in order to provide these new stereotactic coordinates. The retractor mount is loosened so that the retractor can move freely during the movement of the patient's head within the arc-quadrant in order to place this selected part of the tumor at the focal point of the arc-quadrant. When the movement has been completed, the surgeon carefully tightens the set screws of the retractor mount on the arc-quadrant and the collar. This maneuver then orients the stereotactic retractor toward the focal point of the stereotactic arc-quadrant. The configuration of that edge of the tumor with respect to the edge of the retractor is noted on the computer-generated image display before creating a plane between tumor and brain tissue. The actual position of the laser in the surgical field is known in reference to the superimposed computer-generated tumor slice viewed in the "heads-up" display unit of the operating microscope. After this side of the tumor has been separated from brain tissue, attention is now turned to another quadrant of the tumor slice. The relationship between tumor and retractor is again translated on the screen, new coordinates calculated, the other side of the tumor shifted under the retractor, and this side separated from brain.

In this manner, a plane of dissection is developed entirely around the tumor to a depth of about 10 mm beyond the end of the stereotactic retractor. Tumor is then vaporized using 60–100 watts of defocused laser power down to this level at which the plane of dissection between the tumor and brain tissue had been established. The retractor is then advanced 10 mm into the cavity produced and the process described above which develops a plane around the tumor is repeated.

Intraventricular landmarks can be used to maintain surgical orientation in conventional approaches to intraventricular tumors in patients having large lateral ventricles. More difficulty is encountered when attempting to localize lesions in patients having small or normal sized ventricles. A more limited but direct approach to intraventricular lesions can be made stereotactically. Brain and ventricular incisions need to be only large enough to remove the lesion. The surgical approach to a lesion within the lateral ventricle will depend on its location with respect to the central sulcus. In general, anterior lesions are approached anteriorly utilizing a scalp incision behind the hairline, a 1.5-inch diameter trephine, and the superior frontal sulcus. Lesions located posterior to the central sulcus are approached from behind through the superior parietal lobule.

Third ventricular lesions are approached through the right lateral ventricle. Colloid cysts can be removed through the foramen of Monro. Here it is important to approach the more obstructed foramen of Monro. Coronal MRI is most useful in determining if the colloid cyst is leaning forward and dilating one foramen of Monro more than the other. Very large third ventricular lesions can be exposed through the frontal horn of the lateral ventricle. One fornix must be sacrificed to gain the exposure. An internal decompression of the lesion is performed with the laser until only a thin rim of the capsule remains. The computer display of the cross-sections of the digitized tumor volume are extremely useful in this step as the surgeon can be quite aggressive within the tumor with no risk of extending through the capsule and damaging the walls of the

third ventricle. Following this internal decompression, the retractor is withdrawn to the level of the roof of the third ventricle and the capsule is carefully dissected from the walls of the third ventricle. The tumor capsule can be contracted utilizing the defocused laser which facilitates the dissection of the capsule from the wall of the third ventricle.

CONCLUSION

Computer reconstruction of CT and MRI data and intraoperative display provides a mechanism by which a surgeon is able to orient himself to the global lesional volume and have precise feedback information as regards the location of the surgical instruments (stereotactic retractor and CO_2 laser) in relationship to planar contours of the lesion displayed on a monitor in the operating room. With this method and instrumentation, aggressive resection of subcortical lesions is possible with minimal damage to surrounding brain tissue.

Three hundred sixty-two computer-assisted volumetric stereotactic resections for 196 gliomas, 104 nonglial tumors, and 62 nonneoplastic mass lesions were performed at the Mayo Clinic by the author in the five-year period between August 1984 and August 1989. From this experience it is clear that patients having histologically circumscribed lesions such as pilocytic astrocytomas, metastatic tumors, intraventricular lesions, and vascular lesions derive the greatest benefit from this procedure. Postoperative morbidity also depends more on the degree of histologic circumscription than on the location of the lesion. However, in high grade glial neoplasms a maximal reduction of tumor burden can also be achieved by computer-assisted stereotactic resection with better postoperative neurologic results than would be associated with conventional procedures for lesions in central and deep-seated locations.

SAGITTAL SYNOSTOSIS

A. LELAND ALBRIGHT, M.D.

PATIENT SELECTION

Sagittal synostosis restricts transverse skull growth, and infants develop a narrow, elongated skull (dolichocephaly, scaphocephaly) because the normal lambdoid and coronal sutures permit growth in the anterior-posterior axis. Most infants with sagittal synostosis have an unusual head shape at birth and are diagnosed when they are 2–4 months old. The typical child with sagittal synostosis has an elongated head with a palpable bony ridge in the posterior half of the sagittal suture, biparietal narrowing, and occipital bossing. Narrow heads are also seen in premature infants who lay with their heads turned to the side for long times, but these infants lack the typical occipital bossing of sagittal synostosis and the characteristic radiographic finding: skull fusion at the sagittal suture, seen best on the Towne's view. The diagnosis of sagittal synostosis can usually be made on clinical grounds and can be confirmed by skull radiographs. Computed tomography scans, especially those in the coronal projection, demonstrate the sagittal fusion and show compressed cerebrospinal fluid spaces lateral to the cerebral hemispheres, but are not needed to make the diagnosis.

Although a few infants with sagittal synostosis have such mild deformity that an operation is not indicated, almost all have an obviously abnormal head shape and an operation is indicated to normalize that shape. Without an operation, their head shapes subject them to ridicule and name-calling. The optimal time for operation is 3–4 months; at that age, their blood volumes are greater than in newborns, they are past the 8–10-week nadir of physiologic anemia, their skulls have greater pliability than at 6–12 months, and their subsequent brain growth further improves the postoperative skull shape.

Neurologic development is usually normal, with or without an operation. The goal of operations for sagittal synostosis is to normalize skull shape, not to prevent neurologic damage. There is some evidence that intracranial pressure (ICP) is increased in infants with sagittal synostosis: ICP measurements have been higher than normal in several of the few monitored patients, infants are often less irritable postoperatively than they were preoperatively, and in nonoperated children with sagittal synostosis, skull radiographs later in childhood usually demonstrate a beaten-copper appearance.

Operative risks include anesthetic risks, blood loss, infection, dura/sinus tears, and cortical injuries. The likelihood of requiring a transfusion is related to the patient's blood volume, to the compulsiveness of the surgeon to use techniques that minimize blood loss, and to the hematocrit chosen for transfusion (usually 21–24; below that level infants develop tachycardia, tachypnea, diaphoresis, and poor feeding). In my experience with 50 operations for sagittal synostosis, approximately 25% of the patients needed transfusions intraoperatively or within 48 hours postoperatively. The risk of infection is <1% (unless bone edges are lined with Silastic). The risk of dura/sinus tears varies with the technique used but is about 1–2%, and the risk of cortical injury is <1%.

PREOPERATIVE PREPARATION

Neurosurgeons should plan their operations to correct the specific deformities harbored by the individual patient. In my experience, it has not been possible to normalize skull shape—correcting the occipital boss and widening the biparietal diameter—with only a midline strip craniectomy. With current procedures, the use of Silastic and other interposition materials is unnecessary.

The infant's hair can be shampooed and the scalp scrubbed the night before operation. A preoperative blood count should be obtained and blood should be typed and cross-matched. Antibiotics and anticonvulsants are not needed.

OPERATIVE TECHNIQUE

Anesthesia

Communication and trust between the neurosurgeon and the anesthesiologist are imperative because of individual preferences and abilities in these operations. General anesthesia is used. There is no preferred method of induction but anesthesia is usually maintained with inhalation agents because they are more easily reversed than narcotics at the end of the operation. Blood pressure can be monitored adequately with a cuff; arterial cannulation for continuous monitoring is not generally required for sagittal synostosis operations. These operations last less that 2 hours so an indwelling catheter to monitor urinary output is unnecessary.

It is helpful to have two intravenous lines, usually 22- or 24-gauge, so that blood can be infused rapidly if needed. The indications for transfusion are not always clear cut; neurosurgeons and anesthesiologists should discuss the indications preoperatively, considering factors such as preoperative hematocrit, estimated blood volume, ability to adequately oxygenate tissues, the nature of the planned operation, and the risks and benefits of transfusion. Operative blood loss in these operations is difficult to quantitate and transfusions are best begun when the estimated blood loss approaches that volume needed to decrease the hematocrit to 21–24. The risk of clinically important venous air embolism is small and the risk is not worth the additional time (often 45 minutes) required to insert a central venous catheter. The use of Doppler monitoring, etc., is optional.

Operative Positioning

Infants are positioned prone, with the chest elevated by chest rolls and the head resting face down on a foam-padded pediatric horseshoe head holder, with careful inspection to ensure that there is no pressure on the eyes (Fig. 1). Antibiotic ointment should be applied to the corneas and the lids taped closed; tarsorrhaphy sutures are not needed for these operations. The head is positioned with the neck slightly extended, so that there is access anteriorly to the fontanelle and access posteriorly to the undersurface of the occipital prominence. Neurosurgeons who perform only a midline strip craniectomy can position the infant's head in either the prone or lateral position.

Draping

The amount of hair to be shaved and the closeness of drapes to the incision is a matter of personal preference and ranges from shaving and exposing only a 1-cm margin on either side of the incision to a total head shave and exposure of the entire dome of the calvarium.

Skin Incision

The incision depends on the planned procedure. If the neurosurgeon plans to remove the sagittal suture and to alter the abnormal parietal or occipital regions, a transverse incision is used, positioned halfway be-

tween the anterior fontanelle and the bottom of the occipital prominence (Fig. 1). If a midline strip craniectomy alone is planned, a midline sagittal incision is used, extending from the anterior aspect of the anterior fontanelle to just behind the posterior fontanelle. Prior to incising the scalp, 0.5% bipuvacaine containing 1:200,000 epinephrine can be injected intradermally to diminish bleeding and decrease postoperative pain.

Operative Procedure

The scalp edges should be compressed and retracted backward while the epidermis is incised with a knife. Below the epidermis, the scalp can be opened with a needle tip on the unipolar coagulating cautery or with

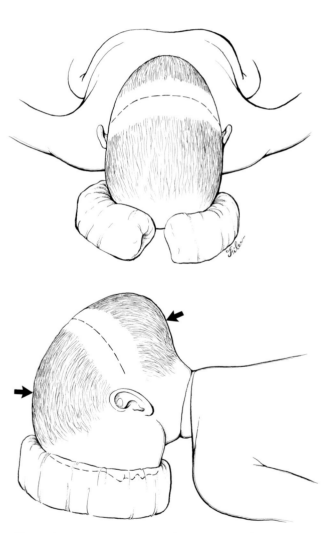

Figure 1. Patient positioning for correction of sagittal synostosis, vertex (*top*) and lateral (*bottom*) views. The incision is marked halfway between the anterior fontanelle and the bottom of the occipital prominence (*arrows*).

the Shaw scalpel, with minimal blood loss. Most neurosurgeons apply hemostatic clips to the scalp margins, and clips are needed if the scalp is not opened with the cautery. The scalp flaps are then elevated away from the underlying periosteum, using the cautery to divide the areolar tissue and vessels between galea and periosteum. Blood loss is increased if the scalp flaps are elevated by the traditional technique of digital dissection. Scalp flaps are mobilized anteriorly until the anteriorly fontanelle is seen and posteriorly until the bottom of the occipital prominence is exposed (Fig. 2).

After the flaps have been mobilized, the first stage of bone work is the sagittal strip craniectomy. Although the sagittal suture is not fused along the entire length of the suture in some infants, it is advisable to remove the entire suture during these operations; it is difficult to normalize head shape if a portion of the suture is left in place. The unipolar coagulating cautery is used to score the periosteum where the skull is to be cut (Fig. 2). Periosteum over the sagittal suture should be left in place; its removal gives no benefit and causes additional blood loss. An Adson periosteal elevator is inserted at the posterior margin of the anterior fontanelle to separate the dura from the bone. Parallel parasagittal cuts are then made in the parietal bones. The width of the strip craniectomy varies inversely with age, from approximately 2.5 cm in a 2-month-old infant to 1.5 cm in a 12-month-old. Bleeding is less if the sagittal strip craniectomy is performed with a high-speed craniotome, e.g., the B-5 attachment of the Midas Rex drill, than by piecemeal removal with rongeurs. The sagittal strip is elevated from anteriorly to posteriorly and the dura, which is usual invaginated into a shallow cleft in the under surface of the bone, is dissected off with an Adson periosteal elevator (Fig. 3A). This dissection needs to be accomplished gently but quickly so that bleeding points on the dura, usually small emissary veins, can be coagulated with the bipolar cautery. The bone edges are then waxed.

The second stage of the procedure addresses the biparietal narrowing. That narrowing can be corrected by bilateral parietal wedge-shaped craniectomies and sutures. Wedge-shaped craniectomies are removed with the craniotome at the sites of maximal parietal narrowing, usually removing wedges 1–1.5 cm at the base and 4 cm in length (Fig. 3B). Two holes are drilled on either side of the craniectomy edges and 2-0 polyglactin sutures are inserted through the holes and tightened to draw the bone edges toward each other enough to visibly widen the biparietal diameter to normal and to shorten the anterior-posterior diameter by 5–10 mm (Fig. 4, A and B). If the infant has no significant occipital bossing, only these two stages are needed, and the wound can then be

closed. Alternative techniques to improve biparietal narrowing include the reverse-pi craniectomy and parietal morcellation.

Most infants have occipital bossing, however, and a third stage of the operation is indicated. I incise the occipital periosteum with bilateral semicircular incisions and then elevate it off the bone with the cautery, leaving periosteum attached at its base below the occipital prominence. An Adson or Cushing periosteal elevator is then inserted at the junction of the sagittal and lambdoid sutures and the dura is separated from overlying occipital bone. The dura is adherent along the lambdoid sutures bilaterally, but rarely adherent at the torcular herophili. A craniotome is then used to remove a circular disc of bone that encompasses the occipital prominence and usually measures 3–4 cm in diameter. Occipital dura should be depressed away from the bone while it is being cut, to minimize the risk of a sinus tear (Fig. 3B). After dural emissary veins are coagulated and the bone margins are waxed, the dura is plicated with either interrupted sutures or by coagulating the dura with the bipolar cautery in parallel vertical rows 5–8 mm apart (Fig. 3C). The occipital bone is then reduced in size by removing a 5–10-mm strip around its periphery and is repositioned with 2-0 polyglactin sutures (Fig. 4A). Occipital periosteum is then drawn back up over the occipital bone and loosely sewn in place with 4-0 polyglactin sutures. The alternative technique, the reverse-pi procedure, removes bilateral rectangular parietal craniectomies just anterior to the lambdoid sutures and parasagittal strip craniectomies and then draws the occipital bone forward with sutures into the parietal bone, anterior to the craniectomy channels. That technique has the advantage of not removing bone over the sinus, but the disadvantage of leaving the occipital prominence.

For the occasional child with marked preoperative frontal bossing, that bossing can be reduced by removing 1-cm rectangular strip craniectomies immediately posterior to the coronal sutures and inserting sutures to draw the frontal bones posteriorly toward the parietal bones.

The traditional parasagittal craniectomy procedure is outdated; it is often followed by refusion and does not correct either the biparietal narrowing, the occipital prominence, or the occasional frontal prominence. With the current procedure, there has been no refusion and the head appearance has been normal in all children operated on at less than 1 year of age. Children operated on at 1–4 years have far less skull mobility, and the neurosurgeon must make additional cuts in the calvarium so that the bones can be put where they should be, without relying on additional brain growth to move them there.

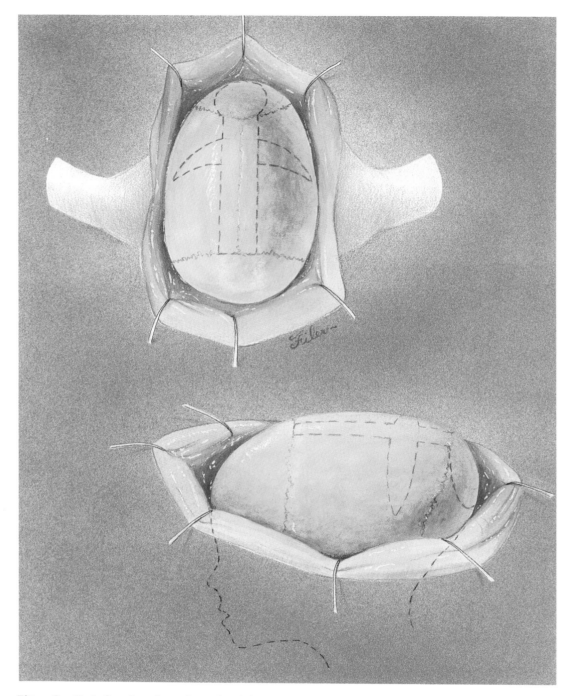

Figure 2.   Scalp flaps have been elevated and the periosteum has been scored with the coagulating unipolar cautery where the skull is to be cut.

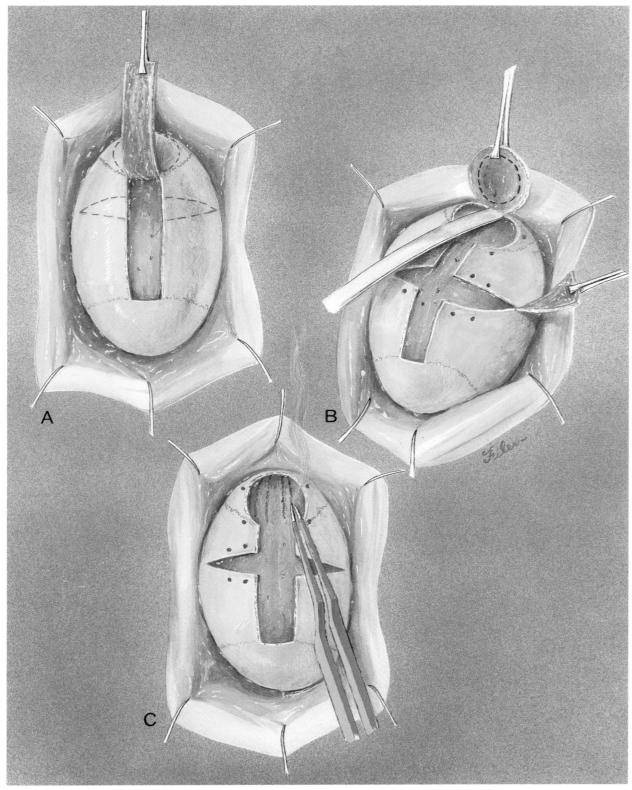

Figure 3. **A,** parasagittal cuts have been made in the parietal bones and the strip craniectomy has been dissected off the dura. Small emissary veins have been coagulated with the bipolar cautery. **B,** the dura has been dissected away from the occipital prominence and the parietal bones. Parietal wedge craniectomies are removed at the sites of maximal biparietal narrowing. The occipital circular craniotomy is removed and reduced in size as indicated by the *dashed line.* **C,** plication of the occipital dura with bipolar cautery.

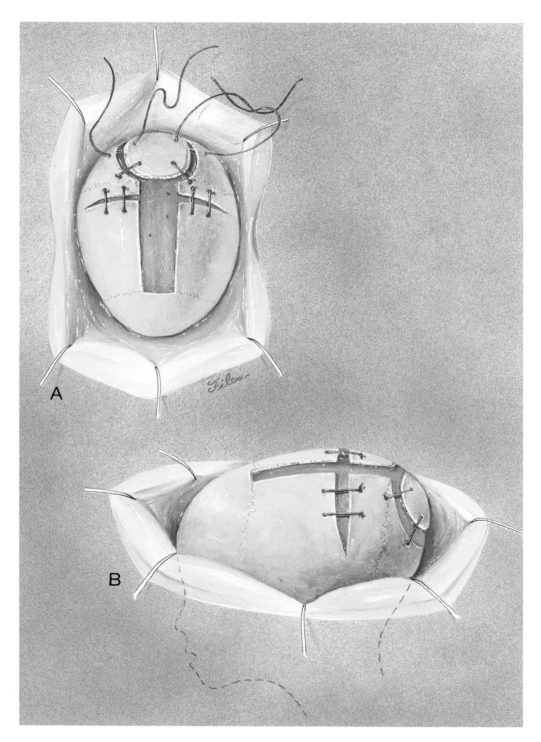

Figure 4. **A,** repositioning of the reduced occipital bone. Parietal sutures have normalized the biparietal diameters and shortened the anteroposterior diameter. **B,** lateral appearance after cranial remodeling is complete.

Closure Techniques

Subcutaneous tissues are irrigated and the scalp is then closed with subcutaneous polyglactin sutures and external nylon sutures. A strip dressing is applied along the incision and the head is wrapped with a 2—3-inch compression bandage to decrease scalp oozing. The scalp always swells substantially for 2—4 days. The use of subcutaneous drains is optional; their use is thought to possibly increase the risk of a wound infection but no data support that postulate. The duration of the operation is generally 60—90 minutes. The sagittal craniectomy channel fills in with bone in approximately 2 months and a protective helmet is not needed postoperatively.

Contributors

CHAD D. ABERNATHEY, M.D.
Neurosurgeon
Department of Neurosurgery
Iowa Medical Clinics
Cedar Rapids, Iowa

OSSAMA AL-MEFTY, M.D.
Professor of Neurosurgery
University of Mississippi Medical Center
Jackson, Mississippi

DANIEL L. BARROW, M.D.
Associate Professor
Department of Neurosurgery
Emory University School of Medicine
Atlanta, Georgia

WILLIAM O. BELL, M.D.
Associate Professor
Department of Neurosurgery
Bowman Gray School of Medicine
   of Wake Forest University
Winston-Salem, North Carolina

EDWARD C. BENZEL, M.D.
Professor and Chief
Division of Neurosurgery
University of New Mexico School of Medicine
Albuquerque, New Mexico

CURTIS A. DICKMAN, M.D.
Chief Resident
Division of Neurological Surgery
Barrow Neurological Institute
Phoenix, Arizona

MARK MAY, M.D.
Clinical Professor
Department of Otolaryngology—Head and Neck
   Surgery
University of Pittsburgh School of Medicine;
Director
Sinus Surgery and Facial Paralysis Center
Shadyside Hospital
Pittsburgh, Pennyslvania

FOAD NAHAI, M.D.
Professor of Surgery
Department of Plastic and Reconstructive Surgery
Emory University School of Medicine
Atlanta, Georgia

BURTON M. ONOFRIO, M.D.
Professor
Department of Neurosurgery
Mayo Clinic/Mayo Medical School
Rochester, Minnesota

MICHAEL P. SCHENK, M.S.
Director of Medical Illustration
University of Mississippi Medical Center
Jackson, Mississippi

ROBERT R. SMITH, M.D.
Professor and Chairman
Department of Neurosurgery
University of Mississippi Medical Center
Jackson, Mississippi

STEVEN M. SOBOL, M.D.
Private Practice
Decatur, Illinois

VOLKER K. H. SONNTAG, M.D.
Vice Chairman
Division of Neurological Surgery
Barrow Neurological Institute
Phoenix, Arizona;
Clinical Associate Professor
Division of Neurosurgery
Department of Surgery
University of Arizona College of Medicine
Tucson, Arizona

TADANORI TOMITA, M.D.
Associate Professor of Surgery (Neurosurgery)
Northwestern University Medical School;
Assistant Head
Division of Pediatric Neurosurgery
Children's Memorial Hospital
Chicago, Illinois

Contents

GLOSSOPHARYNGEAL RHIZOTOMY

BURTON M. ONOFRIO, M.D.

INTRODUCTION

Glossopharyngeal neuralgia is characterized by paroxysms of pain in the sensory distribution of the ninth cranial nerve. Except for the location of the pain and sensory stimuli which induce it, the attacks are identical to trigeminal neuralgia. The attacks are typified by a series of lancinating electric-like jabs of pain in the region of the tonsil or posterior third of the tongue. Radiation to the external auditory meatus or angle of the mandible may make it difficult to differentiate from trigeminal neuralgia involving the third division and pain arising from the nervus intermedius. Occasionally glossopharyngeal neuralgia and trigeminal neuralgia of the third division may coexist and require surgical manipulation of both fifth and ninth cranial nerves. Glossopharyngeal neuralgia occurs with one-seventieth the frequency of trigeminal neuralgia and although trigeminal neuralgia may occasionally be bilateral, this author has never seen a case of bilateral glossopharyngeal neuralgia.

The glossopharyngeal nerve is a mixed nerve. The special visceral efferent fibers, which innervate the stylopharyngeus muscle of the pharynx, originate in the nucleus ambiguus. The general visceral efferent fibers which supply the parasympathetic innervation to the parotid gland arise in the inferior salivatory nucleus and terminate in the otic ganglion. The general somatic afferent fibers supply the sensation to the back of the ear; their cell bodies are in the superior ganglion, and the central connections terminate in the spinal nucleus of the trigeminal nerve. The general visceral afferent fibers supply sensation to the carotid sinus, carotid body, eustachian tube, pharynx, and tongue. The cell bodies are in the inferior (petrosal) ganglion, and the central connections terminate in the tractus solitarius. The special visceral afferent fibers from the taste receptors of the posterior one-third of the tongue, in like manner, have cell bodies in the inferior (petrosal) ganglion and terminate in the tractus solitarius.

The glossopharyngeal nerve emerges from the medulla, dorsal to the inferior olivary nucleus, and

passes through the jugular foramen, in its cephalic portion, being separated from the fibers of the tenth and eleventh cranial nerves by a distinct dural septum. The ganglia of the glossopharyngeal nerve lie within the jugular foramen (Fig. 1A).

When dilemmas arise as to the nerve or nerves of origin of the neuralgia, differential temporary blocks may be employed. Cocainization of the pharynx alleviates the ninth nerve component of the pain while cocainization of the pyriform fossa relieves neuralgia of the superior laryngeal branch of the vagus. Blocking the foramen ovale with bupivacaine determines the component of the pain due to the third division of the trigeminal nerve. A tetracaine block of the jugular foramen will block all afferent impulses via the ninth and tenth cranial nerves and help to discover that rare patient suffering from pain mediated by the nervus intermedius component of the seventh cranial nerve. Obviously, for the blocks to be reliable they must be done when the frequency of the attacks and stereotypic triggers are dependable enough to allow the physician to appreciate an interruption in their occurrence in order to determine the efficacy and dependability of the block in sorting out which nerve or nerves are mediating the pain.

Although the medical treatment of trigeminal neuralgia may give gratifying results for years, this author has not observed the same degree of efficacy of medical treatment in patients suffering from glossopharyngeal neuralgia. While intermittent repetitive alcohol blocks may be very effective in control of the pain of trigeminal neuralgia, the extracranial anatomy of the ninth nerve makes alcohol block of the ninth cranial nerve impossible without incurring unacceptable tenth nerve dysfunction.

PREOPERATIVE CONSIDERATIONS

In determining the type of surgical treatment, the surgeon must be aware of the clinical phenomena associated with the hypersensitivity of the dorsal motor nucleus of the vagus which include cardiac arrest, syncopy, and seizures. Section of the ninth and upper fibers of the tenth cranial nerves causes little or no defineable neurologic deficit. Microvascular decompression risks intraoperative cardiac abnormalities

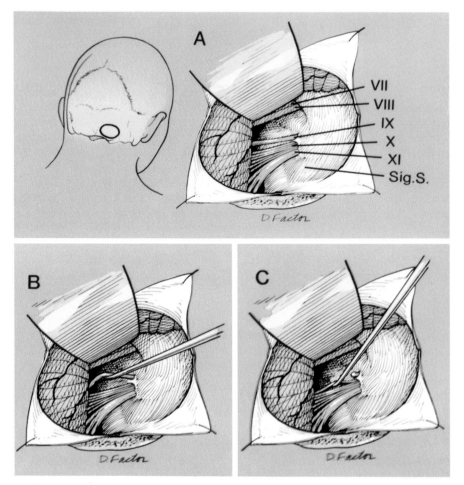

Figure 1. **A,** the head is turned 15° toward the side of the desired ninth nerve visualization. The *inset* to the left shows the initial craniectomy which is then enlarged laterally to, but preferably not into, the mastoid air cells. **B,** the ninth nerve is isolated with a ball-tip dissector. **C,** after sectioning the ninth nerve, the upper one-sixth of the tenth nerve filaments are sectioned.

and invites recurrence of pain postoperatively and seems unwarranted. Authors have described hypertensive crisis and intra- and extracerebellar hemorrhage from ninth and tenth nerve manipulation during microvascular decompression.

Radiofrequency procedures for extracranial destruction of the ninth nerve are unacceptable in that, like extracranial alcohol blocks of the jugular foramen, they invite unacceptable tenth nerve dysfunction. Most surgeons believe, as Dandy did, that there is no other treatment worth mentioning than intracranial section of the ninth and upper one-sixth of the tenth cranial nerves at the jugular foramen.

SURGICAL TECHNIQUE

Anesthesia

The sitting position offers some surgical advantages: ease of surgical exposure and less blood pooling in the operative field. Some anesthesiologists believe that access to the endotracheal tube, the reduction of facial swelling, and the ability to observe facial nerve function are notable advantages of the sitting position in anesthetic management. Hazards to the patient in the sitting position include venous air embolism, arterial hypotension, vital sign changes due to brain stem manipulation, specific cranial nerve stimulation, airway obstruction, and position-related brain stem ischemia. Preoperative identification of a patent foramen ovale cordis may be a relative contraindication to the sitting position. Management should be directed at the prevention, early detection, and treatment of these problems.

At least two intravenous access sites are recommended for posterior fossa procedures. When electroneurophysiologic monitoring is used and an awake baseline is sought, the patient is not sedated prior to the collection of those data. The only exception to that situation is when an awake fiberoptic intubation is done and there is a need to perform somatosensory evoked potential monitoring after the endotracheal tube has been placed.

The anesthesia is induced, and an arterial line is placed. Then, a central venous line is placed from the arm, using electrocardiographic localization, to the high right atrium. Adequate anesthesia is administered for pinion placement, with supplementation by local anesthesia if necessary. If transesophageal echocardiography is to be used, it is placed at this point.

The patient is then placed upright with care to avoid excessive neck flexion in the sitting position. The head is then turned 15° to the side of desired jugular foramen visualization. The awake range of motion tolerated by the patient is now used as a positioning guideline. The arms are carefully padded and, equally important, are carefully supported. With the use of muscle relaxants the weight of the arms themselves is enough in some instances to cause stretch injuries of the brachial plexus. The knees are flexed to avoid sciatic tension and the buttocks are padded to prevent pressure injury to the sciatic nerves. The Doppler monitor is placed and the right atrial catheter is flushed vigorously with saline to confirm correct catheter placement. The blood pressure transducer is placed at the head level. Blood pressure requires some support with vasopressors or lighter anesthesia in about 25% of the cases.

Monitoring for air embolism can be approached from several aspects. Monitors include a precordial Doppler monitor, a right atrial catheter, a capnograph or mass spectrometer, an esophageal stethoscope, transcutaneous O_2 assessment, and echocardiography (ECHO). The most sensitive of these are the ECHO and Doppler, followed by end-tidal CO_2, transcutaneous O_2, expired N_2, right atrial catheter, and (least sensitive) the esophageal stethoscope.

Many surgeons use the park bench position for posterior fossa surgery including that for cerebellopontine angle tumor removal and microvascular decompression of the fifth cranial nerve. Orientation from an anatomic point of view and familiarity with a specific positioning technique are an integral part of minimizing the risk of any operation. For those surgeons familiar with the park bench positioning, the description of the surgical anatomy and orientation of the illustrations are equally as valid as described below for the sitting position by merely rotating the illustrations 90°.

Operative Technique

The patient is placed in the upright sitting position in the pinion headrest, with the head flexed and rotated to the side of the glossopharyngeal neuralgia. A central right atrial catheter for monitoring and aspiration of possible air emboli is placed before the patient is placed in the sitting position. Either an S-shaped or a hockey stick-shaped incision is made over the ipsilateral occipital bone. The 3-cm craniectomy is done inferiorly to incorporate the portion of the occipital bone which lies directly adjacent to the foramen magnum and which is oriented in a transverse plane directly above the lamina of the first cervical segment. If a rongeur is used for the craniectomy, there is increased risk of epidural hemorrhage (Fig. 2, A–C). The high-speed drill obviates the need to introduce a rongeur beneath the inner table of the occipital bone so that there is less chance of a dissecting epidural clot intra- and postoperatively (Fig. 2D). The dural margin remains adherent to the edges of the craniectomy.

The dura is then opened in a cruciate fashion and tacked back over the craniectomy margin to the peri-

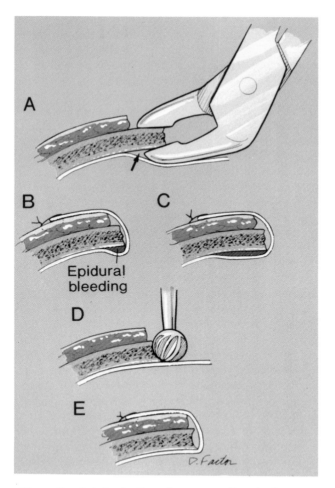

Figure 2. **A,** introduction of a rongeur dissects dura away beyond the limits of the craniectomy. **B** and **C,** this may allow a dissecting epidural hemorrhage to occur. **D** and **E,** a diamond drill (not shown) avoids the dura laceration potential of a cutting burr and allows tight dural bone contact immediate to the craniectomy.

cranium or occipital fascia or muscle layer, preventing a dissecting epidural hemorrhage (Fig. 2E). The cerebellar hemisphere is elevated to expose the arachnoid of the cisterna magna, which is opened, allowing the egress of cerebrospinal fluid and allowing relaxation of the cerebellum. By identifying the sigmoid sinus as it traverses the posterior fossa floor, the surgeon can achieve precise retractor position for identification of the jugular foramen. Once the self-retaining retractor has been fixed in position, illumination by the overhead surgical lights and operating loupes is usually sufficient. The operating microscope may enhance visualization at this point. The ninth cranial nerve in the jugular foramen is always separated by a dural septum from the tenth and eleventh cranial nerves and jugular vein (Fig. 1B).

The ninth nerve and upper one-sixth to one-eighth of the filaments of the tenth nerve are sectioned with the aid of a black spatula or blunt hook and bipolar coagulation (Fig. 1C). The dural opening may then be closed by using pericranium, fascia lata, or homologous dura as a graft, or by closing the dura primarily.

INTRA- AND POSTOPERATIVE CONSIDERATIONS

Although sensation is diminished over the pharynx and the gag reflex is abolished on the side of the divided nerve, and although discrete neurological testing reveals absence of taste over the ipsilateral posterior one-third of the tongue, we, like Dandy, have never noted more than a transient disturbance in swallowing. With sectioning of the ninth and upper rootlets of the tenth cranial nerves, auricular flutter, tachycardia, hypertension, ectopic ventricular contractions, and cardiac arrhythmias have been noted. Most of these events are transient intraoperative events.

OCCIPITOCERVICAL AND HIGH CERVICAL STABILIZATION

VOLKER K. H. SONNTAG, M.D.
CURTIS A. DICKMAN, M.D.

INTRODUCTION

Arthrodesis of the atlas and axis is indicated when instability of these structures becomes clinically or radiographically significant. Atlantoaxial subluxation (AAS) can occur suddenly from traumatic injuries such as upper cervical vertebral fractures or ligamentous disruption, or may develop progressively from rheumatoid arthritis, neoplasm, infection, or os odontoideum. Occipitocervical instability occurs less frequently than AAS and is due to similar pathologic processes.

PATIENT SELECTION

The decision to perform an atlantoaxial or occipitocervical arthrodesis should be individualized, based on the neurologic symptoms and signs, the radiographic extent of AAS, the presence of fractures, the patient's age and medical condition, the specific pathology, and the level of instability. Symptoms or signs of myelopathy from AAS are the most clear indications for arthrodesis. Patients with occipital radicular pain and persistent or progressive radiographic AAS are also surgical candidates. The least well-defined indication is isolated neck pain. In the absence of neurologic deficits, specific pathological and clinical features become more important to the operative decision. Patients at high risk for nonunion of fractures or those with neurologic deficits from progressive AAS may be considered for arthrodesis.

The anatomical features of the atlantoaxial complex should be specifically evaluated in each patient. The odontoid process, spinal cord, and subarachnoid space each normally occupies approximately 1 cm within the spinal canal at the C1 level. These relationships are altered with AAS. The subarachnoid space may be effaced by the subluxed vertebral segments and may be additionally compromised by fracture fragments, inflammation, bony callus, basilar in-

vagination of the dens, or other mass lesions. These features enhance the vulnerability to injury, so that even minor trauma can precipitate deficits. Neurologically intact patients with more than 6 mm of AAS or radiographic progression of AAS are at high risk for neurologic injury or sudden death. Individuals with Type II odontoid fractures with more than 6 mm dens displacement have a high risk of nonunion (60–85%). In these instances, neurologically intact patients may benefit from atlantoaxial arthrodesis.

Radiographic evaluation of patients with AAS should include anteroposterior, lateral, open-mouth odontoid, and oblique roentgenograms. If acute neurologic deficits or acute fractures are absent, lateral roentgenograms in flexion and extension will indicate the extent of AAS. Flexion-extension views are contraindicated with acute unstable fractures because neurologic deficits may be precipitated or exacerbated. Thin-section computed tomography (CT) defines the static relationships of bony abnormalities and the extent of fractures more precisely than plain x-ray films. In selected cases, three-dimensional CT enhances the visualization of osseous pathology. Magnetic resonance imaging (MRI) has replaced myelography for the evaluation of neural compression because of its superb anatomical resolution, high sensitivity, and multiplanar graphic displays. Patients with unstable osseous lesions may be placed in an MRI-compatible halo brace. MRI is most useful for assessing compressive pathology that requires treatment beyond arthrodesis. Flexion and extension MRI (Fig. 1) delineates neural compression and the extent of positional reduction in patients with rheumatoid arthritis and craniovertebral settling, Chiari malformations, or ligamentous AAS.

Patients with irreducible or partially reducible compression of the cervicomedullary junction should undergo decompression. If instability exists after the decompressive procedures, arthrodesis is indicated. Anterior compression from basilar invagination of the dens or from other ventral lesions at the cer-

© 1991 The American Association of Neurological Surgeons

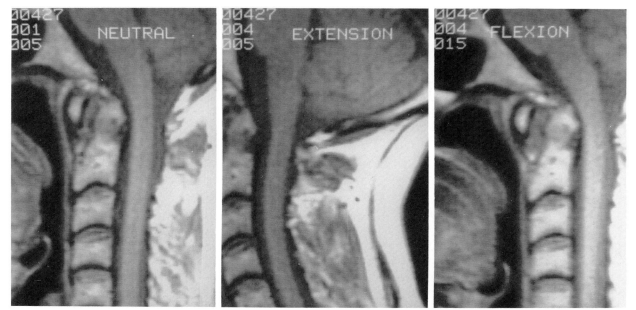

Figure 1. Magnetic resonance imaging study of the cranio-vertebral junction and upper cervical spine. Neutral, extension, and flexion views delineate the extent of atlantoaxial subluxation. Note the effacement of the subarachnoid space and the widening of the predental space with flexion.

vicomedullary junction is best approached trans-orally. Posterior decompressive approaches for Chiari malformations or other lesions may influence the type of arthrodesis needed. Decompression and fusion may be performed simultaneously if necessary.

In most instances of AAS, we prefer to limit the fusion to the atlantoaxial vertebrae. C1-C2 fusion preserves more mobility of the cervical spine compared with occipitocervical fusion, and the rate of nonunion increases when the occiput is included in the fusion. In most cases of AAS, the fusion can be confined to the unstable vertebral segments. If C1 cannot be incorporated into the fusion, then occipitocervical arthrodesis becomes necessary. Other indications for occipitocervical fusion include occipitoatlantal instability or instability at multiple vertebral segments.

Surgery for combination fractures involving the atlas and axis is indicated only if the C2 fracture is unstable or has a high risk of nonunion. In these instances, the extent of the fusion is dictated by the type of C1 fracture. If the atlas fracture involves the anterior portion or lateral ring of C1, then atlantoaxial arthrodesis may be performed. If the C1 fracture involves the posterior ring, then the atlas cannot be wired; an occipitocervical arthrodesis or a C1-C2 screw fixation is required.

PREOPERATIVE PREPARATION

The halo brace is the most rigid form of external immobilization for stabilizing the upper cervical spine. Pre-operative halo placement ensures optimum alignment of subluxed segments and avoids the risk of neurologic injury from cervical manipulation during intubation. A patient in a halo vest should be intubated while awake with nasotracheal, bronchoscopic, or fiberoptic-guided technique. Somatosensory evoked potentials are monitored perioperatively. If an occipitocervical procedure is planned, brain stem evoked potentials are also monitored. Individuals with neurologic deficits are begun on a corticosteroid preparation and an H_2-receptor antagonist at least 24 hours preoperatively.

A patient in the halo brace is placed prone on the operating table. Rolls are positioned to support the chest, to allow adequate respiratory excursion, and to prevent abdominal compression to avoid epidural venous distention. With a Mayfield headholder adaptor for the halo brace (Fig. 2), patients can be secured to the operating table with minimal difficulty. Alternatively, stacked weights can support the anterior bars of the halo brace (Fig. 3). The back plate of the halo vest may be removed to access the posterior cervical region or iliac crest; however, this is often not necessary. The posterior bars of the halo vest function as excellent hand rests when left in place. Securing patients to the operating table with wide cloth tape permits intraoperative table adjustments. Padding avoids compressive neuropathies. The occipital and cervical regions are shaved. Waterproof adherent plastic drapes protect the evoked potential monitoring

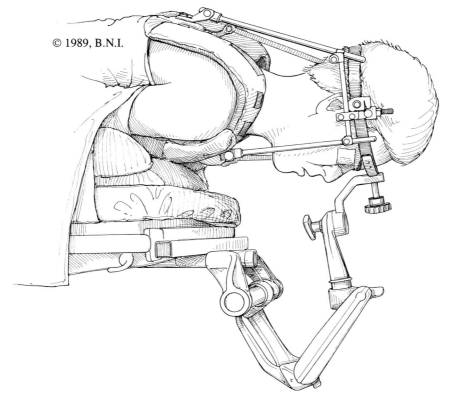

Figure 2. The Mayfield headholder adaptor for the halo brace facilitates patient positioning.

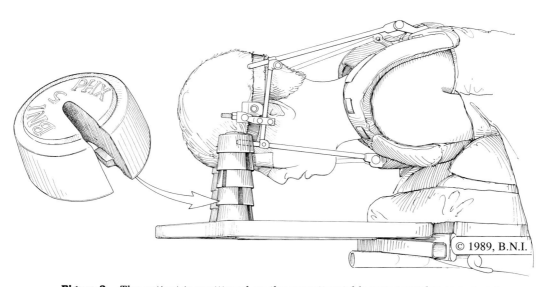

Figure 3. The patient is positioned on the operating table using weights to support the halo brace anteriorly.

leads from moisture. Lateral cervical roentgenograms are obtained to confirm alignment after positioning, and a standard skin preparation is performed.

OPERATIVE TECHNIQUE

Atlantoaxial Arthrodesis

A posterior cervical linear midline skin incision is made, extending from the inion to the spinous process of the vertebra prominens. The incision is deepened to the level of the nuchal fascia. Sharply dividing the fascia and posterior cervical muscles in the midline plane allows a relatively avascular dissection, which is deepened until the posterior arches of C1 and C2 are exposed. The ring of C1 and large spinous process of C2 are palpable landmarks; however, the exploration should be gentle to avoid translocation of C1. The periosteum of the ring of C1 and the tip of the spinous process of C2 are sharply incised, and the paraspinous cervical muscles are swept laterally using careful subperiosteal dissection with lightweight periosteal elevators. This maneuver proceeds from the midline laterally and avoids exposing the vertebral arteries (Fig. 4). Self-retaining angled retractors are inserted to maintain operative exposure.

The soft tissue is removed from the superior and inferior margins of C1 and from the superior margin of C2 with a curette. Along the inferior ring of C1 and the superior surface of the spinous process and laminae of C2, the points of contact of C1 and C2 with the graft are decorticated with a high-speed drill or Kerrison rongeur (Fig. 5). A Kerrison rongeur is used to notch the inferior margin of the spinolaminar junctions of C2 to seat the wire (Fig. 6).

An autologous bone graft (4 cm long × 3 cm high) is obtained from the posterior iliac crest as a curved tricortical segment. Additional cancellous bone is obtained from the iliac crest for use in the fusion.

The graft is prepared by removing its rounded cortical edge with a Leksell rongeur, creating a bicortical curvilinear strut (Fig. 7). The graft is then fitted between C1 and C2 to approximate the curve of the ring of C1. A notch in the inferior margin of the bone graft in the midline matching the contour of the spinous process of C2 enables the graft to fit securely. The graft is temporarily removed to obtain wire placement.

Twenty-four-gauge, double-stranded wire (3 turns/cm) is halved, looped, and passed beneath the posterior arch of C1 in the midline, directed superiorly (Fig. 8). A wire-passer or heavy silk may facilitate the passage. The wire must be simultaneously fed and pulled using a "two-handed" process to avoid traction or manipulation of the atlas and to avoid displacing the wire anteriorly. The graft is then replaced into position

between the atlas and axis. The loop of the wire is passed over the ring of C1 and secured under the base of the C2 spinous process. One free end of wire is passed below the spinous process of C2, and the wires are tightened snugly with a wire twister (Fig. 9). The graft is affixed by wire anteriorly and posteriorly and seated between the posterior-inferior arch of C1 and the posterior-superior arch of C2.

Small areas of the ring of C1, laminae of C2, and cortex of the bone graft are decorticated with a high-speed drill and covered with fragmented cancellous bone (Fig. 10). The wound is closed securely, obliterating all dead space. Muscle and fascia are closed with heavy absorbable sutures in a watertight fashion. Skin closure with nylon suture is preferable.

The halo brace is maintained for 12 weeks postoperatively. The halo ring is then disconnected from the brace. If flexion-extension lateral roentgenograms indicate clinical and radiographic stability, the halo brace is removed and a Philadelphia collar is applied. The collar is weaned according to patient tolerance.

Occipitocervical Arthrodesis

Patient positioning, preparation, and incisions are identical to those described for atlantoaxial fusion. The osseous exposure is more extensive, involving subperiosteal dissection of the squamous portion of the occipital bone, rim of the foramen magnum, and C3 spinous process and laminae. Two burr holes are created in the occipital bone, 0.5 cm superior to the rim of the foramen magnum. The burr holes are waxed for hemostasis, and the dura is separated from the skull using dural elevators, connecting each hole with the foramen magnum. The foramen magnum is enlarged posteriorly with Kerrison rongeurs. Twenty-gauge wires are passed between each of the burr holes and the foramen magnum, and sublaminar at the levels to be fused (C1, C2, and/or C3).

A Steinmann pin, bent into a "U" shape, is fashioned to approximate the contour of the occipitocervical region. The wires are twisted, securing the Steinmann pin to the occiput and cervical laminae (Fig. 11). The threads of the pin prevent excessive mobility of the construct. The bone is decorticated with a high-speed drill, and bone fragments are laid upon the levels to be fused.

When the posterior ring of C1 has been removed or a suboccipital craniectomy has been performed, a plate of cortical iliac crest bone may be wired to the central portion of the Steinmann pin. This plate recreates the osseous contour of the occipitocervical region and provides a template for the subsequently developing fusion mass (Fig. 12). Closure techniques and postoperative care are identical to those described for atlantoaxial fusion.

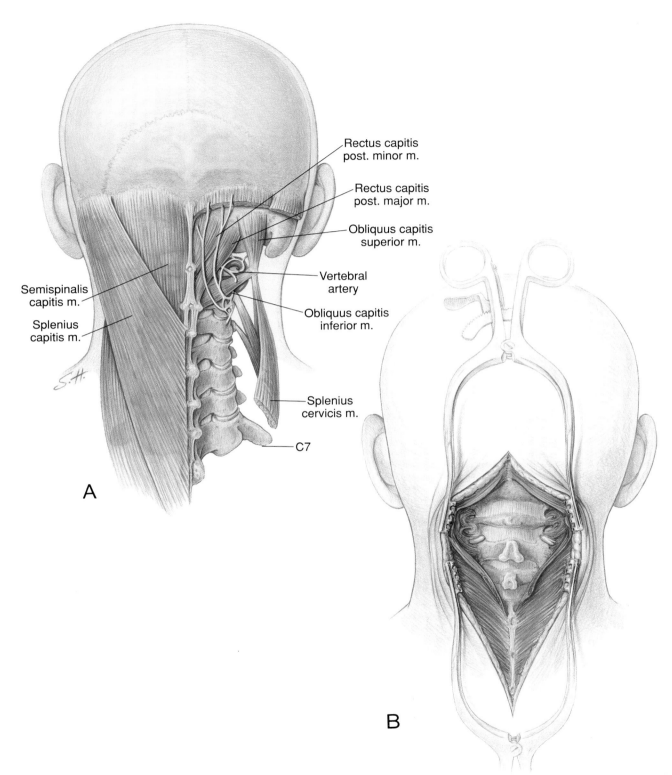

Figure 4. **A,** anatomical relationships of the suboccipital and posterior cervical regions. Note the course of the vertebral artery at the C1 and C2 levels. **B,** illustration of the incision and muscular dissection. The bony exposure is *not* carried laterally enough to expose the vertebral arteries. (© 1990, B.N.I.)

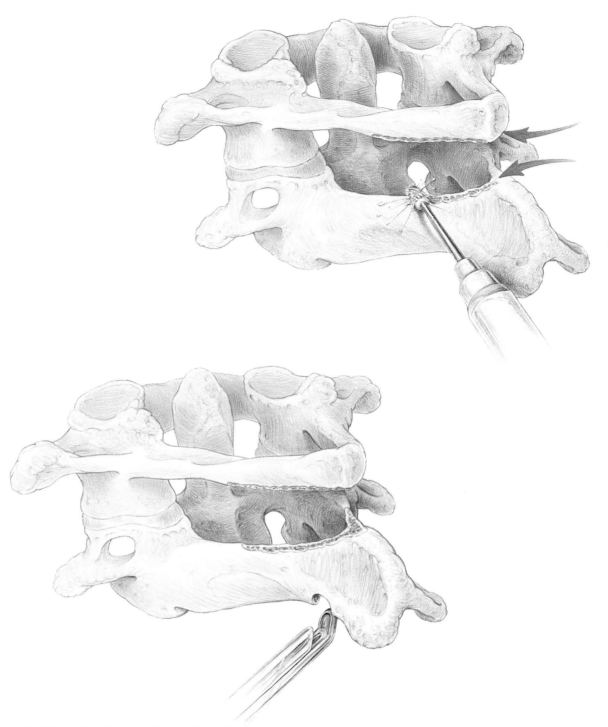

Figure 5. (Top) Decorticating the surfaces of contact of the atlas and axis with the bone graft. (© 1990, B.N.I.)

Figure 6. (Bottom) Notches are created at the inferior spinolaminar junctions of C2 for wire seating. (© 1990, B.N.I.)

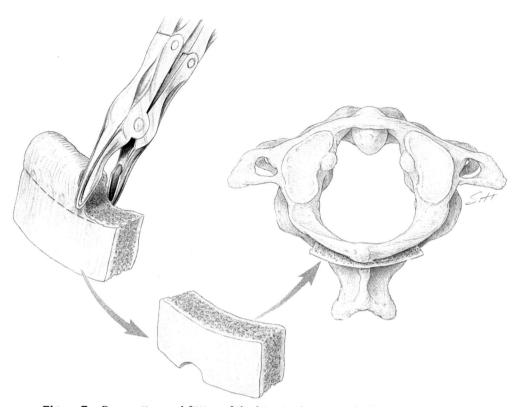

Figure 7. Preparation and fitting of the bicortical strut graft. (© 1990, B.N.I.)

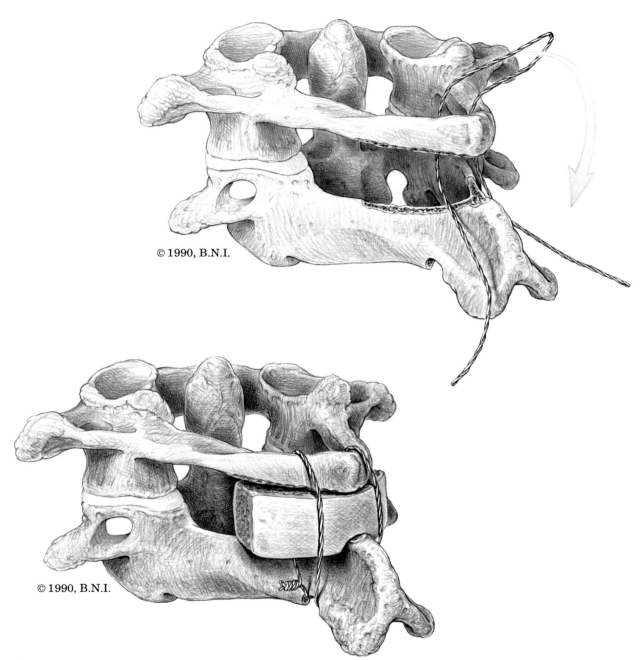

© 1990, B.N.I.

© 1990, B.N.I.

Figure 8. (Top) Sublaminar wire passage at C1. The loop is passed superiorly beneath the atlas.

Figure 9. (Bottom) The fusion construct, demonstrating the relationships of C1, C2, bone graft, and wires.

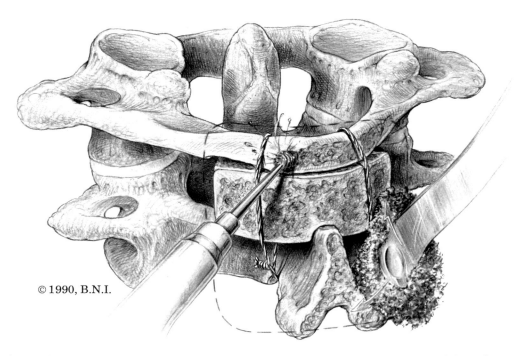

© 1990, B.N.I.

Figure 10. Decortication of the fusion construct. The prepared regions are covered with bone fragments (indicated with *dashed outline*).

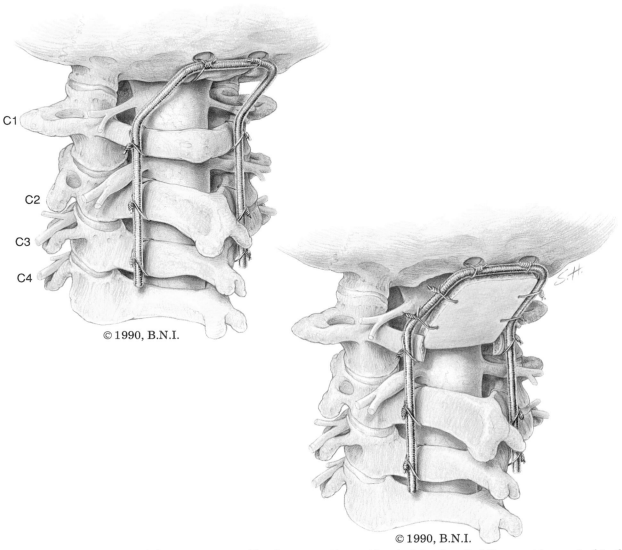

C1

C2

C3

C4

© 1990, B.N.I.

© 1990, B.N.I.

Figure 11. Occipitocervical fusion construct. The Steinmann pin is secured to the occiput and cervical laminae with wires. (© 1990, B.N.I.)

Figure 12. A plate of cortical iliac crest bone wired to the pin can be used as a template to support bone fragments. (© 1990, B.N.I.)

COMPLICATIONS

Wire breakage, inadvertent extension of the fusion mass, or nonunion may occur. The halo brace maintains rigid external immobilization, provides optimal conditions for formation of the fusion, and minimizes the risk of wire breakage. Wire breakage is monitored with intraoperative and postoperative x-ray films. Extension of the fusion is prevented by limiting the subperiosteal dissection to the osseous segments to be fused. If the occiput, C3, or other vertebrae are exposed, they may be inadvertently incorporated into a C1-C2 fusion. This most commonly occurs in children. Osseous union is maximized by sharp subperiosteal dissection, segmentally decorticating small areas of the bone to be fused, and precisely fitting the bone grafts. Monopolar cautery devascularizes bone and may contribute to nonunion. Excessive decortication may weaken the vertebrae. Fibrous union may convert to delayed osseous union with additional halo immobilization. Nonunion must be managed with additional internal fixation.

Neural and dural injuries are prevented by a knowledge of each patient's normal and pathologic anatomy, by avoiding traction or manipulation of unstable osseous segments, and by looping the wires before their sublaminar passage. Evoked potential and postoperative intensive care unit monitoring allow early recognition of neurologic dysfunction.

PETROCLIVAL MENINGIOMAS

OSSAMA AL-MEFTY, M.D.
MICHAEL P. SCHENK, M.S.
ROBERT R. SMITH, M.D.

PATIENT SELECTION

Petroclival meningiomas remain challenging lesions, owing to their rarity, crucial location, insidious growth, and relentless natural progression leading to a fatal outcome. With the advent of advanced imaging, refined approaches, microsurgical techniques, intraoperative monitoring, and modern anesthesia and postoperative care, the previously dismal surgical outcome has been largely overcome. Meningiomas are benign tumors, and the treatment objective is total resection. This is best achieved during the first operation because dissection of neurovascular structures is facilitated by intact arachnoid membranes. Although surgeons should pursue total removal with skill and zeal, their judgment should not be skewed from the goal of preserving or improving neurologic functions. This may require surgeons to accept subtotal removal at times.

The size of the lesion is a significant factor influencing surgical morbidity and mortality. Because these tumors are slow-growing, watchful waiting is justified in elderly patients who are asymptomatic, until evidence of brain stem compression appears. Recently, stereotaxic radiosurgery has offered an alternative for small or residual tumors. The effectiveness and long term results of this modality, however, await further reports.

PREOPERATIVE PREPARATION

Detailed radiological studies are crucial for surgical planning. Computed tomography (CT) scans and magnetic resonance imaging (MRI), in coronal, sagittal, and axial views, are obtained preoperatively for complete definition of the tumor: its location, extension, relation to the brain stem, encasement of vessels, and involvement of the cavernous sinus and the temporal bone (Fig. 1). Angiography remains a necessary preoperative diagnostic study, to identify a vascular lesion, to demonstrate cerebrovascular anatomy and

displacement, to outline the tumor's blood supply, and to confirm the patency and the connection between the two transverse sinuses (Fig. 2). MRI angiography may soon replace conventional angiography in this role.

Dexamethasone is administered preoperatively, and antibiotics are given intraoperatively. The authors' choice of antibiotics is a combination of vancomycin and a third generation cephalosporin.

ANESTHESIA AND MONITORING

Good anesthetic technique is essential for successful removal of petroclival meningiomas. Premedication is usually withheld; induction is rapid and smooth and should be accomplished with an agent that reduces intracranial pressure. Lidocaine, given intravenously after thiopental induction, decreases the intubation-induced hypertensive response. The choice of anesthetic agents should be flexible and tailored to suit the circumstances of each case. Intracranial hypertension should be avoided and adequate cerebral perfusion maintained. The use of intraoperative monitoring of cranial nerve and brain stem evoked potentials necessitates the use of certain anesthetic agents or switching intraoperatively from one to another. Normotension is the goal, and hypotension should be avoided. Should temporary vascular occlusion be necessary during the surgical resection of the tumor, a barbiturate is given for its known cerebral protective effect.

Systemic monitoring is accomplished by means of an arterial line, a double-lumen central venous line (with confirmation of the location of the tip in the right atrium), a Foley catheter, a Doppler monitor, and an oximeter. In addition, end-expiratory PCO_2, arterial blood gas, electrolyte, hemoglobin, and hematocrit values, and coagulation profile are determined as necessary.

Brain stem auditory evoked potentials are recorded bilaterally as are somatosensory evoked potentials. Facial nerve function is monitored by recording an electromyogram (EMG) from several groups of facial muscles on the ipsilateral side.

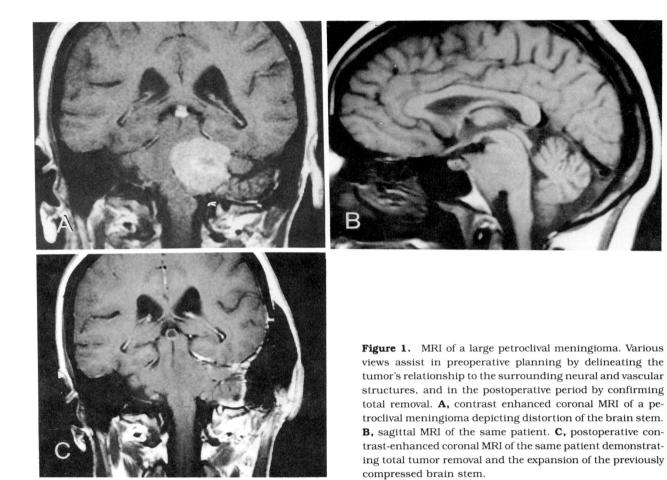

Figure 1. MRI of a large petroclival meningioma. Various views assist in preoperative planning by delineating the tumor's relationship to the surrounding neural and vascular structures, and in the postoperative period by confirming total removal. **A,** contrast enhanced coronal MRI of a petroclival meningioma depicting distortion of the brain stem. **B,** sagittal MRI of the same patient. **C,** postoperative contrast-enhanced coronal MRI of the same patient demonstrating total tumor removal and the expansion of the previously compressed brain stem.

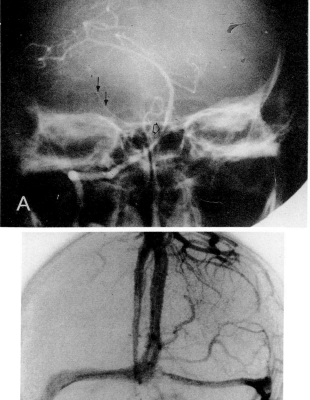

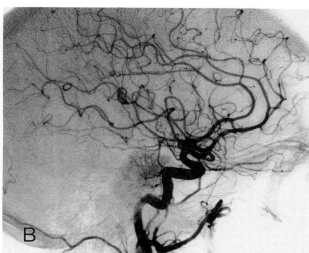

Figure 2. Angiographic views in three different patients revealing important information for surgical planning. **A,** a vertebral angiogram of a large petroclival meningioma showing marked displacement of the basilar artery to the opposite side, stretching of the AICA (*arrows*) and encasement of the basilar artery (*open arrow*). **B,** a lateral carotid arteriogram demonstrating vascular feeders to a meningioma from the intrapetrous segment of the carotid artery. **C,** an anteroposterior angiogram in the venous phase in a patient with a petroclival meningioma. Notice the small left sigmoid sinus that is not connected at the torcular Herophili. Also notice the tumor blush.

OPERATIVE APPROACH

Several approaches or a combination of approaches have been used to remove petroclival meningiomas. These include the frontotemporal, occipital-transtentorial, subtemporal-transtentorial, suboccipital, combined subtemporal and suboccipital, combined subtemporal and translabyrinthine, transcochlear, and the combined suboccipital translabyrinthine approaches. The petrosal approach described herein evolved from refinements of several other techniques. It is centered on the petrous bone, allowing exposure of the tumor extending from the middle fossa to the foramen magnum. This approach is preferred because of the following advantages: (*a*) the cerebellum and temporal lobes are minimally retracted; (*b*) the operative distance to the clivus is shortened by 3 cm; (*c*) the surgeon has a direct line of sight to the lesion and the anterior and lateral aspects of the brain stem; (*d*) the neural and otologic structures, including the cochlea, labyrinth, and facial nerve, are preserved; (*e*) the

transverse and sigmoid sinuses, as well as the vein of Labbé and the basal occipital veins, are preserved; (*f*) the tumor's vascular supply is intercepted early in the procedure; and (*g*) multiple axes for dissection are provided.

Patient Position (Fig. 3)

The patient is placed supine with the patient's head at the foot of the operating table, allowing space and ease of movement for the seated surgeon. The table is flexed to allow 20–30° elevation of the head and trunk. The patient's ipsilateral shoulder is slightly elevated. The head is turned away from the side of the tumor, inclined toward the floor, and tilted toward the opposite side. The position of the neck is inspected to avoid compression of the contralateral jugular vein. The head is fixed in a three-point Mayfield headrest. During the operation, the surgeon's line of sight can be altered by rotating the table from side to side or up and down.

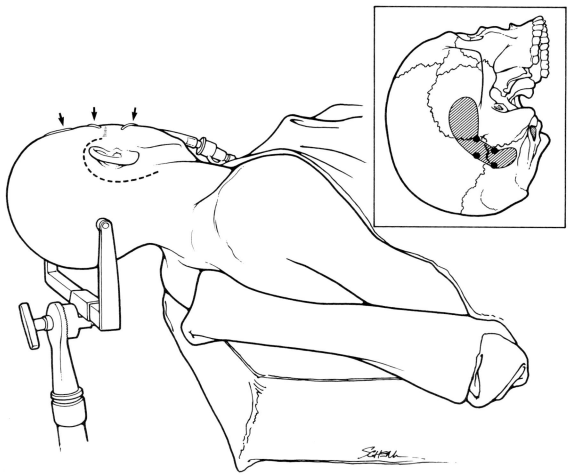

Figure 3. The position of the patient and the skin incision for a right-sided petrosal approach. EMG needle electrodes (*arrows*) are inserted into the muscles innervated by the facial nerve. *Inset*, a skull model depicting the position of the burr holes and outline of the bone flap.

Operative Procedure

Craniotomy Flap (Fig. 4)

A reverse question-mark incision is made starting at the zygoma in front of the ear, circling above the ear, and descending 1 cm medially to (behind) the mastoid process (Fig. 3). The skin flap is elevated and retracted anteriorly and inferiorly. A large triangular pericranial flap with an intact vascular base is elevated and retracted over the skin flap to the level of the external ear canal. This flap is used to cover the drilled surface of the temporal bone at the time of closure. The temporal muscle then is retracted anteriorly and inferiorly while the sternomastoid insertion is detached and retracted posteriorly and inferiorly. The bony surface of the temporal fossa, mastoid, and lateral posterior fossa are thus exposed.

Four burr holes are made, two on each side of the transverse sinus. A hole made just medial and inferior to the asterion opens into the posterior fossa below the transverse sigmoid sinus junction, while a hole located at the squamous and mastoid junction of the temporal bone, along the projection of the superior temporal line, opens into the supratentorial compartment (Figs. 3 and 4). The burr hole at each of these points will exactly flank the sigmoid sinus. The temporal bone and a portion of the occipital bone above the tentorium, as well as the occipital bone below the tentorium, are cut between burr holes using the foot attachment of the Midas Rex drill. The burr holes flanking the lateral sinus are then connected using a thin rongeur, or drilled with the B-1 attachment of the

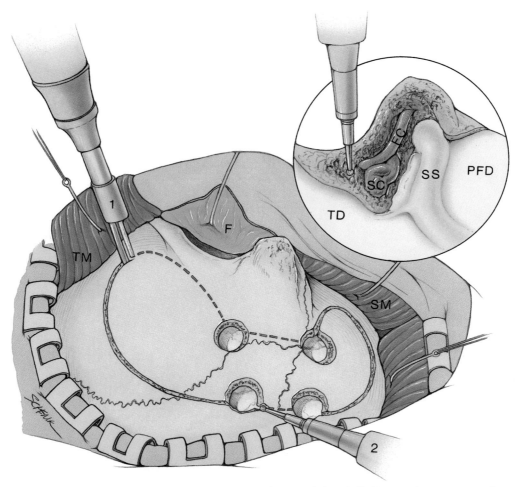

Figure 4. The temporalis muscle (*TM*) and sternomastoid muscle (*SM*) are elevated and retracted on the right side. A pericranial triangular flap (*F*) is elevated and saved for later coverage of the drilled surface of the temporal bone. The position of the burr holes flanking the transverse sigmoid sinus is shown. A craniotome with foot attachment (*1*) is used to make the bony cut in the temporal and posterior fossae, while a drill (*2*) is used to cross over the sinus. *Inset*, the bone flap has been removed, the dura of the temporal fossa (*TD*) and posterior fossa (*PFD*) have been exposed, the right sigmoid sinus (*SS*) has been skeletonized, and the petrous bone has been drilled extensively. The anatomical landmarks in the temporal bone (the facial canal (*FC*) and the semicircular canals (*SC*)) are demonstrated.

Midas Rex drill. Particular attention should be paid to avoid tearing the wall of the venous sinus, which domes into a bony impression on the inner surface of the skull.

The single bone flap is elevated, exposing the transverse and sigmoid sinuses. The bone adheres tightly to the dura at the junction of the sigmoid and transverse sinuses and requires careful dissection and elevation. An alternative to this method of skull-bone removal is to perform a temporal craniotomy, followed by a posterior fossa craniectomy extending over the transverse sinus.

Temporal Bone Drilling (Fig. 4, inset)

The second stage, drilling of the temporal bone, requires a thorough knowledge of the anatomy of the petrous bone and surrounding structures. A Zeiss operating microscope, mounted on a Contraves stand

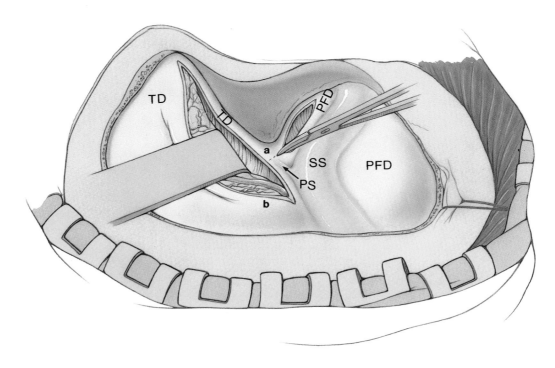

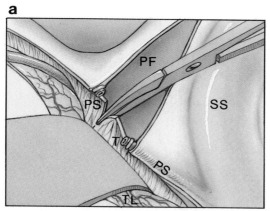

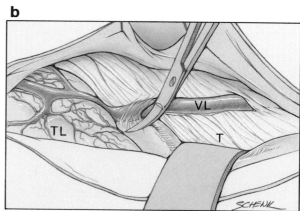

Figure 5. Initial exposure via a presigmoid (retrolabyrinthine) route. The temporal dura is incised along the floor of the temporal fossa. The posterior fossa dura anterior to the sigmoid sinus is incised toward the superior petrosal sinus. The sectioning of the petrosal sinus (*area a*) and the dissection of the vein of Labbé (*area b*) are magnified in *insets a* and *b* (*bottom*). *Inset a*, clipping and sectioning of the superior petrosal sinus and the beginning of the tentorial incision. *Inset b*, dissection of the vein of Labbé in order to retract the temporal lobe and preserve the vein. *SS*, sigmoid sinus; *PS*, superior petrosal sinus; *T*, tentorium; *TL*, temporal lobe; *PF*, posterior fossa; *TD*, temporal dura; *PFD*, posterior fossa dura; *VL*, vein of Labbé.

and equipped with an adjustable-angle eyepiece, is used. The angle of the eyepiece is changed as the field alternates between the subtemporal and suboccipital routes. The surgeon performs a complete mastoidectomy using a high-speed air drill. A diamond bit should be used when drilling is close to vital anatomical structures. The sigmoid sinus is skeletonized down to the jugular bulb. The sinodural angle, Citelli's angle, which identifies the position of the superior petrosal sinus, is exposed. The superficial mastoid air cells behind the posterior wall of the external ear canal, as well as the deep (retrofacial) air cells, are drilled out to expose the facial canal and the lateral and posterior semicircular canals. Drilling is continued along the pyramid to thin the petrous bone toward its apex. The

facial canal as well as the middle and inner ear structures are kept intact, while opened air cells are obliterated with bone wax.

Exposure of the Tumor (Figs. 5–7)

When the surgeon needs a shorter and more lateral access to the petrous apex and clivus, the posterior fossa dura anterior to the sigmoid sinus is opened along the anterior margin of the sinus. The incision is then extended upward toward a supratentorial dural incision made on the floor of the temporal fossa (Fig. 5, *Inset b*). The temporal lobe is gently retracted. The vein of Labbé is preserved by dissection from the cortical surface, allowing retraction of the temporal lobe without tension on the venous wall (Figs. 5 and 6).

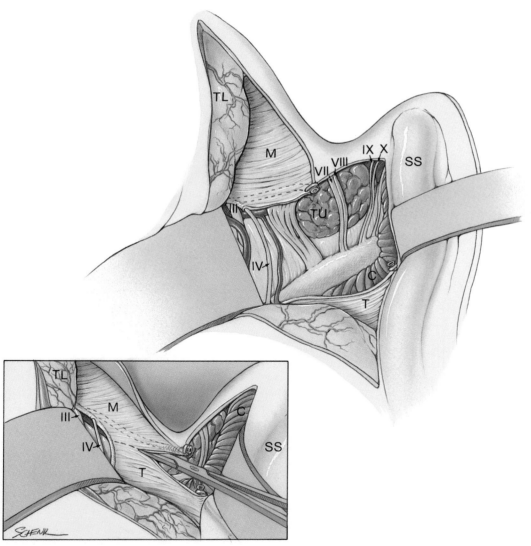

Figure 6. Exposure of the tumor via a presigmoid route. The sigmoid sinus (*SS*) and cerebellum (*C*) are retracted medially while the temporal lobe (*TL*) is retracted superiorly. The tentorium (*T*) is incised along the pyramid, through the incisura. The brain stem, cranial nerves (*III–XI*), and tumor (*Tu*) are visualized. *Inset*, demonstration of tentorial sectioning along the pyramid toward the incisura. *M*, middle fossa floor.

The superior petrosal sinus is clipped or coagulated and transected (Fig. 5, *Inset a*), and the incision is continued on the tentorium, parallel to the pyramid, and extended through the incisura. During this maneuver, the surgeon must make every effort to preserve the trochlear nerve by keeping the incision of the tentorial notch behind the area where the IVth nerve pierces the notch (Fig. 6, *inset*). Opening the tentorium allows excellent exposure to the upper pole of the tumor and the anterior and lateral aspects of the brain stem (Figs. 6, 8, and 9). Trigeminal nerve rootlets, frequently stretched and separated by the tumor, are found under the tentorium (Fig. 6). The retractor is then placed anteriorly, holding medially the sigmoid sinus, the cerebellum, and the cut edge of the tentorium (Fig. 6).

When the tumor is large and extends significantly into both supra- and infratentorial compartments, the dura of the posterior and temporal fossae is then opened along both sides of the sigmoid sinus. The supratentorial incision is continued along the floor of the temporal fossa while the infratentorial incision is extended to the jugular bulb (Fig. 7, *inset*). The dural flaps are left covering the brain for protection. The cerebellar hemisphere, which naturally falls backward, needs little or no retraction. The temporal lobe is elevated gently. There is no need to transect the sigmoid sinus because the fields above and below the tentorium may be exposed alternately.

Tumor Resection

Further relaxation is obtained by opening the arachnoid of the cerebellomedullary cistern and draining

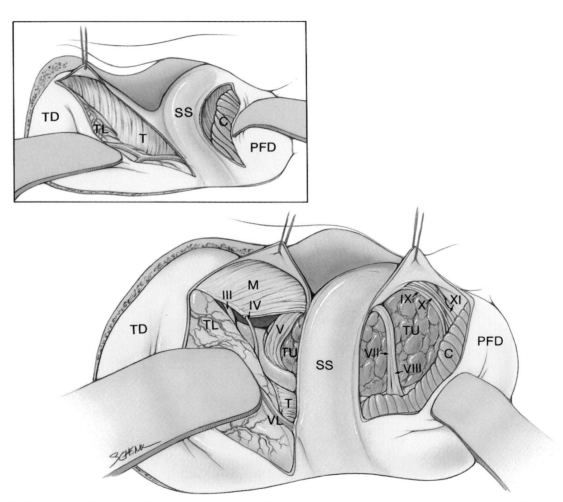

Figure 7. Exposure of the tumor through the suboccipital and subtemporal routes. The cerebellum (*C*) and posterior temporal lobe (*TL*) are held by self-retaining retractors. The tentorium (*T*) is incised around the partially removed supratentorial portion of the tumor (*Tu*). The tumor's relationship to the brain stem and cranial nerves III–XI is demonstrated.

Inset, the dura is opened along both sides of the sinus and extended to the jugular bulb in the posterior fossa and along the floor of the temporal fossa. The sigmoid sinus is kept intact. *SS*, sigmoid sinus; *TD*, temporal lobe dura; *C*, cerebellum; *PFD*, posterior fossa dura; *T*, tentorium; *M*, middle fossa floor.

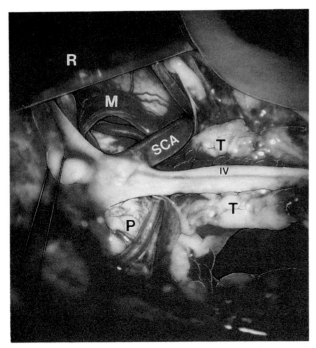

Figure 8. Artist's enhancement of an operative photograph showing removal of a tumor via the petrosal approach after the tentorium has been incised. The debulked tumor lies in front of the midbrain and pons. The IVth nerve is seen on the lateral surface of the brain stem and tumor. *P*, pons; *M*, midbrain; *SCA*, superior cerebellar artery; *T*, tumor; *R*, retractor on the temporal lobe.

11). A cut edge of the tumor should not be allowed to slip away lest the plane of cleavage be lost. Furthermore, gutting the tumor may be necessary before dissection of the thinned-out capsule can be continued.

The lower cranial nerves are dissected off the inferior pole of the tumor. Gentle dissection is required to avoid hypotension and bradycardia from vagal stimulation. The VIIth and VIIIth cranial nerves are carefully dissected from the tumor. The sixth nerve, stretched anteriorly and inferiorly, is dissected free from the tumor and followed distally (Fig. 12). It helps to visualize alternately between the supra- and infratentorial routes while dissecting the tumor capsule carefully away from the brain stem (Figs. 8, 9, and 12). If it is not embedded in the tumor, the basilar artery is usually displaced to the opposite side (Fig. 13). The preservation and careful dissection of the main and small branches of the basilar artery cannot be overemphasized (Fig. 14).

Once the tumor has been excised, all neurovascular structures in the posterior fossa are covered with wet surgical patties, and the area of tumor attachment is vaporized extensively with the laser. If the tumor has extended into the internal auditory meatus, the meatus wall is drilled and the tumor removed. Extension through the jugular foramen is likewise removed.

cerebrospinal fluid (CSF). The tumor is further devascularized by coagulating its insertion on the pyramid and the meningeal feeders over the tentorium. When the tumor is small or moderate in size, the seventh and eighth cranial nerves are usually stretched posteriorly and thus are easily identified (Fig. 6). When the tumor reaches a large size, however, these cranial nerves may well be engulfed in the tumor.

A suitable area on the tumor surface is selected and the arachnoid over the tumor is opened. The tumor is then debulked with extreme caution since the VIIth and VIIIth nerves, as well as the posterior inferior cerebellar artery (PICA) and anterior inferior cerebellar artery (AICA), may be embedded in the tumor. Debulking is performed using suction, laser, Cavitron ultrasonic aspirator, and/or bipolar coagulation and microscissors.

The tumor capsule is then dissected free from the surrounding structures. Maintaining dissection within the arachnoidal planes is crucial to preservation of the vital neural and vascular structures. Cranial nerves and the basilar artery and its branches may, however, be embedded in a large tumor, demanding meticulous and tedious dissection (Figs. 10 and

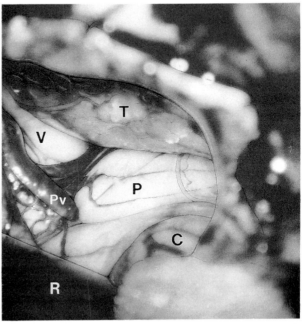

Figure 9. Artist's enhancement of an operative photograph showing tumor exposure via the retrolabyrinthine approach. Notice the direct exposure of the lateral brain stem. *P*, pons; *Pv*, petrosal vein; *T*, tumor; *V*, trigeminal nerve; *R*, retractor; *C*, cerebellum.

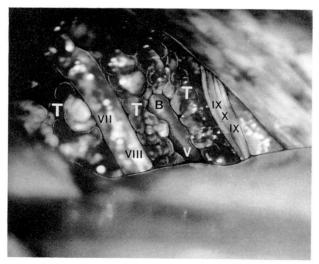

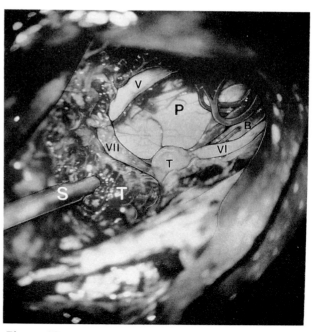

Figure 10. Artist's enhancement of an operative photograph showing the removal of a meningioma encasing the basilar artery, vertebral artery, and cranial nerves VII–XI. *T,* tumor; *B,* basilar artery; *V,* vertebral artery; *VII–IX,* cranial nerves.

Figure 12. Artist's enhancement of an operative photograph showing the upper portion of the tumor dissected from the brain stem and cranial nerves V, VI, and VII. The pons and basilar artery are clearly seen. The lower part of the tumor is still present. *P,* pons; *B,* basilar artery; *T,* tumor; *S,* suction tip; *V–VII,* cranial nerves.

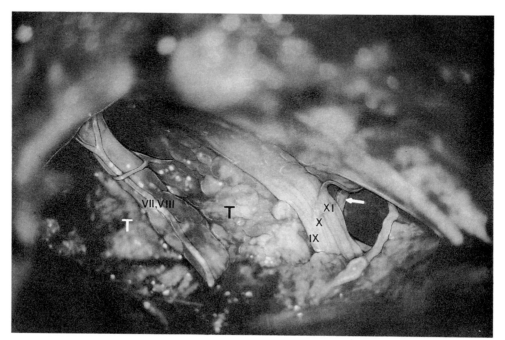

Figure 11. Artist's enhancement of an operative photograph showing cranial nerves (VII, VIII) which were encased by the tumor dissected free with their accompanying nutri- ent vessels. Cranial nerves IX, X, and XI have been dissected free from the lower portion of the tumor. *T,* tumor; *VII–XI,* cranial nerves. *Arrow* points to the PICA.

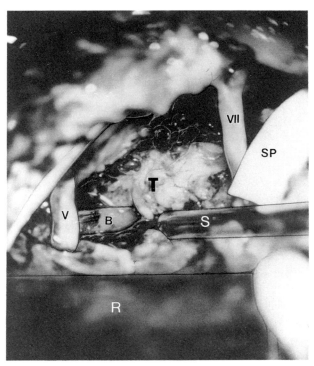

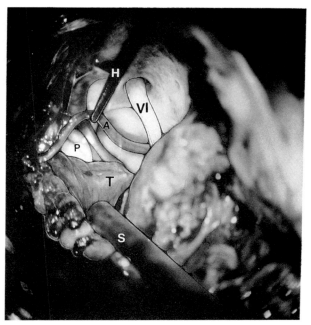

Figure 13. Artist's enhancement of an operative photograph showing the basilar artery displaced by the tumor to the opposite side. Cranial nerves V, VII, and VIII are displaced posteriorly and are easily visualized. Notice the tumor extension across the clivus. *B,* basilar artery; *T,* tumor; *S,* suction tip; *V, VII,* cranial nerves; *SP,* surgical patty.

Figure 14. Artist's enhancement of an operative photograph demonstrating dissection of AICA off the tumor capsule. The VIth nerve and pons are clearly seen. *T,* tumor; *A,* AICA; *P,* pons; *VI,* abducens nerve; *H,* surgical hook; *S,* suction tip.

Closure

The dura is closed in a watertight manner. The periosteum is turned over the petrous bone to avoid a CSF leak, the temporal muscle is rotated over the defect and sewed to the sternomastoid muscle, and the soft tissues are closed in multiple layers.

COMPLICATIONS

Surgery of petroclival meningiomas may entail all potential complications of intracranial surgery. Surgical mortality, usually resulting from manipulation of the brain stem or interference with its blood supply, is high. It was particularly so in the premicroscopic era. Infarction of the lateral tegmental region of the pons results from an occluded AICA. This complication is more likely to occur when the collateral circulation is poor, and the risk is compounded when the AICA loops deeply into the internal auditory canal. Occasionally the appearance of deficit may be delayed during the postoperative period.

Temporal lobe swelling or hemorrhage is a grave potential consequence of the subtemporal exposure, particularly on the dominant hemisphere. It is caused by coagulation or tearing of the vein of Labbé or the basilar occipital veins. Every effort should be made to preserve these veins and minimize temporal lobe retraction. Likewise, cerebellar swelling and an intracerebellar hematoma may follow excessive retraction of the cerebellum. The retrolabyrinthine presigmoid avenue alleviates cerebellar retraction and minimizes the risk of cerebellar swelling. Cerebellar resection is seldom needed nowadays. Posterior fossa hematomas remain a frightening complication because of the resulting rapid and direct brain stem compression. Venous hemostasis is deceptive when the head is elevated and the veins are collapsed. Thus, an induced Valsalva maneuver and jugular compression prior to closure are essential to assure meticulous hemostasis.

Any of the cranial nerves (III to XII) are at risk during surgery of petroclival meningiomas. Injury to the trochlear nerve is a frequent hazard during tentorial splitting, because of its fineness, fragility, and close relationship to the incisura. Morbidity resulting from its paralysis, however, is minimal compared to paralysis of other cranial nerves. Trigeminal nerve deficit is more morbid because of the resulting corneal anesthesia and subsequent keratitis, particularly if the facial nerve is also paralyzed. In these cases, immediate tarsorrhaphy should be performed followed by reconstructive surgery to restore facial nerve function. Trigeminal nerve trauma may result in facial pain, anesthesia dolorosa, and trigeminal neuralgia. Facial pain may develop months or years postoperatively.

Justifiable emphasis has been placed on facial nerve injury. Anatomical preservation, however, does not necessarily mean functional preservation. Tumor size is one of the most decisive factors in preserving facial nerve function. Removal of large tumors is more likely to cause paralysis. The facial nerve is usually displaced posteriorly by petroclival meningiomas, and may actually traverse the tumor. Intraoperative end-to-end direct anastomosis of the facial nerve is feasible, with recovery occurring in 40–80% of cases. Intraoperative nerve grafts may also be performed; however, delayed hypoglossal-to-facial anastomosis is a more common procedure.

Although hearing loss usually exists preoperatively, normal hearing is not infrequent. In the latter instances, loss of hearing becomes a potential complication of surgery. Thus, the VIIIth cranial nerve and the inner ear should be preserved, particularly since improvement in hypoacusis has been reported. Lateral-to-medial retraction of the cerebellum during posterior fossa surgery is more dangerous to hearing than retraction in a caudal-to-rostral direction. When preserving hearing, sparing the cochlear blood supply is as important as preserving the nerve itself.

While emphasis is given to facial nerve preservation, a greater emphasis should be given to preservation of lower cranial nerves. Their deficit is a significant cause of morbidity and mortality. Injury to the lower cranial nerves may be troublesome both intra- and postoperatively. Intraoperatively, dissection of these nerves may produce bradycardia and hypotension. Postoperatively, dysphagia, vocal cord paralysis, and depressed cough and gag reflexes may lead to grave pulmonary complications which could be fatal. Careful dissection of the inferior pole of the tumor and use of nonadherent patties help protect the nerves.

Complications related to disturbed CSF dynamics include CSF leakage, hydrocephalus, and pseudomeningocele formation. Although hydrocephalus may be present prior to surgery and persist despite total removal of the mass, it may also develop postoperatively. Acute postoperative hydrocephalus is usually obstructive and related to mass effect (tumor, edema, hemorrhage) whereas delayed hydrocephalus is usually communicating and related to poor absorption of CSF or scarring of the basal cisterns. A CT scan is diagnostic, and the treatment is shunting.

CSF leakage is a significant risk in the petrosal approach, occurring via the skin or through the middle ear. The leak is best avoided with the following maneuvers: watertight closure of the dura; applying bone wax to the drilled surface of the temporal bone; and placing the pericranial flap over the drilled temporal bone surface.

When a CSF leak occurs, the incidence of meningitis is one in five. Antibiotic coverage during CSF leakage is controversial. Initial management of a CSF leak includes head elevation, repeated spinal taps, or continuous spinal drainage. If the leak does not cease in a few days, or if the area has been previously heavily irradiated, cisternography with water-soluble contrast can determine the leakage site, and may be followed by watertight dural closure with a fascial graft. If hydrocephalus is an underlying factor, shunting is required.

Ligation of the sigmoid sinus is a step used by other surgeons. Although thought to be inconsequential, it has been associated with fatal complications. Assurance of the patency of the opposite sigmoid sinus and normal connection through the torcular herophili is a prerequisite to ligation of the sigmoid sinus. The above described approach preserves the sinus and eliminates the risk associated with its ligation.

FACIAL REANIMATION WITHOUT THE FACIAL NERVE

MARK MAY, M.D.
STEVEN M. SOBOL, M.D.

INTRODUCTION

Combining a clinical experience with over 1430 facial reanimation procedures with well-established neuroscientific principles, the authors have established guidelines for the rehabilitation of facial paralysis which stress restoration of facial symmetry and facial function. The choice of the most appropriate rehabilitation procedure is dependent on a number of factors, including: 1) cause of paralysis; 2) extent of paralysis and functional deficits; 3) duration of paralysis; 4) likelihood of recovery; 5) presence of concomitant cranial nerve deficits; 6) life expectancy; and 7) patient needs and expectations.

It is generally accepted that restoration of facial nerve continuity is the preferred approach whenever possible, provided it can be established ideally within 30 days and not greater than 1 year following injury. When the central stump of the facial nerve is not available, and the facial muscles can still be innervated, a hypoglossal-facial anastomosis is the favored approach, albeit not without drawbacks. This procedure is most effective when performed within two years of injury and not later than four years. However, when the facial nerve is unavailable, or when the facial muscles are deficient, other methods of facial reanimation must be selected. This might include situations in which an attempt to preserve the facial nerve or grafting has failed, and the critical time frame of two years has been exceeded. After this period, sufficient collagenization of the distal facial nerve may prevent any significant amount of useful axonal reentry regardless of the proximal nerve's ability to regenerate.

In the absence of the facial nerve, both dynamic and static procedures may prove useful. Dynamic procedures which we have found most valuable include regional muscle transposition using the temporalis muscle and occasionally the masseter, and certain eyelid reanimation procedures including gold weight lid loading and eyespring implantation. Static procedures serve predominantly an adjunctive role, and will thus not be discussed in any great detail in this chapter. Those which we have found most helpful include fascial and alloplastic slings, brow lift, rhytidoplasty, canthoplasty, and lid-tightening procedures. Our overall experience suggests that an approach which 1) divides the face into upper and lower segments (i.e., looks at the eye and mouth separately), 2) individualizes patient needs, and 3) combines both static and dynamic procedures provides the best results in terms of optimizing regional reanimation.

EYELID (UPPER FACIAL) REANIMATION

The goals of an ideal procedure aimed at reanimating the paralyzed facial muscles about the eye are to: 1) provide corneal protection; 2) avoid restriction of the visual field; 3) be cosmetically acceptable; 4) restore dynamic blink; 5) be reversible in the event of nerve recovery; and 6) be technically reproducible. Our preferred procedures are the gold weight lid implant and the open eyelid spring. Both techniques are thought to be superior to traditional tarsorrhaphy which is often cosmetically unappealing, restricts the visual field, and fails to reanimate dynamically. Our experience with over 280 gold weights and 250 eye springs has allowed us to formulate criteria for patient selection, and develop techniques which provide reproducible results.

Gold Weight Implantation

Gold weight implantation is best for patients with paralysis associated with minimal lid retraction, and those with reversible or partial paralysis. Eyelid closure is augmented by the force of gravity acting on the gold weight. Eyelid closure is therefore best when the head is in an upright or semiupright position. Implant extrusion and migration are rare if the weight is properly inserted and secured. The procedure is potentially reversible and may be performed under local anesthesia. Success in terms of satisfactory eyelid closure and patient satisfaction is better than 90%. Occasionally, mild ptosis or bulging of the implant will be problematic.

The operative field is prepared and draped in the usual manner, topical anesthetic is placed in the eye, and a scleral shield is placed over the cornea for protection. One percent Xylocaine with 1:100,000 of adrenalin is injected into the tarsal-supratarsal fold. An incision is made with a razor blade knife in the fold about 1 cm in length (Fig. 1A). The incision is extended through skin, subcutaneous tissue, and orbicularis oculi muscle and through the levator aponeurosis down to and on top of the tarsus. A pocket is created to accommodate the gold weight (Fig. 1, B and C). A 1-g weight is sufficient for the majority of patients. At times a lighter (0.75 g) or heavier (1.2 g) gold weight is used. The optimal weight is determined prior to surgery by pasting the gold weight on the eyelid and selecting the proper weight by trial and error. The gold weight is approximately 1 mm thick, 5 mm high, and 1 cm long; it has three holes in it. The gold is 24 carats and polished so that there are no rough edges. The gold weight is placed in the pocket and secured with an 8-0 permanent monofilament suture through each of the three holes in the gold weight (Fig. 1D). The two upper openings are sutured to the orbital septum and the lower one is sutured to the tissue just lateral to the tarsus. It should be noted that the suture is not passed through the tarsus. Figure 1E demonstrates the gold weight in its position about 3 mm from the lash line and camouflaged under the supratarsal fold when the eyelid is open (Fig. 1F).

Open Eyelid Spring Implantation

The open eyelid spring is most effective in patients with complete and/or permanent facial paralysis associated with significant lid retraction and/or a poor Bell's phenomenon. When properly designed and positioned, the spring affords the best degree of restoration of normalcy to rapid, spontaneous, and voluntary blink, compared to the gold weight. Potential problems with the spring include: 1) the technical mastery required; 2) ptosis if the spring is open too far; 3) the bulge created by the Dacron cuff over the distal wire in thin-skinned individuals; 4) the increased difficulty associated with spring removal compared with removal of the gold weight; and 5) the increased extrusion rate in inexperienced hands. Despite these potential drawbacks, success has been achieved in over 85% of carefully selected patients.

The operative field is prepared and draped in the usual manner and 1% Xylocaine with 1:100,000 of adrenalin is infiltrated along the supratarsal-tarsal upper lid fold. The injection is extended along the lateral orbital rim to the periosteum. A razor blade knife is used to make an incision through the skin, subcutaneous tissue, and orbicularis oculi muscle to the tarsus (Fig. 2A). Bleeding is controlled with a bipolar forceps and the tarsus is uncovered with scissors. Next, the periosteum over the lateral orbital rim is exposed through a separate incision (Fig. 2B). A spring is fabricated prior to surgery, when the patient is evaluated in the office setting. The spring is made of 0.01-inch round orthodontic wire; it is prepared as illustrated in Figure 2, C–F, using orthodontic instruments. The final configuration is determined by making the spring conform to the natural curvature of the patient's orbit (Fig. 2, G–H). The proper tension is adjusted in order to provide adequate opening and closing of the eyelid. A 19-gauge spinal needle is passed just lateral to the tarsus within a tunnel of soft tissue and brought out at the lateral orbital rim pocket just lateral to the periosteum (Fig. 2, I–J). The stylet from the spinal needle is removed (Fig. 2K). The wire is then placed into the spinal needle and the spinal needle is withdrawn (Fig. 2L). The lower limb of the spring that is now in place is secured with a 5-0 Supramid suture to the periosteum (Fig. 2, M and N). Two or three sutures are placed around the fulcrum to the periosteum in the area of the lateral canthus. This fixes the fulcrum to the periosteum just above and lateral to the lateral canthus. The upper limb of the wire is looped and sutured with two 5-0 Supramid sutures along its shaft (Fig. 2O), and then the lower limb is looped (Fig. 2P) and enveloped in Dacron as noted in Figure 2Q. The Dacron is closed over the loop with 8-0 monofilament sutures. The wound is closed in layers using 7-0 Vicryl for the deep layer and 6-0 chromic catgut for the skin (Fig. 2R).

Comments

Both the gold weight and eye spring implantation are preferred techniques because they allow for eyelid closure, independent of mouth movement. Since neither the gold nor the spring relieves the lack of lower lid tone, paralytic ectropion, and brow ptosis associated with the paralysis, each may be combined with static procedures aimed at correcting these defects. Our preferred method of lower lid tightening has been the Bick procedure or a modification known as a lateral tarsal strip. In either of these procedures a lateral wedge of the lower lid is removed and a tongue of tarsus is developed, resutured, and anchored to the lateral orbital rim, thus shortening and tightening the lower lid to correct the paralytic ectropion. Care must be exercised in either technique not to excise too much lower lid tissue since this can result in pulling the puncta away from the globe, resulting in increased epiphora. In cases in which the lower lid tends to pull away from the globe resulting in increased epiphora, we have found that implantation of autogenous auricular car-

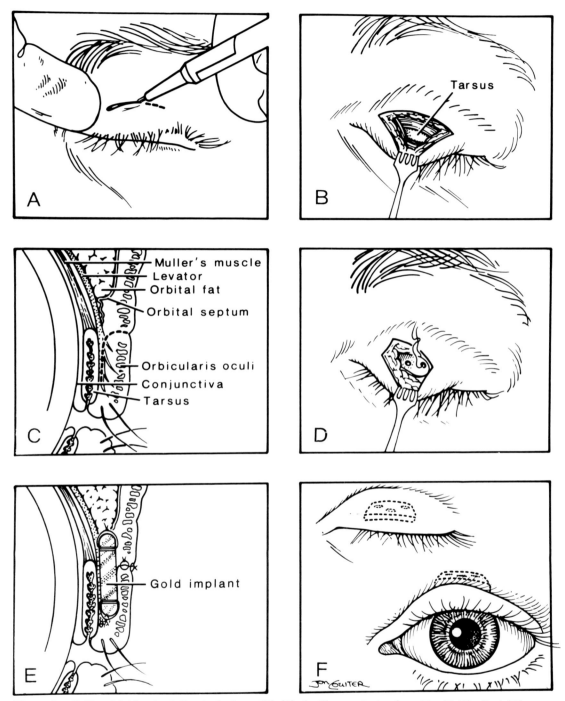

Figure 1. Gold weight implantation technique. (Modified with permission from May M. The Facial Nerve. New York: Thieme-Stratton, 1985).

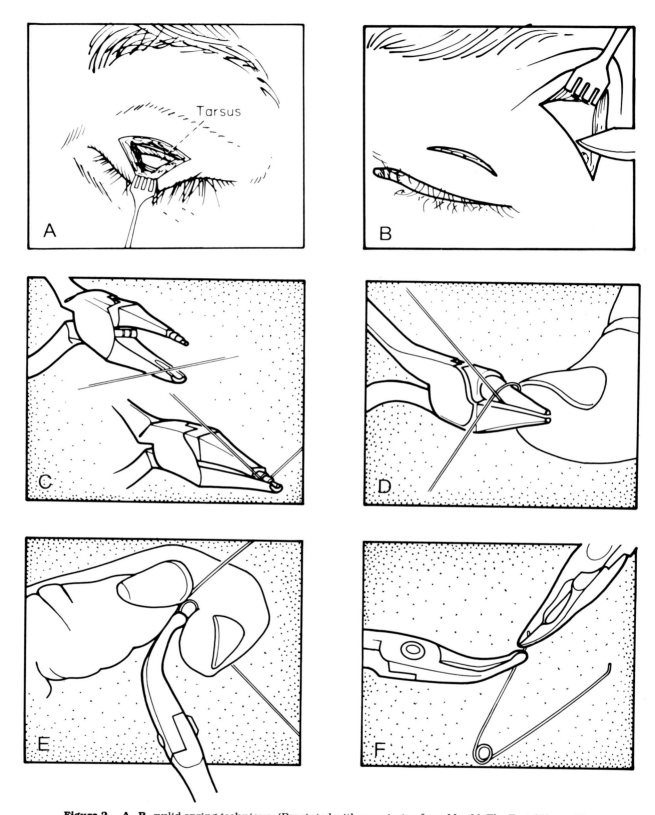

Figure 2. **A–R,** eyelid spring technique. (Reprinted with permission from May M. The Facial Nerve. New York: Thieme-Stratton, 1985).

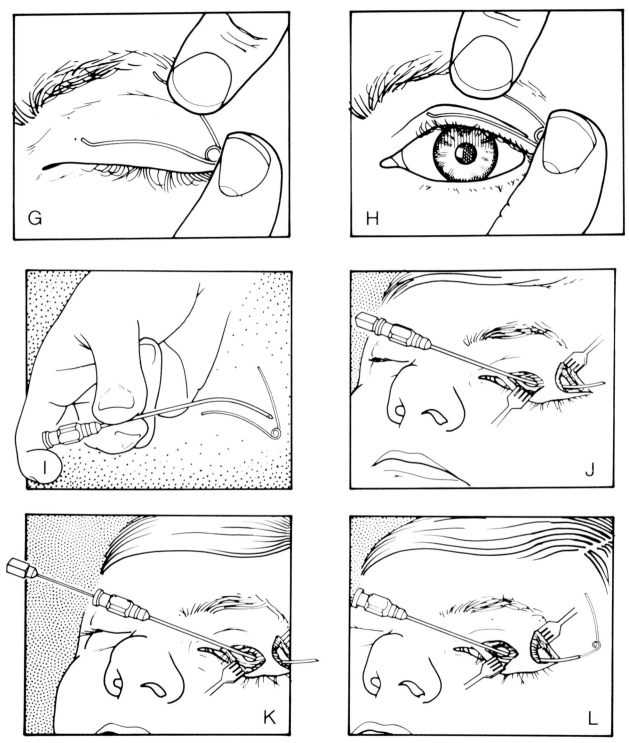

Figure 2. (*Continued*)

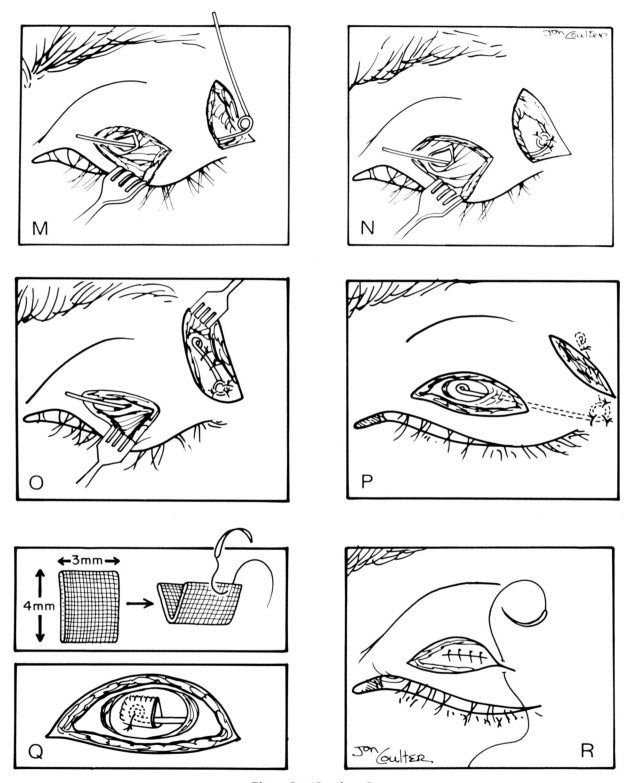

Figure 2. (*Continued*)

tilage to the midportion of the lower lid deep to the tarsus in a subconjuctival plane is a very useful procedure. Brow ptosis and supratarsal fold hooding may be corrected with a brow lift (with or without blepharoplasty) in an effort to further improve the quality of eyelid reanimation and cosmetic appearance. Caution must be exercised not to excise too much tissue in this area, however, for fear of compromising eyelid closure.

MOUTH (LOWER FACIAL) REANIMATION

In the absence of a usable facial nerve, reanimation of the mouth and lower face has been achieved using the temporalis muscle transposition. It is useful in patients with long-standing facial paralysis and has also been employed in selected cases to augment the results following a nerve graft or hypoglossal-facial nerve anastomosis. Our experience with over 200 temporalis muscle transpositions has yielded satisfactory results in approximately 90% of the cases. Early improvement in symmetry and a limited volitional smile may be achieved in three to six weeks with continued expected improvement with proper exercises over a period of one year. Motivated patients may further enhance their results through motor sensory reeducation. In approximately 10% of patients, facial movements in response to emotional stimuli have been observed.

Temporalis Muscle Transposition

The patient is prepared and draped in the usual fashion. The hair is parted and, using scissors, hair is removed through a narrow path over the region of the proposed incision in the scalp (Fig. 3A). The areas of the incisions in the vermillion and in the scalp are infiltrated with 1% Xylocaine and 1:100,000 of adrenalin for hemostasis. After waiting 5–10 minutes, the incision in the scalp is made with a cutting cautery down to the superficial musculoaponeurotic system (SMAS). SMAS is divided with scissors, exposing the fascia over the temporalis muscle. The temporalis muscle is elevated in its midportion in a strip approximately 4 cm wide extending from above the fascia-periosteal attachment superiorly to the level of the zygomatic arch inferiorly (Fig. 3B). The cutting cautery is used to outline the flap and an elevator to lift the muscle-periosteum from the skull (Fig. 3, C and D). The layer between the subcutaneous tissue and SMAS is identified and a pocket is made between the two with scissors (Fig. 3E). This ensures that any residual function that might be present via the facial nerve will be preserved since the facial nerve fibers lie in or deep to SMAS. Then an incision is made in the vermillion exposing the orbicularis oris muscle (Fig. 3F). The layer just deep to the subcutaneous tissue and lateral

to SMAS is established using scissors (Fig. 3G). The pocket started in the scalp lateral to SMAS and that in the vermillion region are connected with scissors and then enlarged to accommodate two fingers (Fig. 3H). The temporalis muscle that was elevated is bisected and 3-0 Prolene sutures are passed through each of the pedicles in a figure eight fashion (Fig. 3I). The sutures are then brought through the tunnel using a Kelly clamp (Fig. 3J). With the muscle pulled through the pocket (Fig. 3K), it is sutured to the submucosa (Fig. 3L) and subcutaneous layer (Fig. 3M). This double closure sandwiches the muscle between the submucosa and the subcutaneous layers. The corner of the mouth is overcorrected in order to ensure a pleasing result (Fig. 3N). The overcorrected smile will begin to normalize over a period of three to six weeks. The defect created by transposing the temporalis may be refilled by implanting a soft Silastic implant. A drain is placed through the scalp into the cheek and hooked to wall suction for two days.

Comments

Although the temporalis muscle has been used by others to reanimate the entire face including the eye region, we have found that using it exclusively for the mouth offers better regional reanimation by separating eye and mouth function. A variety of modifications have been introduced to eliminate many of the problems encountered by others using this technique, which may have contributed to the lack of uniformly high-quality results. The prominent bulge in the cheek often noted by many performing this procedure has been reduced by creating an adequate tunnel which allows the transposed muscle to lie flat. Moreover, since only the middle one-third of the temporalis muscle is used, there is less bulk in the cheek and less tendency toward temporal depression. The depression which is created is remedied using a soft Silastic implant placed at the time of transposition. Facial symmetry is further enhanced by close attention to proper positioning of the muscle slips to the mouth in an effort to achieve a mirror image of the muscle pull seen on the normal contralateral side. Using Conley's modification of raising periosteum attached to the superior aspect of the temporalis muscle, rather than repositioning and suturing the temporalis fascia to the muscle as proposed by Rubin, has given more consistent results. The method of attachment to the oral region has also been modified. Access is gained through a vermillion-cutaneous incision rather than a nasolabial incision which further reduces the visible scar. Multiple sutures placed in the muscle-submucosal layer at the level of the superior and inferior-lateral aspect of the orbicularis oris, creating a substantially overcorrected smile have afforded the most

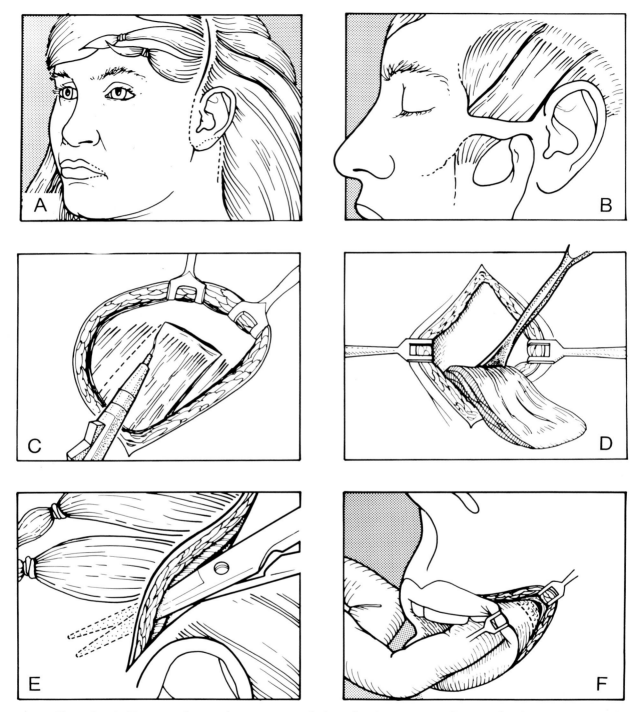

Figure 3.   A–N, temporalis muscle transposition for lower facial reanimation. (Reprinted with permission from May M. The Facial Nerve. New York: Thieme-Stratton, 1985).

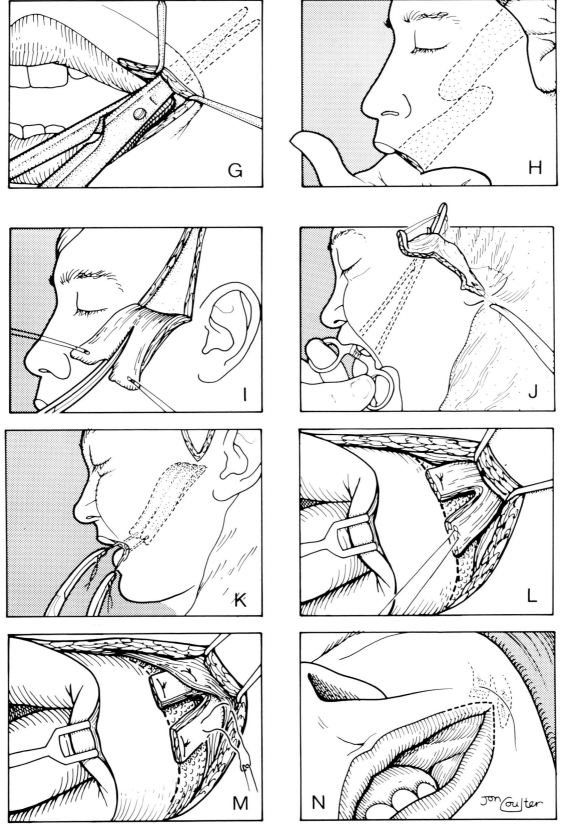

Figure 3. *(Continued)*

consistent results. The importance of overcorrection cannot be overemphasized.

Although the masseter muscle has been used alone or in combination with the temporalis muscle by some surgeons, our experience has been less satisfactory. We have found it less optimal in terms of vector forces, and, moreover, it adds little to the effect of the temporalis muscle.

Complications of the temporalis muscle transposition have included hematomas, seromas, infection, and suture granulomas. Using both a temporal-facial suction drain as well as a small suction lip-cheek drain reduces the incidence of these complications. By avoiding penetration of the oral mucosa with the suspension sutures, the incidence of the suture granulomas is reduced. Prophylactic antibiotics are given routinely. Using the soft Mentor prefabricated temporal implant has reduced our early experience with implant extrusion noted with the hard carved Silastic implants.

The temporalis muscle itself creates a moderate degree of static suspension in addition to providing dynamic reanimation to the mouth area. However, if sufficient overcorrection is not achieved at the primary procedure, or if the anchoring sutures pull out, the overall static suspension effect may diminish with time. The temporalis muscle may be tightened by plication utilizing the same vermillion incision or augmented with the use of fascia or alloplastic material (i.e., Gortex). When prestretched Gortex is utilized, the suspensory effect should be permanent if the Gortex is securely anchored to a fixed bony structure cephalad. We prefer a mini lag screw technique. A rhytidoplasty (face lift) may be combined with a temporalis muscle transposition in patients with long-standing facial paralysis accompanied by loss of skin tone and sagging.

CONCLUSIONS

Without a useful facial nerve, facial reanimation can only be achieved using methods other than nerve grafting and nerve substitution procedures. Separate eyelid reanimation using the gold weight implant or eyelid spring, combined with regional temporalis muscle transposition to the mouth, provides the best opportunity for independent eye and mouth movement. By combining appropriate static procedures aimed at correcting brow ptosis, lower lid ectropion, epiphora, and facial sagging, facial symmetry and function are improved dramatically in the majority of patients. As innovative surgeons strive for perfection, improvement in overall results can be expected.

OMENTAL AND MUSCULOCUTANEOUS FREE FLAPS FOR COVERAGE OF COMPLICATED NEUROSURGICAL WOUNDS

DANIEL L. BARROW, M.D.
FOAD NAHAI, M.D.

INTRODUCTION

Extensive areas of traumatic or neoplastic tissue loss involving the face, scalp, skull, and dura present formidable problems in reconstruction. Successful reconstructive surgery should protect vital structures and restore form and function. In planning any reconstructive effort, the surgeon should utilize the simplest method to provide adequate coverage and aesthetic results. The least complex means of repair on the "reconstructive ladder" is direct closure. When direct closure is not feasible, one must consider more complex methods of wound closure. Split-thickness skin grafts are usually not sufficient to cover exposed cranium. When the wound includes loss of cranium, the problem is compounded by the risk of cerebrospinal fluid leakage and subsequent infection. Local rotation of scalp flaps is often sufficient if the extent of the wound permits use of this method. With more extensive loss of scalp, local rotation flaps cannot provide adequate coverage. Staged distant flaps have been used in this situation but require multiple operations carried out over long intervals.

Following the loss of a large area of full-thickness scalp, including periosteum, the bare bone of the cranium requires coverage as soon as possible. Often the outer table of the skull will have to be removed or perforated and time allowed for granulation before applying a flap.

The development and refinement of microvascular surgical techniques has led to the use of heterotopic transfer of free vascularized grafts to cover distant areas of the body that are devoid of skin and subcutaneous tissue. Early use of musculoskeletal flaps involved transposition of muscle locally on its vascular pedicle. A prerequisite for the use of a transposed flap is the presence of a dominant vascular pedicle on which the flap can be rotated through an arc. This arc of rotation is based on the length of the dominant pedicle.

With the advent of microvascular techniques, the area to be reconstructed is no longer limited by the arc of rotation of the vascular pedicle. Instead, the muscle and overlying skin that is best suited for adequate coverage may be dissected out as a free flap, with microvascular anastomosis of an arterial supply and venous drainage to locally existing vessels. In certain clinical situations involving primarily soft tissue loss, replacement by a free omental graft is, in our opinion, the procedure of choice. Distant flaps, examples of which are musculocutaneous and omental free flaps, represent the highest rung on the reconstructive ladder. Wounds of the face and head, especially those involving the cranium or dura, frequently require these more complex methods of reconstruction.

Optimal results are achieved in these complex reconstructive procedures through the cooperative efforts of the neurosurgeon and the plastic and reconstructive surgeon.

INDICATIONS

Latissimus Dorsi Musculocutaneous Free Flap

In the majority of situations, when a distant composite flap is required for reconstruction, the musculocutaneous free flap is ideal. The latissimus dorsi muscle provides the most versatile musculocutaneous flap for reconstructive microsurgery. The muscle and the cutaneous territory overlying it represent the largest single flap available. Furthermore, its sacrifice presents minimal functional deficits. The latissimus dorsi is supplied by a consistent proximal vascular pedicle of generous length and caliber. The vascular supply allows the muscle to be split to individualize each reconstruction or to preserve some function at the donor site, where a viable, innervated segment of the muscle may be retained.

This flap is excellent for providing coverage under circumstances when the wound requires a flat, broad, malleable flap. As such, it is ideal for the coverage of scalp, cranial, and dural defects as well as those that result from orbital exenteration with maxillectomy.

Omental Free Flap

In certain clinical situations involving primarily soft tissue loss, replacement by a free omental graft is, in our opinion, the most appropriate procedure. When the defect involves primarily subcutaneous tissue loss resulting in an abnormal contour, an omental free flap provides effective coverage and restoration of contour. In addition, the inherent capability of this tissue to combat infection and furnish an ideal bed for establishment of skin or bone grafts provides further indications for its use. Therefore, there are three basic uses for omentum in reconstruction at a distant site: 1) to provide contour when there is soft tissue loss (in this circumstance, especially if the face is involved in the wound, a musculocutaneous flap is too bulky and muscle atrophy unpredictable); 2) to fill a cavitary wound and establish an appropriate defense against infection; and 3) to provide a vascular bed for grafts of bone and skin.

The greater omentum has a characteristic ability to repair defects through cellular proliferation, fibrous tissue formation, and adhesion production. It has a rich vascular and lymphatic supply, which probably accounts for its ability to rapidly absorb exudate or edema fluid and combat infection. Another major reason for the ability of omentum to cope with infection is related to the large number of macrophages within its areolar tissue. The inherent ability of omentum to control infection and provide a vascular bed for skin or bone grafts is retained when omentum is used as a transplant.

SURGICAL PROCEDURE

Latissimus Dorsi Musculocutaneous Flap

Surgical Anatomy

The latissimus dorsi muscle takes its origin from the lower six thoracic, the lumbar, and the sacral vertebrae and from the posterior crest of the ilium (Fig. 1). There is also a muscular origin along the anterior lateral border of the lower four ribs. The insertion of the muscle is into the intertubercular groove of the humerus. The latissimus dorsi extends, adducts, and

rotates the arm medially. It also draws the shoulder downward and backward. Mathes and Nahai have classified the vascular anatomy of muscles based on variables in the anatomical configuration of their vascular pedicles. Muscles of Type I, II, III, and V are usually suitable for free-flap transplantation because of their dominant vascular pedicle. The latissimus dorsi is a Type V muscle, the major vascular pedicle of which is the thoracodorsal artery, a terminal branch of the subscapular artery. The thoracodorsal artery and nerve, along with one or two venae comitantes, enter the muscle at the neurovascular hilum on the deep surface, approximately 10 cm from the insertion of the muscle.

The thoracodorsal motor nerve to the latissimus dorsi muscle is derived from the posterior cord of the brachial plexus. The nerve is intimately associated with the thoracodorsal vascular pedicle and branches into the muscle in conjunction with the blood vessels. The muscle also receives the segmental innervation of intercostal nerves T2 to T6. The thoracodorsal nerve is traditionally sacrificed during free tissue transfer to the head and neck to prevent inappropriate motor function postoperatively. The denervation of the muscle also results in a variable reduction in muscle bulk up to 50% over the ensuing 12 months, which yields an ever-improving wound contour.

Preoperative Preparation

Preoperatively, the surgeon must ascertain the presence of a functional latissimus dorsi muscle on the side from which transfer is anticipated. This is most easily accomplished by having the patient place his or her hands on both iliac crests and apply pressure. The muscle should become visible and palpable in the posterior axillary fold. The night before surgery, the back, shoulder, face, neck, and head are washed with Betadine solution; also at that time, a broad spectrum antibiotic or antibiotic appropriate to the flora of the wound is given parenterally.

Surgical Procedure

The patient is securely positioned on the operating table in a lateral decubitus position. The ipsilateral arm should be included in the sterile field to facilitate dissection of the pedicle (Fig. 2). The exact position of the head may vary according to the local pathology. Occasionally, the patient may have to be repositioned after the latissimus dorsi is harvested.

After local excision of the scalp and cranial or intracranial pathology, the recipient vessels are exposed. Branches of the external carotid system such as the superior thyroid, facial, and occipital arteries are suitable recipients for the thoracodorsal artery. The superficial temporal artery may be used but is often much

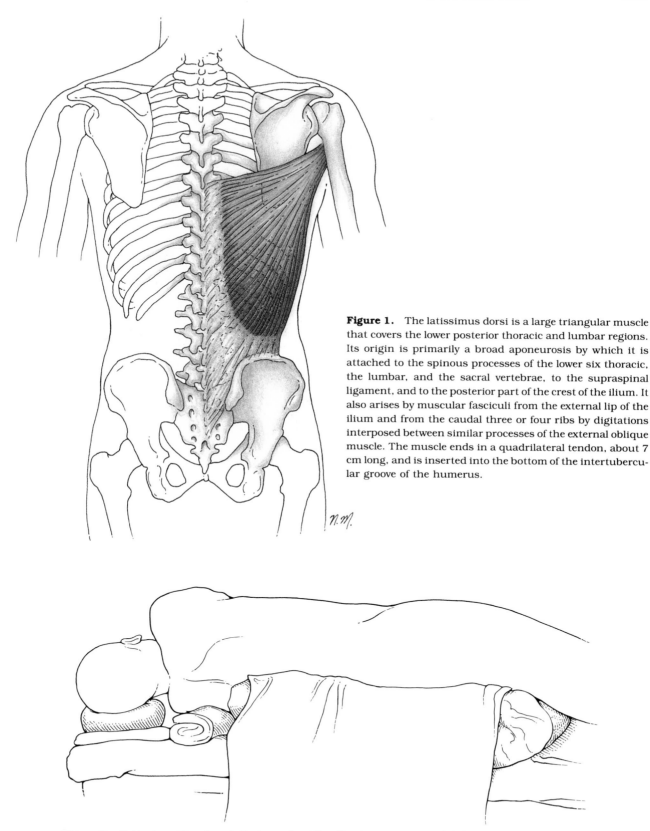

Figure 1. The latissimus dorsi is a large triangular muscle that covers the lower posterior thoracic and lumbar regions. Its origin is primarily a broad aponeurosis by which it is attached to the spinous processes of the lower six thoracic, the lumbar, and the sacral vertebrae, to the supraspinal ligament, and to the posterior part of the crest of the ilium. It also arises by muscular fasciculi from the external lip of the ilium and from the caudal three or four ribs by digitations interposed between similar processes of the external oblique muscle. The muscle ends in a quadrilateral tendon, about 7 cm long, and is inserted into the bottom of the intertubercular groove of the humerus.

Figure 2. Patient position for a latissimus dorsi free flap to cover a cranial defect. The ipsilateral arm is included in this sterile field to facilitate dissection of the vascular pedicle.

smaller than the thoracodorsal artery and is frequently damaged by the local pathology or previous cranial surgery. Venous drainage may be accomplished by preserving the external jugular vein during neck dissection or by anastomosis to the posterior facial vein or the internal jugular vein.

A limited incision is performed transversely across the lower axilla and carried down along the posterior axillary fold. The subcutaneous tissue over the entire portion of the muscle to be transferred is elevated. For musculocutaneous flaps, the skin island is designed and then incised down to the fascia of the latissimus dorsi muscle.

The thoracodorsal artery can be easily visualized on the deep surface as the vascular pedicle enters the ventral aspect of the muscle approximately 10 cm below its humeral insertion. Here the thoracodorsal vessel divides into a lateral branch to the anterior portion of the muscle and a medial branch to the posterior portion.

The anterior border of the latissimus dorsi muscle is identified and the plane between it and the underlying serratus anterior muscle is bluntly dissected toward the posterior midline. The muscle is then transected distally and elevated to visualize the vascular pedicle on the deep surface (Fig. 3). Crossing branches of the thoracodorsal artery to the serratus anterior muscle are divided as are the muscular branches to the teres major. The vascular pedicle is dissected circumferentially and then protected during the transection of the tendinous humeral insertion of the muscle as well as when transecting the thoracodorsal nerve. Thus, the muscle remains attached only by the vascular pedicle and dissection proceeds toward the axilla to obtain the desired pedicle length. The vascular pedicle may be dissected all the way to the axillary artery and vein, if necessary (Fig. 3).

As dissection proceeds upward, care must be taken not to injure the intercostobrachial sensory nerve to the inner aspect of the upper extremity. This nerve courses across the axilla inferior to the axillary artery. Likewise, the long thoracic nerve which courses the length of the chest wall superficial to the serratus anterior muscle must be preserved; otherwise a winged scapula will result.

After preparation of the recipient vessels, the thoracodorsal artery and vein are transected and irrigated with heparinized saline. The flap is then transferred to the area to be reconstructed and temporarily sutured in place. Under the operating microscope, the open proximal ends of the recipient vessels are held secure by microvascular clamps and the adventitia is excised. The thoracodorsal artery and vein are placed in microvascular approximating clamps after the ad-

ventitia is removed. Under magnification of an operating microscope, end-to-end anastomoses are made using interrupted sutures of 9-0 or 10-0 Prolene. Once the vascular anastomoses are completed, the clamps are removed. The flap is sutured or stapled to the local tissue and, if necessary, the muscle may be grafted with a split-thickness skin graft from the thigh.

A suction drain is placed in the back and the donor wound is closed primarily (Fig. 4). Any musculocutaneous flap wider than 10–12 cm will not allow a primary closure of the donor site, and a skin graft will be required. To improve the aesthetic appearance of bulky flaps, the muscle is transferred without overlying skin and fat and is skin grafted. This is our preferred method as it leaves a more acceptable donor defect.

Postoperative Care
The suction drain is removed three to four days postoperatively when drainage has decreased to less than 50 ml in 24 hours. The axilla should be checked daily for the development of a hematoma or seroma. Physical therapy consisting of passive range of motion of the shoulder and upper arm is initiated on the third or fourth postoperative day. Active exercises are initiated one week after surgery.

In the immediate postoperative period, the free flap should be closely observed for evidence of vascular compromise. Early signs of vascular impairment include flap cyanosis or the development of vascular petechiae associated with sudden swelling of the flap. When the muscle is covered by a skin graft, the most reliable check of vascular patency is obtained by piercing the flap with a 21-gauge needle. Arterial blood should be seen. Rapid flow of venous blood may indicate venous obstruction. Early detection of thrombosis of the vascular pedicle may enable successful revision of the vascular anastomoses, especially if implemented within the first 12 hours of the time of vessel thrombosis. Success is less likely if thrombosis occurs more than 48 hours after initial transfer of the free flap.

Illustrative Case
A 22-year-old man suffered a full-thickness electrical burn of the scalp and skull. After failure of a free flap performed at another institution, the exposed skull was covered by expanding the existing hair-bearing scalp with rotational flaps. This coverage also broke down, leaving exposed cranium and dura (Fig. 5). The wound was covered with a latissimus dorsi muscle free flap covered by a split thickness skin graft, and the patient experienced good functional and aesthetic results (Fig. 6).

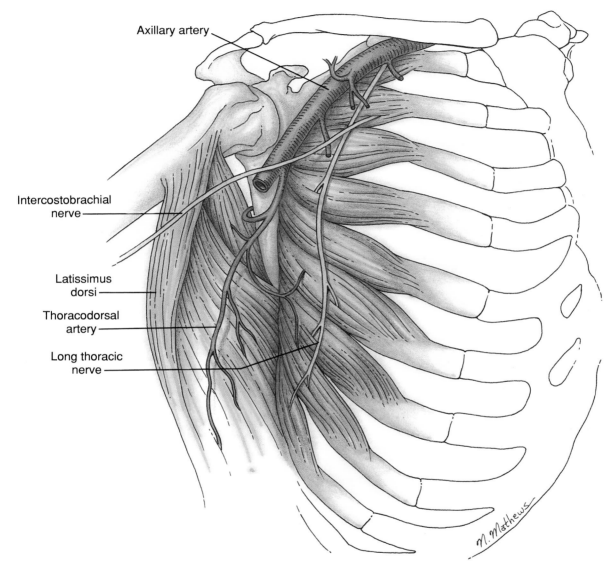

Axillary artery

Intercostobrachial
nerve

Latissimus
dorsi

Thoracodorsal
artery

Long thoracic
nerve

Figure 3. The latissimus dorsi has been separated from the underlying serratus anterior muscle. The vascular pedicle is identified on the inferior surface of the muscle. Vascular pedicles crossing to the serratus anterior and teres major are divided. Dissection of the latissimus dorsi and the thoracodorsal artery is extended toward the axilla as far as necessary to obtain an adequate pedicle length.

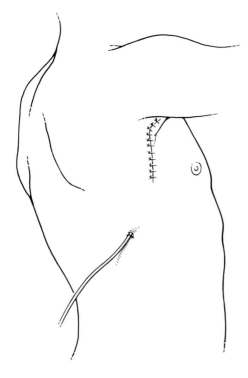

Figure 4. Illustration of wound closure with a drain in place.

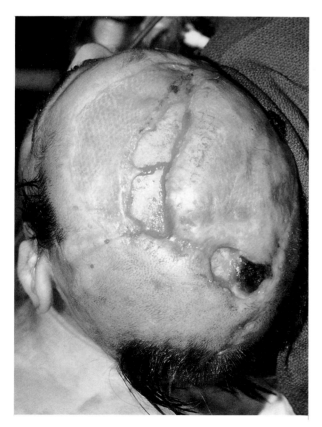

Figure 5. Preoperative photograph of full thickness loss of scalp and skull following an electrical burn. Note the breakdown of previous rotation flaps used to provide coverage.

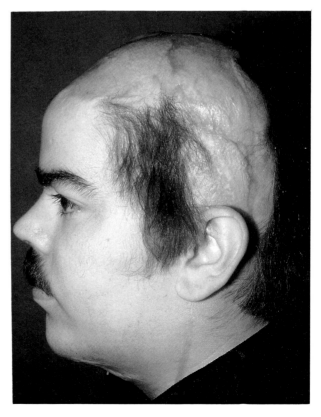

Figure 6. Postoperative appearance following latissimus dorsi musculocutaneous free flap coverage.

Omental Free Flap

Surgical Anatomy

The greater omentum is a double layer of peritoneum that arises from the greater curvature of the stomach. It lies over the abdominal viscera and folds posteriorly over the transverse colon. It is based on the right and left gastroepiploic arteries, which join to form the gastroepiploic arch (Fig. 7). From the main arch a variety of vascular arcades then distribute the blood throughout the omentum. There are usually three main omental vessels that arise from the gastroepiploic arcade. These vessels are 1.5–3.0 mm in diameter, providing adequate size for microvascular anastomoses. Although the omental flap can be based on either pedicle, we generally prefer the right gastroepiploic pedicle because it is larger than the left and dissection in the region of the spleen is avoided.

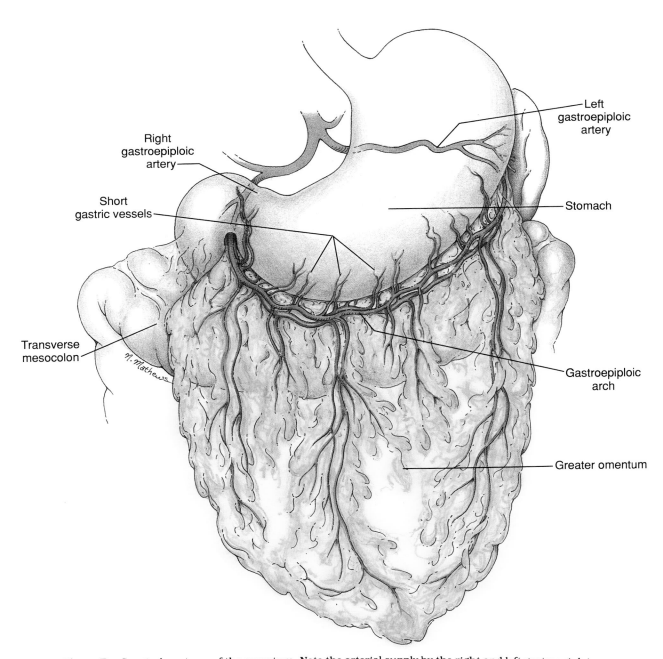

Figure 7. Surgical anatomy of the omentum. Note the arterial supply by the right and left gastroepiploic arteries, which join to form the gastroepiploic arch.

Preoperative Preparation

One day before surgery the patient is placed on a clear liquid diet and the bowel is mechanically prepared. The abdomen, face, neck, and head are washed with Betadine solution the night before operation. Either a broad spectrum antibiotic or an antibiotic appropriate to the flora of the wound is started by parenteral administration on the night before surgery.

Surgical Procedure

The patient is placed in the supine position. An incision is made in the head or neck to isolate the vessels to be used for microvascular anastomosis. The incision will vary with the particular local wound or pathology. Branches of the external carotid artery and internal or external jugular vein are preferred as recipient vessels. Normal vessels outside the field of previous resection, trauma, or radiation therapy are selected.

A second team of surgeons with separate instruments and scrub team simultaneously performs an abdominal exploration through a midline celiotomy (Fig. 8). The omentum is separated from the transverse mesocolon, proceeding from left to right, by dividing the translucent nonvascular attachments (Fig. 9). The omental flap is usually based on the right

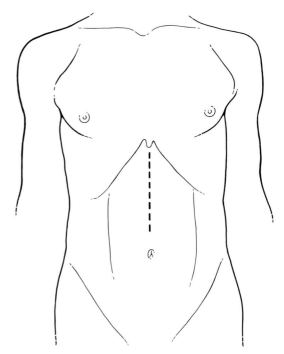

Figure 8.   Incision used for harvesting an omental free flap.

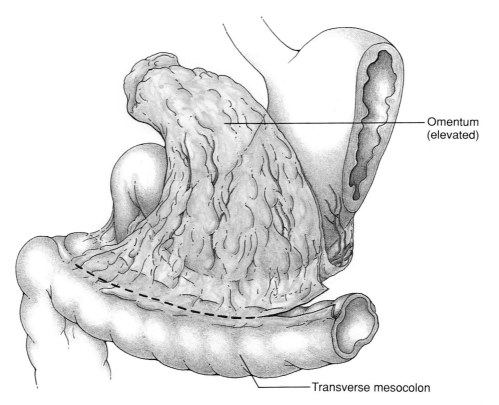

Omentum (elevated)

Transverse mesocolon

Figure 9.   Separation of the omentum from the transverse mesocolon by division of the translucent nonvascular attachments.

gastroepiploic vessels. The omentum is then divided from the peripheral margin toward the gastroepiploic arcade at a point that would leave a suitable volume of tissue based on the right gastroepiploic vessels. The short gastric vessels are isolated, clamped, cut, and ligated, proceeding along the greater curvature of the stomach to the pylorus (Fig. 10). The right gastro-

epiploic vessels are isolated, freed of surrounding fat, and dissected separately as artery and vein toward the gastroepiploic artery, thereby developing a vascular pedicle 6–10 cm long with a diameter of 1.5–2 mm.

When the recipient vessels in the neck have been prepared, the right gastroepiploic artery and vein are clamped and divided and the omentum is removed

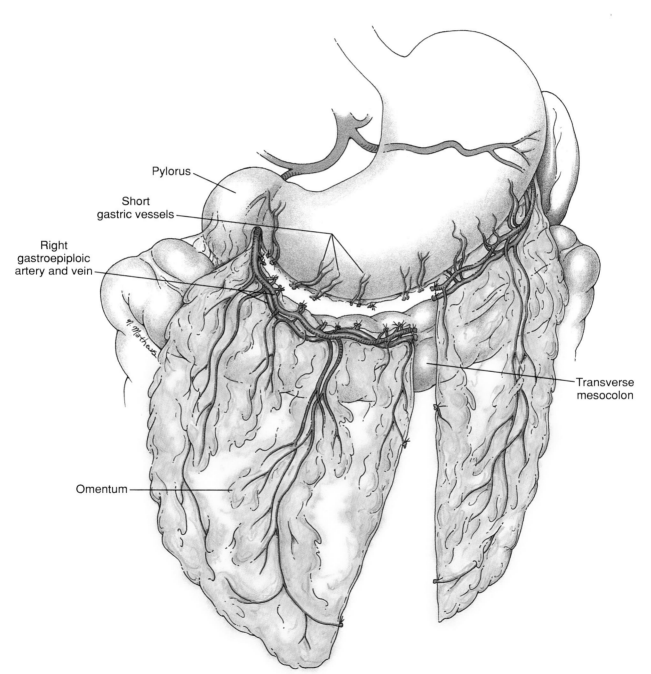

Figure 10. The short gastric vessels are isolated, clamped, cut, and ligated along the greater curvature of the stomach to the pylorus. The omental flap is based on the right gastro-epiploic artery and vein.

from the peritoneal cavity. The vessels are tied and the abdominal wall, subcutaneous tissue, and skin closed. No drains are used. Once the omental tissue is harvested and the closure is completed, that surgical team is excused.

Because no resorption of omentum occurs, it is necessary to trim all tissue and use only that amount necessary to reconstruct the wound. The vascular anatomy of the omentum permits the isolation of multiple small flaps or fingers within the major omental graft to restore contour to the forehead, eyelids, cheek, lips, or scalp. Any portion of the exposed omentum that cannot be covered with adjacent skin undergoes immediate grafting with a split-thickness skin graft.

The omentum is transferred to the area of reconstruction, temporarily sutured or stapled in place, and covered with a moist sponge. Under the operating microscope, the open proximal ends of the recipient vessels are held by microvascular clamps, and the adventitia is excised. A standard microsurgical anastomosis of the vessels is performed. Once the vascular anastomoses are completed, the clamps are removed. There should be immediate flow into the omentum with a visible pulse in the gastroepiploic arcade.

Postoperative Care

As with the muscle flap, the omental flap should be closely observed for evidence of vascular compromise. The patient is given clear liquids and the diet is advanced once bowel sounds are present.

Illustrative Cases

Figure 11: A 52-year-old man presented with a chronic open frontal sinus infection following trauma. Multiple surgical attempts to heal the wound had failed. The wound was debrided and reconstructed with free vascularized omentum. The sinus was filled with omentum and the wound closed, producing a good aesthetic result and a healed wound.

Figure 12: A 34-year-old man developed an infiltrating squamous cell carcinoma at the site of a 20-year-old injury to his scalp. At his initial operation, the tumor extended through the cranium and involved the outer layer of the dura and sagittal sinus. A wide resection of the scalp and cranium was performed and free margins obtained. The surgical defect was filled with a latissimus dorsi free flap and skin graft. The patient did well for one year following this procedure but developed a recurrence of his tumor that extended through the muscle flap. At reoperation, the tumor was found to invade the dura, falx, sagittal sinus, and brain. The entire muscle flap was removed and the dura excised along with the occluded sagittal sinus. The tumor invading the brain was removed as totally as could be determined grossly. The defect was then covered with an omental free flap and skin graft.

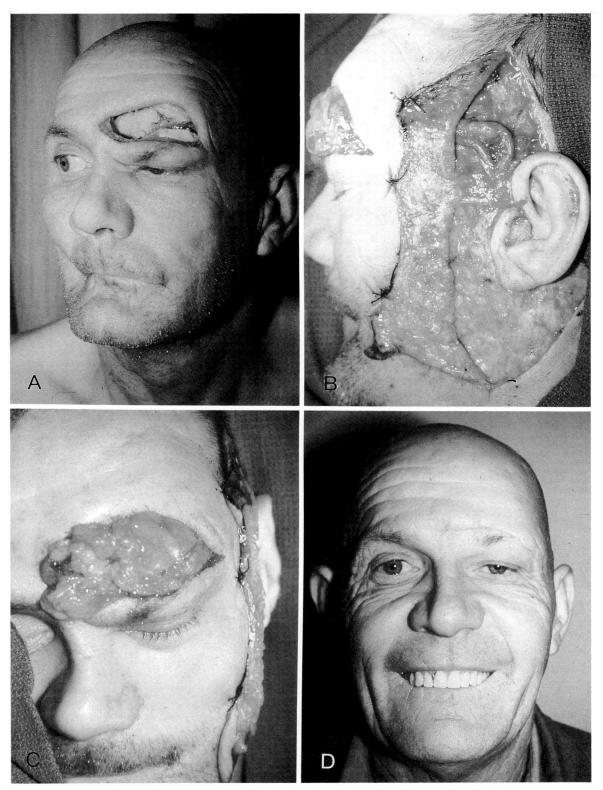

Figure 11. **A,** the appearance of an open left frontal sinus infection following multiple attempts to close the wound. **B,** an intraoperative photograph demonstrates the anastomosis of the gastroepiploic artery and vein to the superficial temporal artery and vein with the omental flap tunneled under the scalp to the area of the wound. **C,** front view of the omental flap before wound closure. **D,** final result.

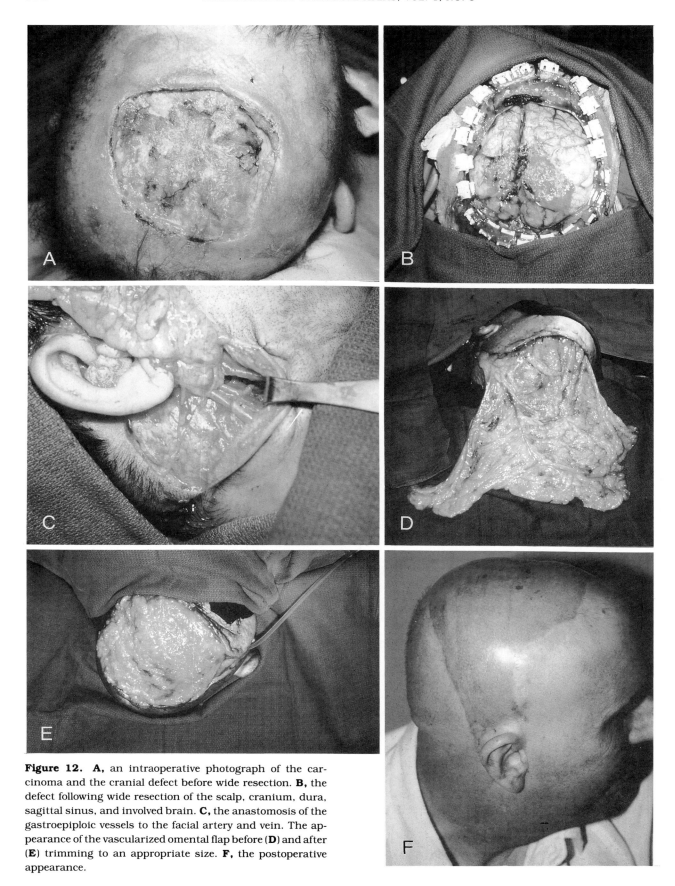

Figure 12. A, an intraoperative photograph of the carcinoma and the cranial defect before wide resection. **B,** the defect following wide resection of the scalp, cranium, dura, sagittal sinus, and involved brain. **C,** the anastomosis of the gastroepiploic vessels to the facial artery and vein. The appearance of the vascularized omental flap before (**D**) and after (**E**) trimming to an appropriate size. **F,** the postoperative appearance.

REPAIR OF "GROWING" SKULL FRACTURE

TADANORI TOMITA, M.D.

INTRODUCTION

Growing fracture is a rare complication of skull fracture occurring in infancy and early childhood. This late complication of skull fracture is also known as a leptomeningeal cyst. "Growing" fracture is somewhat of a misnomer, but it is characterized by progressive diastatic enlargement of the fracture line. Although skull fracture is a common occurrence in the pediatric age groups, the incidence of growing fracture is only 0.05–1% among skull fractures in childhood.

The usual presentation of the growing fracture is a progressive, often pulsatile, lump on the head. Neurologic symptoms such as seizure, hemiparesis, and mental retardation are less frequent. However, not infrequently, these patients may be perfectly asymptomatic, and a palpable mass or widening of the fracture line is the sole sign noted incidentally by the parents. Usually a growing fracture develops within several months following the initial skull fracture, but it may not be recognized for many years.

Growing skull fractures usually occur during the first three years of life (most often during infancy), and almost never occur after eight years of age. Although fractures occur in any part of the skull, the most common site for growing fracture is over the skull vault in the parietal region. Dural laceration is always present along the fracture line, and it is an essential factor for the development of a growing fracture. The dural laceration enlarges and grows larger with the growing fracture. Computed tomography (CT) or magnetic resonance imaging (MRI) often demonstrates a focal dilatation of the lateral ventricle near the growing fracture. Lack of resistance of both dura and skull leads to focal amplification of the pulse wave of the intracranial pressure, causing herniation of the brain or subarachnoid space through the fracture line and the dural defect. The "growth" of the fracture line is owing to bone resorption due to continuous pulsatile pressure at the edge of the fracture line. A rapidly developing infantile brain and associated pathologic conditions such as brain edema or hydrocephalus also contribute an outward driving force to cause brain herniation through the dural and skull defect. This pulsatile force of the brain during the period of its maximum growth produces the brain herniation through the dural laceration and fracture line, causing the enlargement of the fracture line of the thin skull.

One of the risk factors for the development of a growing fracture is the severity of head trauma. A linear skull fracture with underlying hemorrhagic contusion of the brain suggests a severe injury, significant enough to cause a dural laceration. Initial CT scans for the evaluation of head trauma in patients who ultimately develop a growing fracture usually reveal significant hemorrhage or contusion subjacent to the skull fracture. When a growing fracture is inspected at the time of surgical repair, the herniated brain is seen to be developing a cerebromeningeal cicatrix. In some cases, loculated subarachnoid cerebrospinal fluid (CSF) cyst(s) may be noted with underlying gliotic, atrophic brain. Although the loculated subarachnoid space may become cystic (leptomeningeal cyst), true leptomeningeal cysts are rare. The cystic changes in the growing fracture usually represent cystic encephalomalacia.

Depressed fractures usually do not cause growing fractures, but a linear fracture extending from the depressed fracture can lead to a growing fracture. The child who on initial x-ray films of the skull has diastasis of the fracture more than 4 mm is considered to be at risk for future development of a growing fracture. Diastasis of a cranial suture, however, is an unusual site for a growing fracture.

A growing fracture at the skull base can occur in an older age group, especially where the bone is thin such as the orbital roof, if a linear fracture is accompanied by a dural laceration. Growing fracture and a meningoencephalocele can develop with a similar mechanism as those occurring in the skull vault of the young patient.

RADIOLOGIC STUDIES

X-ray films of the skull show a wide diastasis of the fracture line. If initial skull films are available, one can compare the films to confirm "growth" of the fracture line during the interval. When multiple fractures are noted in the same patient, healing of the fracture in one area may be noted as opposed to a growing fracture in another area (Fig. 1, A and B). The fracture line can cross the coronal or lambdoid sutures but is usually limited to one parietal bone.

CT scanning provides information regarding the contents within the growing fracture and any intracranial pathological changes. Furthermore, if CT scans are available from the time of initial trauma, it should be possible to demonstrate progressive changes. It is not unusual that the initial CT scans show hemorrhagic contusion, or subarachnoid or extraparenchymal hemorrhage. At the time of discovery of the growing fracture, CT demonstrates the diastasis of the fracture line and often a hypodense lesion near the fracture site. This hypodensity may rep-

resent encephalomalacia, a loculated arachnoidal cyst, or cortical atrophy. The ipsilateral ventricle tends to show focal porencephalic dilatation with ipsilateral shift of the midline structure. This phenomenon may not only be due to lack of dural resistance but due to cerebral atrophy. MRI provides further information as to pathological processes in association with the growing fracture.

MANAGEMENT

Surgical intervention is indicated with a growing fracture line, seizure disorder, or progressive neurologic deficits. A progressive cystic degeneration in the brain that has herniated through the dural and cranial defects can occur; therefore, surgical correction is recommended in young children even when seizures or other neurologic symptoms or signs are absent. However, incidental, asymptomatic, and stable fractures in late childhood or adulthood probably do not require surgery. The purpose of surgery for growing skull fracture is to repair the dural laceration and cranial defect,

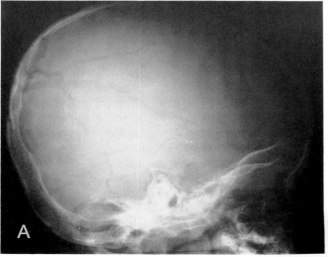

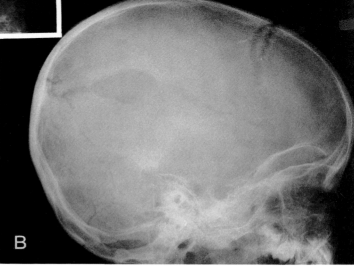

Figure 1. **A,** an x-ray film of the skull made shortly after head trauma showing multiple linear fractures in both parietal bones. **B,** a film obtained four months later showing a growing skull fracture with a resolving fracture on the contralateral side.

and to resect seizure foci. Growth of the growing fracture may arrest after CSF diversion shunting by a decrease of the CSF pulse pressure, but this does not correct a seizure disorder. Placing a shunt for primary treatment of these patients is not advised unless hydrocephalus is present. Shunting for nonhydrocephalic patients creates undesirable shunt dependence.

Preoperative medications include anticonvulsant and antibiotic drugs. In a patient who is not already receiving an anticonvulsant, Dilantin should be given at a dosage of 15 mg/kg of body weight. Nafcillin in a dose of 50 mg/kg of body weight is given intravenously in the operating room just prior to surgery.

General anesthesia with an endotracheal tube is used. For a parietal or frontal lesion, the patient is in a supine position with the ipsilateral shoulder elevated about 30° (Fig. 2). For an occipital lesion, a prone position is used. Because a young child has a thin skull, a U-shaped head holder is preferable to head pins.

SURGICAL TECHNIQUE

The scalp incision should be large enough to expose the entire length of the skull defect. An S-shaped or semicircular skin incision is made, and the scalp flap is turned subgaleally, leaving the underlying periosteal tissue intact (Fig. 3A). By palpation, the entire length of the cranial defect covered by pericranium is exposed to surgical view. The site of the cranial defect is bulging and may be accompanied by a bluish appearance due to an underlying subarachnoid cyst. As the cranial defect is covered by the overgrowth of the pericranium, the edge of the cranial defect is dissected by incising the pericranium along the edge of the bony defect (Fig. 3B). Soft tissues adherent to the edge of the cranium defect are scraped off by a sharp dissector.

One should remember that the dural edge is usually retracted under and adherent to the inner table of the skull (the dural defect is invariably larger than the cranial defect), and that the pericranium is directly adherent to the underlying cerebral tissue at the cranial defect. An effort to expose the dural edge by removing the cranial edge should not be undertaken as this procedure is often complicated by removing the dura simultaneously with the skull bone due to the adhesive nature of the dural edge. In order to identify the dura, several burr holes are made away from the skull defect with a distance of at least 50% of the width of the cranial defect. At this time, a large enough amount of pericranium is removed from the neighboring skull in order to use it for repair of the dural defect. Once the dura is identified at each burr hole site, the dura is separated from the inner table of the skull toward the defect (Fig. 3C). A craniotomy is made around the skull defect by connecting the burr holes with a craniotome. Two pieces of the craniotomy flap are obtained, one from each side of the growing fracture.

After the craniotomy is completed (Fig. 4A), reactive

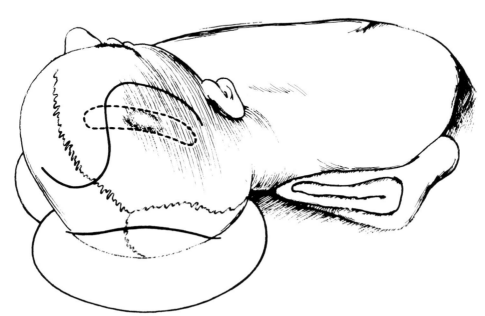

Figure 2. Operative position. The patient is placed in a supine position with the ipsilateral shoulder elevated for a frontal or parietal lesion. If the lesion is located in the occipital region, a prone position is preferable. The scalp incision should be large enough to expose the entire length of the fracture line and surrounding cranium.

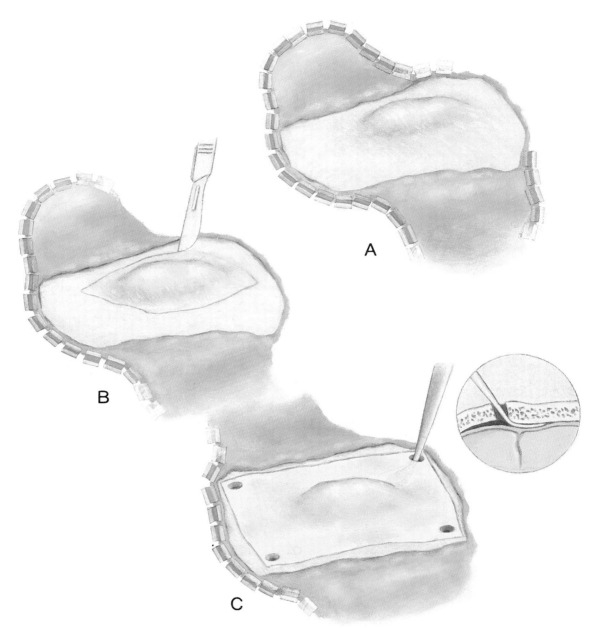

Figure 3. **A,** the scalp flap is turned subperiosteally. The cranial defect is usually covered by the pericranium. **B,** the pericranium is incised along the edge of the cranial defect. Then, the edge of the cranial defect is exposed by scraping off the soft tissues adherent to it. **C,** the pericranium is removed from the surrounding skull surface and preserved for dural repair. Four burr holes are made in the surrounding skull for a craniotomy. After the confirmation of intact dura mater under the burr hole, the dura is separated from the burr hole toward the cranial defect. One should not attempt to identify the dura by removing the bone from the edge of the cranial defect. The craniotomy is carried out on both sides of the growing fracture. The two bone flaps are removed and preserved for autologous bone cranioplasty.

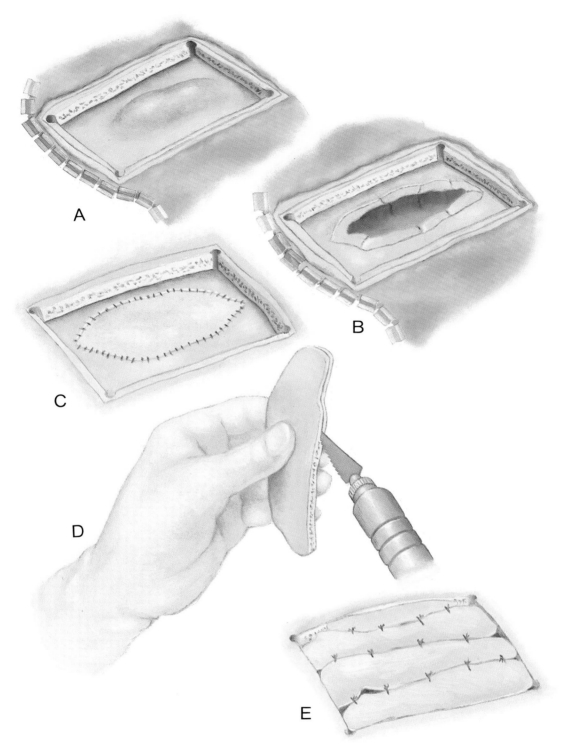

Figure 4. **A,** after the craniotomy, the intact dura mater is exposed around the dural defect which is covered by the periosteum. Underneath the overgrowing periosteum is a cerebromeningeal cicatrix which is removed using bipolar cautery and sharp dissection until healthy white matter is exposed. **B,** after all pathological tissues have been removed, the edge of the surrounding dura is separated from the intact cortical surface. **C,** the previously removed periosteum is used to repair the dural defect. A watertight closure is achieved with 4-0 sutures. **D,** the bone grafts are split at the diploic space between the inner and outer tables by means of an osteotome. **E,** the obtained split bone flaps are used to repair the cranial defect. The bone flaps are secured to each other and to the edge of the cranial defect with nylon sutures or stainless steel wires.

periosteal tissue and the cerebromeningeal cicatrix at the cranial defect should be removed. There is a relatively well demarcated plane between the cicatrix and the white matter. Under magnified vision by means of surgical loupes, the cicatrix including the periosteal tissue is lifted, and all abnormal tissue is separated and transected using a bipolar cautery until normal white matter is exposed (Fig. 4B). The edge of the dura is separated from the cerebral tissue, carefully avoiding trauma to the cerebral blood vessels. In this region, abnormal tissue such as cystic changes or xanthochromic discoloration due to previous hemorrhage is often noted.

After adequate debridement of the cicatrix at the growing fracture and freeing the intact dural edge from the cortical surface, the dural defect is closed using the periosteal graft (Fig. 4C). Autologous pericranium is preferable to cadaver dura. A watertight closure of the dura is important to avoid a recurrence of the growing fracture or postoperative CSF leakage.

Each of the obtained craniotomy flaps is split at the diploic space with an osteotome, separating it into inner and outer tables (Fig. 4D). The cranial defect is then repaired by laying in the split autologous skull grafts. Usually four pieces are laid next to each other side by side to fill the cranial defect. These flaps are secured to each other with either nylon sutures or stainless steel wires through drill holes (Fig. 4E). These flaps are further secured to the craniotomy edge. If the defect of the skull is too large or the skull is too thin to separate into inner and outer tables, one may consider autologous rib grafts. These autologous bone grafts are well incorporated and healing is excellent. Foreign materials such as methyl methacrylate should be avoided for cranioplasty in the growing skull.

SPECIFIC CONSIDERATIONS

The growing fracture may extend toward a dural venous sinus such as the superior sagittal or lateral sinus. Although these venous sinuses were spared from direct injury at the initial trauma, direct exposure of them is not advised or necessary. When the fracture line extends perpendicularly to these sinuses, the closest end to the sinus does not need dural repair. However, if the growing fracture is parallel and near to the sinus, dural repair may be difficult due to the lack of enough dural edge next to the sinus. In these cases, one may repair the dural defect with a periosteal graft sutured to the periosteum of the skull above the sinus.

CSF diversion shunting has been recommended for persistent postoperative CSF leakage from the craniotomy wound. It is justified if coexisting hydrocephalus is evident, or if CSF leakage occurs despite adequate repair of the growing fracture. A lumboperitoneal shunt or temporary lumbar CSF drainage is to be considered under these circumstances.

OCCIPITAL ENCEPHALOCELES

WILLIAM O. BELL, M.D.

INTRODUCTION

Encephaloceles are uncommon congenital malformations of the central nervous system (CNS) occurring in approximately 1–3 of every 10,000 live births in Western civilization. Seventy to eighty percent of all encephaloceles occur in the occipital area, with the remainder located anteriorly or at the base of the skull. In the Far East, anterior and skull-base encephaloceles are the most common, and cranial CNS malformations are more common than spinal malformations.

Occipital encephaloceles range in size from quite small (1–2 cm) to larger than the neonate's head. Almost all are covered with partial-thickness skin, although the skin over smaller defects may be of full thickness. Identification of these anomalies is usually easy, because they are almost always quite obvious. However, a few may be small, sessile, and nearly planar with the surrounding skin, thereby making their identification more difficult. Operative closure of these very small encephaloceles is not necessary, but their presence can have broad prognostic implications, especially if hydrocephalus is also present.

The occurrence of hydrocephalus in the presence of encephalocele is due to aberrant development of the brain stem and cerebrospinal fluid (CSF) pathways. Hydrocephalus may be present at birth or develop following repair of the encephalocele. Up to 50% of infants with an occipital encephalocele will require a CSF shunt for control of hydrocephalus.

PREOPERATIVE CONSIDERATIONS

Operative closure of an occipital encephalocele is usually straightforward, as long as certain important points are kept in mind. A computed tomography (CT) or magnetic resonance imaging (MRI) scan should be obtained preoperatively in order to assess the intracranial contents for gross brain structure and ventricular size. I prefer a CT scan using 3-mm cuts, because the information sought can be obtained easily by this procedure and monitoring the infant during

an MRI scan may be problematic. Very often, there are striking brain abnormalities that will affect subsequent management, and these should be discussed with the parents before the repair is begun.

The majority of occipital encephaloceles are located infratentorially. The exact locations of the major venous sinuses and their relationship with the encephalocele can be determined accurately with MRI if needed.

All except the very smallest encephaloceles must be repaired, but because the majority are covered with skin, there is no emergent need to take the child to surgery within 24–48 hours of birth. This delay allows adequate time for preoperative planning and a full discussion of the implications of an encephalocele with the infant's parents. Although the risk of seizures after repair is high, I do not begin prophylactic anticonvulsants preoperatively, but wait for seizures to occur before starting these drugs.

OPERATIVE TECHNIQUE

A general anesthetic is required for this surgery. In the vast majority of instances, an inhalational anesthetic such as halothane combined with nitrous oxide is sufficient. The anesthesiologist may or may not elect to use neuromuscular junction blocking agents such as vecuronium.

The infant must be positioned prone (Fig. 1). If the encephalocele is large, this positioning will result in undue pressure being placed on the globes unless appropriate care is taken to keep the area of the orbits free from any encumbrance. I use umbilical tape around the padded horseshoe headrest at the level of the orbits for this purpose (Fig. 1). For lesions at the vertex, the neck may be placed in a neutral position, but for lesions in the suboccipital area, the neck must be flexed as much as possible in order for the surgeon to work effectively. The anesthesiologist must be made aware that the neck will be flexed and that this maneuver may change the position of the endotracheal tube. Extraordinary care must be taken to ensure that the endotracheal tube is securely taped to avoid its dislodgement during the procedure.

The child's torso is placed on soft rolls oriented

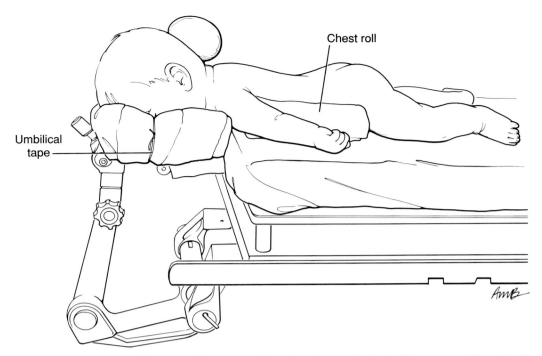

Figure 1. The patient's position for repair of an occipital encephalocele. Note the umbilical tape around the horseshoe headrest at the level of the eyes and the rolls placed beneath the child.

either vertically or horizontally and care is taken to avoid any pressure points. I usually do not place an arterial line or a Foley catheter, because these operations are neither bloody nor lengthy.

I use the 3M 1010 drapes, because they nicely establish the perimeter of the area to be draped and reduce the amount of exposed skin, thereby allowing the infant to retain body heat during the procedure. In addition, these drapes prevent the skin preparation solution, blood, and irrigation fluid from dislodging the tape holding the endotracheal tube in place.

For skin-covered defects, I prepare the skin using diluted Betadine scrub, tincture of iodine, and alcohol in that order. For defects with exposed tissue, I use Betadine scrub and Betadine solution, followed by a normal saline rinse. This avoids applying alcohol to the exposed tissue.

I open the encephalocele sac either vertically or horizontally with a scalpel and then use Metzenbaum scissors (Fig. 2, A and B) in order to obtain a direct view of the interior of the sac. The walls of the sac may be resected or they may be everted with stay sutures (Fig. 2C), whichever provides the greater exposure. Frequently, there are multiple concentric layers of arachnoid that need to be opened with forceps in order to expose the neural tissue that is located at the base of the encephalocele sac (Fig. 2C).

What to do with neural tissue located outside the cranial cavity remains controversial. Some have advocated pushing it back inside the cranium; others have suggested first performing electroencephalographic or evoked potential recordings to determine whether it is functional neural tissue. Whether the externalized tissue is functional or not, forcing it inside a cranium that has not been housing it may exacerbate hydrocephalus or disrupt intracranial dynamics. Histologic sections of this external neural tissue invariably show disorganized neural tissue without layered cerebral or cerebellar cortex. The neurons are usually interspersed in a glial background in what appears to be a random manner.

My usual practice is to excise the exposed neural tissue (Fig. 3, A and B). Frequently, there are reasonably large vascular channels (both arterial and venous) coursing through the tissue, and these must be electrocoagulated carefully with the bipolar forceps (Fig. 3A) before the scissors are used to excise the tissue (Fig. 3B). If the location of the major venous sinuses is known beforehand and reasonable care is taken during the excision, the torcular herophili and transverse sinuses are rarely encountered.

There is always a dural defect, and it is always somewhat smaller than the associated skull defect. In order to obtain a watertight dural closure, I use the

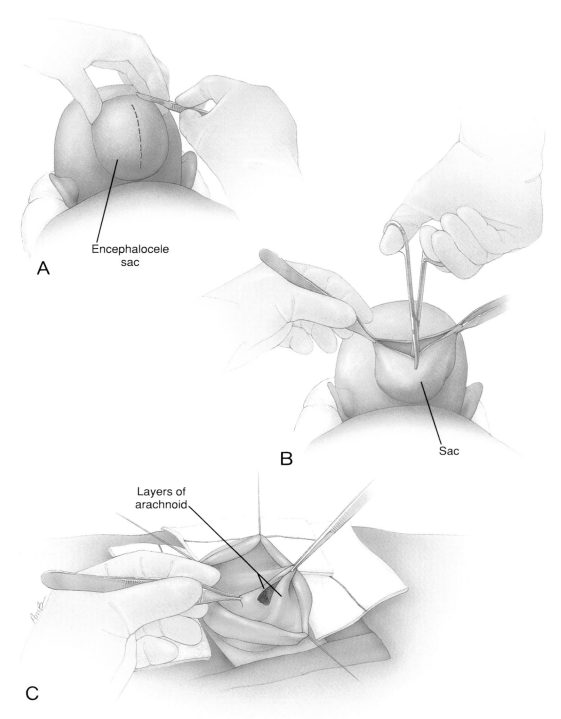

Figure 2. The initial incision may be made vertically or horizontally (**A**) and then opened further with the scissors (**B**). Generally, there are arachnoidal layers that must be opened with forceps so that the abnormal neural tissue at the base (**C**) can be identified.

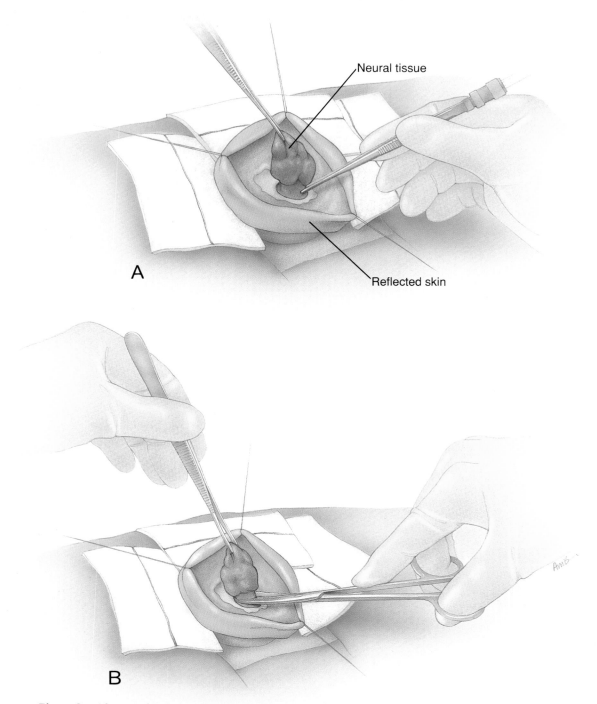

Figure 3.   After careful electrocoagulation with the bipolar forceps (**A**), the abnormal tissue is then excised with the scissors (**B**).

surrounding periosteum (Fig. 4, *A–C*). A No. 15 blade scalpel is used to incise the periosteum, which is then reflected with an elevator, such as the Dingman periosteal elevator (Fig. 4, *A* and *B*). The periosteum/dura is then closed with an interrupted or running absorbable suture such as 4-0 Vicryl in a "vest-over-pants"

fashion (Fig. 4*C* and 5*A*). Because dura and periosteum have been used, this type of closure may allow some ossification of the skull defect, but complete ossification has been rare in my experience. If the skull defect is large, a piece of adjoining skull can be used to cover the defect, sutured in place with absorbable 3-0

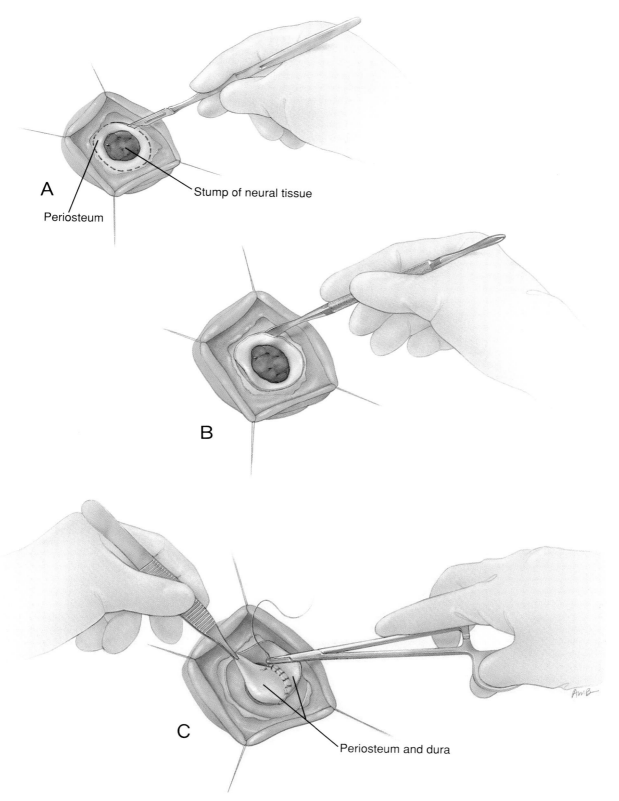

A

Stump of neural tissue

Periosteum

B

C

Periosteum and dura

Figure 4. The periosteum is incised with a scalpel (**A**) and then reflected using a periosteal elevator (**B**). The dura is closed in a "vest-over-pants" fashion using absorbable suture (**C**).

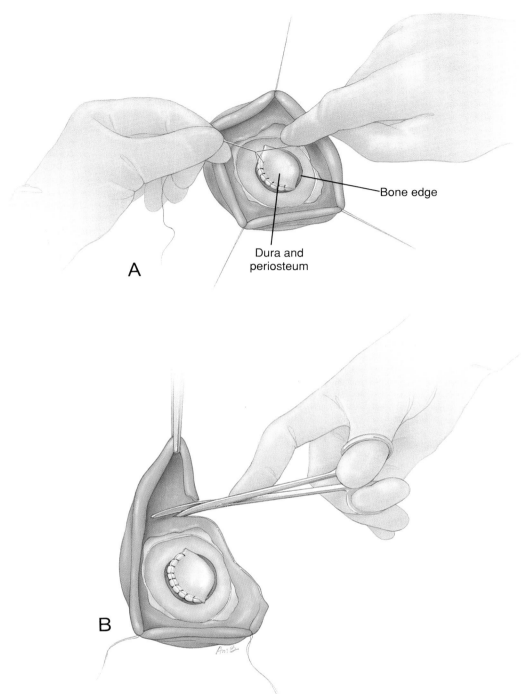

Figure 5. Once this closure has been completed, the bone edges of the defect will be identified (**A**). The excess partial-thickness skin may then be trimmed (**B**).

or 4-0 sutures. The area from which the graft is taken will reossify in one to three months.

The skin may be closed in a vertical, horizontal, or oblique direction. The first step toward closure is to trim away excess partial-thickness skin (Fig. 5B) and

then to begin blunt dissection in the subgaleal space (Fig. 6A). The most distance for skin closure is obtained in the cephalocaudal direction, and it is for this reason that I usually choose a horizontal skin closure (Fig. 6B). The galea is closed with interrupted, buried

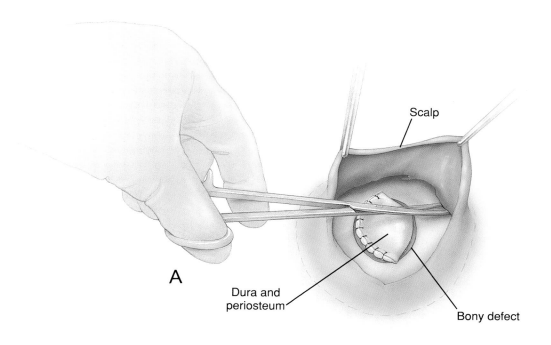

A

Scalp

Dura and
periosteum

Bony defect

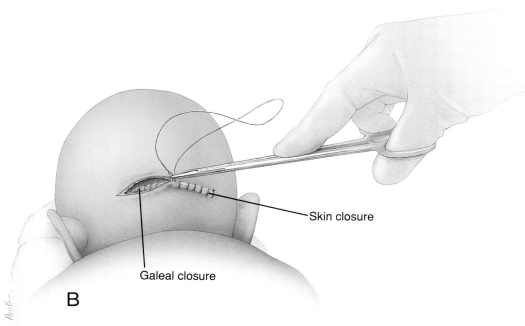

B

Skin closure

Galeal closure

Figure 6. Undermining is done in the subgaleal space to allow for skin mobilization sufficient for closure (**A**). After the galea is closed, the skin is closed using a running monofilament suture (**B**).

4-0 Vicryl sutures and the skin with a running 4-0 monofilament suture. I prefer Prolene for skin closure because of its low tissue drag and ease of removal.

POSTOPERATIVE CONSIDERATIONS

Postoperative care is routine, with the only admonition being that the infant be kept from lying directly on the incision until adequate healing has occurred, and that one be vigilant for developing hydrocephalus. Before the infant is discharged from the hospital, if overt hydrocephalus has not developed, a follow-up CT scan or ultrasound study should be obtained for a baseline measurement.

FORAMEN MAGNUM MENINGIOMAS AND SCHWANNOMAS: POSTERIOR APPROACH

CHAD D. ABERNATHEY, M.D.
BURTON M. ONOFRIO, M.D.

INTRODUCTION

Approximately one-third of all foramen magnum region neoplasms are benign extramedullary tumors. The majority are surgically removable meningiomas and schwannomas occurring in a ratio of roughly three to one. By definition, foramen magnum tumors include those lesions which extend into both the posterior fossa and the upper cervical canal. Further subdivision into craniospinal and spinocranial types may be made based upon the primary location of the tumor mass. Most schwannomas are of the spinocranial variety, with the majority arising from the C-2 nerve root. Two-thirds of the meningiomas are also of the spinocranial type and occur in the anterolateral aspect of the foramen magnum. Tumors to be excluded from the designation of foramen magnum neoplasms are those which arise in or adjacent to the cerebellopontine angle, jugular foramen, vermis, and high cervical spinal cord.

There is a female preponderance (3:2), with the median age of onset occurring in the fifth decade. Due to the capacious nature of the subarachnoid spaces in the vicinity of the foramen magnum, these tumors may reach immense proportions before producing clinically identifiable symptomatology. Making the diagnosis by clinical means is difficult due to the protean nature of the symptoms and signs caused by tumors in this location. The most common presentation is suboccipital or cervical pain with or without associated dysesthesias in the hands. Progression usually involves weakness and atrophy of the intrinsic hand muscles, especially in anteriorly placed tumors. Other symptoms and signs include astereognosis and incoordination of the hands, sensory or motor deficits of all four extremities, nystagmus, lower cranial nerve palsies, and long tract signs. There is typically a chronic progression. However, a remitting course may occur which can confuse the clinical impression. Differential diagnoses based on clinical grounds include cervical spondylosis, multiple sclerosis, syringomyelia, intramedullary tumor, type I Chiari malformation, normal pressure hydrocephalus, amyotrophic lateral sclerosis, and subacute combined degeneration.

PREOPERATIVE EVALUATION

Prior to the advent of computed tomography (CT) and magnetic resonance imaging (MRI), the diagnosis of a foramen magnum meningioma or schwannoma was often delayed or missed entirely. This was due to the paucity of findings on routine radiographs and the fact that Pantopaque myelography was often not done in the supine position to diagnose posteriorly placed lesions or that the foramen was inadequately imaged in the prone position due to technical difficulties in holding the contrast medium optimally across the foramen magnum.

At present, CT myelography and MRI are mutually complementary studies (Fig. 1, A and B). CT myelography allows precise delineation of the tumor-cord interface and the cephalad-caudal extent of the pathologic process. However, bony artifact may occur at the craniovertebral junction. MRI is able to avoid this artifact and provide high resolution and detailed anatomical information including vascular anatomy (Fig. 2, A and B). A tumor, especially a meningioma, may contain proton density comparable to that of the nearby nervous tissue, and not be seen by routine MRI imaging techniques. If a tumor is expected, intravenous gadolinium-enhanced MRI imaging is recommended.

NEUROSURGICAL OPERATIVE ATLAS, VOL. 1, NO. 5

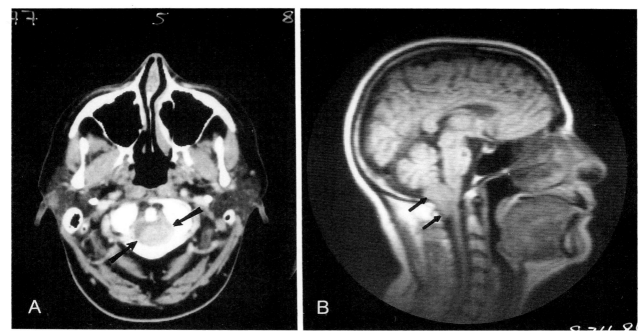

Figure 1. **A,** a CT scan with intrathecal contrast shows a large posteriorly placed meningioma extending from the foramen magnum to C-2 (*arrows*). **B,** a T1 weighted non-contrasted MRI scan of the same patient shows the tumor (*arrows*).

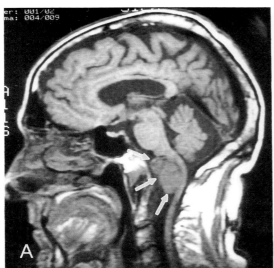
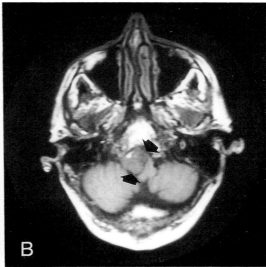

Figure 2. **A,** an anteriorly placed meningioma (*arrows*) at the foramen magnum is well seen with a T1 weighted MRI midline sagittal section. **B,** an axial MRI view accurately displays the tumor location anteriorly (*arrows*) and the degree of brain stem rotation and displacement.

SURGICAL TECHNIQUE

The decision to administer steroids and diuretics is determined by the severity of clinical findings and the amount of cord compression demonstrated on the neurodiagnostic studies. Intraoperative electromyographic recording of the lower cranial nerves and somatosensory evoked potential monitoring of the posterior columns are warranted. In the sitting position, Doppler sonography is used to detect air embolism and preoperative placement of a right atrial catheter is used to monitor cardiac function and for the withdrawal of air emboli. A preoperative echocardiogram will define a patent foramen ovale and allow the surgeon to determine the most prudent surgical position, either prone or sitting. If the sitting position is chosen, the degree of neck flexion from the neutral position is limited by 1) the degree of osteoarthritic spurring of the cervical interspaces and associated risk of anterior spinal cord compression, and 2) body habitus, i.e., short or elongated neck with the risk of carotid and jugular compression varing with each individual patient. The head is secured in a pinion fixation device and the surgical area prepared and draped from the inion to the upper thoracic vertebrae. The attitude of the neck and lateral flexion are tailored to the position of the tumor as related to the brain stem and upper cervical cord. If it is anterior to the stem and cord, head rotation to the side of the lesion maximizes tumor visualization and decreases the need for brain stem retraction.

A linear midline incision is made from the inion to the level of the C-5 spinous process (Fig. 3). The inci-

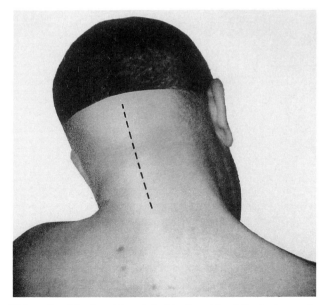

Figure 3. The head is rotated to the side of the lesion and slightly flexed to visualize the tumor depicted in Fig. 2, *A* and *B*.

sion is carried to the fascia of the paraspinous muscles and hemostatic clips are placed along the skin margins. The muscles are then separated from the spinous processes and swept laterally, being held in position by self-retaining retractors. The attachments of the trapezius, semispinalis capitis, and splenius capitis muscles are elevated from the occipital squamae in a subperiosteal fashion. With the deep occipital triangle thus exposed, the remaining muscular attachments to the posterior rim of the foramen magnum, arch of C-1, and spinous process and laminae of C-2 are dissected free utilizing sharp, blunt, and electrocautery dissection. The subperiosteal dissection of the arch of C-1 is carried laterally until a pocket of loose areolar tissue is encountered, which is in close proximity to the vertebral artery. The dissection of the spino-occipital musculature may be carried laterally on the occipital squamae until the mastoid processes are encountered (Fig. 4).

The arch of C-1 is then removed by rongeur resection and/or the use of a diamond drill. Commonly, the inferior extension of the tumor necessitates a complete laminectomy of C-2 as well. Care must be taken to identify the venous plexus that exists between the C-1 and C-2 vertebrae. This plexus may be entered unknowingly, especially laterally, and act as an occult source of air emboli. The suboccipital craniectomy is performed by placing multiple burr holes and rongeuring away the intervening occipital bone or by utilizing a diamond burr. The majority of tumors will arise in the anterior portion of the foramen magnum along the basilar groove. For tumors in this location, the lateral extension of bony removal along the arch of C-1 and the rim of the foramen magnum must be taken as far laterally as possible to allow adequate exposure of the tumor and its vascular supply. Extensive lateral exposure also permits decreased manipulation of the medulla and cervical spinal cord as the tumor is evacuated.

The dura is opened in a standard Y shape with the superior flap reflected upward and secured to the bony margin or muscle. The lateral dural margins are tacked to the paraspinous musculature. After opening the arachnoid, the tumor will be identified as arising primarily from an anterior or posterior origin in relationship to the medulla and cervical spinal cord. The majority of tumors lying in the anterolateral position will be meningiomas. Conversely, schwannomas will more commonly be found in the posterolateral location. Initial assessment of the vascular supply to the tumor is imperative. Tumors arising in the posterior portion of the foramen magnum typically derive their vascular supply from the posterior meningeal artery which is a branch of the vertebral artery just below the foramen magnum. Anteriorly located tumors will obtain their blood supply from the anterior meningeal branch of the vertebral artery which arises immediately inferior to the initial genu of the vertebral artery. This is roughly at the level of the axis. This artery tends to course medially and superiorly along the midline, supplying the dura mater of the anterior foramen magnum. Great effort must be made to preserve the vertebral, posterior inferior cerebellar, anterior spinal, and posterior spinal arteries.

Posteriorly located tumors are approached directly. However, anteriorly positioned tumors tend to push and rotate the cord and medulla posteriorly, stretching the dentate ligaments, first and second cervical roots, and the eleventh nerve over the tumor (Fig. 5). Division of the dentate ligaments allows access to the anterior arachnoidal cisterns as well as providing a means of supporting the spinal cord during the tumor dissection. On occasion it will be necessary to sacrifice the first or second cervical roots and possibly the motor rootlets of the accessory nerve. The mass is delivered piecemeal by means of sharp dissection and aspiration techniques. The ultrasonic aspirator and the

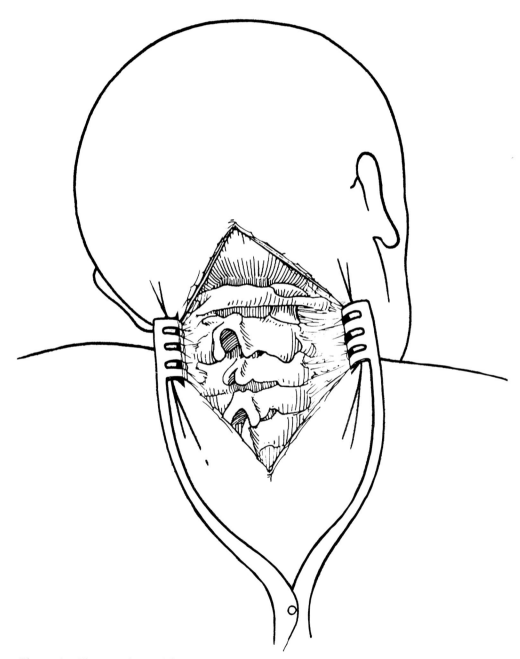

Figure 4. The muscles and fascia have been dissected, leaving the occiput and upper cervical laminae in view.

CO₂ laser may be useful in accomplishing tumor removal. If possible, the tumor-dural interface is developed with the aid of bipolar coagulation, leaving the tumor as its own retractor of the lower brain stem and upper cervical cord (Fig. 6). When that is impossible or can be incompletely performed, then gutting of the tumor using bipolar coagulation and sharp dissection may be necessary. Leaving the spinal cord/brain stem-tumor plane intact until the tumor has been devascu-

larized and debulked will allow separation of the tumor from the anterior spinal artery. Large tumors often parasitize blood supply from the pial vasculature and care should be taken to identify these arteries (Fig. 7). Undue traction on these with rupture will make identification of the source of bleeding difficult or impossible and, if attendant with occult subpial hemorrhage, will herald a potentially tragic result.

Posterolaterally positioned meningiomas require a

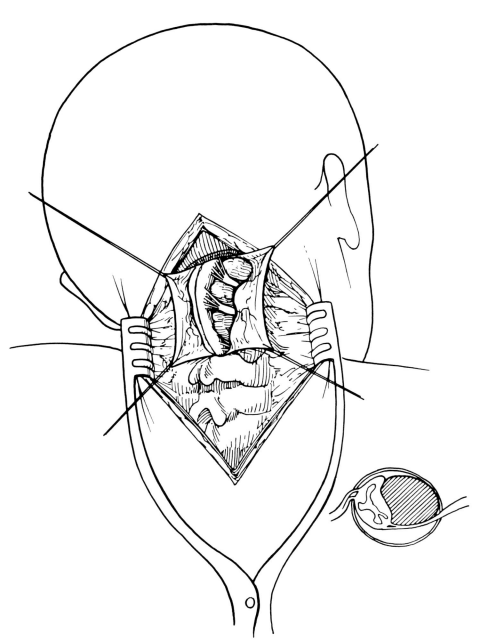

Figure 5. In anteriorly placed lesions, the upper cervical roots and spinal portion of the eleventh cranial nerve are displaced over the posterior aspect of the tumor and often will need to be sectioned to permit access to the tumor. The vertebral artery will be anterior to the tumor in most instances.

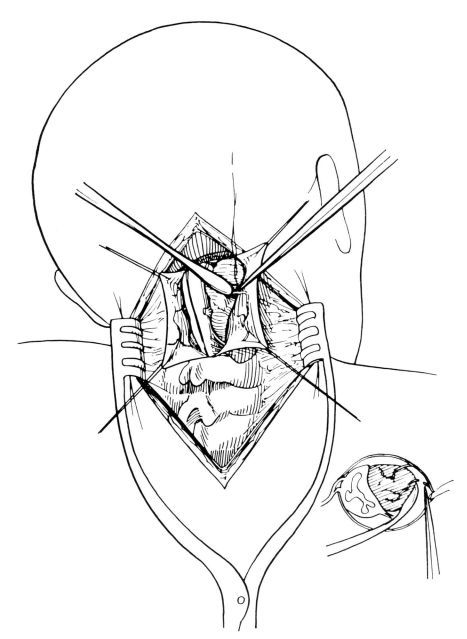

Figure 6. Obtaining hemostasis by devascularizing the dural-tumor interface will allow debulking of the tumor at a later stage while using the tumor judiciously as a brain stem retractor.

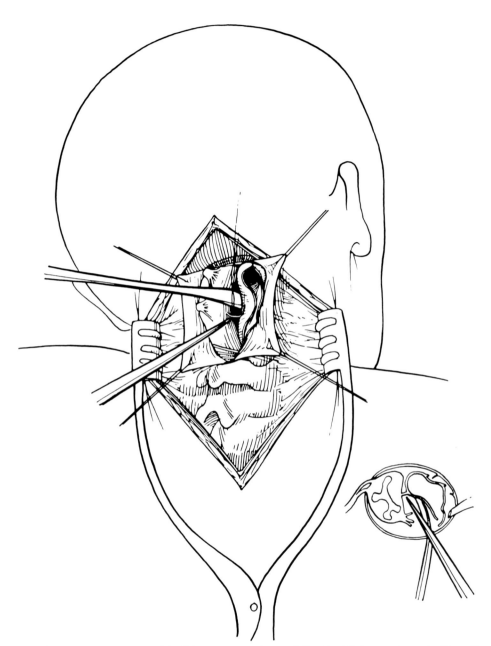

Figure 7. The last and most important post-debulking procedure is gently retracting the tumor away from the brain stem while identifying and controlling the arterial and venous supply common to the tumor and the brain stem.

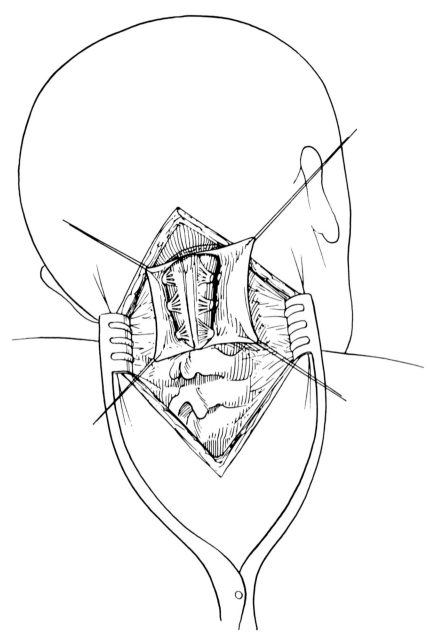

Figure 8. The tumor has been removed and the brain stem achieves a more normal position.

dural resection which encompasses the tumor's origin. The dura will necessarily be left intact on anteriorly located meningiomas but must be cauterized to decrease the chances of recurrence. For foramen magnum schwannomas, the nerve root of origin should be sacrificed with adequate proximal and distal margins to encompass the tumor extension along the root.

Upon completion of the tumor removal, complete hemostasis must be obtained (Fig. 8). A watertight closure of the dura is mandatory, either primarily or with a fascia lata graft. The capitis and trapezius musculature is then reapproximated in the midline in layers with taut suture lines. One should begin at the base of the incision and work superiorly with each successive suture line, ensuring that the muscles do not compress either the cerebellum, brain stem, or cervical cord. The suture line is carried superiorly until apposition of the musculature is no longer possible. The most important layer is the ligamentum nuchae inferiorly and the galea superiorly. This layer must be closed meticulously as a single structure. The subcutaneous tissues are then reapproximated and finally the skin is closed.

COMPLICATIONS

Perioperative complications are largely preventable with compulsive attention to detail during the procedure. Complications include postoperative hemorrhage in the region of the cervicomedullary junction and cerebrospinal fluid leakage from the wound. If either of these should occur, the treatment of choice is re-exploration of the wound with improved closure technique. Infection is a potential sequela of this operation and must be differentiated from aseptic meningitis. Finally, one must be prepared for the development of an air embolus which can occur at any juncture of the procedure, particularly during opening of the dura mater and sectioning of the circular sinus.

PENETRATING WOUNDS OF THE SPINE

EDWARD C. BENZEL, M.D.

INTRODUCTION

The treatment of penetrating wounds of the spine is controversial. Some advocate surgery in the majority of cases while others advocate a nonsurgical approach in nearly all cases. This controversy is fueled by a clinical situation in which neurologic improvement often ensues, regardless of the treatment administered to the patient. Treatment efficacy is, thus, difficult to assess. Because the majority of penetrating wounds of the spine are gunshot wounds and because the majority of surgical indications are for gunshot wounds, the ensuing discussion will address them directly. Other penetrating wounds of the spine are relatively uncommon and seldom lead to surgical intervention. The indications for surgery, however, are similar.

Complications of surgical therapy for gunshot wounds of the spine are predominantly related to infection, cerebrospinal fluid (CSF) leakage, and/or neurologic injury incurred via surgical trauma. The potential for an adverse outcome from surgery must be weighed against the chance that surgery might confer a neurologic improvement to the patient in addition to that expected with nonsurgical treatment alone. A number of authors have documented the relative safety of surgery for gunshot wounds. The advantages of surgery, however, are based upon anecdotal information and a few retrospective series only. The true efficacy of surgery, therefore, is not known.

INDICATIONS FOR SURGERY

There are two fundamental indications for spine surgery following trauma: neural element compression and spinal instability. Neural element decompression may be necessary under the following circumstances: 1) infection (including osteomyelitis, disc interspace infection, and epidural or intradural abscess) and 2) extra- or intradural compression from the missile, bone, soft tissue, or blood clot. In many clinical situations, a combination of these indications may exist simultaneously. In addition to these indications, the

location and the type of injury affect the decision-making process regarding the utility of surgery. Several anatomical/clinical spinal gunshot injuries which may benefit from surgery, therefore, exist. These include: 1) A through and through injury to the spinal cord which has resulted in a complete cervical myelopathy or an incomplete cervical, thoracic, or lumbar myelopathy (Fig. 1A); 2) a dorsal injury to the spine which has resulted in a compressive mass lesion without dural penetration and an incomplete myelopathy (Fig. 1B); and 3) a ventral injury to the spine which has resulted in a compressive mass lesion without dural penetration and an incomplete myelopathy (Fig. 1C). Obviously, clinical indications for any planned treatment supersede radiographic indications under most circumstances.

In this regard, patients who are candidates for surgery include: 1) patients in whom computed tomography (CT), myelogram, or magnetic resonance imaging (MRI) evidence of neural compression exists and in whom an incomplete myelopathy is present; 2) patients with a complete cervical myelopathy in whom the trajectory of the missile does not explain a higher neurologic (motor and/or sensory) level or loss of function with an accompanying radiographic evidence of neural compression; 3) those patients who harbor migratory or potentially migratory intradural missiles or missile fragments and in whom intermittent neurologic worsening is encountered or is probable; 4) those patients who have incurred an unstable spine secondary to disruptive forces imparted to the spine by the missile; and 5) patients in whom infection is present.

Patients with a complete myelopathy who 1) are not deteriorating neurologically, 2) do not have an unstable spine, 3) do not have a paraspinal or intraspinal abscess, 4) do not have a significant neurologic deficit above that expected by the trajectory of the missile alone, and 5) do not have radiographic evidence of neural compression above the level of the injury are *not* candidates for surgery. Therefore, regarding patients with a complete myelopathy, only those with cervical injuries who have a neurologic impairment which is one or more segmental levels higher than that expected by the missile's trajectory should even be considered for surgery. The remainder of the surgical can-

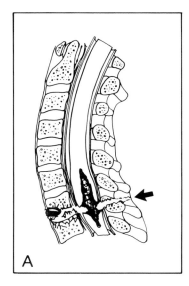

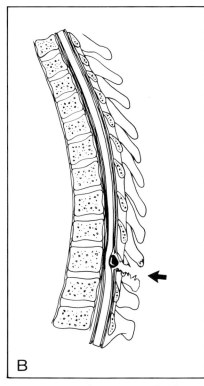

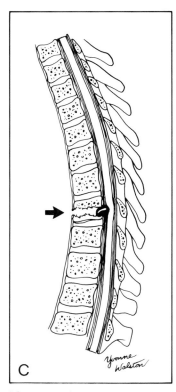

Figure 1. Illustrations depicting the major injury types and locations which are amenable to surgery. **A,** a through and through injury to the cervical spinal cord has resulted in a complete myelopathy. In this circumstance, surgery is indicated if spinal instability ensues or if the neurologic level of injury is significantly higher than the spinal level of injury and if there coexists imaging evidence of either an extramedullary or intramedullary mass effect. **B,** a dorsal extrinsic mass effect has resulted from missile impingement upon the dural sac. If an incomplete myelopathy is present, surgical decompression via laminectomy is indicated. **C,** a ventral extrinsic mass effect has resulted from missile impingement upon the dural sac. Ventral dural sac decompression is indicated if an incomplete myelopathy exists. Ventral decompression of the thoracic or lumbar dural sac requires a more thoughtful surgical approach.

didates have an incomplete myelopathy, combined with either an extrinsic dural sac compressive lesion or an intradural mass lesion. It is emphasized that the indications for surgery, therefore, are relatively uncommon.

Although surgery for spinal instability is included in the discussion above, its treatment will not be addressed here. The discussion, instead, will focus on the treatment of injuries to or compression of the dural contents.

In view of the variability of injuries and injury patterns, a multitude of surgical approaches may be applied to the treatment of spinal gunshot wounds. The surgeon must use a rational and often creative approach and must be armed with the ability to exercise many of a multitude of available options. The most common approaches will be discussed and illustrated here.

TIMING OF SURGERY

Early surgery (surgery within the first five to seven days following injury) is associated with a relatively high complication rate, predominately related to infection and cerebrospinal fistula formation. It is therefore suggested that few, if any, patients undergo early surgery (within the first week following injury) for penetrating missile injuries of the spine. The rare exception to this policy pertains to the patient with progressive neurologic deterioration. This might be caused by a migrating missile, infection, or vertebral column instability or malalignment. The complications of early surgery are often secondary to contamination incurred at the time of injury (infection) and difficulties related to obtaining a tight wound closure following operative intervention (CSF fistula formation). If surgery is delayed, the contamination inoculum incurred at the time of injury will have decreased significantly by virtue of the patient's own defense mechanisms and via medical therapy, i.e., the administration of antibiotics. Furthermore, tissue friability is increased immediately following missile injuries and tissue integrity is decreased. Wound healing capacity is, therefore, diminished.

PREOPERATIVE PREPARATION

Patients are prepared for surgery in a routine manner. Broad spectrum antibiotic coverage should have been administered for three to five days immediately following the injury. Prophylactic antibiotic administration should again be utilized prior to, during, and perhaps for one to two days following surgery. Under most circumstances, the patient should be positioned in the prone position (although the lateral decubitus and the three-quarters prone position may occasionally be used, depending upon the operative approach used).

Care should be taken to avoid abdominal compression during the surgical procedure. The patient is prepared and draped in a routine manner with the draping including the upper and lower extremes of possible surgical exposure.

DORSAL APPROACH

Most surgical approaches for the treatment of penetrating wounds of the spine involve a dorsal exposure of the spine. For these patients, a midline incision and subperiosteal exposure of the spine is performed. The surgical treatment of spinal gunshot wounds via this approach usually is undertaken through a laminectomy or laminotomy approach (Fig. 2, A and B). If an intradural exploration is indicated, a longitudinal dural incision is usually made, thus exposing the injured segment of the spinal cord (Fig. 2C)). A midline myelotomy of the spinal cord is appropriate when an intramedullary mass effect and a corresponding neurologic deficit are present (Fig. 3, A and B). Great care needs to be taken to not waver from the midline when performing the myelotomy. Injury to longitudinal ascending tracts (posterior columns) may result if deviation from the midline is excessive. Removal of blood clot which should be liquified at the time of surgery is then performed (Fig. 3B).

Dural closure should be attempted aggressively. Care should be taken to not compromise the intradural contents by constriction by the dural closure. Accessible dural holes, in addition, should be closed. Ventral dural holes which are not accessible through the posterior approach are, in most circumstances, best left alone. Dorsal dural defects may be closed with dural patch grafting (Fig. 3C). It is my preference that autogenous material be used: either locally obtained fascia (such as thoracodorsal fascia) or fascia lata. Previously reported experiences with fascia lata dural repairs have illustrated its strength and utility, as well as its association with few complications. Patch grafting the dura mater should prevent spinal cord compromise.

Dorsal compressive injuries, which do not penetrate the dural sac, are best removed via laminectomy and generous exposure of the injured region. Following such an exposure, the offending lesion may simply be removed (Fig. 4A). The exposure needs to be wide enough to allow for a safe dural sac decompression. However, it should not be so extensive that it compromises stability. This is particularly the case with facet joint disruption. Care should be taken to preserve the integrity of the facet joints when possible.

POSTEROLATERAL AND ANTERIOR APPROACHES

The posterolateral approach to spinal gunshot

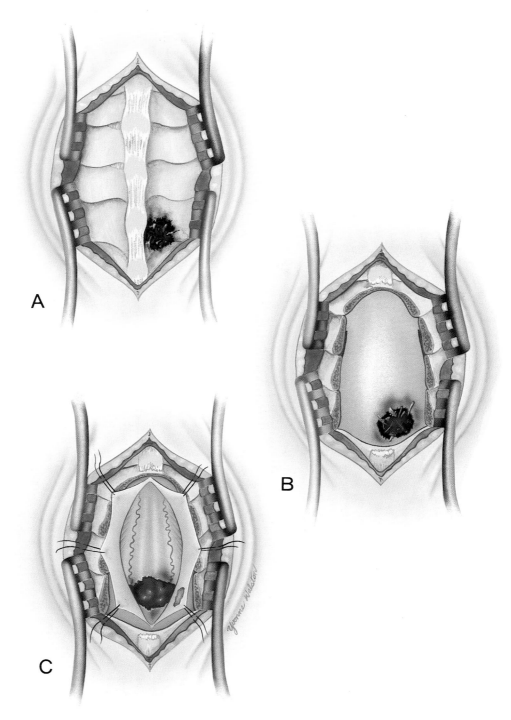

Figure 2. A dorsal through and through injury to the cervical spine and its treatment are illustrated, **A,** a subperiosteal exposure of the spine has allowed observation of the missile's site of entrance into the spinal canal. Care should be taken during the subperiosteal dissection. Inadvertent plunging into the spinal canal may be avoided by simply being cognizant of this possibility and by simultaneously taking appropriate precautions. **B,** a generous laminectomy has been performed, thus exposing the site of missile entrance through the dorsal dural sac. **C,** a dural opening has allowed visualization of the spinal cord. Note that the spinal cord was generously exposed both superiorly and in a limited manner inferiorly. This allows for the decompression of the cervical spinal cord cephalad to the injury site in the case of a patient whose neurologic level is higher than that expected by the trajectory of the missile. Also note the hole in the dural sac through which the missile passed.

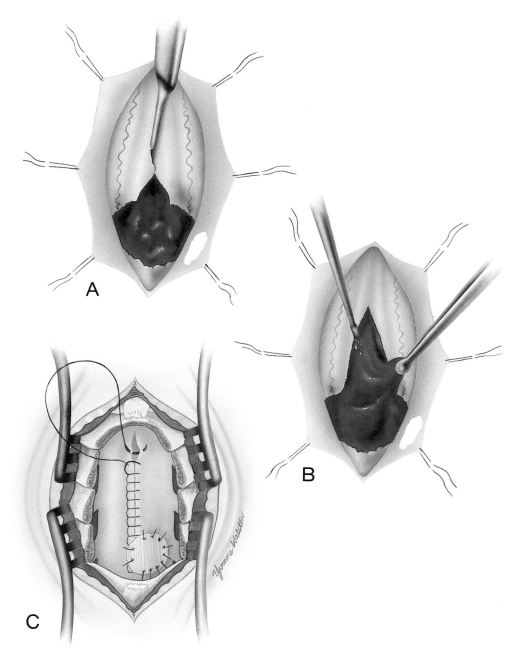

Figure 3. An illustration of the intradural and intramedullary decompression of a cervical spinal cord injury, as depicted in Figure 2. **A,** a midline dorsal myelotomy is made with a sharp knife, such as a No. 11 blade. Bipolar cautery with a microforceps is emphasized so that minimal posterior column injury is incurred. Care must be taken to not waver from midline while performing the myelotomy for similar reasons. **B,** the exposure of an intramedullary blood clot and its removal are illustrated. Care must be taken to avoid spinal cord tissue manipulation. The timing of the surgery to ensure that the clot is at least semiliquified may help minimize surgical trauma. **C,** the dural sac closure is illustrated. A running suture closure of the dural incision and a fascial patch grafting of the missile penetration hole have been performed. Fascia may be obtained locally (i.e., from thoracodorsal fascia), by harvesting fascia lata, or by utilizing nonautogenous material. The ventral dural sac hole usually does not need to be closed.

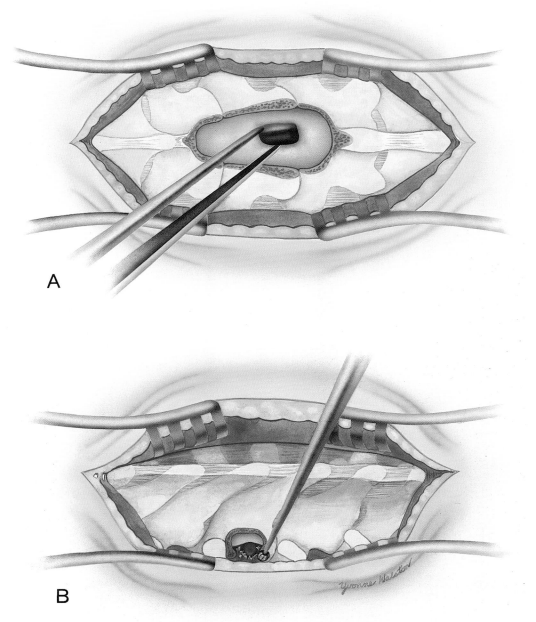

Figure 4. An illustration depicting two types of extrinsic dural sac compression. **A,** a dorsal injury has resulted in extrinsic compression of the dural sac. A simple generous laminectomy allows treatment of this problem. **B,** a ventral injury has resulted in anterolateral compression of the dural sac. In this case, a posterolateral approach has allowed an adequate exposure of the missile and should allow for its safe removal and dural sac decompression. It is emphasized, however, that oftentimes a more anterior approach may be more effective and simultaneously safer.

wounds is most appropriate for anterolateral and lateral extrinsic mass lesions. This approach utilizes an exposure gained by a wide lateral retraction of the paraspinous tissues, which, in turn, offers the surgeon a view of the facet joints, transverse processes, and pedicles (following a laminectomy or laminotomy). This approach, therefore, might be more appropriately termed a transpedicular approach.

It is useful, almost exclusively, for ventral and/or lateral lesions which are compressing the dural sac. The exposure gained allows for a simple decompression. Figure 4B illustrates the exposure gained by this approach, following lateral soft tissue retraction. More extensive decompressive operations, especially for lesions involving the ventral dural sac, might be best approached via a variety of available anterior approaches. These include the anterior approach to the cervical spine, as well as the anterior, anterolateral, and lateral extracavitary approaches to the thoracic spine and lumbar spine. It is emphasized that these latter approaches are rarely indicated and that they *do not* offer a wide exposure of the dural sac. Therefore, injuries which are associated with dural sac penetration and which require intradural exploration and dural sac closure are fraught with difficulty when approached from an anterior direction. It is also emphasized, however, that no other approaches for truly ventral lesions are feasible. Therefore, if such an approach is truly indicated, its degree of difficulty must be understood by both the surgeon and the patient prior to surgery. The anterior approaches are best suited for extrinsic lesions resulting in dural sac compression such as is illustrated in Figure 1C.

WOUND CLOSURE

Closure of the wound should be performed in multiple layers, usually with absorbable sutures. A tight closure is emphasized. This should minimize the chance for cerebrospinal fluid leakage. Patients with penetrating spinal gunshot wounds are at a relatively high risk for fistula formation. It is my preference to not utilize drains, unless absolutely necessary. Careful attention to hemostasis should, under most circumstances, minimize the indication for drains. Intraoperative evoked potential monitoring should seldom play a role in the surgical management of patients with spinal gunshot wounds.

COMPLICATIONS

Complications of surgery for penetrating wounds of the spine are usually secondary to infection, iatrogenic exaggeration of a neurologic deficit, or cerebrospinal fluid leakage. Spinal instability may occasionally present as a problem. These complications are minimized by paying careful attention to surgical technique and the use of appropriate antibiotics. Patient selection for surgery should be relatively strict, as well. This will minimize the chance for complications resulting from surgical intervention. Abdominal injuries in which the bullet may have penetrated contaminated viscera prior to entering the spine should be treated with antibiotics following general surgical consultation.

The proximity of the vertebral and carotid arteries to the cervical spine is of significance. Patients with penetrating injuries of the cervical spine should almost always undergo angiography shortly following admission to the hospital. The passage of the vertebral arteries through the foramina transversaria is of even greater significance. Bone or disc fragments, as well as missile fragments, may disrupt vessel integrity and alter flow through or occlude these vessels. It is emphasized that neither the external visual examination of an artery nor its palpation can define the presence or absence of endothelial injury, including intimal flap formation, dissection, and even occlusion.

NEUROSURGICAL
OPERATIVE ATLAS
Volume 1

NEUROSURGICAL OPERATIVE ATLAS
Volume 1

AANS PUBLICATIONS COMMITTEE

Editors

SETTI S. RENGACHARY, M.D.

Professor and Chief
Section of Neurological Surgery
University of Missouri at Kansas City
Kansas City, Missouri

ROBERT H. WILKINS, M.D.

Professor and Chief
Division of Neurosurgery
Duke University Medical Center
Durham, North Carolina

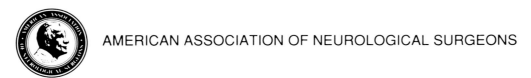

AMERICAN ASSOCIATION OF NEUROLOGICAL SURGEONS

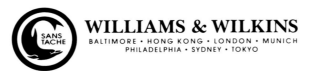

WILLIAMS & WILKINS
BALTIMORE · HONG KONG · LONDON · MUNICH
PHILADELPHIA · SYDNEY · TOKYO

Editor: Charles W. Mitchell
Managing Editors: Marjorie Kidd Keating, Victoria M. Vaughn
Copy Editor: Janet Krejci
Designer: Dan Pfisterer
Illustration Planner: Wayne Hubbel
Production Coordinator: Raymond E. Reter

Copyright © 1991
The American Association of Neurological Surgeons
Park Ridge, Illinois

This publication is published under the auspices of the Publications Committee of the American Association of Neurological Surgeons (AANS). However, this should not be construed as indicating endorsement or approval of the views presented, by the AANS, or by its committees, commissions, affiliates, or staff.

Printed in the United States of America

Library of Congress Cataloging-in-Publication Data
Neurosurgical operative atlas / AANS Publications Committee ; editors, Setti S. Rengachary, Robert H. Wilkins.
     p.   cm.
   Includes index.
   ISBN 0-683-07234-X (v. 1)
    1. Nervous system—Surgery—Atlases. I. Rengachary, Setti S.
  II. Wilkins, Robert H. II. AANS Publications Committee.
  [DNLM: 1. Nervous System—surgery—atlases.   WL 17 N494]
RD593.N43 1991
617.4′8′00222—dc20
DNLM/DLC
for Library of Congress   90-14551
                               CIP

91 92 93 94 95
1 2 3 4 5 6 7 8 9 10

Foreword

I am honored to write this foreword to the American Association of Neurological Surgeons' *Neurosurgical Operative Atlas*. The list of operations is impressive and covers almost every detail of neurosurgery. The authors selected to present these operations are even more impressive, representing, as they do, outstanding individuals in the United States and Canada who are respected and admired by everyone in the medical profession.

This is not the first effort the former Harvey Cushing Society has made in this field—more than 25 years ago the Board of Editors of the *Journal of Neurosurgery* agreed that it was important to publish a section, entitled *Neurosurgical Techniques*, of select operative drawings with brief explanatory text that would be published as fascicles over the ensuing years.

Most of us in neurosurgery at that time had depended on the volume devoted to the nervous system in Bancroft and Pilcher's *Surgical Treatment*, the responsibility for which had been that of Cobb Pilcher, then at Vanderbilt. Although *Surgical Treatment* was not specifically a "techniques" book, it had much technique in it and was widely used. The editorial board of the *Journal of Neurosurgery* hoped that *Neurosurgical Techniques* would serve as a more up-to-date version of that volume of *Surgical Treatment*.

Emphasis in *Neurosurgical Techniques* was given to the artists' depictions of established, safe techniques. The editors of the Journal realized that a procedure might be done sucessfully in more than one way, but at least one good and safe technique was to be described, and it was assumed that the more skilled and experienced surgeons would utilize other methods they found suitable.

The basis of the decision to focus on the drawings and to have relatively little associated text was a previous atlas, the *Atlas of Surgical Operations* (1). Many of the editors of the Journal had become familiar with this atlas during their general surgical training. Mildred Codding, who had been the artist for Harvey Cushing, had developed an effective technique of drawing the stages of operative procedures that had been and remains an effective teaching aid.

The fascicles of *Neurosurgical Techniques* in the *Journal of Neurosurgery* were to be bound together, but, due to changes in publishers, this was never done. Fortunately, some of the plates were preserved and given to me, as editor of the fascicles. Three of these are shown to provide a historical perspective.

The first two figures illustrate a technique by Dr.

James Greenwood of Houston, Texas (2), who pioneered the complete removal of ependymomas in the cervical spinal cord and developed unique bipolar Bovie forceps with suction at the tips. Use of his Bovie forceps enabled him to carry out detailed dissections with magnifying lenses before the advent of the operating microscope. Figure 1 shows the spinal cord split, the tumor being removed, and a line of cleavage being developed; Figure 2 shows a further removal with the suction bipolar forceps in the field.

Figure 3 shows a cervical fusion technique (3) and is published to give due credit to Mr. George Lynch, the artist who approved of and often redrew illustrations that were published in *Neurosurgical Techniques*. Figure 3 illustrates the final stages of cervical fusion for dislocation of C-3, C-4, using bone and wire for the fusion process. This technique was used before the development of the acrylic fusion technique, which came to replace the bone grafting procedure.

As was expressed in the final paragraph of the introduction to *Neurosurgical Techniques* (4), neurosurgery was evolving rapidly, and often the procedure described had not originated with the person who wrote about it. Then, as now, surgery was a combination of new knowledge with old. Since knowledge is freely shared among surgeons nationally and internationally, original techniques and ideas are passed from teacher to student, from surgeon to surgeon, and

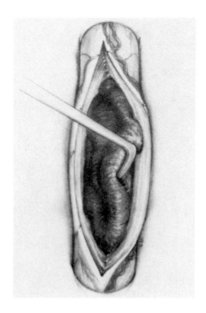

Figure 1.

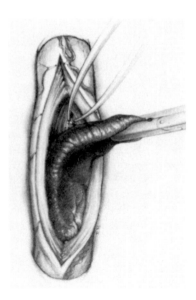

Figure 2.

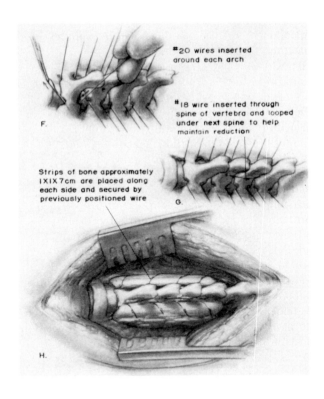

Figure 3.

altered with changing developments and experience. A procedure well-established today may seem naive or useless a few years hence. One can make valid judgments only on the basis of data that become available. Thus, it is my great pleasure to introduce this ambitious project by Dr. Wilkins and Dr. Rengachary. Not only will it update neurosurgical techniques, but it is also a further development of the effort made by the editors of the *Journal of Neurosurgery* 25 years ago. We hope it will surpass that effort.

EBEN ALEXANDER, Jr.

References
1. Cutler EC, Zollinger R. Atlas of surgical operations. Illustrated by Mildred B. Codding. New York: Macmillan, 1939.
2. Greenwood J, Jr. Surgical removal of intramedullary tumors. J Neurosurg 1967;26:275–282.
3. Alexander E, Jr, Davis CH, Jr, Forsyth HF. Reduction and fusion of fracture dislocations of the cervical spine. J Neurosurg 1967;27:587–591.
4. Alexander E, Jr. Neurosurgical techniques introduction. J Neurosurg 1966;24:817–819.

Preface

Man has always had an innate urge to depict his activities in drawings, as the paintings of cave dwellers would attest. Surgical atlases perhaps represent a formalized version of such an urge; the atlases, in addition to documenting the work, have instructional value as well—being able to teach generations of trainees the craft of surgery as practiced by the masters of the trade. Although electronic images have greatly advanced the instructional process, printed artwork remains the backbone of the media for teaching.

There has been a perception among all neurosurgeons for some time that a contemporary atlas in neurosurgery is due. To fill this void, the Publications Committee of the American Association of Neurological Surgeons has undertaken the task of producing a comprehensive atlas. The atlas will be published at bimonthly intervals in the form of fascicles containing up to six operations each. To allow timely publication, topics are included in a random fashion.

The *Neurosurgical Operative Atlas,* we believe, is unique in several respects. It is comprehensive. When completed, it will contain descriptions of up to two hundred operative procedures. It is multiauthored. Given the complexity of the field and the explosive advances in techniques, it is impossible for any one individual to be skilled enough to describe the entire spectrum of techniques authoritatively. In many instances, the chosen authors are those who developed a technique originally or have used the technique so extensively as to be an authority on it. Many illustrations are depicted in full color despite the high costs involved in preparing the artwork and printing. In many instances where there is more than one way to approach a problem, two different authors have been requested to write on the same subject so that the reader will benefit from knowing alternative surgical techniques.

The atlas has been possible in large measure due to the efforts and sacrifices of the contributing authors. In addition to sharing their knowledge and expertise, they have incurred large expenses in getting the artwork done; they have spent long hours with their illustrators to achieve the accurate and esthetically pleasing depiction of the procedures. One can also see the spectrum of artistic talent that made this work possible.

We thank George T. Tindall, M.D., for forming the Publications Committee; Eben Alexander, Jr., M.D., for preparing the Foreword; Carol-Lynn Brown and Marjorie Kidd Keating of the Williams & Wilkins Company, and Carl H. Hauber and Gabrielle J. Loring of the American Association of Neurological Surgeons for coordinating various phases of the project; Sherylyn Cockroft and Gloria K. Wilkins for secretarial help; members of the Publications Committee for innumerable suggestions; and Diane Abeloff for overseeing the entire artwork.

SETTI S. RENGACHARY
ROBERT H. WILKINS

Contributors

CHAD D. ABERNATHEY, M.D.
Neurosurgeon
Department of Neurosurgery
Iowa Medical Clinics
Cedar Rapids, Iowa

A. LELAND ALBRIGHT, M.D.
Associate Professor
Department of Neurosurgery
University of Pittsburgh School of Medicine
Pittsburgh, Pennsylvania

OSSAMA AL-MEFTY, M.D.
Professor of Neurosurgery
University of Mississippi Medical Center
Jackson, Mississippi

RICHARD P. ANDERSON, M.D.
Chief Resident
Department of Neurosurgery
West Virginia University Hospitals
Morgantown, West Virginia

EHUD ARBIT, M.D.
Associate Attending Surgeon
Neurosurgery Service
Department of Surgery
Memorial Sloan-Kettering Cancer Center
New York, New York

ISSAM A. AWAD, M.D.
Vice Chairman
Department of Neurological Surgery
The Cleveland Clinic Foundation
Cleveland, Ohio

DANIEL L. BARROW, M.D.
Associate Professor
Department of Neurosurgery
Emory University School of Medicine
Atlanta, Georgia

JOSHUA B. BEDERSON, M.D.
Resident
Department of Neurosurgery
University of California, San Francisco
San Francisco, California

WILLIAM O. BELL, M.D.
Associate Professor
Department of Neurosurgery
Bowman Gray School of Medicine
    of Wake Forest University
Winston-Salem, North Carolina

EDWARD C. BENZEL, M.D.
Professor and Chief
Division of Neurosurgery
University of New Mexico School of Medicine
Albuquerque, New Mexico

DERALD E. BRACKMANN, M.D.
Clinical Professor of Otolaryngology
University of Southern California
    School of Medicine
Los Angeles, California

MICHAEL N. BUCCI, M.D.
Resident
Section of Neurosurgery
University of Michigan Medical Center
Ann Arbor, Michigan

KIM J. BURCHIEL, M.D.
Professor and Head
Division of Neurosurgery
Oregon Health Sciences University
Portland, Oregon

AANS Publications Committee

PAUL J. CAMARATA, M.D.
Resident
Department of Neurosurgery
University of Minnesota
Minneapolis, Minnesota

CHRISTOPHER E. CLARE, M.D.
Chief Resident
Department of Neurosurgery
Emory University School of Medicine
Atlanta, Georgia

RALPH B. CLOWARD, M.D.
Clinical Professor
Department of Neurosurgery
John A. Burns School of Medicine
University of Hawaii
Honolulu, Hawaii

CURTIS A. DICKMAN, M.D.
Chief Resident
Division of Neurological Surgery
Barrow Neurological Institute
Phoenix, Arizona

DONALD F. DOHN, M.D.
Chairman
Department of Neurological Surgery
The Cleveland Clinic Florida
Fort Lauderdale, Florida

JAMES FICK, M.D.
Resident
Department of Neurosurgery
University of Cincinnati Medical Center
Mayfield Neurological Institute
Cincinnati, Ohio

EUGENE S. FLAMM, M.D.
Charles Harrison Frazier Professor and Chairman
Division of Neurosurgery
University of Pennsylvania School of Medicine
Philadelphia, Pennsylvania

EDDY GARRIDO, M.D.
Private Practice
Lancaster, Pennsylvania

SARAH J. GASKILL, M.D.
Resident
Division of Neurosurgery
Duke University Medical Center
Durham, North Carolina

FRED H. GEISLER, M.D., PH.D.
Clinical Assistant Professor
Department of Surgery
Division of Neurosurgery
The Shock Trauma Center of the Maryland
    Institute for Emergency Medical Service
    Systems and the University of Maryland
Baltimore, Maryland
Chief of Neurosurgery
Department of Neurosurgery
Patuxent Medical Group
Columbia, Maryland

ATUL GOEL, M.CH.
Fellow
Center for Cranial Base Surgery
Department of Neurosurgery
University of Pittsburgh School of Medicine
Pittsburgh, Pennsylvania

JAMES T. GOODRICH, M.D., PH.D.
Director, Division of Pediatric Neurosurgery
Leo Davidoff Department of Neurological Surgery
Albert Einstein College of Medicine
Montefiore Medical Center
Bronx, New York

DAVID J. GOWER, M.D.
Assistant Professor
Division of Neurosurgery
University of Oklahoma Health Sciences Center
Oklahoma City, Oklahoma

STEPHEN J. HAINES, M.D.
Associate Professor
Division of Pediatric Neurosurgery
Department of Neurosurgery
University of Minnesota
Minneapolis, Minnesota

CRAIG D. HALL, M.D.
Institute of Plastic and Reconstructive Surgery
Albert Einstein College of Medicine
Montefiore Medical Center
Bronx, New York

SAMUEL J. HASSENBUSCH, M.D., PH.D.
Section Head
Neuro-Pharmacologic Oncology
    and Pain Management
The Cleveland Clinic Foundation
Cleveland, Ohio

PATRICK W. HITCHON, M.D.
Professor
Division of Neurosurgery
The University of Iowa Hospitals and Clinics and
    Department of Veterans Affairs Medical Center
Iowa City, Iowa

JULIAN T. HOFF, M.D.
Professor and Chair
Section of Neurosurgery
University of Michigan Medical Center
Ann Arbor, Michigan

HAROLD J. HOFFMAN, M.D.
Professor of Surgery
Division of Neurosurgery
University of Toronto;
Chief of Neurosurgery
The Hospital for Sick Children
Toronto, Ontario, Canada

ROBERT S. HOOD, M.D.
Clinical Assistant Professor
Division of Neurosurgery
University of Utah College of Medicine
Salt Lake City, Utah

EDGAR M. HOUSEPIAN, M.D.
Professor
Department of Clinical Neurological Surgery
College of Physicians & Surgeons
Columbia University;
Attending Neurosurgeon
New York Neurological Institute
Columbia-Presbyterian Medical Center
New York, New York

JOHN A. JANE, M.D.
Professor and Chairman
Department of Neurosurgery
University of Virginia Health Sciences Center
Charlottesville, Virginia

HOWARD H. KAUFMAN, M.D.
Professor and Chairman
Department of Neurosurgery
West Virginia University Hospitals
Morgantown, West Virginia

PATRICK J. KELLY, M.D.
Professor
Department of Neurologic Surgery
Mayo Medical School
Rochester, Minnesota

LEE KESTERSON, M.D.
Assistant Professor
Division of Neurosurgery
University of New Mexico School of Medicine
Albuquerque, New Mexico

PHYO KIM, M.D.
Resident
Department of Neurologic Surgery
Mayo Clinic/Mayo Medical School
Rochester, Minnesota

MILAM E. LEAVENS, M.D.
Associate Professor and Chief
Department of Neurosurgery
The University of Texas M.D. Anderson
    Cancer Center
Houston, Texas

MICHEL F. LEVESQUE, M.D.
Division of Neurosurgery
UCLA Center for the Health Sciences and
    School of Medicine
Los Angeles, California

ARTHUR E. MARLIN, M.D.
Chief, Pediatric Neurosurgery
Vice Chairman, Pediatric Surgery
Santa Rosa Children's Hospital
San Antonio, Texas

MARK MAY, M.D.
Clinical Professor
Department of Otolaryngology—Head and
    Neck Surgery
University of Pittsburgh School of Medicine;
Director
Sinus Surgery and Facial Paralysis Center
Shadyside Hospital
Pittsburgh, Pennsylvania

DAVID C. McCULLOUGH, M.D.
Chairman
Department of Neurological Surgery
Children's Hospital
Washington, D.C.

DENNIS E. McDONNELL, M.D.
Associate Professor
Department of Surgery
Section of Neurosurgery
Medical College of Georgia
Augusta, Georgia

ARNOLD H. MENEZES, M.D.
Professor and Vice Chairman
Division of Neurosurgery
The University of Iowa Hospitals and Clinics
Iowa City, Iowa

FREDRIC B. MEYER, M.D.
Consultant
Department of Neurologic Surgery
Mayo Clinic
Rochester, Minnesota

FOAD NAHAI, M.D.
Professor of Surgery
Department of Plastic and Reconstructive Surgery
Emory University School of Medicine
Atlanta, Georgia

W. JERRY OAKES, M.D.
Associate Professor
Division of Neurosurgery
Department of Surgery;
Assistant Professor
Department of Pediatrics
Duke University Medical Center
Durham, North Carolina

BURTON M. ONOFRIO, M.D.
Professor
Department of Neurologic Surgery
Mayo Clinic/Mayo Medical School
Rochester, Minnesota

JOHN A. PERSING, M.D.
Professor
Department of Neurosurgery;
Associate Professor and Vice-Chairman
Department of Plastic Surgery
University of Virginia Health Sciences Center
Charlottesville, Virginia

JOSEPH H. PIATT, JR., M.D.
Head, Pediatric Neurosurgery Section
Division of Neurosurgery
Oregon Health Sciences University
Portland, Oregon

PREM K. PILLAY, M.D.
Consultant
Singapore General Hospital
Singapore
Fellow
Department of Neurological Surgery
The Cleveland Clinic Foundation
Cleveland, Ohio

JOSEPH RANSOHOFF, M.D.
Professor and Chairman
Department of Neurosurgery
New York University Medical Center
New York, New York

MICHAEL P. SCHENK, M.S.
Director of Medical Illustration
University of Mississippi Medical Center
Jackson, Mississippi

SYDNEY S. SCHOCHET, M.D.
Professor of Pathology, Neurology, and
    Neurosurgery
Department of Pathology (Neuropathology)
West Virginia University Hospitals
Morgantown, West Virginia

LALIGAM N. SEKHAR, M.D.
Associate Professor
Center for Cranial Base Surgery
Department of Neurosurgery
University of Pittsburgh School of Medicine
Pittsburgh, Pennsylvania

JATIN SHAH, M.D.
Attending Surgeon
Head and Neck Service
Department of Surgery
Memorial Sloan-Kettering Cancer Center;
Professor
Cornell University Medical College
New York, New York

ROBERT R. SMITH, M.D.
Professor and Chairman
Department of Neurosurgery
University of Mississippi Medical Center
Jackson, Mississippi

STEVEN M. SOBOL, M.D.
Private Practice
Decatur, Illinois

VOLKER K. H. SONNTAG, M.D.
Vice Chairman
Division of Neurological Surgery
Barrow Neurological Institute
Phoenix, Arizona
Clinical Associate Professor
Division of Neurosurgery
Department of Surgery
University of Arizona College of Medicine
Tucson, Arizona

THORALF M. SUNDT, Jr., M.D.
Professor and Chairman
Department of Neurologic Surgery
Mayo Medical School
Rochester, Minnesota

EDWARD TARLOV, M.D.
Department of Neurosurgery
Lahey Clinic Medical Center
Burlington, Massachusetts

JOHN M. TEW, Jr., M.D.
Professor and Director
Department of Neurosurgery
University of Cincinnati Medical Center
Mayfield Neurological Institute
Cincinnati, Ohio

GEORGE T. TINDALL, M.D.
Professor and Chairman
Department of Neurosurgery
Emory University School of Medicine
Atlanta, Georgia

TADANORI TOMITA, M.D.
Associate Professor of Surgery (Neurosurgery)
Northwestern University Medical School;
Assistant Head
Division of Pediatric Neurosurgery
Children's Memorial Hospital
Chicago, Illinois

VINCENT C. TRAYNELIS, M.D.
Assistant Professor
Division of Neurosurgery
The University of Iowa Hospitals and Clinics and
    Department of Veterans Affairs Medical Center
Iowa City, Iowa

ROBERT H. WILKINS, M.D.
Professor and Chief
Division of Neurosurgery
Duke University Medical Center
Durham, North Carolina

CHARLES B. WILSON, M.D.
Tong-Po Kan Professor and Chairman
Department of Neurosurgery
University of California, San Francisco
San Francisco, California

ERIC J. WOODARD, M.D.
Assistant Professor
Department of Neurosurgery
Emory University School of Medicine
Atlanta, Georgia

RONALD F. YOUNG, M.D.
Professor and Chief
Division of Neurological Surgery
University of California, Irvine
Irvine, California

Contents

PERCUTANEOUS RADIOFREQUENCY RHIZOLYSIS FOR TRIGEMINAL NEURALGIA

JAMES FICK, M.D.
JOHN M. TEW, JR., M.D.

INTRODUCTION

Medically intractable trigeminal neuralgia, an incapacitating pain, can be eliminated by a percutaneous stereotactic rhizotomy. A review of 1000 procedures performed by the senior author documents that 91% of patients obtain complete relief of their pain with mild to moderate sensory loss.

The facial pain caused by this disorder is likened to an electrical current coursing through the nerve. This excruciating sensation occurs in regions innervated by the trigeminal nerve. The characteristic lancinating bursts of pain are provoked by speaking, a change in facial expression, or even a gentle breeze striking the face. The pain is intense. It may strike with the fury of a summer thunderstorm. It is common for patients to withdraw to a sheltered environment, shunning food and conversation. In the worst cases, despair builds to the point that threats of suicide are common.

The initial treatment of patients with trigeminal neuralgia is pharmacologic. Drugs with anticonvulsive properties rather than analgesic ones are most effective. Carbamazapine (Tegretol) can provide partial to complete resolution of the symptoms in most patients for several months. Diphenylhydantoin (Dilantin) is a less effective option. Patients treated with these drugs should be followed closely because hematologic abnormalities, hepatic dysfunction, and allergic reactions occur with variable frequency. A patient who does not tolerate one of these medications should be tried on the other or on baclofen (Lioresal). Serum levels should be monitored especially if high doses of drug are needed to control the pain.

The pain of trigeminal neuralgia is characterized by a fluctuating course which, in the early stages, often spontaneously resolves. The medication can then be tapered and discontinued. Drug therapy should be reinstituted during periods of exacerbation. The pain is easily controlled initially, but symptoms become more intractable to medication as remissions become less frequent. Relief can be achieved only by larger volumes of drugs and drug combinations. Unwanted side effects (lethargy and confusion) or toxic complications ultimately lead most patients to consider other forms of treatment. For most patients, selective interruption of the nociceptive fibers is the best form of surgical therapy. Our experience documents that radiofrequency thermocoagulation of the pain fibers at the level of the posterior root is a very safe and effective procedure. The percutaneous stereotactic rhizotomy (PSR) should be the first procedure considered for patients with proven trigeminal neuralgia. Structural causes of trigeminal neuralgia should be excluded by an imaging procedure. Magnetic resonance imaging or high resolution computed axial tomographic scanning are the preferred techniques for evaluation.

Patients are frequently evaluated for this procedure while they are suffering from incapacitating pain. They may have been unable to eat or sleep for several days and often appear exhausted and dehydrated. They may demonstrate symptoms of excessive narcotic consumption or of toxic levels of the anticonvulsant medication. In these circumstances, hospital admission for a careful assessment of the general medical condition may be required.

OPERATIVE PROCEDURE

Oral intake is restricted six hours prior to the procedure. Atropine (0.4 mg intramuscularly) to reduce the oral secretions and prevent bradycardia during sedation is administered one hour prior to the procedure. An intravenous line is required for the injection of an anesthetic medication.

The procedure is performed in the diagnostic radiology suite. Figure 1 demonstrates how the equipment and personnel are arranged. The patient lies on the table in a supine position. The surgeon stands to the patient's right and must be able to control the radiofrequency generator and view the fluoroscopy monitor. A qualified nurse or anesthesiologist stands on the opposite side of the surgeon in order to administer the intravenous anesthetic agent methohexital (Brevital) and observe the blood pressure utilizing an external monitor.

A reference electrode is placed over the deltoid region of the arm. Alternatively, a 21-gauge spinal needle may be inserted in the subcutaneous tissue. Rare reports of skin burns occurring with the use of a needle has led some authorities to recommend grounding pads with an area of 150 cm² for use as the reference electrode. The cheek of the affected side is prepared with an antiseptic solution.

The procedure is begun with a lateral cinefluorography (cine) radiographic view of the skull base. This view should clearly demonstrate the sella turcica and the clivus. A bolus of methohexital (Brevital) (30–50 mg) is injected intravenously prior to placing the needle into the foramen ovale. A 19-gauge stainless steel needle insulated to the tip with Teflon is shown in Figure 7.

Three anatomical landmarks are used to guide the needle placement. Marks are placed on the skin: 1) 3 cm lateral to the oral commissure; 2) on the lower eyelid at the medial aspect of the pupil; and 3) 3 cm anterior to the external auditory meatus. These landmarks are shown in the *inset* of Figure 2. In learning how to perform this procedure, the junior author has found it helpful to use these landmarks to plot the proper trajectory for the placement of the needle into the foramen ovale. This anterior approach allows the surgeon to place the needle in the medial aspect of the foramen ovale by aiming at the intersection of the coronal plane 3 cm anterior to the external auditory meatus with the sagittal plane centered at the medial aspect of the pupil. Figure 2 depicts how these planes intersect at the foramen ovale at the base of the skull. On the *inset* of Figure 2 the *vertical hatched line*

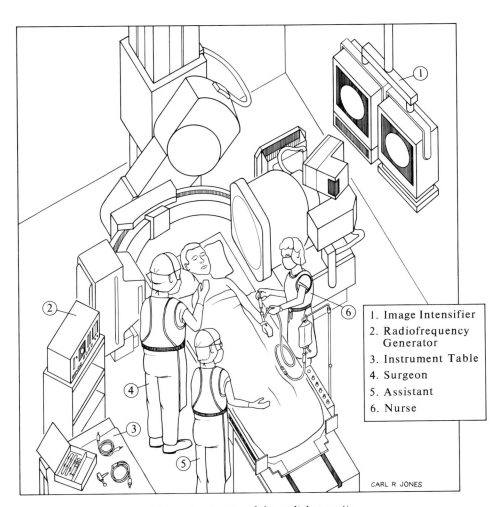

1. Image Intensifier
2. Radiofrequency Generator
3. Instrument Table
4. Surgeon
5. Assistant
6. Nurse

CARL R JONES

Figure 1. Set-up of the radiology suite.

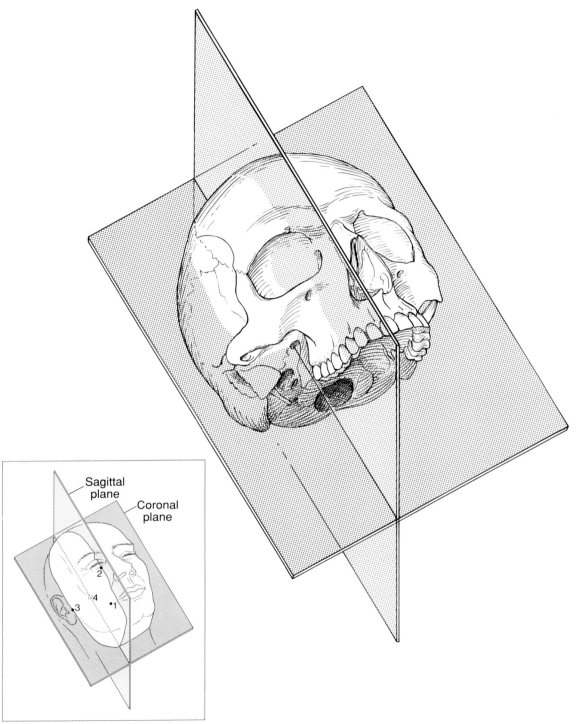

Figure 2. Artistic depiction of the method used to plot the location of the foramen ovale at the point of the intersection of the sagittal plane projecting from the medial aspect of the pupil and the coronal plane projecting from 3 cm anterior to the external auditory meatus. The *vertical hatched line* is the intersection of the planes at the foramen ovale which is labeled *4. Inset, 1* needle entry point; *2,* medial pupillary point; *3,* a point 3 cm anterior to the external auditory meatus; *4,* foramen ovale.

represents the intersection of these planes and depicts the relationship of the landmarks on the skin to the foramen ovale. This helps a surgeon who has not performed a large number of these procedures to visualize where the needle tip is to be directed.

Figures 3 and 8 illustrate how the needle is inserted. The cannula enters the skin 3 cm lateral to the oral commissure, as depicted in Figure 2, and is guided along the buccal surface toward the target. The surgeon's gloved index finger, placed in the patient's mouth with its tip inferior to the lateral pterygoid wing, is used to guide the cannula into the foramen ovale. The finger prevents penetration of the oral mucosa by the tip of the cannula, the occurrence of which would introduce the risk of meningitis.

A lateral view of the skull base is obtained with an image intensifying device to assist in the needle placement. The tip is directed toward the clival line as depicted in Figure 4. This trajectory permits the needle to be advanced into the foramen ovale which is signaled by a brief contraction of the masseter muscle. This results from a motor response when the needle stimulates the motor fibers of the mandibular nerve at the entrance of the foramen ovale. The needle placement is confirmed by a lateral image. The tip of the needle should be located along the clivus at a point 5–10 mm below the floor of the sella turcica. Figure 5 is a demonstration of this fluoroscopic view with the needle properly positioned. This approach of utilizing the lateral skull view to direct the needle tip toward a

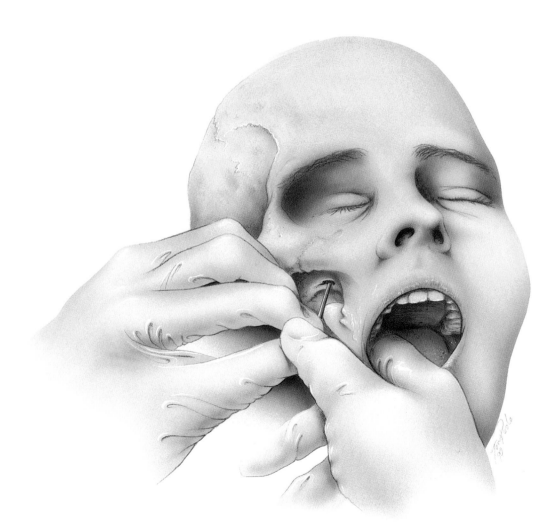

Figure 3. Demonstration of the technique used to place the needle in the foramen ovale. The surgeon's finger is shown inferior to the lateral pterygoid wing and guides the needle tip toward the foramen while preventing penetration of the oral mucosa.

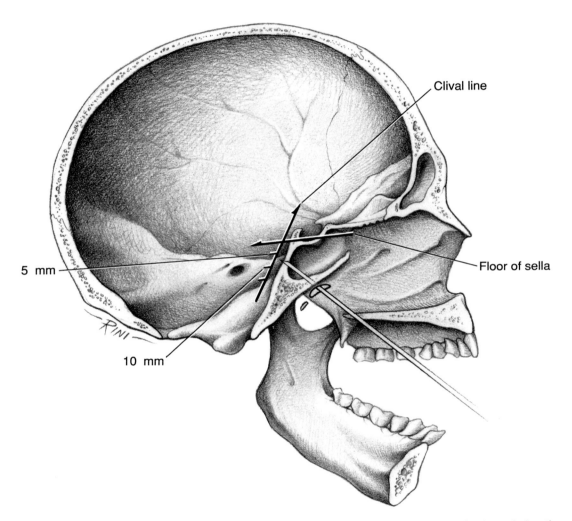

Figure 4.   This depicts how the needle should be directed at a point on the clival line 5–10 mm below the floor of the sella turcica.

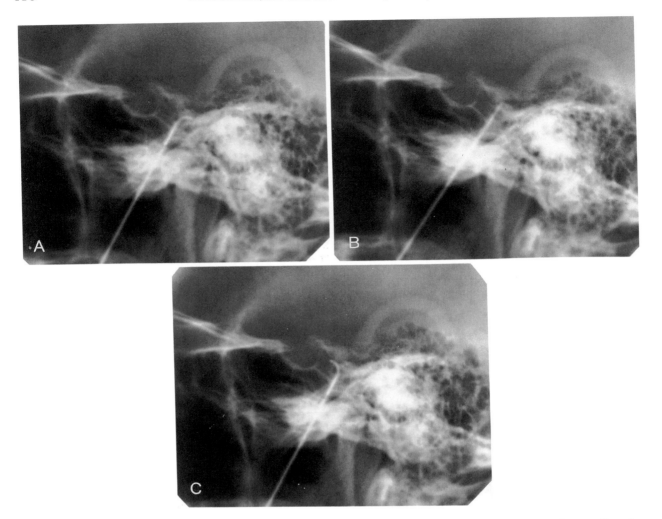

Figure 5. Fluoroscopic images used to guide the electrode placement. The electrode tip is shown positioned in each of the three divisions: mandibular division (**A**); maxillary division (**B**); ophthalmic division (**C**).

selected point along the clivus is preferred by the senior author. The proper needle trajectory can be aimed and the needle then reliably placed in the foramen ovale by using the landmarks obtained from the lateral skull image (Fig. 6).

The stylet is removed to ensure that the carotid artery has not been penetrated. If pulsatile blood flow is obtained, the needle is withdrawn and manual pressure is applied over the posterior pharyngeal space. During this phase of the procedure the carotid artery can be injured at three locations: 1) In attempting to penetrate the foramen ovale, a posteromedial deviation can result in the needle piercing the cartilaginous covering of the foramen lacerum. 2) Upon entering the middle cranial fossa, an inferior and medial trajectory of the needle can penetrate the carotid artery where it lies behind the mandibular nerve. 3) Finally, if the cannula is directed in the region of the first 5 mm of the clival line below the floor of the sella turcica, the

carotid can be pierced in the cavernous sinus where a carotid cavernous fistula may be created.

The needle is advanced to a point even with the profile of the clivus. Removal of the stylet will allow the egress of cerebrospinal fluid (CSF) unless the subarachnoid space has been obliterated by a previous rhizotomy or chemical injection (Fig. 9). A flexible electrode is inserted into the cannula. The Radionics TEW KIT cannula permits the use of either a straight or curved-tip electrode. The curved-tip electrode allows one to refine the lesion production during the procedure and has resulted in a substantive reduction of the side effects of this procedure. The curved electrode tip is a coil spring which carries a thermocouple, a stimulator, and a lesion-generating probe into the tissue at the end of the cannula. An insertion tool is used to insert the electrode into the cannula (Fig. 7). The guide of the insertion tool is aligned with the slot in the cannula (Fig. 9). The curved-tip electrode is guided

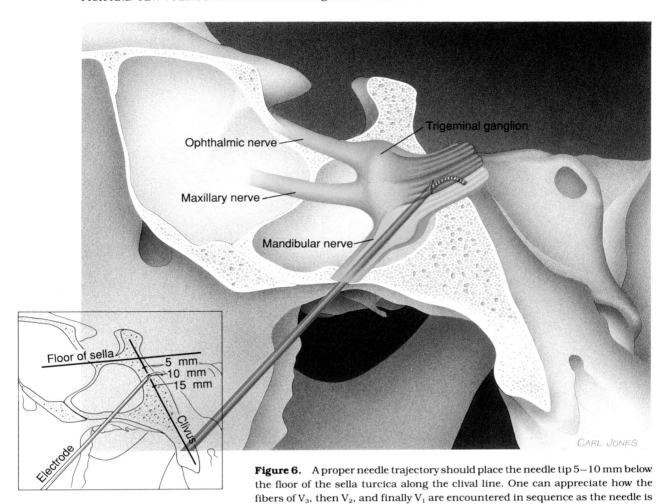

Figure 6. A proper needle trajectory should place the needle tip 5–10 mm below the floor of the sella turcica along the clival line. One can appreciate how the fibers of V_3, then V_2, and finally V_1 are encountered in sequence as the needle is advanced toward the clivus.

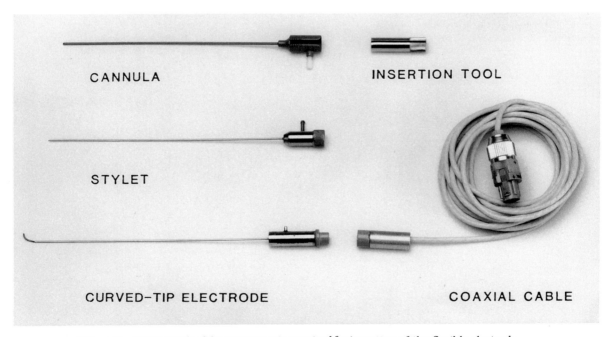

Figure 7. Photograph of the components required for insertion of the flexible electrode.

into the cannula (Fig. 10). The insertion tool is removed and the electrode is pushed to the hub of the cannula (Fig. 11). The exposure of the electrode tip can be controlled by a millimeter scale on the cannula's hub. A plastic clip is attached to the cannula where it enters the skin to prevent advancement of the cannula into the cranium. The electrode is then connected to the radiofrequency generator by a coaxial cable (Fig. 12).

Several models of the radiofrequency generator are available for use. The specific operation procedures for each model should be obtained from the operator's manual. Each model provides the ability to measure stimulation parameters (frequency, pulse wave) and lesion data (voltage, amperage, and temperature) at the tip of the electrode during the administration of the radiofrequency current to the nerve. The older models require a thermocouple adapter if the Tew curved electrode is to be used. The newest digital model, RFG-3C, is currently used (Fig. 13).

Physiologic localization of the electrode tip is determined by the patient's response to electrical stimulation. The needle is located, for descriptive purposes, in relationship to the profile of the clivus. Generally, the mandibular division of the root is encountered 5 mm proximal to the clivus, V_2 is located at the clivus, and V_1 is 5 mm distal to the clivus (Fig. 6). The precise placement is confirmed by stimulus-provoked paresthesia and provocation of pain. The pain and paresthesias originate from the characteristic trigger point and radiate into the dermatome where symptoms occur. This response can be elicited by a stimulus with the following parameters: 1 ms, 100–400 mV, and 50 Hz. A higher voltage, 0.5–1.5 V, may be required in patients who have undergone previous rhizotomy procedures or chemical injections. Increas-

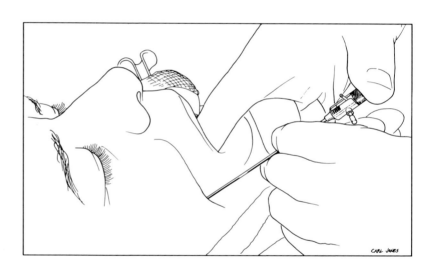

Figure 8. The technique of needle placement. A gauze-padded bite block is shown.

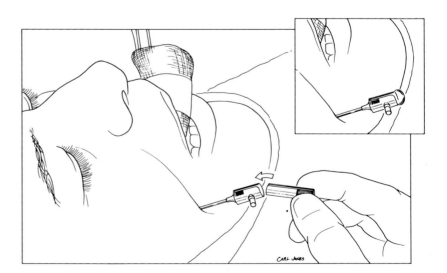

Figure 9. Placement of the insertion tool into the cannula. The *inset* demonstrates how CSF may drip from the cannula when the stylet is removed.

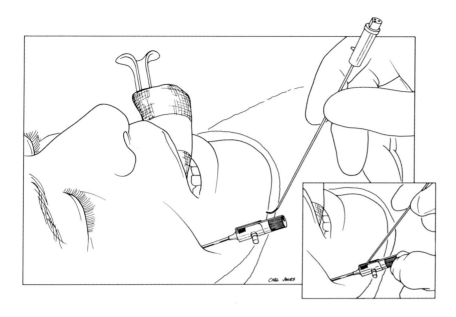

Figure 10. Placement of the curved tip electrode into the cannula.

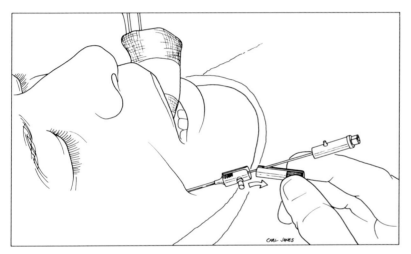

Figure 11. Removal of the insertion tool.

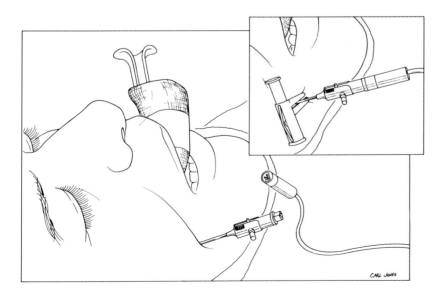

Figure 12. Connection of the coaxial cable to the electrode. The *inset* demonstrates how the electrode is secured against the skin with a plastic clip.

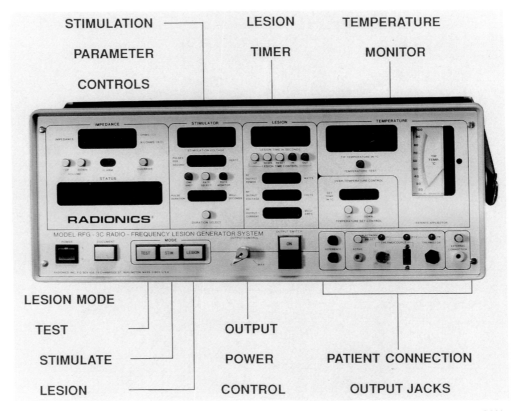

Figure 13. Photograph of the RFG-3C radiofrequency generator (Radionics Inc., Boston, MA).

ing stimulus voltage can reliably reproduce both the character and location of the pain. Pain or paresthesia should be obtained, sequentially, in the third, the second, and finally the first division of the nerve. This sequential response ensures the best chance of alleviating the pain without producing undesired sensory loss in unaffected regions of the face.

If paresthesia or pain is not provoked in the expected distributions when a low stimulus threshold is used, the cannula should be advanced, the electrode reinserted, and the stimulation repeated. The flexible tip electrode provides distinct advantages over the straight tip electrode during the needle localization for stimulation. Rotation of the flexible tip 180° along the long axis of the electrode enables one to reposition the tip to the V_3 division fibers caudally or to the V_1 division fibers by rotating the cannula cephalad. This maneuver can be accomplished without requiring that the cannula be withdrawn or advanced (Fig. 14).

Contractions of the masseter and pterygoid muscles may occur at a low stimulation threshold. The needle should be repositioned in a more lateral trajectory to limit the involvement of the motor fibers. Stimulus-evoked facial contractions indicate that the electrode is either too deep or is inclined too low on the clivus, or the stimulation level is too high.

If movements of the eyes occur during stimulation, the needle is too deep and the oculomotor, trochlear, and abducens nerves are at risk for injury if a lesion is produced. Diplopia can result from injury to these nerves along their course in the cavernous sinus at the medial aspect of Meckel's cave. This complication should be avoided if the needle is not advanced more than 5 mm beyond the clival line. Movement of the eyes indicates that the cannula is too deep in the cavernous sinus or too near the brain stem. The electrode must be repositioned and the stimulation performed again.

When an acceptable electrode placement is confirmed by stimulation, a second dose of intravenous anesthetic is injected and a preliminary lesion is produced at 65°C for 60 seconds. During the heating of trigeminal rootlets a facial blush will frequently appear in the trigeminal division which is being heated. Although this observation does not permit the precise localization of the site of sensory denervation, the observation can help to avoid unwanted sensory loss in an adjacent division. This concept is particularly important in preventing denervation of the corneal surface if the neuralgia has not involved the ophthalmic division.

After the intravenous anesthetic agent dissipates in 120–180 seconds, a careful sensory examination of

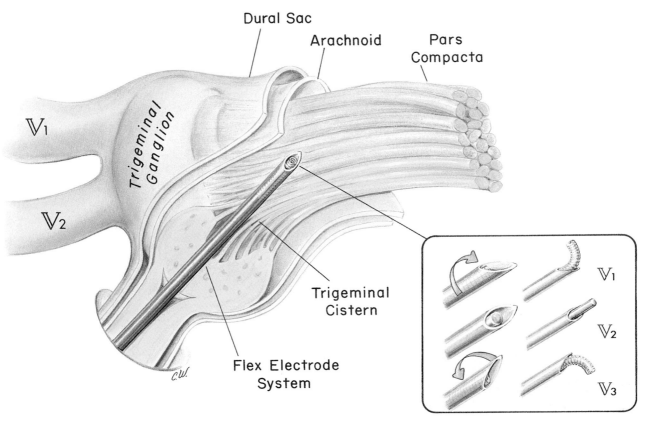

Figure 14. Artistic demonstration of the trigeminal ganglion which demonstrates how the curved-tip electrode can be positioned in each division of the nerve without changing the depth of the cannula.

the face should be performed. The targeted area for sensory impairment is determined by the division of the trigeminal nerve involved, the severity of the symptoms, and preoperative discussions with the patient. These considerations enable us to determine the extent of deficit best suited for each clinical situation. The lesion should be extended if pain persists after the initial coagulation, even if sensory deficits have been produced. Sequential lesions, produced by 60- to 90-second applications, are performed by increasing the temperature by 5°C increments until the desired result is achieved. This goal can frequently be achieved without additional intravenous anesthesia. Consequently, it is possible to have the patient's cooperation with the sensory examination in order to monitor the sensation of the cornea and face and to prevent the spread of sensory loss to undesired locations.

The results of the cranial nerve examination are recorded immediately after the procedure and at the time of dismissal, which usually occurs within 24 hours. Patients are allowed to resume normal activities following the procedure. A diet consisting of soft food and liquids is advisable for several days while the patient becomes accustomed to any change of oral and facial sensation or weakness of the muscles of mastication. Occasionally a hematoma of the cheek may occur at the needle insertion site. Corneal sensitivity is protected with artificial tears and frequent observation.

Detailed instructions concerning early symptoms of corneal abrasion and concerning eye care are given to each patient. Every patient and family must understand that any symptoms of corneal abrasion require prompt ophthalmologic evaluation. Anticonvulsant medication should be gradually withdrawn to avoid symptoms of agitation.

CONCLUSIONS

Percutaneous stereotactic rhizotomy is a very effective procedure for eliminating the painful symptoms of medically intractable trigeminal neuralgia. The goal is to coagulate the nerve fibers responsible for generating the pain impulses while minimizing sensory loss over the areas of the face not involved with the neuralgia. Using technical developments such as the curved electrode and increasing experience, the complications can be limited to a very acceptable level. The precision of lesion production and minimal surgical complications allow this procedure to be offered as a valid option for all patients with trigeminal neuralgia. The low morbidity and effective results justify selection of this procedure for most older patients for whom major intracranial procedures offer greater risk.

EXTENDED COSTOTRANSVERSECTOMY

EDDY GARRIDO, M.D.

INTRODUCTION

Thoracic spinal cord compression due to lesions located anteriorly or anterolaterally in the spinal canal cannot safely be managed with the standard laminectomy approach because any significant manipulation of the spinal cord will likely lead to paraplegia. Other surgical approaches have been developed over the years to enter the spinal canal from an anterior or posterolateral direction. Thoracotomy, costotransversectomy and its various modifications, and the transpedicular approach are the different ways in which these lesions can be removed with a low risk of spinal cord damage. Each one of these approaches has advantages and disadvantages and its selection depends on the experience of the surgeon. It is not within the scope of this paper to compare each of these surgical procedures.

I have had experience with a modification of the costotransversectomy approach to the thoracic spine in a series of 18 patients. The lesions surgically treated were as follows:

Herniated thoracic disc	8 cases
Fracture, vertebral body	4 cases
Large neurofibroma	2 cases
Metastatic tumor	3 cases
Epidural abscess	1 case

The radiographic diagnosis is made with x-ray films of the thoracic spine, computed tomography (CT) scans, and magnetic resonance imaging (MRI) scans. The MRI scan is probably the best imaging modality for the thoracic cord and has, for the most part, replaced the use of myelography.

SURGICAL PROCEDURE

The procedure is done with the patient under general anesthesia. A Foley catheter is inserted. Ancef (cefazolin), 1 g intravenously, is given just prior to beginning surgery as a prophylactic antibiotic. The patient is placed in the prone position on the operating table with the chest and abdomen resting on rolls. The arms are tucked along the sides of the patient. The procedure is usually done on the patient's left side unless the lesion is to the right of the midline which mandates a right-sided approach. The approach from the left is technically easier for the right-handed surgeon. The operating table should permit the use of anteroposterior x-ray films or fluoroscopy for localizing purposes.

After the patient has been positioned on the operating table, the appropriate rib to be resected is identified by radiography and/or fluoroscopy and marked with methylene blue. One needs to remember that the lower rib will lead to the desired disc space. For instance, the head of the 8th rib will articulate with the T7-T8 disc space; however, the 11th and 12th ribs articulate just below the disc space (Fig. 1).

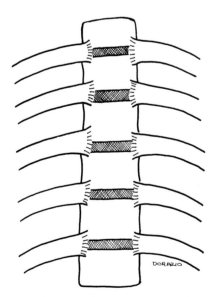

Figure 1. This diagram shows a segment of the thoracic spine to indicate the anatomic relationship of the ribs with the vertebral bodies and intervertebral discs. The 11th and 12th ribs, however, attach to the vertebral body just below the disc space.

Either of two types of skin incision can be used depending on the lesion to be dealt with (Fig. 2). An oblique incision following the rib to be resected and extending across the midline is preferred for relatively localized lesions such as herniated discs or neurofibromas or other focal neoplasms. In more extensive lesions and particularly in traumatic cases with fractured vertebral bodies where there is the need to do a fusion procedure with instrumentation, then a T-shaped incision is best. This will allow the surgeon to resect several ribs and expose the spinal column at multiple levels.

With either incision, the surgeon continues by transecting the trapezius or latissimus dorsi muscle depending on the level of the thoracic spine. The paraspinal muscles are exposed, separated subperiosteally from the laminae, and transected and retracted superiorly and inferiorly. To minimize bleeding, the muscle section is best done with the electrosurgical knife. The ribs, laminae, facet joints, and transverse processes are visualized at this point (Figs. 3 and 4). The proximal 5–6 cm of the selected rib is resected after stripping off the periosteal covering as well as any other soft tissues. The transverse process and the head of the rib

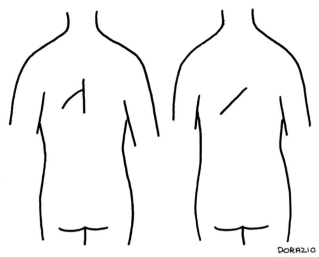

Figure 2. This diagram shows the patient positioned prone on the operating table. **Left,** the T-shaped incision is used when a more extensive exposure is needed such as for those cases requiring anterior decompression of the canal and a posterior fusion with instrumentation. **Right,** the oblique incision is used more frequently and gives adequate exposure for removal of herniated discs, dumbbell neurofibromas, and localized epidural abscesses.

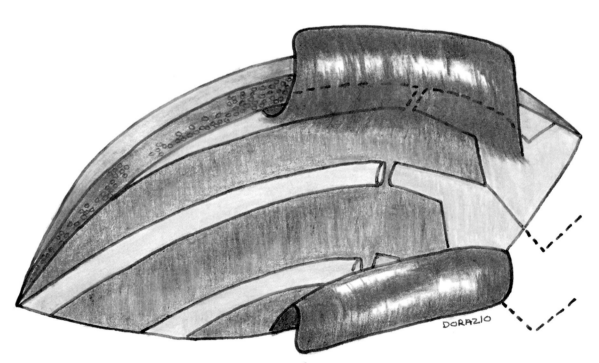

Figure 3. This drawing illustrates the initial approach with section of the trapezius or latissimus dorsi muscle and the paraspinal muscles and exposure of the laminae, transverse process, and rib.

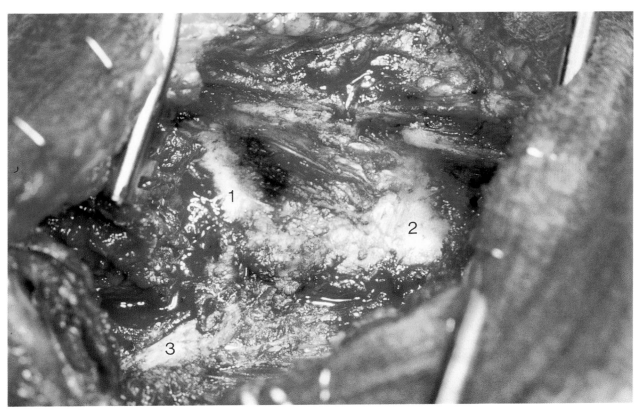

Figure 4. Operative photograph showing the exposed laminae (*1, 2*) and the rib (*3*). A right-sided approach was made in this case.

are then removed. The spinal canal is exposed by doing a complete unilateral hemilaminectomy of the two adjacent laminae. The facet joint is removed entirely. The lateral aspect of the dural sac and spinal cord is seen at this point (Figs. 5 and 6). The disc space can be seen and palpated. The pleura is easily separated from the lateral wall of the vertebral bodies and disc space and is retracted laterally (Fig. 6). The nerve root and intercostal neurovascular bundle which has been separated from the rib is left intact whenever possible.

The operation then proceeds according to the pathological lesion (Fig. 7). For a herniated disc, it is best to drill out the pedicles and adjacent vertebral bodies next to the disc, therefore creating a cavity where the disc material could be curretted down and extracted without manipulation of the spinal cord (Fig. 8). Similarly, bony fragments in the anterior aspect of the spinal canal can be removed by thinning it down with the high-speed drill and by downward pressure with downward angled currettes. Tumors can also be easily removed under direct visualization of the dural sac. In cases of neurofibroma, the dura should be opened to remove the intraspinal portion of the tumor. With this exposure there is a clear view of the anterior and lateral aspects of the dural sac, the nerve root, the disc, and the vertebral bodies. The operating table can be rotated 10–15° away from the surgeon to facilitate the view under the dural sac. After removal of the herniated disc or vertebral body fragments one could use the ultrasound imaging equipment to check

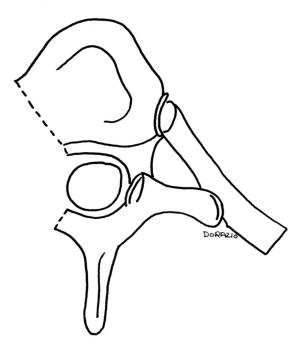

Figure 5. Axial view of the thoracic spine which demonstrates the unilateral removal of the rib, transverse process, pedicle, laminae, facet joint, disc, and part of the adjacent vertebral bodies.

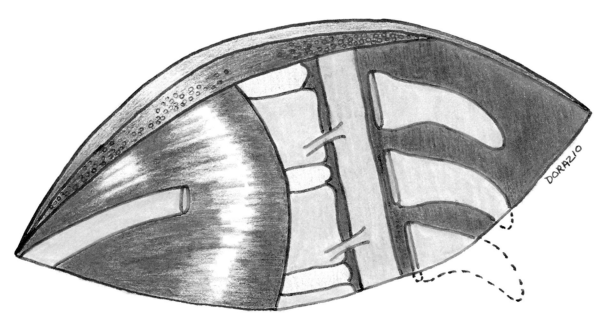

Figure 6. This drawing shows the lateral wall of the dural sac, part of the vertebral bodies, and the intervertebral discs. At this stage of the operation the laminae, facet joint, transverse process, and part of the rib have been resected. The pleura is easily retracted from the lateral wall of the spine.

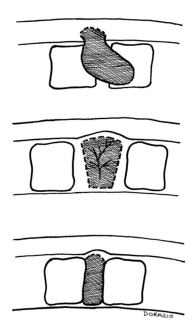

Figure 7. This illustration shows the three most common lesions that are managed with the extended costotransversectomy approach. **Top,** dumbbell neurofibroma. **Middle,** fractured vertebral body with bone fragments in the spinal canal. **Bottom,** herniated disc.

the area to be certain that no disc or bone fragments have been missed. The arthroscope with an angle camera can also be used to look under the dural sac. A fiberoptic headlight and $\times 3.5$ magnifying surgical glasses are extremely useful for adequate visualization. The high-speed air drill is essential.

Spinal cord evoked potential monitoring has not been used in any of these patients during surgery. The value of such monitoring is somewhat controversial. This surgical exposure gives such a clear, direct view of the dural sac that the surgeon does not have to move or manipulate the spinal cord to remove the pathological lesion.

To close the wound, the different muscles and fascial layers are approximated with heavy sutures. A Jackson-Pratt drain is used for 24 hours postoperatively. No problem with wound healing has been encountered in any case.

COMPLICATIONS

Possible complications are wound infection, pneumothorax, spinal cord damage from direct manipulation or from ischemia due to ligation of a radicular artery, and spinal instability. The only complication in this group of 18 cases has been that of a wound infection which was treated with drainage and appropriate antibiotics.

If there is a significant tear in the pleura, it would be best to use a chest tube for 24 hours. Neurologic deficits are avoided if one is careful not to manipulate

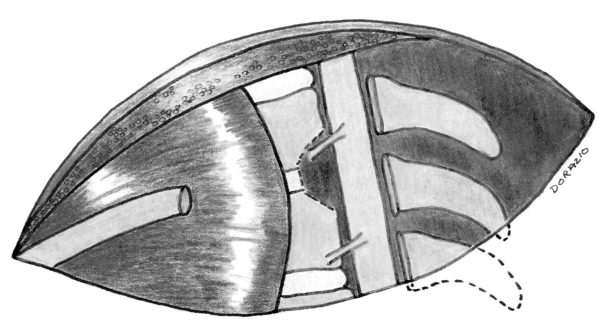

Figure 8. This illustration shows the defect left after removal of the disc and adjacent areas of the vertebral bodies. The nerve root is left intact in most cases.

the spinal cord. Ischemic neurologic complications could occur if a major radicular artery to the spinal cord is ligated along with the nerve root. Given the extensive and multiple radicular blood supply to the spinal cord, the potential for this complication to occur is low and it is not necessary to sacrifice the nerve root and radicular blood supply in most cases. No instances of spinal instability have occurred from the limited bony removal with this procedure.

SUMMARY

The extended costotransversectomy or posterolateral approach to the thoracic spine is an excellent way to treat pathological lesions anterior to the spinal cord. There is no need to enter the thoracic cavity; therefore, a chest surgeon's assistance is not necessary. Herniated thoracic discs, large dumbbell neurofibromas, metastatic spinal cord tumors, abscesses, and traumatic bone fragments are the usual pathologic lesions that can be managed with this surgical approach. In traumatic cases where a posterior fusion with instruments is needed, it is done at the same time as the decompression.

SURGICAL RESECTION OF POSTERIOR FOSSA EPIDERMOID AND DERMOID CYSTS

LEE KESTERSON, M.D.

INTRODUCTION

Intracranial epidermoid and dermoid tumors are uncommon lesions that account for less than 2% of intracranial tumors in most series. The ratio of intracranial epidermoids to dermoids is 4:1 with epidermoid tumors typically becoming symptomatic during the third and fifth decades whereas dermoids tend to occur in the pediatric age group.

Aberrant closure of the dorsal neural tube is thought to account for the occurrence of these congenital, histologically benign lesions. Epidermoid tumors tend to occur off the midline in a more lateral location while dermoid tumors occur near the midline. In the posterior fossa the typical location of epidermoid tumors is the cerebellopontine angle, petrous apex, cerebellum, and fourth ventricle. Dermoids are reported to occur more frequently in the region of the fourth ventricle and may communicate with the skin via a sinus tract. The midline location of these tumors is due to the fact that the neuroectoderm separates dorsally along the midline. The lateral occurrence of epidermoid tumors is possibly due to proliferation of multipotential embryonic cell rests or the transplantation of epithelial rests carried laterally with the migrating otic vesicles or developing neurovasculature.

Dermoid and epidermoid tumors are frequently referred to as inclusion tumors because their growth occurs by progressive desquamation of the capsular components. Generally these are considered benign lesions; however, there have been rare instances of malignant degeneration. The only difference between these two lesions is the histology. The cyst lining of an epidermoid is composed of a capsule of stratified squamous epithelium. Dermoid cysts not only contain this element but also dermal derivatives such as hair and sebaceous glands. Because of the presence of these latter elements, dermoids are firmer and lack the pearly appearance that is characteristic of epidermoid tumors.

These lesions are confined to the extraparenchymal area and can literally "flow" into any available subarachnoid space, crossing cisternal and compartmental boundaries. These masses can insinuate themselves between cranial nerves and vascular structures, and into the exit foramina of the fourth ventricle, sulci, and fissures. Because the growth is slow and the included elements are soft and pliable, an inclusion cyst tends to conform to the shape of the cavities it enters, with symptoms resulting from compression, distortion, and/or obstruction occurring long after the mass has attained a very large size. Furthermore, the neurologic symptoms initially may be vague and nonspecific with periods of waxing and waning similar to those described for demyelinating disease.

Epidermoid and dermoid tumors of the posterior fossa present with headaches, disequilibrium, and/or cranial nerve involvement. These lesions may also present with the classic symptoms and signs of hemifacial spasm or trigeminal neuralgia. Another form of presentation is that of cyst rupture which allows spillage of keratinous material into the cerebrospinal fluid (CSF) spaces with the subsequent development of aseptic meningitis.

PREOPERATIVE EVALUATION

The main radiologic imaging modalities utilized now are computed tomography (CT) and magnetic resonance imaging (MRI). Contrast agents are generally used as is the case in the evaluation of most intracranial masses. The use of these modalities is complementary because of the effectiveness of MRI in demonstrating anatomical detail in the posterior fossa and CT for its value in delineating bone anatomy.

With CT the attenuation value of an epidermoid cyst is usually very low (-20 to $+30$ Hounsfield units); however, there have been some lesions reported with attenuation values somewhat higher (80–120

Hounsfield units). This range of attenuation values has been thought to be due to varying amounts of low-density lipid and high-density keratin in the desquamative debris of the tumor. Certainly, this debris can be visualized in the subarachnoid space if the cyst has ruptured. Very uncommonly, calcification is noted in the capsule of an epidermoid tumor. Dermoid tumors have similar radiologic findings but have a greater range of attenuation values with more frequent association with calcification and with developmental anomalies of the skeleton. Neither tumor enhances to a great extent with contrast infusion.

Epidermoids usually have prolonged relaxation times on both T_1 and T_2 weighted images on MRI. On the other hand, dermoid tumors have variable relaxation times depending upon the amount of fat present but commonly have short T_1 and prolonged T_2 relaxation times. The extent of tumor growth is probably better detected by MRI because of the lack of bone artifact.

PREOPERATIVE PREPARATION

The occurrence of postoperative aseptic meningitis following resection of posterior fossa tumors, especially inclusion tumors, is well known; consequently, the routine perioperative use of steroids for resection of these lesions seems reasonable. However, the use of perioperative antibiotics continues to be controversial in clean neurosurgical procedures. Although the mastoid air cells are frequently entered when attempting to gain far lateral exposure, these air cells are usually considered to be sterile. The use of antibiotics is probably justified in those cases involving reoperation, when there has been a history of mastoid disease, or following radiation therapy. If an antibiotic is used, a third generation cephalosporin may be considered because of its ability to cross the blood-brain barrier and also provide broad-spectrum antibacterial coverage.

OPERATIVE PROCEDURE

The best positioning for the surgical procedure depends on the experience of the surgeon and anesthesiologist, the location of the lesion, and the medical condition of the patient. I utilize the prone and lateral positions for resection of almost every posterior fossa lesion except for midline lesions for which I tend to use the sitting position (Fig. 1A). In the sitting position it is important to have a precordial Doppler monitor to detect venous air emboli as well as to have central venous access to aspirate such emboli.

When resecting lesions in proximity to the seventh nerve, it is important to consider monitoring seventh nerve function intraoperatively. There are monitoring devices on the market which make an audible tone when the nerve is being manipulated. This provides an on-line monitoring system so that the surgeon can be warned on his proximity to the nerve.

The placement of the scalp incision and the craniectomy site is predicated by the location of the mass. Midline lesions are typically resected via a medial suboccipital craniectomy whereas lesions occurring in the cerebellopontine (CP) angle can be resected via a lateral retromastoid suboccipital craniectomy. Because of the growth characteristics and the consistency of these lesions, a single-staged operation is all that is required for resection. For example, as the tumor grows it expands the subarachnoid space; consequently, a "channel" is created as the center of the tumor is removed which allows further exposure allowing easier resection even in regions not routinely available via a specific approach. A single-staged resection, however, requires careful preoperative planning with the aid of modern imaging modalities.

Fourth Ventricular Tumors

Midline lesions, particularly those located in the fourth ventricle, are best approached by the classically described suboccipital craniectomy (a craniotomy can often be performed easily instead of a craniectomy, especially in younger patients). Because of the superiorly directed angle of the axis of the fourth ventricle, fourth ventricular tumors are frequently best approached with the patient in the sitting position, which allows both surgeon comfort and adequate visualization. The scalp incision of the midline suboccipital craniectomy extends approximately 3–4 cm superior to the inion with the inferior extension to the level of approximately C-4 (Fig. 1B). To achieve scalp hemostasis, disposable Raney clips are used. Placement of these clips above the level of the superior nuchal line is relatively easy; however, sharply undermining the subcutaneous tissue below this level aids in their application.

The median avascular plane is then dissected with the aid of a needle tip cautery. Although initial dissection of the soft tissues in this region is performed with a needle point cautery, a broad, flat periosteal elevator and Metzenbaum scissors are used in the latter aspects of the exposure. It must be emphasized that only 1.5 cm of lateral exposure is required at the level of C-1 and the foramen magnum, which lowers the risk of vertebral artery injury.

During the dissection in the region of the occipital bone, foramen magnum, and C-1 lamina, venous bleeding is commonly encountered, requiring bone wax, gentle tamponade, or meticulous use of the bipolar cautery for control. It is imperative to properly address each bleeding source because one cannot safely operate in this region under a "pool" of blood. Furthermore, sources of air embolism must be elimi-

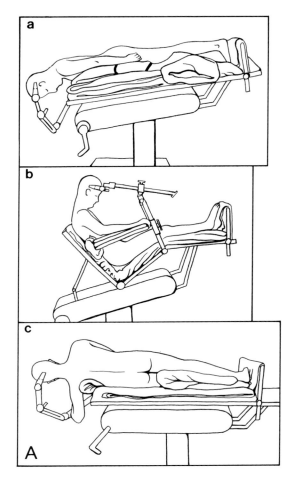

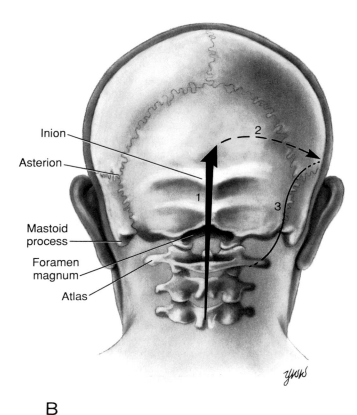

Figure 1. **A,** the various positions that are available for resection of a posterior fossa lesion. The prone position (a) is good for caudally located posterior fossa and craniocervical junction lesions; the sitting position (b) is especially good for vermian lesions; and the lateral ("park-bench") position (c) is good for laterally located hemispheric lesions and cerebellopontine angle lesions. in the lateral position, the vertex of the head should not be angled toward the floor too greatly be- cause of the potential for venous obstruction. Note the importance of padding pressure points and avoiding excessive neck flexion (the latter is also important in preventing venous obstruction). **B,** the various scalp incisions that are available for approaching the different regions of the posterior fossa. One incision not depicted is a vertical incision that is located midway between the inion and mastoid, which gives good visualization of laterally located lesions.

nated whether the patient is in the prone or sitting position.

As this region is progressively exposed, Weitlaner (curved) self-retaining retractors are utilized to provide adequate exposure and the delineation of dissection planes. Once the soft tissue dissection is completed, one Miskimmons cerebellar self-retaining retractor usually provides adequate exposure. To begin the craniectomy, burr holes are created with either an air-powered perforator or a Hudson brace—at least one being placed on each side of the midline which will avoid encountering a persistent occipital dural sinus. Then double-action (Leksell) and/or single-action (Adson) rongeurs are used to perform the craniectomy. The craniectomy is carried to the level of the transverse sinus superiorly, through the foramen magnum inferiorly, and near the mastoid process on each side. The removal of the bone in the region of the superior nuchal line is facilitated by thinning the cranium with the use of a Midas Rex pneumatic drill. For the vast majority of lesions located superior to the foramen magnum, a C-1 laminectomy is not required.

A Y-shaped dural incision is then created with the superolateral incisions being carefully carried to the level of the transverse sinus bilaterally and with the caudal extent of the midline incision being carried to near the level of the superior ring of the atlas (Fig. 2A). A persistent occipital sinus may be encountered when making this incision; consequently, it must be appropriately suture-ligated (with new imaging modalities, metal ligature clips should be avoided; furthermore, good suture techniques are usually easier to use).

Once the dura has been adequately opened and retracted, the cisterna magna is incised to allow drainage of CSF and brain relaxation. Once the incision of the arachnoid of the cisterna magna is completed, lateral retraction of the cerebellar tonsils will allow entrance into the caudal region of the fourth ventricle (Fig. 2B). Not infrequently the lesion is directly visualized at this point; however, completion of the exposure requires the incision of the caudal vermis providing access to the cephalad aspect of the fourth ventricle. It must be emphasized that total circumferential exposure of the lesion is not required at this point, but the lesion's relationship to the floor of the fourth ventricle must be identified. It is at this point that a cottonoid is *laid* onto the floor of the fourth ventricle to provide protection and to maintain identification of this cleavage plane during tumor dissection. At this point a "ribbon" retractor (0.5–0.75 inch in width) is attached to a Leyla retractor arm as a self-retaining retractor. Moreover, it frequently is easier to perform resection of a midline tumor if two Leyla retractors are utilized, with each providing retraction of a cerebellar tonsil and the adjacent lateral vermis to

the ipsilateral side. At this point the tumor capsule is opened generously and the "debulking" of the lesion is initiated (Fig. 3A). The debulking process allows the tumor mass to be more mobile and allow for a more atraumatic circumferential dissection. Debulking of an inclusion cyst can usually be performed adequately with a conventional sucker but the use of an ultrasonic aspirator will further facilitate this activity. The subsequent routine is not unlike the removal of other tumor types located adjacent to other vital neural and vascular structures in that the debulking process is repeatedly alternated with gentle circumferential dissection until the lesion is removed. In this particular instance, cottonoids are placed repeatedly as the cleavage plane with the floor of the fourth ventricle is extended. It cannot be overemphasized that the cottonoids are *not* to be used as dissecting tools; on the contrary, the lesion is either gently pulled away or sharply incised from its attachments (Fig. 3B).

Once the lesion is removed, the attainment of hemostasis is easily achieved with gentle tamponade with either cottonoids alone or in combination with Surgicel. When operating in the ventricular system, little or no Surgicel should be left in the tumor bed.

For lesions with lateral extension, a scalp incision that is a variant of the midline craniectomy incision is utilized. This involves an extension of the superior limb to a position at the level of the posterior aspect of the pinna with the cephalad extent being 1–2 cm superior to the superior nuchal line (Fig. 1B). This scalp incision gives excellent lateral exposure while maintaining access to the midline. A craniectomy is then created that extends from the midline to the sigmoid sinus laterally, with the superior extent being the exposure of the transverse sinus.

Cerebellopontine Angle Tumors

The removal of a cerebellopontine angle lesion is achieved by utilizing a paramedian retromastoid incision located 2–3 cm posteromedial to the mastoid process. This is a vertical incision that extends 3–4 cm cephalad to the superior nuchal line with the cephalad extension forming a gentle curve anteriorly to a level at the posterior aspect of the pinna. The caudal limb extends 7–8 cm inferior to the superior nuchal line with the caudal extension forming a gentle curve medially (Fig. 1B). The gentle curves in the incision create an S-shape which allows more lateral exposure than a conventional straight vertical incision. Again, the tissue is undermined approximately 1 cm on each side of the incision to allow placement of Raney clips. The periosteum and superficial muscles are dissected with the electrocautery and a periosteal elevator (a pericranial graft can be obtained easily at this time for later use for dural closure). The superficial muscula-

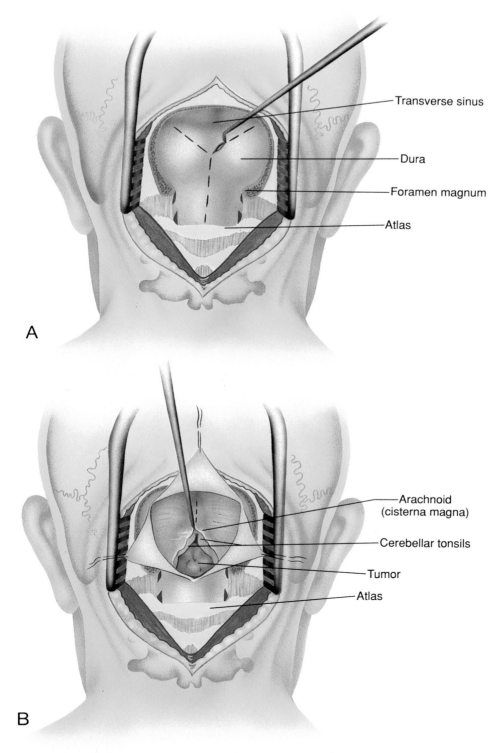

Figure 2. A, a suboccipital craniectomy has been performed and a Y-shaped dural incision is depicted with the superior limbs extending to the inferior aspect of the transverse sinus. The ring of the atlas is intact, with the posterior aspect of the foramen magnum having been removed. Note that one Miskimmons retractor is all that is usually required to provide soft tissue retraction. **B,** the dural incision has been completed and the dural leaves are retracted. The cisterna magna is opened with the fourth ventricular tumor visualized between the cerebellar tonsils.

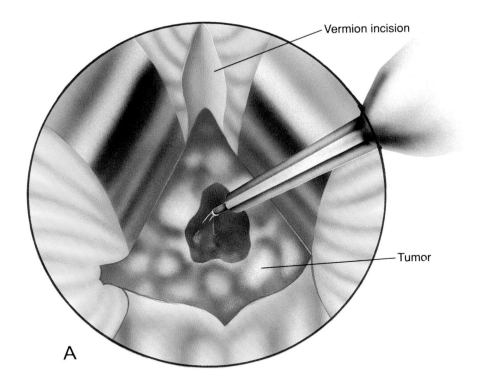

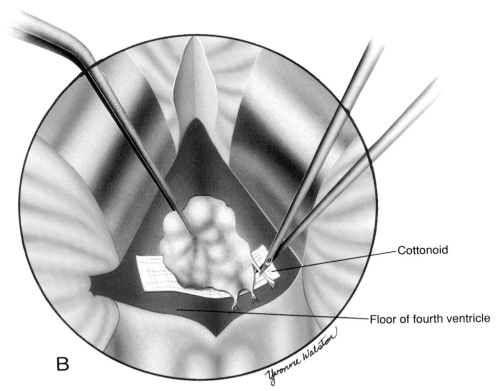

Figure 3. **A,** the debulking process has begun, with two retractors in place that retract the cerebellar tonsils. This process allows the mass to be more mobile, making its later dissection off of the floor of the fourth ventricle more atrauma-tic. **B,** the debulked mass is removed sharply from the floor of the fourth ventricle. Note the presence of a cottonoid that has been laid in the cleavage plane between the lesion and the fourth ventricular floor.

ture below the superior nuchal line (splenius capitis, trapezius, and sternocleidomastoid) are all that need be incised, with dissection of the deeper musculature (obliques and rectus capitis) being reserved for lesions at the level of the foramen magnum. The bony landmark for the inferior aspect of the soft tissue dissection is a small ridge that is referred to as the inferior nuchal line. The extracranial vertebral artery is located in a fatty triangle posterior to the arch of the atlas and usually is not exposed. A single Weitlaner retractor is usually all that is required for retraction of the soft tissues.

A craniectomy is created with the superior aspect of bone removal being carried to the asterion, the bony landmark of the junction of the transverse and sigmoid sinuses. The lateral extent of the bony removal involves exposure of the sigmoid sinus even if significant removal of the mastoid process is required. Generous use of bone wax is required to occlude the mastoid air cells and prevent CSF leakage. The medial extent of the bony removal is approximately 4–5 cm medial to the mastoid process.

A K-shaped dural incision is created with the base of each limb again based on a venous sinus (Fig. 4A). This incision is created in such a way that the cerebellar hemisphere remains covered with dura. The dura is sutured to the surrounding musculature to provide retraction.

With the aid of the operating microscope, the inferior cerebellopontine cistern is easily visualized by placing a retractor blade along the inferolateral aspect of the cerebellar hemisphere and retracting cephalad and slightly medially (Fig. 4B). The inferior cerebellopontine cistern is readily identified by following the spinal accessory nerve to the jugular foramen. The arachnoid is initially incised with a Beaver 5910 knife, with the extension of the dissection with bayoneted microscissors (the use of scissors is probably less traumatic than the use of the knife alone). There is no need to cauterize the arachnoid layer because it is avascular. The opening of this cistern provides brain relaxation as well as early identification of the lower cranial nerves (IX, X, and XI).

The capsule of the tumor is incised and debulked in a similar manner to that described for the resection of a fourth ventricular lesion (Fig. 5A). It is important to systematically identify the vascular and neural structures as the removal progresses because of the tendency of these lesions to insinuate themselves among these elements, making their location unpredictable (Fig. 5B). As the mass is made to be increasingly more mobile as the debulking process is performed, these critical structures are protected by laying a cottonoid onto them. It must be emphasized that the literature is unclear as to how much tumor or capsule removal is required to prevent the patient from having recurrent clinical problems. Even the most aggressive surgeons occasionally leave remnants of capsule behind. Consequently, aggressive dissection around the neural and vascular structures (especially the basilar artery and its small perforators) should be tempered by this fact.

In closing the wound, a watertight closure of the posterior fossa dura should be attempted, which may require the use of a patch graft. A multilayer closure of the paravertebral musculature and fascia is performed with an interrupted suturing technique.

OTHER SURGICAL ALTERNATIVES

There are multiple approaches to the resection of CP angle lesions. One that has been quite popular for almost three decades is the translabyrinthine approach, primarily used in the resection of acoustic neuromas. This is impractical, however, if the preservation of hearing is desired. Variations of this approach, such as the retrolabyrinthine trans-sigmoid approach, may be quite advantageous in those instances where a significant portion of the mass is located anterior to the brain stem. One of the limiting aspects of this approach is the continued need to dissect and remove tumor between cranial nerves VII and VIII.

Another modification that may be required of the standard paramedian suboccipital craniectomy is in the situation where there is significant tumor extending through the tentorial incisura. This lesion can be readily dealt with by extending the scalp incision and craniectomy a few centimeters above the transverse sinus. The dural opening will include incisions into both the supra- and infratentorial spaces, ligation of the transverse sinus, and incision of the tentorial incisura. Without a lot of work, this modification gives a tremendous amount of exposure to the incisura.

Another limitation of both of the previously described approaches is the sacrifice of the ipsilateral venous drainage. Consequently, a preoperative angiogram must be performed to delineate the collateral venous drainage before either of these maneuvers can be performed safely.

Petrous apex lesions may present a dilemma in regard to surgical approaches. The transcochlear approach could be an appropriate consideration if hearing is absent. If hearing is present, however, the transzygomatic-middle cranial fossa approach could be used, but the cochlea and the internal carotid artery must be avoided.

POSTOPERATIVE MANAGEMENT

It should be noted that even in the best of circumstances, a CSF fistula (usually presenting with rhinorrhea) or pseudomeningocele may occur and require an

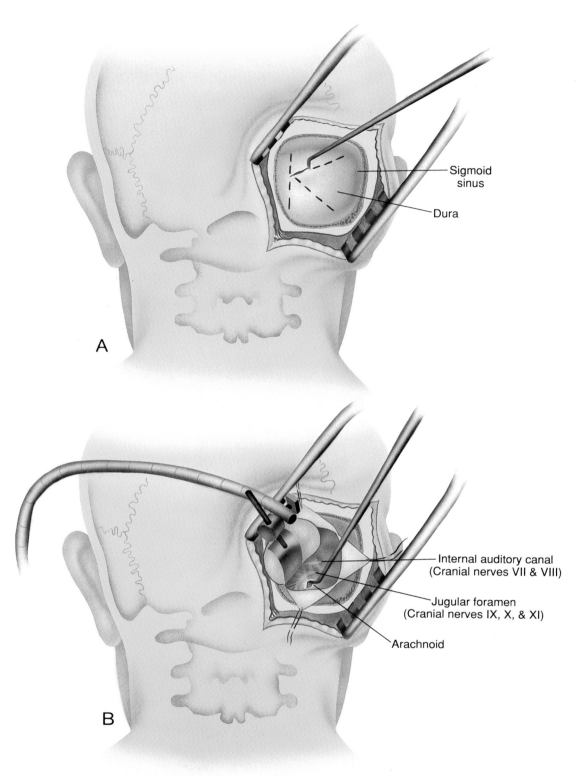

Figure 4. **A,** a lateral suboccipital craniectomy has been performed and a K-shaped incision has been initiated. The base of each limb is located at a venous sinus. Note that only one Weitlaner retractor is required to provide soft tissue retraction. **B,** a self-retaining Leyla retractor is lifting the cerebellar tonsil cephalad and slightly medially to expose the inferior cerebellopontine cistern. This is readily located by identifying the spinal accessory nerve and following it to the jugular foramen. This cistern is opened early in the dissection because it allows brain relaxation and identification of the lower cranial nerves. Note the caudal to cephalad direction of the arachnoid incision.

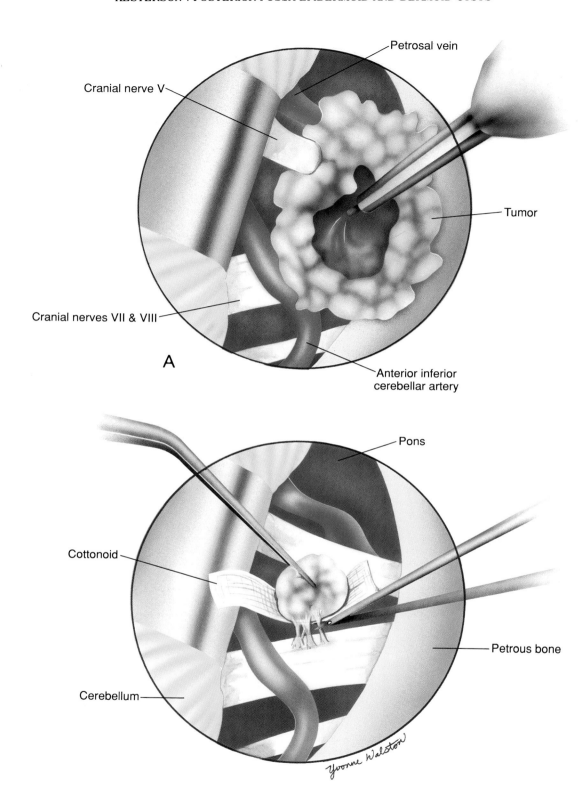

Figure 5. A, the debulking process has been initiated with the cranial nerves and vascular structures already identified as much as possible. The petrosal vein is usually cauterized and transected early in the procedure to prevent its inadvertent avulsion during the retraction of the cerebellum. **B,** the late stage of tumor removal is shown. At this point, the tumor has been debulked and is very mobile, allowing it to be sharply incised from the cranial nerves and arteries. Note that a cottonoid has been laid in the cleavage plane to maintain anatomical orientation as well as to provide protection to the neural and vascular structures.

open surgical repair. Whenever one of these two complications occurs, the presence of hydrocephalus must be considered. An initial trial of CSF drainage may be utilized for either problem because the impairment of CSF circulation that may occur after a posterior fossa tumor operation can be transient. Because each of these complications may allow enough CSF decompression to prevent the development of ventriculomegaly, the possibility of hydrocephalus developing following repair should also be considered.

The most frequency source of CSF leakage is the failure to completely occlude the mastoid air cells coupled with the lack of a good dural closure. When operating to repair a CSF fistula, the surgeon should address both aspects of the problem to minimize the need for further intervention.

Pseudomeningocele formation occurs most frequently because of a small dural rent where there is a "ball-valve" effect with the subsequent formation of an extradural collection of CSF. The repair of these lesions usually requires an open operation but this can be delayed if the suture line is not compromised.

Postoperative follow-up evaluations will always be required, particularly for those patients with a tumor of the cerebellopontine angle where fragments of the tumor capsule were left attached to cranial nerves and arteries. Because of the ability of these lesions to attain a large size prior to causing clinical symptoms, imaging studies must be incorporated into the follow-up evaluations. There has been no proven benefit to the adjuvant use of radiation therapy following resection of these inclusion cysts.

LUQUE ROD SEGMENTAL SPINAL INSTRUMENTATION

EDWARD C. BENZEL, M.D.

INTRODUCTION

The instrumentation of the unstable thoracic and lumbar spine has been revolutionized by the introduction of universal spinal instrumentation techniques. The surgeon's ability to rigidly instrument the spine in a relatively safe manner has thus been greatly enhanced. Specific circumstances exist, however, in which neither the "traditional approaches" such as Harrington distraction rod instrumentation techniques nor the "newer" universal spinal instrumentation techniques are ideal.

Sublaminar wire augmentation of Harrington distraction rod techniques has occasionally proven to be useful in some of these situations. It has been successfully applied in circumstances where the chance for instrumentation failure was high and simultaneously where the risk of application was outweighed by the benefits of increased stability. The sublaminar wire fixation allows for the acquisition of substantial "supplemental" stability and rigidity over that obtained with the Harrington distraction rod system alone. Anterior migration of sublaminar hooks into the spinal canal induced by ventral migration of the rod into approximation with the lamina by the sublaminar wires, however, can result in dural sac compression. This obviously decreases the impetus to place such a construct. Therefore, it may only be indicated when both distraction *and* multiple level segmental fixation are truly necessary.

Luque rod spinal instrumentation techniques, however, may be utilized effectively in patients in whom substantial spinal instability exists preoperatively and in whom the intraoperative acquisition of significant structural stability is desired. This technique usually requires the application of a long moment arm (lever arm) to the unstable segment in order to be effective. This dictates that the construct be fixed at least two to three spinal segments above and two to three spinal segments below the unstable segment.

The operative procedure, therefore, involves significant surgical manipulations at multiple levels. This, in turn, may require a prolonged operative time. These factors must be considered in advance of the surgery.

OPERATIVE INDICATIONS

Patients considered to be appropriate candidates for a Luque rod spinal segmental instrumentation procedure are those with thoracic and/or lumbar spine trauma or cancer who harbor a grossly unstable spine. Patients with substantial spinal deformities which defy correction by routine techniques are also candidates. The patient with a complete myelopathy (loss of all motor and sensory function below the level of the injury) and an accompanying unstable spine is a prime candidate for the Luque rod technique. This latter patient has both the structural criteria for the procedure (gross instability) and simultaneously is subjected to minimal neurologic risk from the placement of sublaminar wires (a complete myelopathy already exists). The risks of sublaminar wire placement are small but, nevertheless, ever present. The passage of the wire under the lamina obviously exposes the underlying dura mater to inadvertent compression. Furthermore, following the sublaminar passage of the wire, its manipulation prior to obtaining its security via twisting around the rod may result in ventral protrusion of the wire. This may result in wire impingement upon the dura mater. Great care, therefore, must be taken throughout nearly the entire operation with regard to wire manipulation and the potential for injury to the dural contents.

A patient with a fracture that is difficult to reduce is similarly an ideal candidate for the Luque instrumentation technique because it offers a better advantage for deformity correction than any other available technique. This advantage, however, is at the expense of its degree of difficulty and risk.

PREOPERATIVE PREPARATION

The patient is prepared for surgery and anesthesia is administered in a routine manner. The patient is positioned in a prone position on the operating table (although the three-quarters prone or lateral decubitus position may occasionally be used). Care should be taken to prevent abdominal compression. The utilization of generous rolls, special frames, or a variety of alternative positioning techniques may be helpful. The back is scrubbed and draped in a manner that allows both the exposure of the spinal midline and of the bone graft donor site (if necessary).

It is recommended that the anesthetic technique not include pharmacologic muscle paralysis. This allows for the detection of muscle contraction induced by iatrogenic neural trauma. If such is observed intraoperatively, the surgical manipulation which induced the event (such as the overaggressive passing of a sublaminar wire) should be avoided.

OPERATIVE TECHNIQUE

Preparation for Sublaminar Wire Passage

The desired length of the dorsal spinal midline is exposed in a subperiosteal manner. The interspinous ligaments, both above and below each lamina to be instrumented, are removed with a rongeur. This exposes the underlying ligamentum flavum. This structure, at each intersegmental level, is then penetrated. A curved curette is useful for this purpose. The underlying epidural fat and dura mater are thus exposed. A Kerrison rongeur is then used to enlarge the interlaminar space. The bone removal should not be extensive enough to weaken the construct by excessively diminishing the amount of laminar bone available for purchase by the construct. It, however, must be extensive enough to allow for a safe passage of the wire underneath the lamina itself. All potentially interfering soft tissue must be removed from the area so that the wires may be passed with ease and without interference from rough bony edges or soft tissue. This minimizes the chance for passing the wire onto the dural sac and its contents. Palpation for rough spots which may impede passage of the wire with a large nerve hook or Woodson instrument is recommended prior to passing the wires.

Sublaminar Wire Passage

A 10-inch length of 1.2-mm wire is looped to form two 5-inch double strands. The looped wire is then passed underneath the lamina in a caudad to cephalad direction (Fig. 1A). The passage of the wire is facilitated by using a sturdy needle holder. As the wire emerges from underneath the superior aspect of the lamina, its continued passage may be further facilitated by first gripping the wire with a sturdy nerve hook or Woodson instrument and then by using a second sturdy needle holder to pull the wire through. The wire is then cut with a wire cutter (Fig. 1B). This allows the utilization

of one-half of the wire on each side of midline. One must remember that the cutting of wires and the leaving of jagged metal edges increases the chances of glove tears or perhaps even skin cuts.

Two double strands of wire may be passed at each level so that the complete double strand may be used on either side of midline. This may occasionally be indicated if the wire is thought to be the weakest link in the construct complex.

It is my preference to always pinch the wires together over the lamina as illustrated in Figure 1C (*center*), so that inadvertent bumping of the wire does not cause its protrusion ventrally into the dural sac (Fig. 1C, *left*). It is also recommended that the surgeon develop a convention when placing the wires around the rods. My convention is that the cephalad aspect of the wire is located most medially and the caudal aspect of the wire most laterally, such that the wires go around the rods similarly at every level of the spinal column as illustrated in Figure 1D.

Fixation of the Rod to the Lamina

The rod on each side of midline is cut to the appropriate length with a bolt cutter and placed along the lamina. The wires are twisted around the rods (Fig. 1D). "L"-shaped rods are routinely used. The "L" shape aids in spine settling and prevention of rod rotation.

Reduction of Spinal Deformity

In fractures that are difficult to reduce, the Luque rod system is a particularly appropriate choice, especially in those situations where neither distraction nor compression is desired. Figure 2 illustrates a technique where the rod on one side of the spine is initially tightened at its caudal end and the rod on the contralateral side is simultaneously tightened at its cephalad end (the L end of the rod is the end which is initially tightened with this technique). The rods are then gradually secured by subsequently tightening the wires in sequence (Fig. 2B). As the wires are sequentially tightened, spinal alignment is gradually attained (Fig. 2, C and D). The most difficult of spinal deformities to reduce can be aligned with such a technique.

Special Considerations and Techniques

L-shaped rods should always be used. The L should pass across the midline though an interspinous space and underneath the straight aspect of the opposing rod (Fig. 3A). This prevents the dorsal protrusion of the L aspect of the rod and minimizes the chance that it will subsequently migrate.

Following the completion of the tightening of all wires, the bone fusion is placed. A ventral interbody

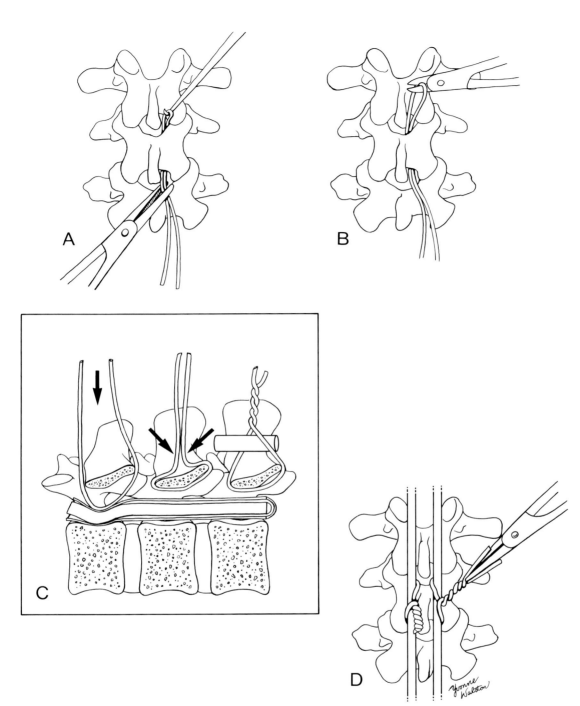

Figure 1. An illustration of some fundamentals of the application of Luque rod instrumentation. **A,** the passage of the looped 1.2-mm wire is facilitated by using a blunt-nosed needle holder, while its retrieval is facilitated by the use of a sturdy nerve hook or Woodson instrument. **B,** the cutting of the looped wire with a wire cutter is illustrated. This is performed in order to allow one-half of the wire to be used on each side of the midline. **C,** the potential for wire impingement onto the dural sac and its contents is illustrated on the *left* (*arrow* denotes the potential for ventral wire migration prior to tightening). This potential for neural compromise is present from the time the wire is passed underneath the lamina until it is tightened (twisted) around the rod (*right*). The wire may be crimped around the lamina in order to minimize its chance for causing injury during this aspect of the operation (*center; arrows* denote the crimping of the wire). **D,** a dorsal view of the relationship of the twisted wires to the rods. Note that superiorly the wires arise medial to the rods and caudally the wires arise laterally.

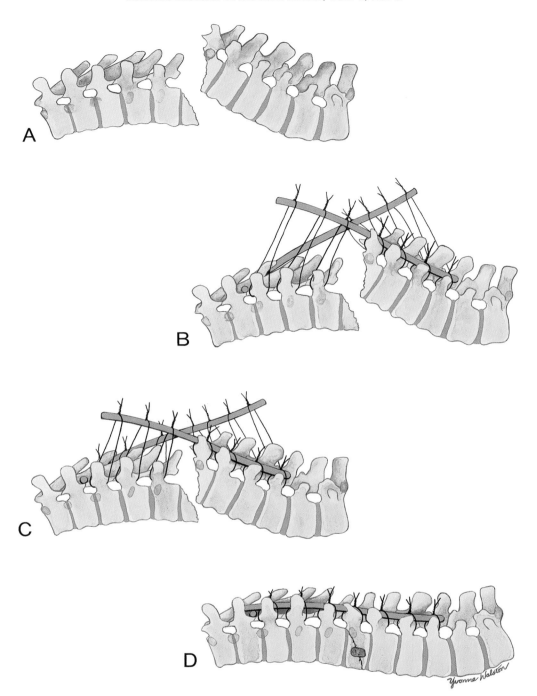

Figure 2. An illustration of the Luque rod technique as applied to the correction of gross spinal deformities. When a significant spinal deformity is present, as illustrated in **A,** closed or even open reduction of the spine may be very difficult. The open reduction of the deformity with the Luque rod instrumentation technique is facilitated, under these circumstances, by bone and soft tissue removal. This destabilizes the spine enough to allow for reduction. Subsequent fusion allows for the eventual acquisition of bony stability. Following the removal of the impediments to reduction and the passage of the sublaminar wires, the L rods are placed along the spine and cut to the appropriate length with a bolt cutter. The L end of each rod is placed through the most superior and inferior interspinous spaces, respectively. The wires are then twisted around the rods as illustrated in **B.** Beginning at the L end of each rod, the wires are gradually tightened (**C**) until acceptable alignment is obtained (**D**). Usually, a bony fusion is then performed. In **D,** an anterior fusion is illustrated. In patients with cancer, bony fusion may not be an acceptable alternative. In these cases, the chance for the acquisition of a solid bony fusion may be nil. An acrylic strut may be placed in selected cases. In others, no fusion at all may be appropriate.

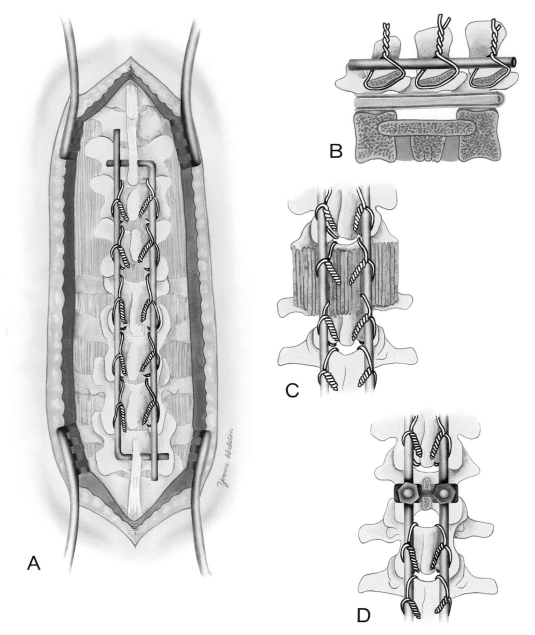

Figure 3. An illustration of some "final touches" with regard to the application of Luque rod instrumentation. A dorsal view of a Luque rod system in place is illustrated in **A.** Note the convention of the wires passing from caudad to cephalad in a lateral to medial direction. An opposite convention would be equally appropriate. Also note that the L aspect of each rod lies underneath the straight end of the contralateral rod. This prevents the dorsal rotation of the L end of the rod which could easily result in its cephalad or caudad migration. In **B,** the placement of a ventral interbody fusion is illustrated. The surgical approach used allowed for a more than adequate decompression of the dural sac prior to placement of the bony fusion. The extent of dissection also allowed for the destabilization of the spine prior to placement of the Luque rod system, thus facilitating the acquisition of appro- priate spinal alignment. Subsequent stability is initially gained via the acquisition of bony fusion. In **C,** a posterior fusion has been placed. A posterior fusion is used when ventral decompression of the dural sac is not necessary or when a more aggressive surgical approach (i.e., a ventral dural sac decompressive operation) is not warranted. In **D,** the placement of a rigid Luque Crosslink is illustrated. This allows for the acquisition of a more rigid construct. Of greater importance with the Luque rod technique, however, is that it virtually eliminates the chance for significant rod migration or rotation. Collapse of the Luque rod construct with time may occasionally occur secondary to the rods slipping through the wires. The Crosslinking technique prevents this.

fusion may be placed, either via an anterior, anterolateral, or lateral extracavitary approach (Fig. 3B). If a dorsal fusion is placed, the wires may be turned over the graft in order to assist in the attainment of its position and security (Fig. 3C). For most neurosurgical applications, the fusion of a short segment of the spine is indicated. Only if multiple level instability is present should a more extensive fusion be entertained. The wound is then closed in multiple layers, usually with absorbable sutures. It is the author's preference to not place a drain. A drain is not a substitute for the adequate acquisition of hemostasis. Furthermore, it encourages wound infection by allowing an avenue for the entrance of contaminating microorganisms. This is of particular significance in patients who have undergone the placement of hardware.

Evoked potential monitoring may be useful during the application of Luque rods, especially in cases where significant deformity correction is planned. It must be emphasized, however, that many surgeons (including the author) believe that the monitoring of intraoperative evoked potentials does not confer an element of safety. It, in fact, may be the source of anxiety for the surgeon, which, in turn, may lead to a suboptimally performed surgical procedure. Furthermore, once an alteration or obliteration of the evoked potential is observed, the neurologic injury is almost always already incurred. Further intervention is, therefore, unlikely to alter the outcome.

High-speed burrs may be used to assist in denuding the cortex of the dorsal spine in preparation for bone graft placement. Specialized wire twisters are useful for the uniform twisting of the wire. A rongeur or high-speed burr may be used to perform facetectomies at the level(s) of planned fusion. The greater the surface area for bony fusion, the greater the chance for the acquisition of bony union.

COMPLICATIONS

Infection, neurologic injury, non-union, and the inadequate acquisition of deformity correction are complications which may occur with any spinal instrumentation procedure. Strict adherence to standard neurosurgical operative techniques and to the specific techniques outlined here should minimize, but not eliminate, the incidence of these complications.

Loss of height of the construct is a complication which is particularly unique to Luque rod spinal instrumentation. The neutral nature of the Luque rod construct implies that it applies neither distraction nor compression to the spine. It, however, does allow for the sliding of the rods through the wire loops. This, in turn, allows for the sliding of each rod past its counterpart and a resultant settling of the spine. This latter phenomenon may be prevented by the application of Crosslinks (Fig. 3D). The Luque Crosslinking System is rigid and, therefore, eliminates the sliding action of the rods by making the right and left rod into a single functional unit. The application of Crosslinks also allows for the acquisition of a quadrilateral frame construct which substantially augments its rigidity.

EN BLOC ANTERIOR TEMPORAL LOBECTOMY FOR TEMPOROLIMBIC EPILEPSY

MICHEL F. LEVESQUE, M.D.

INTRODUCTION

The "Falconer-Crandall" resection of the anterior temporal lobe is performed in patients with medically intractable epilepsy of temporal lobe origin. This procedure has been demonstrated previously to be sufficient to achieve seizure control independent of intraoperative interictal spiking activity. The validity of this approach is based on the excellent seizure outcome after resection based on presurgical criteria of focal structural and functional abnormalities and, in selected patients, the results of invasive monitoring studies. The advantage of this technique is that it allows surgery under general anesthesia with the surgical microscope using sharp dissection to provide a "standard" surgical specimen. This approach has permitted scientific analysis of pathophysiological changes in temporolimbic structures and correlation with neuropsychological and seizure outcome.

PATIENT SELECTION

The majority of patients with medically intractable epilepsy will present with a focal seizure disorder. This group usually has stereotypical complex partial seizures with rare secondary generalization. Advances in neuroimaging and invasive neurophysiological studies with stereoelectroencephalography (SEEG) have led to a better understanding of the underlying focal epileptogenesis and focal pathology amenable to surgical treatment. Criteria for patient selection have thus been widened to include patients with several types of partial simple, partial complex, and secondarily generalized seizures. However, patients with chronic psychosis or severe mental retardation are usually excluded from surgical consideration. Surgery is performed in patients whose seizures have been medically intractable for at least two years unless there is evidence of a structural abnormality on magnetic reso-

nance imaging (MRI) which may indicate the site of seizure origin.

The en bloc anterior temporal lobectomy is one of several surgical approaches to temporolimbic and temporal lobe neocortical epilepsies. Patients with a documented seizure onset within the mesial temporal lobe may benefit from a smaller resection such as an amygdalohippocampectomy. Patients who present with evidence of an extrahippocampal structural lesion may in some cases benefit from resection of the lesion only. In most cases, however, the mesial temporal structures are involved in the seizure onset and propagation and present evidence of pathological changes. The most significant damage occurs in the hippocampus.

A potential risk of this surgery is to operate on a temporal lobe without sufficient evidence of seizure localization or without clearly documenting the ability of the contralateral hemisphere to support memory function. The purpose of the initial noninvasive evaluation (Phase I) aims at providing presumptive evidence of a focal cerebral origin of the seizure disorder. The strongest evidence is provided by recording stereotypical seizures by videotelemetry with scalp and sphenoidal electroencephalograms (EEGs). Several types of seizure onset are suggestive of temporal lobe involvement. The EEG can show an initial focal onset (Fig. 1), a delayed focal onset, or a regional pattern. A structural abnormality within the same temporal lobe seen with MRI is also a strong factor in the surgical decision-making process. Evidence of a focal functional deficit suggested by an area of hypometabolism using 18-fluorodeoxyglucose positron emission tomography also strongly suggests a limbic seizure to originate within the temporal lobe (Fig. 2). The results of neuropsychological tests demonstrating lateralized dysfunction have also been correlated with the site of seizure origin. The intracarotid amytal test (Wada test) helps to define the language representation in the cerebral hemispheres and also documents mem-

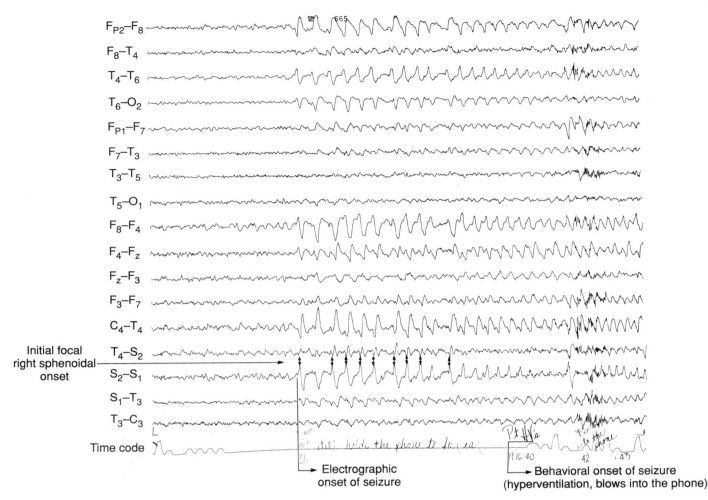

Figure 1. A spontaneous seizure captured on scalp and sphenoidal EEG leads in a patient with complex partial seizures. There is an initial focal onset at the right sphenoidal electrode.

ory deficit within the lobe involved and the ability of the contralateral lobe to support memory function. If the patient fails the memory test he is at an increased risk of developing global amnesia after resection of the epileptogenic focus.

If all evidence points to the same temporal lobe, the patient is then a candidate for an en bloc temporal lobectomy. However, if there is conflicting evidence from electrophysiological, radiological, or psychological testing, then the patient may have to undergo invasive intracranial recording (Phase II) to confirm the lateralized temporal lobe dysfunction. Because there is frequently evidence of bilateral temporal lobe involvement in seizure propagation and bilateral underlying pathological hippocampal changes, one single investigation should not be relied upon as the basis for a surgical decision.

PREOPERATIVE PREPARATION AND OPERATIVE PROCEDURE

After a complete neurological examination has been conducted and informed consent has been obtained, all documented evidence is reviewed with the patient and his or her family. Anticonvulsant levels are verified and maintained at an appropriate therapeutic value. In some cases, an additional load of anticonvulsants becomes necessary due to a decrease in levels postoperatively following anesthesia or due to decreased intake. Diphenylhydantoin is not routinely used as a loading agent prior to surgery.

Once of the patient is called to the operating room, he is given a dose of 10 mg of dexamethasone to decrease postoperative brain swelling. In addition, the patient receives a course of prophylactic antibiotic medication for the next 48 hours. After induction, the

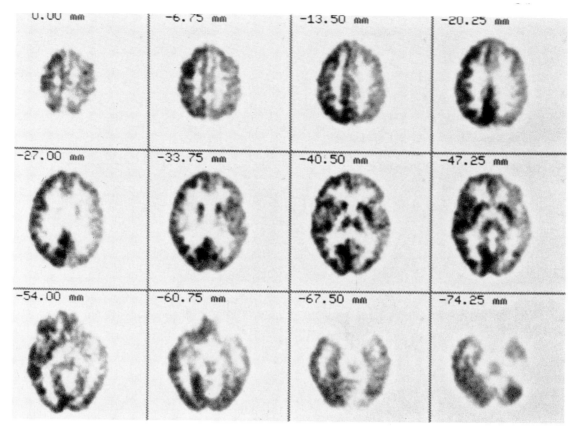

Figure 2. Interictal 18-fluorodeoxyglucose positron emission tomography in a patient with complex partial seizures of left temporal origin. There is significant relative hypometabolism involving the left temporal lobe and extending into the whole left hemisphere.

patient is given general anesthesia. An arterial line and Foley catheter are inserted. The patient is positioned supine with a small bolster under the ipsilateral shoulder, and the head turned to the side contralateral to the temporal lobe to be removed. The head is turned approximately 30° from the horizontal and the vertex is tilted inferiorly to bring the zygoma slightly above the level of the vertex (Fig. 3). The head is also maintained above the level of the right atrium to facilitate unobstructed venous drainage. The patient's hair is shaved in the operating room over the temporal, frontal, and parietal regions. A 10-minute scrub using slow-releasing iodophor solution is then applied. Sterile draping is placed in a standard fashion.

The incision line is then infiltrated with 1% lidocaine with 1/200,000 epinephrine. A question mark incision is used beginning 5 mm in front of the tragus at the level of the zygoma (Fig. 3). The incision is then curved at approximately 1 cm above the ear and extends posteriorly to the anterior aspect of the mastoid to curve superiorly toward the parietal region at approximately 5 cm from the midline. The incision is then carried anteriorly toward the frontal region just above the temporal line.

At first the scalp and galea are dissected and an attempt is made to preserve the superficial temporal artery. A subgaleal plane is easily defined and a skin flap is elevated and wrapped in a moist laparotomy sponge. The scalp is reflected forward with the use of fishhooks. The temporalis muscle is then incised longitudinally along the length of its fibers (Fig. 3). This allows a smaller amount of muscle bulk anteriorly at the area of the craniectomy and appears to minimize local jaw pain postoperatively. The temporalis muscle is detached anteriorly and posteriorly along its attachment to the superior temporal line. The muscle flaps are then reflected anteriorly and posteriorly and also retracted with fishhooks. Both frontal and temporal origins of the zygomatic arch are exposed.

A craniotomy is then created over the temporal and inferior frontal and parietal regions using a high-speed drill and craniotome. Two burr holes are usually placed, above and below the pterion, respectively. An

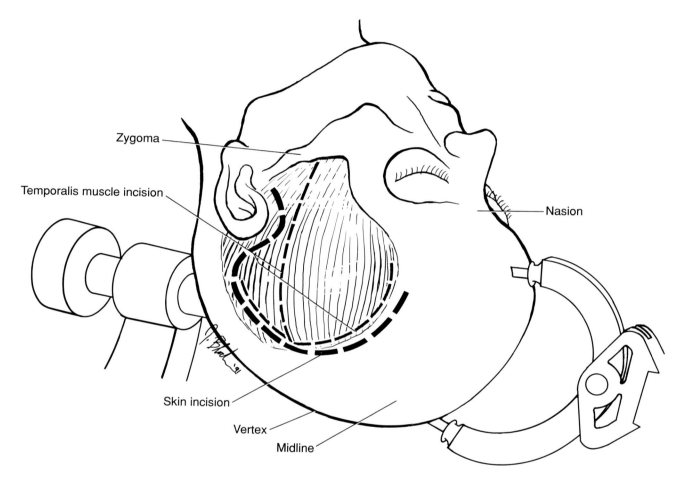

Figure 3. Positioning of the patient for a left frontotemporoparietal craniotomy. The nose is tilted 30° from the horizontal plane and the vertex is lowered 30° from the midline. The skin incision is shaped in a question mark fashion within the hairline. The temporalis muscle is split longitudinally, detached from the temporal line, and reflected anteriorly and posteriorly.

additional burr hole may be needed at the most superior and posterior aspect of the craniotomy. The bone is freed from the dura using a No. 3 Penfield dissector and a free bone flap is created. Suture holes are placed through the bone along the perimeter of the craniotomy as well as through the bone flap. The inferior aspect of the temporal craniotomy may be extended anteriorly and inferiorly with the use of rongeurs. This allows satisfactory exposure of the anterior temporal area and usually reaches the floor of the middle fossa. Care is taken not to enter the air cells along the mastoid bone and bone wax is placed if such a cell is entered. Dural retention sutures are placed at the perimeter of the bony opening using 4-0 Nurolon.

At this stage dural tension is assessed. Intravenous mannitol (1 g/kg) is given routinely at the time of incising the skin, and hyperventilation is used to create an end-tidal CO_2 of approximately 30 mm Hg. Before the dura is opened, saline irrigation is used over the exposed area and bone dust or dried blood is washed from the surgical gloves. Bacitracin-soaked sponges are also placed at the perimeter of the exposure, followed by sterile towels. A semicircular incision is placed through the dura which is reflected anteriorly and held with a suture. The posterior dura is incised perpendicular to the C-shaped incision and the dural leaves are then reflected superiorly and inferiorly. These leaves are covered with moist cotton to prevent desiccation, thus allowing an easy dural closure.

The cortical surface is at first inspected and any localized atrophy or lesion is noted. The vascular drainage of the temporal lobe is also studied, in particular the location of the vein of Labbé. The sylvian fissure is easily identified as well as the sylvian veins. The extent of resection is measured from the tip of the temporal lobe at the level of the anterior wall of the middle fossa along the second temporal convolution. On the dominant side, the plane of resection lies about 4.5–5 cm posterior to the tip, and on the nondominant side, about 5–6 cm posterior to the tip (Fig. 4). The posterior margin may vary with the location of the vein of Labbé which is usually behind the planned resection plane.

The posterior (inferior) incision is made at approximately 45° to the anterior (superior) incision to spare primary auditory cortex and possible speech-sensitive cortex over the superior temporal gyrus (Fig. 4). The initial pial incision is placed approximately 5 mm inferior to the sylvian veins and continues anteriorly parallel to the curvature of the sphenoid wing until the floor of the middle fossa is reached. The pia and bridging vessels are coagulated and sharply divided with microscissors. The superior aspect of the cut pia is then elevated and subpial dissection is made with the use of a small-bore aspirator and small retractor. Dissection of the mesial aspect of the superior temporal gyrus is then carried along the sylvian cistern, preserving the arachnoid layer over the branches of the middle cerebral artery (Fig. 5, Step 1). The cortex is progressively lifted until the level of the insula is reached at the limen insulae (Fig. 5, Step 2).

The surgeon's attention is then turned to the posterior margin of the dissection where the incision is deepened vertically with a bipolar coagulator and suction. The plane is progressively deepened into the temporal stem and inferiorly along the floor of the middle fossa (Fig. 5, Step 3). At this level the pia is gently elevated to avoid injury to the underlying fourth cranial nerve. Dissection is then carried medially until the edge of the tentorium is identified. An orthostatic Greenberg retractor may be used at this point to elevate the anterior portion of the temporal lobe. Retraction over the posterior aspect of the temporal lobe is avoided to decrease the amount of brain swelling and, on the dominant side, postoperative speech impairment.

The draped surgical microscope is then brought over the surgical field posteriorly and the ependyma of the temporal horn is carefully opened (Fig. 5, Step 4). A gush of clear cerebrospinal fluid usually emerges from the opening and a micro-cotton is placed in the opening to avoid any entry of blood or debris into the ventricle. However, hemostasis has been achieved at each step of the dissection and the surgical field at this point is usually very dry. Once within the ventricle, the dorsal aspect of the hippocampus is clearly visible and the orientation of the ventricle is studied. The roof of the ventricle is identified in relation to the limen insulae. By progressively thinning the roof of the ventricle, complete exposure of the anterior ventricular horn is achieved, until the tip is reached. A retractor is then positioned to elevate the temporal lobe laterally; the horn is then dissected off the lateral amygdala which is located anterior to the tip of the temporal horn. This dissection bridges the initial exposure of the first temporal gyrus and is made subpially at the level just inferior to the sphenoid ridge. This will allow exposure of the carotid cistern as well as the oculomotor nerve, which is preserved. A small cottonoid is left at this site for future reference.

The microscope is then brought back to the level of the posterior exposure. The third temporal convolution inferiorly as well as the parahippocampal gyrus are then dissected to reach the floor of the middle fossa. The pia is progressively dissected until the edge of the tentorium is reached. At this level the dissection is carried in a subpial fashion more mesially and another cottonoid is left in place for future reference. The surgical microscope is then brought over the mesial

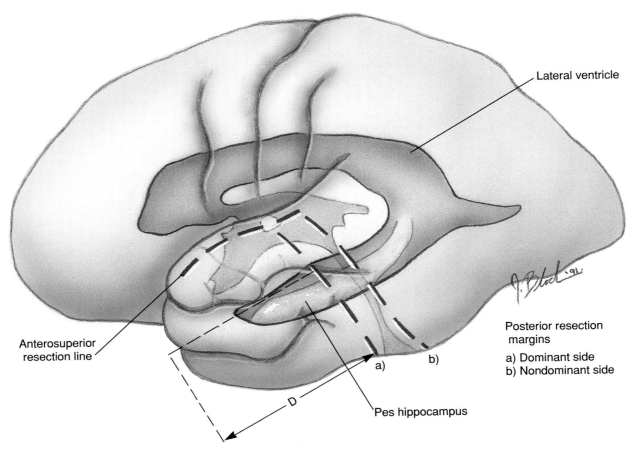

Figure 4. Lateral view of the left hemisphere showing the extent of resection of a standard anterior temporal lobectomy. A distance of 4.5–5 cm is measured over the second temporal convolution from the anterior wall of the middle fossa of the dominant side (5–6 cm for a nondominant resection). The hippocampal resection extends at least to the level of the lateral incision and usually reaches 3 cm.

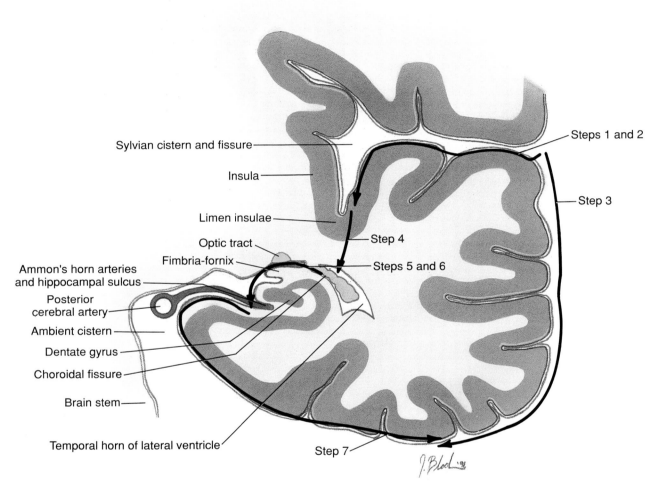

Sylvian cistern and fissure

Insula

Limen insulae

Optic tract

Fimbria-fornix

Ammon's horn arteries
and hippocampal sulcus

Posterior
cerebral artery

Ambient cistern

Dentate gyrus

Choroidal fissure

Brain stem

Temporal horn of lateral ventricle

Steps 1 and 2

Step 3

Step 4

Steps 5 and 6

Step 7

Figure 5. Coronal representation of the anterior temporal lobe showing the different steps completing the en bloc anterior temporal lobe resection. A key landmark is the temporal horn of the lateral ventricle which will give access through the choroidal fissure to the ambient cistern.

aspect of the hippocampus where the choroid plexus is elevated to expose the choroidal fissure as well as the fimbria-fornix (Fig. 5, Step 5). This last structure is usually very thin and can be dissected with a micro-probe or a microbipolar forceps. In some cases, it can just be peeled off to give access to the ambient cistern. At this point, a second retractor is positioned over a nonadhesive pledget to maintain the elevation of the choroid plexus. Gentle retraction is applied. The for-nix is dissected longitudinally for a distance of approx-imately 3–3.5 cm. At this posterior level the hippo-campus is transected in the coronal plane using microbipolar forceps and a microaspirator until the mesial hippocampal pia is identified. The subpial dis-section is then carried inferiorly and laterally to reach the posterior cotton left previously.

In the ambient cistern, perforating vessels originat-ing from the posterior cerebral artery are seen within the hippocampal sulcus and are dissected from the main feeding vessels (Fig. 5, Step 6). These small per-forators, called Ammon's horn arteries, are then taken progressively from posterior to anterior to allow access to the presubiculum and parahippocampal gyrus re-gions. The hippocampus is gently retracted laterally and the pia is incised longitudinally over the parahip-pocampal gyrus which is then peeled off progressively from posterior to anterior (Fig. 5, Step 7). Anteriorly, some arteries may originate from the anterior choroi-dal artery but the major medial branches are pre-served. No attempt is made to identify the superiorly placed optic tract to prevent injury. Because of the curvature of the hippocampus at the level of the uncus, the anterior dissection is carried more mesially in front of the brain stem. Subpial dissection is then completed and the hippocampus can be elevated off the pia within the ambient cistern. The whole speci-men is elevated superiorly until the edge of the ten-torium is identified (Fig. 6). There, the anterior cot-tonoid is again identified and usually a small remnant of the pia has to be cut over the tentorial edge to obtain an en bloc specimen. The specimen is immediately placed into a cold solution of artificial cerebrospinal fluid (CSF). The hippocampus will again be measured and dissected from the temporal lobe and sent for further studies.

The resection cavity is then inspected and hemo-stasis is completed, usually at the margin of the pial resection. Care is taken not to coagulate over the ten-torium itself or close to the cranial nerves. Layers of oxidized cellulose may be left over the pial surface of the insula and sylvian cistern. Hemostasis proceeds from inferior to superior levels of the dissection. The resection cavity is filled with saline irrigation followed with bacitracin irrigation. The surgical cavity is filled with fluid and the dura is closed in a watertight fash-

ion using interrupted and continuous sutures. The bone flap is sutured back in place with large more absorbable sutures and central tack-up sutures. No drains are left in place. The temporalis muscle and fascia are then closed using 3-0 Vicryl sutures along the temporal line. The skin is closed in two layers and a local dressing is applied.

The patient is sent to the recovery room after ex-tubation and is subsequently monitored in the inten-sive care unit overnight. Hourly neurologic checks and vital sign measurements are carried out. A postopera-tive computed tomography (CT) or MRI scan is ob-tained the following day (Fig. 7).

COMPLICATIONS AND OUTCOME

The most frequent side effect of the temporal lobec-tomy is the production of a superior quadratic homon-ymous field defect that is innocuous to the patient. This "pie in the sky" defect varies with the posterior extent of the dissection; a temporal lobectomy rarely produces a complete homonymous hemianopia. This is usually prevented by limiting the posterolateral dis-section just above the ventricle and avoiding the optic tract and optic radiation.

A second complication is the production of aseptic meningitis. This occurs in approximately 10% of oper-ated patients and typically begins with a spiking fever, neck stiffness, and photophobia on the fourth to sev-enth postoperative day. Typically the lumbar puncture will show xanthochromic CSF with significant leuko-cytosis and a decreased glucose content. However, all cultures remain negative. These patients are treated by increasing the steroid dosage and using wide spec-trum antibiotic therapy until it is determined that the cultures are negative. The best preventive measures are to achieve complete methodical hemostasis and to leave the pia layer above the ambient cistern.

Extraocular nerve paresis may also occur if care is not taken with the dissection in the region of the third and fourth cranial nerves. This is usually transient and extraocular movements are back to normal within the first six weeks.

"Manipulation hemiplegia" has been described af-ter temporal lobectomy. This has been attributed to traction on the sylvian branches over the insula, or to delayed vasospasm of one of these branches. Another possible cause is damage to the mesial branch of the anterior choroidal artery which supplies the lateral part of the cerebral peduncle.

Another frequent side effect is a short-term mem-ory impairment. This has been found to affect verbal memory on the dominant side and nonverbal memory on the nondominant side. However, 30% of patients present with such a deficit prior to surgery, with tran-sient worsening postoperatively which then improves

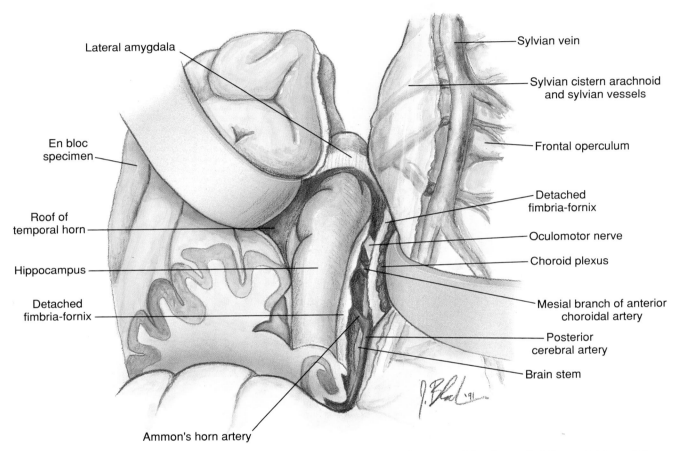

Lateral amygdala

En bloc
specimen

Roof of
temporal horn

Hippocampus

Detached
fimbria-fornix

Ammon's horn artery

Sylvian vein

Sylvian cistern arachnoid
and sylvian vessels

Frontal operculum

Detached
fimbria-fornix

Oculomotor nerve

Choroid plexus

Mesial branch of anterior
choroidal artery

Posterior
cerebral artery

Brain stem

Figure 6. Surgeon's view of an en bloc specimen after a left anterior temporal lobectomy. The fimbria-fornix has been detached and the ambient cistern is reached to expose the Ammon's horn arteries reaching the hippocampal sulcus. The lateral retractor lifts the roof of the ventricle and the medial retractor is gently positioned over the choroid plexus and insula.

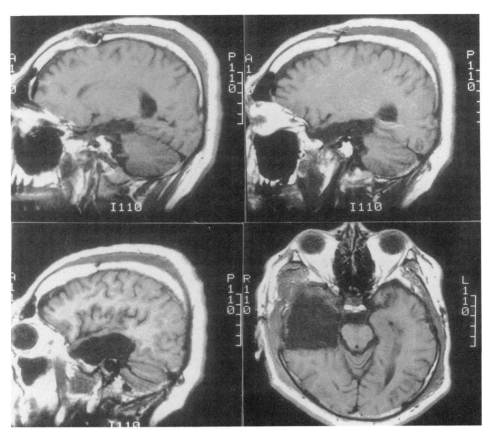

Figure 7. Postoperative MRI views (T1-weighted images) showing the mesial and posterior extent of the hippocampal resection on the sequential sagittal views. The *lower right* view is an axial image showing the posterior extent of a nondominant right anterior lobe resection.

during the following year. More severe global amnesia is usually prevented by documenting preoperative memory function with the intracarotid Amytal test. Patients who fail this test usually have evidence of bilateral hippocampal damage and should not undergo mesial temporal lobe resection. Receptive aphasia or dysphasia may occur on the second to fourth day after an operation on the dominant side. This is related to the degree of brain edema and resolves when the edema disappears. When the epileptogenic lesion appears to arise from the neocortex close to or within Wernicke's area, surgery should be performed under local anesthesia to obtain a complete mapping prior to resection.

The overall morbidity of the procedure is below 5% and there have been no deaths following this procedure at our center. The outcome of this procedure has been excellent (Class I and II of Engel) for at least 80% of patients and with additional functional criteria, the success rate now reaches above 90%.

CINGULOTOMY FOR INTRACTABLE PAIN USING STEREOTAXIS GUIDED BY MAGNETIC RESONANCE IMAGING

SAMUEL J. HASSENBUSCH, M.D., PH.D.
PREM K. PILLAY, M.D.

INTRODUCTION

Pain relief in cancer patients can be difficult to achieve and maintain. Oral narcotics remain the mainstay of treatment but can be limited by the development of tolerance to relatively large doses. Side effects, especially somnolence, nausea, and vomiting, often limit the degree to which the dose of systemic (e.g., oral, rectal, subcutaneous, intravenous) narcotics can be increased. These problems are particularly true of the terminal cancer patient with unresectable, disseminated disease. Frequently all treatment options, both medical and operative, will have been exhausted in these patients without provision of adequate comfort and the ability to perform simple daily activities.

Operative options in these patients have included nerve blocks, implantable morphine (or other narcotic) pumps, and various surgical ablative operations. The list of neurosurgical ablative operations in these patients is a lengthy one: neurectomy, rhizotomy, myelotomy, cordotomy, medullary tractotomy, mesencephalotomy, thalamotomy, and cingulotomy, among others. The usefulness of these operative options is often limited by the cardiopulmonary risks of a major operation under general anesthesia in these debilitated patients. The added risk of a neurologic deficit with these open operations is also an important consideration. For these reasons, major ablative operations are often not recommended in such patients.

In search of a safe, effective operation for cancer patients with intractable pain, the procedure of cingulotomy has been modified using stereotaxis guided by magnetic resonance imaging (MRI) (Fig. 1). Although lesions of the cingulate gyrus have been created in the past, the lesions have been placed using ventriculogram guidance. This required ventricular puncture with the possible risks of meningitis and hemorrhage. Ventriculogram guidance to the cingulate gyrus was also indirect and potentially inaccurate. The operation was somewhat cumbersome and usually required general anesthesia.

A new technique for the placement of these lesions using MRI guidance in conjunction with a stereotactic localizing system is presented. The operation can be performed under local anesthesia, is effective, and involves minimal risk to the patient. Since most neurosurgeons are more familiar with and more likely to have access to the Brown-Roberts-Wells (BRW) and Cosman-Roberts-Wells (CRW) systems, the technique was initially developed with these systems. The technique can also be easily adapted to the Compass Stereotactic (Kelly-Goerss) System which allows a simple and reproducible ring reapplication.

PATIENT SELECTION

Following its development, this technique has been usually applied to patients who: 1) have terminal cancer with midline, bilateral, and/or diffuse body pain; 2) are ineligible for resection of any tumor; 3) have had inadequate pain control by non-narcotic medications (e.g., antidepressants, nonsteroidal anti-inflammatory agents, non-narcotic analgesics); 4) have had inadequate pain control by oral, rectal, and/or intravenous preparations of narcotics without significant side effects (e.g., nausea, vomiting, somnolence, headache, respiratory depression); 5) have no significant pain components that would be amenable to special nerve block or denervation procedures; 6) have an expected survival time of at least one month; 7) have received maximal radiation therapy to the pain sites or have such extensive disease that radiation therapy is not practical; 8) have no contraindications to an intracranial ablative operation (e.g., previous craniotomy and brain resection, significant untreated hydrocephalus, intracranial vascular malformation, significant abnormal anatomy (as shown by computed to-

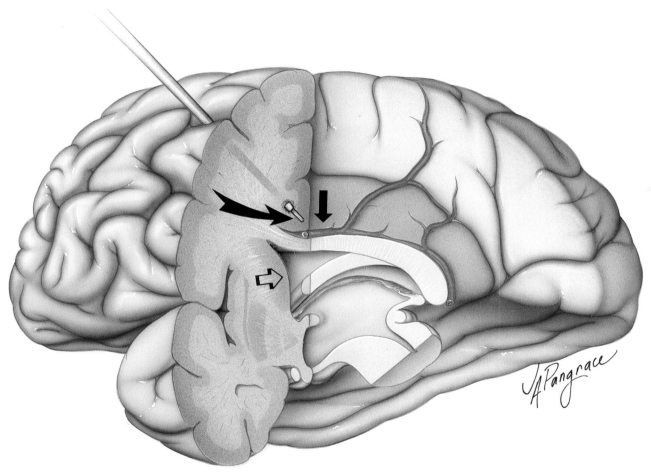

Figure 1. Graphic illustration of the placement of the cingulotomy electrode through the cortex so that the electrode tip is located in the center of the left cingulate gyrus. Note the relative positions of the 10-mm exposed tip of the electrode (*curved arrow*), the distal portion of an anterior cerebral artery (*closed arrow*), and the lateral ventricle (*open arrow*).

mography (CT) or MRI) in the cingulate gyri, or infection in the scalp, skull, or brain); and 9) have no significant psychiatric illness that would interfere with the treatment.

As can be seen from the above list, these patients are often the type for whom long-term intraspinal (e.g., epidural, intrathecal) infusions of narcotics (often with an implanted programmable infusion pump) would be considered. In such a situation, both options are often offered to allow the patient to choose according to individual preference between an essentially one-time intracranial ablative operation and an intraspinal operation requiring postoperative pump refills and rate adjustments. It should also be noted that the use of one of these options does not preclude a later use of the other option should pain control become more difficult as the underlying neoplasm progresses.

The patients are usually evaluated and treated by a multidisciplinary team composed of a neurosurgeon, psychiatrist, anesthesiologist, palliative care oncologist, and nurse clinician. Evaluation of the patient's pain, both preoperatively and postoperatively, is a very important aspect of this technique. A pain scale (e.g., a visual analog or a verbal digital scale) is usually utilized to quantitate the degree of pain preoperatively and at multiple points after the operation. The verbal digital scale, which is more facile for routine visits, consists of asking the patient to rate the pain on a scale of 0 to 10, where 0 represents no pain and 10 the worst imaginable pain. The second part of pain assessment consists of the use of a McGill Pain Questionnaire to assess differential improvements in the sensory (Groups 1–10 on the questionnaire) or the affective (Groups 11–15) categories.

PREOPERATIVE PREPARATION

Because of the relatively simple and noninvasive nature of this technique, very little preoperative preparation is required. A preoperative CT or MRI scan with contrast (iohexol (300 mg of iodine/ml), or gadolinium DTPA (0.1 mmol/kg), respectively) is usually performed to confirm the absence of significant vascular or anatomical abnormalities that would preclude accurate and safe stereotactic localization in the cingulate gyri. A prophylactic antibiotic is routinely given with one dose, usually of cefamandole nafate, in the operating room immediately prior to the skin puncture for stereotactic electrode placement. Postoperative antibiotic therapy is continued every six hours for four more doses. Anticonvulsants are not given unless there is a previous history and treatment of seizures. Steroids are also not given because the lesions, using the present technique, cause very little perilesional edema.

OPERATIVE PROCEDURE

Anesthetic Technique

The major advantage of this technique for pain control in terminally ill patients with cancer is that it can be easily performed under local anesthesia with some intravenous sedation. Xylocaine (1% without epinephrine) is usually utilized for local anesthesia of the scalp where the pins of the stereotactic arc are screwed into the outer table of the skull. Similarly, 1% Xylocaine without epinephrine is also sufficient for the scalp where the puncture site is made for the insertion of the radiofrequency electrode. The use of a twist drill to make the small hole in the skull and the puncture of the underlying dura mater are usually painless or minimally painful and do not require anesthesia. The actual passage of the electrode through the brain is likewise painless.

To facilitate patient cooperation and comfort, the operation is routinely done with the presence of an anesthesiologist who administers intravenous sedation. A combination of midazolam HCl and fentanyl citrate is usually given as needed to ensure patient comfort. Because of the medical condition of the usual patient, the dosages of these medications are limited as much as possible although it is not required that the patient be awake at any point during the operation.

In the MRI suite, monitoring of the patient consists of an automated blood pressure monitor and a pulse oximeter with an anesthesiologist or anesthetist present. In the operating room during creation of the actual lesion, an electrocardiogram monitor is also added. Further specialized monitoring is usually not necessary.

Specialized Instrumentation

This procedure utilizes standard BRW-CRW stereotactic equipment for all parts. Each of the pieces of equipment is labeled by letter in Figure 2. Specifically, the MRI head ring with MRI head ring posts and MRI head fixation screws (A), MRI localizer cage (B), CT head ring (C), Mayfield adaptor and screws (D), and the BRW stereotactic arc (E) are all standard equipment for any stereotactic procedure under MRI guidance utilizing the BRW system. A standard block (F) is placed in the holder at the top of the arc. A standard guide tube (G) is secured in the block. The bone drill bit (H) and the BRW arc system pointer (I) which are used to make a hole in the skull and the dura mater are also standard pieces. The actual electrode (J) is a thermistor (type TM) straight radiofrequency electrode with a 10-mm exposed tip. It is connected to a standard radiofrequency wire (K) which is then connected to the radiofrequency generator.

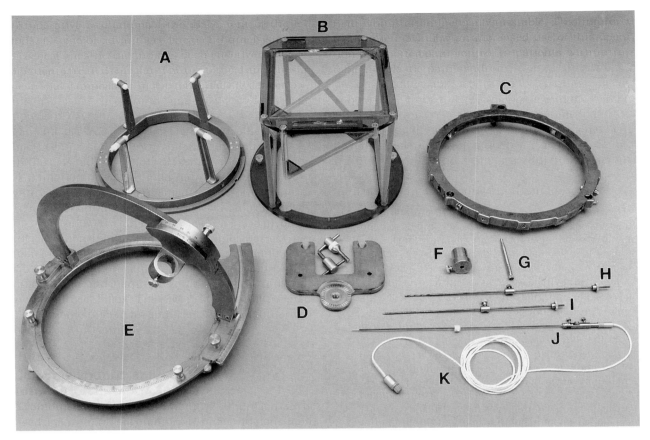

Figure 2. Equipment used for stereotactic cingulotomy. Shown are: MRI-compatible head ring with head ring posts and head fixation screws (**A**); MRI-compatible localizer ring (**B**); CT-compatible head ring (**C**); Mayfield adaptor with attachment screws (**D**); BRW stereotactic arc (**E**); standard block for the arc (**F**); standard needle holder (**G**); bone drill bit (**H**); BRW arc system pointer (**I**); thermistor (type TM) straight radiofrequency electrode with 10-mm exposed tip (**J**); and standard electrode wire for connection to the radiofrequency generator (**K**).

Operative Technique

Target Data Acquisition

A standard MRI-compatible BRW head ring (with MRI-compatible head fixation screws) is applied to the patient's head under local anesthesia (Fig. 3A). As the nylon head fixation screws are applied to the MRI-compatible head ring, an assistant holds the head ring steady, making sure that the ring is placed symmetrically on the patient with minimal or no rotation or inclination to one side. It is important to be sure that the ring is located so that the BRW arc has sufficient clearance over the top of the patient's head to allow movement of the arc and the block holder over the head. The MRI localizer ring is then applied to the head ring (Fig. 3B). This part of the operation takes place in a small induction room adjacent to the scanner suite.

The MRI scan is performed using a GE Sigma 1.5 Tesla MR scanner with a 32-cm scan circle. A T1 signal (TR 500 ms, TE 15 ms) in the coronal plane, without intravenous contrast, is utilized with 5-mm-thick sections spaced every 6 mm. The location for the coronal sections is chosen from a scout midline sagittal scan with the most anterior section located in front of the corpus callosum (Fig. 4A). A total of approximately 11 slices is required. The most anterior coronal slice containing any portion of the frontal horns of the lateral ventricles is determined (Fig. 4B). The coronal slice that is four sections more posterior is then chosen as the target slice (Fig. 4C). This gives a cingulate gyrus target that is 24 mm posterior from the tips of the frontal horns.

On this target slice, the coordinates of the fiducials are determined using a software program (resident on the MRI scanner) with the ability to translate any cursor-labeled point on the MRI screen into cartesian coordinates. The fiducial coordinates are determined

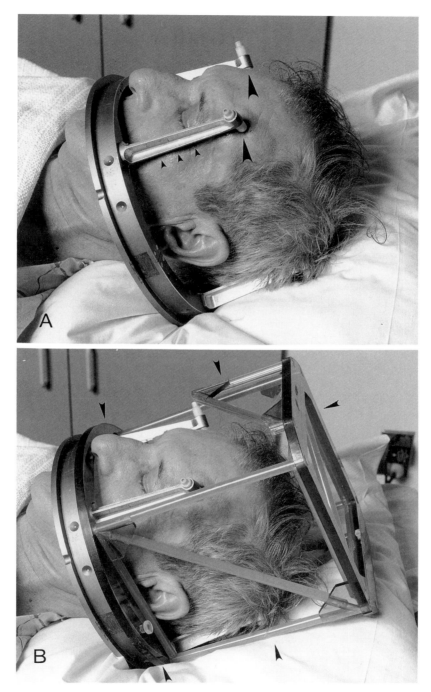

Figure 3. **A,** placement of the MRI-compatible BRW/CRW head ring on the patient's head. Note the head ring posts (*small arrowheads*) and head fixation screws (*large arrowheads*) securing the ring to the outer table of the skull. This is usually performed using local anesthesia but can be carried out under general anesthesia. **B,** the MRI-compatible BRW/CRW localizer ring (*arrowheads*) is attached to the head ring prior to the performance of the MRI scan.

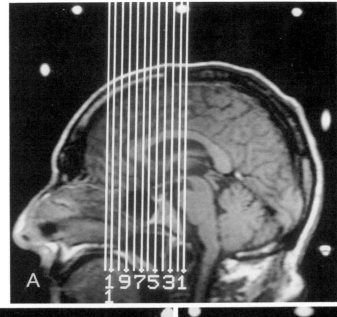

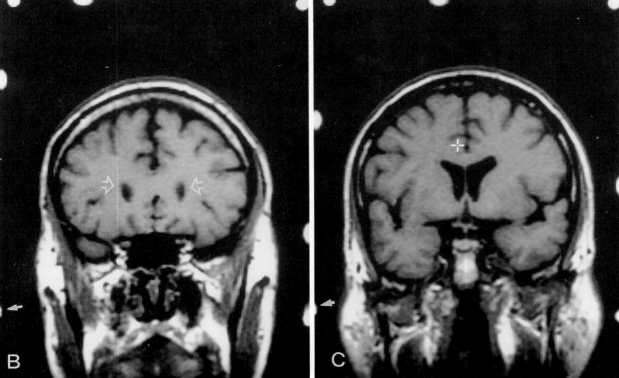

Figure 4. An MRI scan (without intravenous enhancement) using a T1 signal (TR 300 ms, TE 15 ms). The scan was performed using a GE Sigma 1.5 Tesla MR scanner with a 32-cm scan circle. **A,** a scout sagittal midline view: the location for the coronal sections is chosen with the most anterior section located in front of the corpus callosum. A total of approximately 11 slices is required. **B,** the most anterior coronal slice containing any portion of the frontal horns of the lateral ventricles (*open arrows*) is shown. Coronal sec-tions were 5 mm thick and spaced every 6 mm (i.e., 1 mm between each slice). **C,** the coronal slice that is four sections more posterior to that shown in **B** is chosen as the target slice and gives a cingulate gyrus target that is 24 mm posterior from the tips of the frontal horns. The cursor (*shown*) is placed on the center of the right cingulate gyrus. The fiducial points for the MRI localizer ring are seen on the scan. The hollow point fiducial (*closed arrow*) is the first fiducial point.

beginning with the hollow-point fiducial (Fig. 4C, arrow) and continuing to the next nearest fiducial. The center of each cingulate gyrus (right and left) is chosen as a target and appropriate coordinates are likewise determined (Fig. 4C, cursor). On completion of the MRI study, the patient is transferred to the operating room.

Calculation of Target Point Coordinates

The coordinates for the fiducials of the MRI localizer cage and for the right and left cingulate gyrus targets are then entered into the BRW system laptop computer, which is an Epson HX-20 portable computer. The actual coordinates obtained from the MRI scanner software are entered into the Epson computer using the TMRI-86A program and selecting the coronal MRI option in the main menu. This produces a set of BRW system coordinates (anteroposterior, lateral, and vertical numbers) for each target (cingulate gyrus) site. These numbers are then entered into the Target Menu of the Epson computer using the STAX-84K program. By proceeding then to the Approach Menu of the same program and using the Azimuth/Declination Method, the actual approach parameters (alpha, beta, gamma, delta, and target depth) of the targets (right and left cingulate gyri) can be obtained. For the right cingulate gyrus, an azimuth of 45° and a declination of 45° is used. For the left gyrus, an azimuth and declination of 315° and 45°, respectively, are specified. The actual approach parameters are then set on the BRW stereotactic arc. The phantom base is then used as a double-check for correct arc settings with the BRW arc. BRW system coordinates (anteroposterior, lateral, and vertical) are set on the phantom base. The arc is then placed on the phantom base and the arc's settings verified with a probe placed through the block in the BRW arc. The depth of the probe (and subsequent electrode) is calculated from the depth given by the actual approach parameters added to the height (usually 10 mm) of the block on the arc added to the further height of the guide tube in the block for the probe or electrode.

The CRW arc can also be used in a somewhat more simple and shortened method. BRW system coordinates (anteroposterior, lateral, and vertical) can be directly set on the CRW arc without the need for using the STAX-84K program to obtain approach parameters. The CRW arc can then be placed on the patient's head and the entry point adjusted to use a point located behind the hairline, in front of the coronal suture, and at least 3 cm lateral to the sagittal sinus. For safety, it is recommended that the arc be tested against the phantom base, which is set up as described above for the BRW arc. The depth of the probe (and subsequent electrode) is calculated from 160 mm

(a standard value for the CRW system) added to the height (usually 10 mm) of the block on the arc added to the further height of the guide tube in the block for the probe or electrode.

Creation of Lesions

In the operating room, the patient is placed in the supine position, with the head slightly flexed and the nose pointing upward without rotation. The CT-compatible head ring is then placed on top of the MRI-compatible head ring that is attached to the patient. This CT head ring is necessary both for stabilization of the patient's head to the operating room table as well as for attachment of the actual BRW arc to the patient. The CT head ring is then connected by the Mayfield adaptor (an attachment plate) to a Mayfield head holder apparatus (Fig. 5, A and B, closed arrow) that is secured to the operating table.

Both frontal scalp areas are then shaved, cleaned, and prepared with an iodine solution. A iodophor-impregnated plastic craniotomy sheet (Ioban2 Antimicrobial Film) is draped over the top of the patient's head and over the head rings. For the purposes of this procedure, no further sterile drapes are needed over the patient. Openings are made in the Ioban sheet for the CT head ring's three holes which are used to secure the BRW arc to the patient. The BRW arc, after being sterilized, is placed over the patient's head and the three pegs on the underside of the arc are secured to the CT head ring. The block and the guide tube (Fig. 5A, curved arrow) are then added to the top of the arc (Fig. 5, A and B).

On the left side, the skull entry point is marked on the scalp and a small skin puncture created down to the periosteum with a No. 15 scalpel blade. A 3-mm twist drill hole is made in the skull at the same site by placing the drill bit through the guide tube in the BRW arc. The dura mater is then gently perforated with a trocar or the BRW arc system pointer.

A thermistor (type TM) straight radiofrequency electrode with a 10-mm exposed tip is then passed through the guide tube in the BRW arc (Fig. 5, A and B, open arrow indicates electrode hub). It is directed through the hole in the skull so that the center of the exposed electrode tip is centered at the target, namely, the center of the cingulate gyrus (Fig. 1). This electrode is connected by wire (Fig. 5B, double arrows) to a radiofrequency generator (Fig. 6).

A lesion is made using an electrode temperature of 75° C for 60 seconds. The exact same operation is then performed in the right hemisphere. A single stitch is placed in each scalp puncture site. The patient is observed overnight and discharged the next morning. Follow-up MRI scans using a T1 signal (TR 600 ms, TE 30 ms) and a spin density signal (TR 2000 ms, TE 32

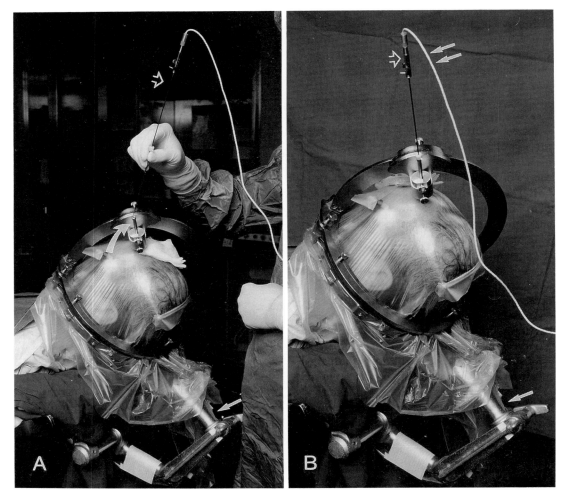

Figure 5. Intraoperative pictures during the actual creation of the lesions. The head ring is attached by a Mayfield adaptor (covered by the drape) to a Mayfield holder (*solid straight arrow*) which is connected to the operating table. **A,** the insertion of the electrode (*open arrow*) into the guide tube (*curved arrow*) of the stereotactic arc. **B,** after insertion of the electrode and at the time of actual lesion creation, the hub of the electrode (*open arrow*) is connected by wire (*double arrows*) to the radiofrequency generator.

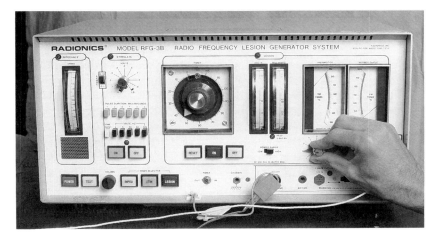

Figure 6. A radiofrequency generator showing the settings during the actual lesion production. The temperature is maintained at 75 °C for 60 seconds.

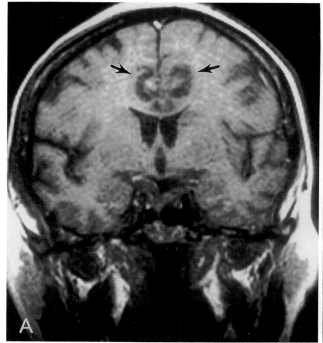

Figure 7. Postoperative MRI scans without contrast, using a T1 signal (TR 600 ms, TE 30 ms). This patient had no postoperative neurologic deficits. **A,** coronal view: the location of the lesions (*arrows*) corresponds closely with the stereotactic targets (center of each hemisphere's cingulate gyrus). **B,** sagittal view: the right-sided lesion (*arrow*) is shown in this slice.

ms) are performed in the coronal and sagittal planes without contrast one week later to evaluate placement of the lesions (Fig. 7).

COMPLICATIONS

One of the major strengths of this operation is the relative safety of the cingulate gyrus area when creating lesions. In our experience, this operation using MRI guidance and the radiofrequency settings described above has been without complications in these terminally ill cancer patients with intractable pain. One early patient, treated with three overlapping lesions created in each gyrus using a higher electrode temperature (85° C) for a longer time (90 seconds) than described above, did experience global aphasia for five days which then resolved over the next five days without subsequent problems. Despite the close proximity of the electrode tip to the anterior cerebral arteries and the lateral ventricles (Fig. 1), no complications have occurred in relation to either of these structures.

Cingulotomy using ventriculogram guidance has been previously reported in many older studies involving a total of more than 1000 patients. The studies included both neurologic and cortical function (psychometric) testing. In these reports, the mortality rate was 0.09% and one-sided paralysis rate (caused by bleeding) was 0.36%. A study from the Massachusetts Institute of Technology indicated that, in 137 patients undergoing bilateral cingulotomy, the only lasting behavioral deficit seen after the operation consisted of difficulty in copying a complex drawing on the Rey-Taylor Complex Figure Test. This change was seen in a small minority of patients and was of minimal clinical significance to the patients.

Because these patients have usually been on long-term large doses of narcotics and because the operation often gives marked, almost immediate, pain relief, great care has to be exercised in ensuring an adequate and slow narcotic detoxification to avoid withdrawal symptoms in the postoperative period.

CONCLUSIONS

The adaption of stereotaxis using MRI guidance for the creation of cingulate gyrus lesions is an improvement that potentially allows the routine creation of these lesions in cancer pain management. The direct visualization on MRI scanning of the cingulate gyri, both for stereotactic localization of the lesions and for postoperative evaluation of the placement of the lesions, is a major advantage. The technique is simple, uses local anesthesia, and has been effective and safe in patients treated thus far. The use of local anesthesia is especially important in the terminally ill cancer patient who is often medically unstable. This improved technique may allow an increased use of this operation and better pain control in patients with intractable neoplastic pain syndromes.

CEREBELLAR ASTROCYTOMAS

A. LELAND ALBRIGHT, M.D.

PATIENT SELECTION

Cerebellar astrocytomas occur in the cerebellar hemispheres and in the vermis, and in either site frequently cause hydrocephalus, which causes recurring headaches, vomiting, and drowsiness. Astrocytomas in the cerebellar hemispheres often cause appendicular ataxia or tremulousness; those in the vermis may cause truncal ataxia or no cerebellar signs. On computed tomography (CT) and magnetic resonance imaging (MRI) scans, astrocytomas enhance brightly after contrast injection and are often partially cystic (Fig. 1).

Operations are performed to diagnose and remove the tumor. Cerebellar astrocytomas are perhaps the most surgically curable tumors; there is no role for subtotal resection and postoperative irradiation unless the tumor cannot be excised safely. The timing of operation depends primarily on the severity of the associated hydrocephalus: the greater the hydrocephalus, the greater the urgency. Children who are lethargic from hydrocephalus secondary to a posterior fossa tumor should be operated on within 48 hours.

Potential risks of operation include death (~0.5%), wound infection (1%), ventriculitis/meningitis (2–3%), cerebrospinal fluid (CSF) leakage (1%), cerebellar signs (permanent 10%, transient 25%), and the pseudobulbar posterior fossa syndrome (3–5%).

PREOPERATIVE PREPARATION

Patients are usually treated for at least 24 hours preoperatively with corticosteroids, which decrease peritumoral edema and may improve symptoms of hydrocephalus. Seizures are an infrequent problem in treating either cerebellar astrocytomas or their associated hydrocephalus, and prophylactic anticonvulsants are not needed. Preoperative antibiotics are not needed; several studies have demonstrated that intraoperative antibiotics effectively decrease the risk of infection.

In the past, hydrocephalus was often treated with a

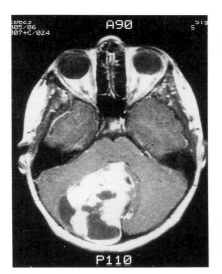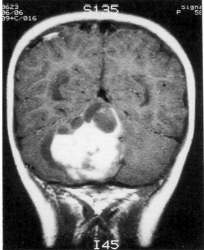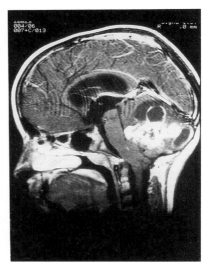

Figure 1. Axial, coronal, and sagittal magnetic resonance images of a partially cystic juvenile pilocytic astrocytoma.

CSF shunt several days before the craniotomy. That is infrequently appropriate now, because hydrocephalus is treated effectively by an external ventricular drain—inserted intraoperatively just prior to tumor removal—and postoperative shunts are needed in only 25% of patients after removal of cerebellar astrocytomas.

SURGICAL TECHNIQUE

Anesthesia

Preoperative sedation is usually not given to patients with posterior fossa tumors, especially those with hydrocephalus, because sedatives may depress respirations, causing arterial pCO_2 and intracranial pressure to rise. After patients are in the preoperative "holding area" and are under continuous close observation, intravenous sedation may be given, often with midazolam. Two peripheral venous catheters provide the customary venous access. There is debate about the role of central venous catheters: they provide information about intravascular volume and allow aspiration of some air in case of venous air embolism, but their insertion via the internal jugular or subclavian vein risks a hematoma that may compress the vein and increase venous and intracranial pressure, risks a pneumothorax, and they probably do not permit the aspiration of adequate volumes of air. Pulse oximeter monitoring is standard. An arterial catheter is commonly inserted for continuous blood pressure monitoring and for withdrawal of blood samples.

Anesthesia is usually induced with thiopental and maintained with a mixture of intravenous fentanyl plus nitrous oxide or with an inhalation agent such as isoflurane. The chest should be auscultated after the head is in its final position; the neck is commonly flexed in either the prone or sitting position and the endotracheal tube may advance into the right mainstem bronchus after the neck is flexed. A precordial Doppler monitor is often applied to detect air embolism, which causes a characteristic washing-machine sound. If air is detected, the operative field can be flooded with saline and the venous pressure can be increased, either by lowering the head of the operating table or by jugular venous compression.

Operative Positioning

If the patient has hydrocephalus or if hydrocephalus is likely to develop in the postoperative period, an external ventricular drain (EVD) should be inserted before the craniotomy is performed. That drain can be inserted into the frontal horn of the lateral ventricle through a small hole at the junction of the coronal suture and the pupillary line, aiming in an anteroposterior trajectory 1 cm anterior to the ear and a transverse trajectory so that the catheter ends at the midline. The

distance from the skull to the foramen of Monro can be estimated from the CT scan and is usually 5–6 cm. The distal end of the catheter should be drawn several centimeters subcutaneously before it exits through a stab wound and is then connected to a closed drainage system. The system is closed during positioning of the patient for craniotomy but is set to drain at approximately 10–15 cm above the lateral ventricles; the EVD is opened during the craniotomy if the dura is tense.

Surgeons who prefer the patient in a sitting position may insert the EVD catheter via the occipital approach once the patient is in position, inserting it through a burr hole 6 cm above the inion and 2.5 cm lateral to the midline, aiming at the ipsilateral inner canthus. This technique is usually successful if the ventricles are large, but otherwise there may be difficulty entering the ventricle.

The prone (angulated Concorde) position (Fig. 2) is the position used most commonly to remove cerebellar astrocytomas. The risk of air embolism is low and there is less risk of tearing bridging veins between the cerebellum and tentorium than in the sitting position. The patient orientation is direct and the surgeon can stand comfortably. The sitting position (Fig. 3) is the second most frequently used position. For tumors in the lateral cerebellar hemisphere, operations are often done with the patient in the lateral or "park bench" position (Fig. 4), with a roll under the axilla and the head fixed in the Mayfield head holder.

For the prone position, patients are positioned at the surgeon's side of the operating table and are supported on chest rolls that extend from the shoulders to the pelvic crest, with no compression of the abdominal viscera. Head support varies with the age of the patient: less than 10–12 months, the skull is usually too soft to permit reliable pin fixation and the head is therefore supported in the foam-padded pediatric horseshoe head holder; pediatric pins are used in 1–2 year olds, and adult pins are used thereafter. The head is fixed in the three-pin (Mayfield) head holder and angled about 30° away from the midline, turning the posterior fossa toward the surgeon. The neck is flexed approximately 30°; a distance of one to two finger breadths must be left between the chin and the chest.

The sitting position is used by some neurosurgeons for removal of midline and paramidline posterior fossa astrocytomas. Its advantages include direct orientation of the patient/tumor position and the removal of blood and CSF by gravity, but its disadvantages include the risk of air embolism and the fatigue of the surgeon's elevated arms. For the sitting position, patients are positioned on the operating table with their shoulders at the end of the main portion of the table. The head is fixed in the three-pin head holder and the crossbar is attached to side rails near the foot of the

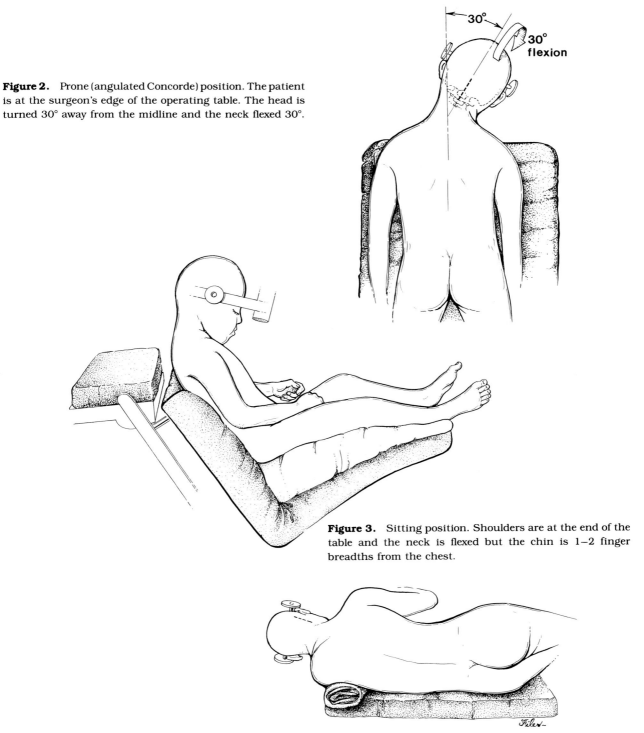

Figure 2. Prone (angulated Concorde) position. The patient is at the surgeon's edge of the operating table. The head is turned 30° away from the midline and the neck flexed 30°.

Figure 3. Sitting position. Shoulders are at the end of the table and the neck is flexed but the chin is 1–2 finger breadths from the chest.

Figure 4. Lateral position. The vertical retromastoid incision is centered over the maximal tumor volume.

table. The table is maximally flexed; folded blankets may be placed under the buttocks to keep the shoulders at the desired height. The table back is flexed upward, the head holder is connected to the crossbar, and the table's headrest is folded downward to a position comfortable for the surgeon's elbows to rest on. The head is kept in the midline for midline and paramedian tumors.

Skin Incision

To approach midline and paramidline tumors, a midline incision is made from the inion to the C1-2 interspace. For lateral hemispheric tumors, a vertical incision is made between the midline and mastoid, centered over the maximal volume of the tumor.

Operative Procedure

The epidermis can be opened with a No. 15 blade and the subcutaneous tissues opened in the midline with the needle tip of the coagulating monopolar cautery. If the cautery is not used, scalp clips (Raney, Leroy, or Children's Hospital clips) must be applied to the scalp margins. Tissues are opened in the midline with the cautery down to the occipital bone. A Weitlaner or posted Jannetta retractor is inserted and periosteum is dissected off the occipital bone with the cautery or with a broad periosteal elevator laterally for 3–4 cm from the midline; the bony and dural exposure must be sufficient to permit the hemispheres to be retracted away from the tumor. Venous emissary channels must be immediately and meticulously waxed to minimize air embolism. Tissues need to be dissected away from the C1-foramen magnum space and off the C1 spinous process and lamina. An Adson periosteal elevator is inserted to dissect dura away from the the posterior rim of the foramen magnum. The completed exposure is shown in Figure 5A.

The traditional method of occipital bone removal is by a craniectomy, removing bone with Kerrison and Leksell rongeurs from the foramen magnum upward until the inferior margin of the transverse sinus is seen. Equivalent exposure can be achieved with a craniotomy, which avoids the postoperative concavity so common after a craniectomy. Two burr holes are made in the occipital bone just below the expected level of the transverse sinus. Bone is often much thinner over the tumor than elsewhere. Dura is dissected away from the bone in three directions: from the burr holes downward to the foramen on either side and across the midline between the holes. Craniotomy cuts are made first from the burr holes down to the foramen magnum and then across the midline; the likelihood of a dural tear is decreased if dura is depressed with a Penfield dissector inserted from the opposite side while the bone is being cut across the midline. Bone margins

are waxed. A C1 laminectomy does not have to be performed in the majority of these operations, but may be needed if the cerebellar tonsils have herniated to the C1-2 interspace. If the dura is tense, the EVD should be opened and CSF drained until the dura is slack before it is opened.

To approach midline and paramidline tumors, the dura is opened in a Y-shaped manner (Fig. 5B), beginning with the lateral limbs of the Y and incising toward the midline. As the opening nears the midline, the occipital sinus must be occluded before the dura is divided. That occlusion can be accomplished by: (a) temporary occlusion with hemostats while the dura is cut (Fig. 5C), then coagulating/ligating the sinus, or (b) permanent occlusion with Weck clips, which may distort the postoperative MRI scan. The inferior limb of the Y is then opened down to C1. Dural tackup sutures, usually 4-0 Nurolon, are inserted and the dural leaves are retracted backward over 0.5 × 2-inch cottonoid strips, kept moist during the procedure to prevent dural drying and shrinkage. The arachnoid over the cisterna magna is opened. Cottonoid patties are inserted at the foramen magnum to lessen caudal migration of blood during the operation and, if appropriate, are inserted between the tonsils and onto the floor of the fourth ventricle to protect the brain stem. Blades are attached to a retractor system (Jannetta, Greenberg, Yasargil).

If the outer surface of the astrocytoma is not visible, folia overlying the tumor are usually thinned and widened. At this point in the operation, neurosurgeons in the past would insert a blunt needle into the tumor cyst to decompress the posterior fossa; that is infrequently needed now if the associated hydrocephalus has been treated by an EVD. Pia is coagulated with bipolar forceps (Fig. 5D) and opened with a No. 15 blade and fine-tipped scissors. Underlying white matter along that line is suctioned away down to the tumor surface and retractor blades are inserted to hold the parenchymal surfaces apart. Once the tumor is visible, many neurosurgeons elect to biopsy the tumor for a frozen section diagnosis, although the subsequent resection is infrequently altered by that information. If a diagnosis of cerebellar (juvenile pilocytic) astrocytoma (JPA) is made, meticulous attempts to achieve a complete removal are indicated because the tumor is generally surgically curable. JPAs have a fleshy appearance and frequently have a distinct plane demarcating them from surrounding cerebellum. Small tumors can be excised en toto, dissecting in that plane with Penfield or microdissectors to extract them from surrounding tissue. Larger tumors are internally debulked with the ultrasonic aspirator (Fig. 5E), then their exterior is dissected out (Fig. 5F). For JPAs that have a "mural nodule" and an associated cyst, removal

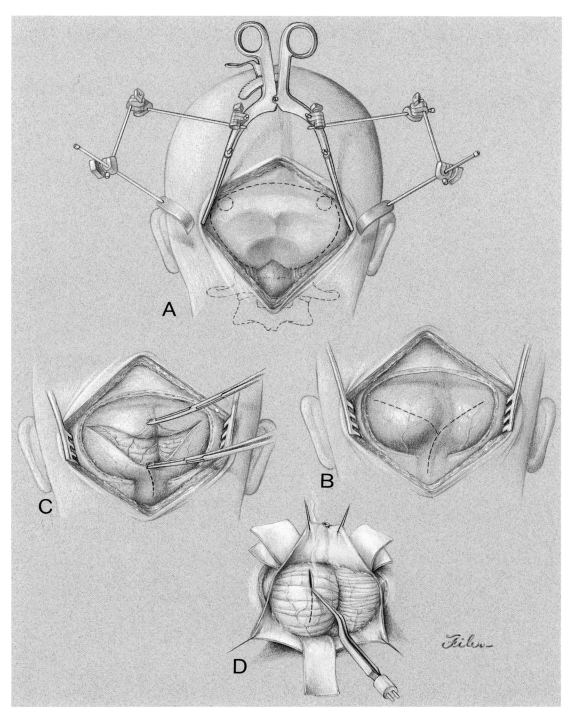

Figure 5. A, completed exposure of the occipital bone and C1 lamina. The sites for burr holes and for the craniotomy are depicted. A posted Jannetta retractor and blades are demonstrated. **B,** completed craniotomy, exposing dura from the inferior aspect of the transverse sinus down to the C1 lamina. A left hemispheric tumor and the planned dural incisions are shown. If the tumor has a major cystic component and if the dura is tense, the cyst can be aspirated via a 14–16-gauge blunt (Cone) needle, inserted before the dura is opened. **C,** lateral dural incisions have been made. The midline occipital sinus is occluded temporarily by hemostats before the midline is divided. The sinus is subsequently coagulated and ligated and the inferior limb of the Y is then opened. **D,** dural leaflets are sutured backward over the moist cottonoid strips. A cottonoid strip is inserted into the cisterna magna to prevent blood from entering the cisterna magna/foramen of Magendie. Cerebellar folia overlying the tumor can be opened transversely or vertically, depending on the maximal diameter of the tumor and thinness of the folia. Pia is coagulated with a bipolar cautery and opened with microscissors.

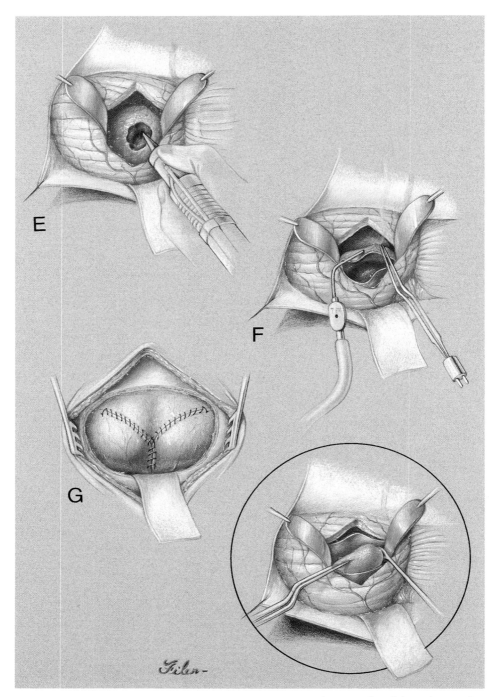

Figure 5. (*Continued*) **E,** cerebellum is retracted away from the pial opening and tumor with blades attached to a posted Jannetta retractor or to a Greenberg retractor. The ultrasonic aspirator is used to decompress the interior of predominantly solid astrocytomas. **F,** after the majority of the interior of the tumor has been removed, the periphery of the solid tumor is dissected away from adjacent cerebellum, retracting with the suction tip and coagulating small bridging vessels with the bipolar cautery. *Inset,* for cystic astro-cytomas with a mural nodule and a membranous cyst wall, the nodule can be dissected out with Penfield dissectors or the bipolar cautery. Membranous cyst walls need not be removed; walls 1–2 mm thick because of tumor infiltration must be dissected out. **G,** primary dural closure is usually possible if the dura is kept moist. If primary closure is not possible, a small graft of fascia or lyophilized dura is inserted. The bone flap is held in place with 2-0 Vicryl sutures.

of the tumor is usually curative (Fig. 5, *inset*). Cyst walls that are membranous and translucent are typical; the cyst margin infrequently contains tumor cells. If there is suspicion about the presence of tumor in the wall, a frozen section biopsy should be obtained. For astrocytomas without a clear peripheral dissection plane, the ultrasonic aspirator is used to remove tumor, beginning in its core and proceeding toward the periphery until normal tissue appears.

After the resection is complete, the cerebellar tonsils should be inspected and, if herniated, lifted above the foramen magnum. Meticulous hemostasis is obtained with bipolar cautery in the tumor bed and hemostasis is checked by Valsalva's maneuver, performed for approximately 10 seconds. The walls of the cavity are often lined with Surgicel to aid hemostasis; Gelfoam is less appropriate because it swells postoperatively and may be confused with residual tumor on the immediate postoperative CT scan.

Closure Techniques

The dura is closed by an initial single central suture to approximate the three corners of the dural flaps together, followed by either a running suture or multiple interrupted sutures to close the dura (Fig. 5G). If the dura cannot be closed primarily or if the primary closure is tight because of edema of the underlying cerebellum, a dural patch graft is indicated. Small grafts can be obtained from adjacent fascia; larger grafts are of lyophilized dura or fascia lata.

The bone flap is sewn back in place with 2-0 Vicryl or silk sutures rather than wire, which distorts postoperative scans. If there is no bone flap, some neurosurgeons lay a piece of Gelfoam over the dura in the hope of reducing the risk of a CSF leak and some insert calvarial fragments removed during the opening. The various layers (deep fascia, superficial fascia, subcutaneous tissues, and skin) are closed individually with either running or interrupted sutures. Subcutaneous drains are not needed.

MONITORING

Intraoperative monitoring is probably not indicated if the tumor is located in a cerebellar hemisphere, because evoked potentials cannot evaluate cerebellar pathways. For tumors that may invade the brain stem, monitoring somatosensory or auditory evoked potentials and direct potentials from the sixth and seventh nerves may add a measure of safety. Intraoperative ultrasonography is infrequently useful; tumor margins are usually evident and many ultrasound probes are inappropriately large.

SPECIALIZED INSTRUMENTATION

High-speed drills such as the Midas Rex drill have facilitated posterior fossa craniotomies; they are more maneuverable than traditional drills and cut through thick occipital bone more rapidly and with less effort. The ultrasonic aspirator is a more efficient tool than the laser for removing most astrocytomas. Posterior fossa astrocytomas were traditionally removed without magnification or perhaps with loupes, but the operating microscope provides illumination and clarity of vision which may increase both the safety and completeness of tumor resection.

COMPLICATIONS

Postoperative pseudomeningoceles and CSF leaks are usually due to inadequate drainage of CSF and are better prevented than treated: EVDs should be kept 5–10 cm above ventricular level for the first 2–3 days postoperatively, then increased by 5 cm/day until the drip chamber is 25–30 cm above ventricular level—a process that takes 5–6 days—and then clamped for 12–24 hours and removed if the patient has no symptoms of increased pressure. Pseudomeningoceles have been treated by repeated percutaneous aspirations which are sometimes effective but risk introducing bacteria.

The likelihood of a postoperative hematoma—in the resection cavity or the epidural space—large enough to produce signs of increased pressure and to warrant removal, is small, approximately 1–2%, if the techniques described above are used. The risk of postoperative wound infection is similar in spite of intraoperative antibiotics. The likelihood of staphylococcal infection of the EVD is 5–10%. CSF samples should be cultured daily from the EVD; the infection rate may be decreased by the daily instillation of vancomycin, 10–20 mg, into the EVD catheter.

The risk of postoperative cerebellar deficits depends on the tumor location and on the trauma of its removal, and ranges from 10 to 25%. Corticosteroids are usually given in high doses for 2–3 days postoperatively, and then tapered over 3–7 days. Postoperative edema is not a conspicuous feature of most posterior fossa astrocytomas.

The presence of residual tumor is important since JPAs are usually surgically curable tumors. A CT scan should be obtained if possible within the first 48 hours postoperatively. If the scan demonstrates residual tumor that appears to be safely excisable, it is appropriate to return to the operating room and remove it.

The posterior fossa pseudobulbar syndrome occurs in 3–5% of patients. It is characterized by the delayed onset (12–48 hours after operation) of confusion, agitation, aphasia, and at times, ataxia, or hemiparesis. Its cause and treatment are unknown. CT, MRI, and cerebral blood flow scans have been normal.

EXTREME LATERAL LUMBAR DISC HERNIATION

ROBERT S. HOOD, M.D.

INTRODUCTION

The development of high-resolution computed tomography (CT) scans allowed reliable identification of extraforaminal or extreme lateral lumbar disc herniations for the first time. It is now apparent that extreme lateral disc herniation occurs more frequently than once appreciated, perhaps representing up to 10% of clinically significant disc herniations. Surgical techniques were poorly adapted to manage these herniations and surgeons were less familiar with the operative anatomy in this region. Extreme lateral disc herniations, when inadequately removed, represent one cause of failed back surgery. Operative techniques needed to be modified so the surgeon could approach this area more easily without the necessity of exploring within the spinal canal. The technique described herein allows easy access to the extreme lateral and neural foraminal region under direct visualization, with the option of spinal canal exploration, while avoiding instability due to facet destruction.

The clinical syndromes associated with extreme lateral disc herniation differ from typical intraspinal herniation, in that extreme lateral herniations seem to occur with equal frequency at L3-4, L4-5, and L5-S1. Because the pedicle of the vertebra below the disc prevents caudal migration of fragments, cephalad migration of fragments usually occurs, making midlumbar radicular syndromes much more likely. Herniations occurring within the spinal canal typically produce a radicular syndrome affecting the nerve root exiting below the disc space, in contrast to the extreme lateral herniation which affects the nerve root above (e.g., the L4 nerve root with extreme lateral herniation at L4-5). The clinician should thus be alert that pain or sensory, motor, or reflex deficit in the anterior thigh may well be caused by an extreme lateral disc herniation.

High-resolution CT or magnetic resonance imaging (MRI) scans are the diagnostic procedures of choice for extreme lateral lumbar disc herniation. Myelography with postmyelogram CT is occasionally helpful to exclude concurrent intraspinal or axillary herniation or stenosis. Myelography alone and discography have generally not been helpful or necessary.

Unless major neurologic deficit has occurred, all patients are treated conservatively with an initial period of rest, limited activity, use of anti-inflammatory agents (nonsteroidal or steroids), and, occasionally, physical therapy. Conservative treatment is undertaken for a minimum of approximately three weeks. If the patient is not sufficiently improved, such that there remains significant limitation from radicular pain or neurologic deficit, then more aggressive treatment is warranted.

In addition to long-term conservative treatment, both chemonucleolysis and automated percutaneous lumbar discectomy may be alternatives. However, since extruded migrated fragments occur in 95% of extreme lateral disc herniations, and the nerve is significantly displaced near the site of usual needle or cannula placement for each of these procedures, they seem less likely to give satisfactory relief. These alternatives may also have a higher risk of nerve injury than when they are used for herniation within the spinal canal.

Several surgical alternatives exist. Traditional laminotomy risks failure, because the annular defect and the fragments cannot be visualized directly or reached easily with standard instrumentation. Extension of the laminectomy to include facetectomy allows adequate exposure, but entails more bone removal than is necessary and risks instability. The approach to the extreme lateral space by undermining the lamina with medial facetectomy from an intraspinal direction allows exposure to the medial neural foramen, but less easily to the extreme lateral portion of the vertebral body and disc. It also has the disadvantage that the nerve the surgeon is trying to protect and decompress is not visualized until after the disc herniation is removed, risking nerve injury. The far lateral region can be reached satisfactorily using a paramedian approach through the paraspinal muscles, which allows good lateral access. However, the target is deep and the approach is more disorienting. The paramedian approach also does not allow exploration within the spinal canal for caudally migrated fragments, if present, because the pedicle below limits lateral access.

The following surgical approach is used for extreme lateral or foraminal herniations, which may include some herniations in the axilla above. It is also useful where extreme lateral foraminal and intraspinal herniation coexists with foraminal stenosis.

OPERATIVE PROCEDURE

The patient is operated upon under general inhalational anesthesia. An intraoperative antibiotic irrigation solution is used, but neither antibiotics nor steroids are given systemically during the pre- or intraoperative period. The patient is placed prone on the operating table, on chest rolls or a lumbar frame, with the table flexed and the patient's legs flexed at the knees. Standard draping techniques using paper drapes with an adherent plastic drape on the skin are used.

The first portion of the procedure is performed using operating loupes and a high-intensity headlight, with an operating microscope brought into use later. The skin incision is in the midline, about 4–5 cm in length, and is centered slightly more cephalad than the usual incision for a typical intraspinal disc herniation, because the neural foramen lies at and above the disc space and extruded fragments tend to migrate cephalad (Fig. 1). A small subcutaneous fat graft is excised and preserved in saline for later use. An ipsilateral fascial incision is made about 1 cm lateral to the midline. The paraspinal muscles are cleared with a periosteal elevator and curettes over the superior articular process, centered over the neural foramen, which is then easily visualized. At this point a portable, lateral x-ray film is made with a marker placed at the foramen to localize the dissection accurately. Muscle exposure should be carried far enough lateral to include the articular processes both above and below the foramen and should extend caudal to but not beyond the lamina unless intraspinal exploration is also necessary. A self-retaining retractor, usually a single-bladed long Williams retractor, is inserted, centered over the neural foramen (Fig. 2). Exposure does not need to include the transverse processes.

The edge of the foramen is identified and the ligamentum flavum, which extends even lateral to the foramen, is separated from the bony edge using a small angled curette (Fig. 3). A high-speed drill is then used to unroof the foramen from lateral to medial, extending from the pedicle above to the pedicle below such that the full extent of the foramen and disc are visualized adequately (Fig. 4). Adequate bone removal

for exposure is essential for both visualization and adequate decompression. The extent of medial bone removal is dependent on the exact location of the herniation as shown on the preoperative studies and at surgery. Bone removal is completed with rongeurs and can be carried medially to visualize the main thecal sac, which is necessary when dealing with axillary or medial foraminal herniation. Bone removal must also include the cephalad one-quarter to one-third of the facet below, which always overhangs the far lateral portion of the disc. Preoperative studies occasionally suggest the presence of disc fragments both far lateral and within the spinal canal below the disc space. If exploration in both places is warranted, then partial hemilaminectomy can also be performed, leaving at least a strut of laminar bone to the facet, in order to avoid potential instability.

The operating microscope is then brought into place and is used for the remainder of the procedure. Use of the microscope at an earlier stage is acceptable but can slow the procedure and may lead the surgeon to the pitfall of inadequate bone decompression, with a greater possibility of overlooking residual pathologic changes, due to the limited focus as a result of magnification.

The first step in dissection is to find and thus protect the nerve, which is always easily located at the

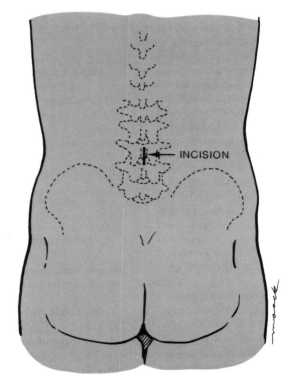

Figure 1. A midline incision, oriented adjacent to the neural foramen, slightly cephalad to the disc space.

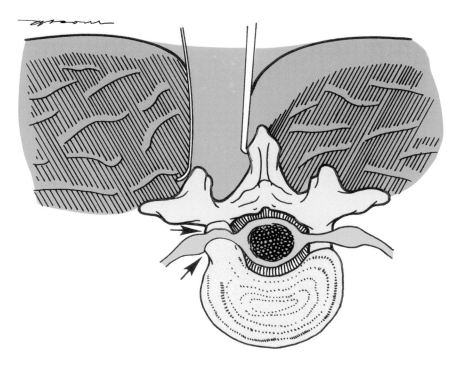

Figure 2. A paramedian approach with a self-retaining retractor exposing the neural foramen and facet joint.

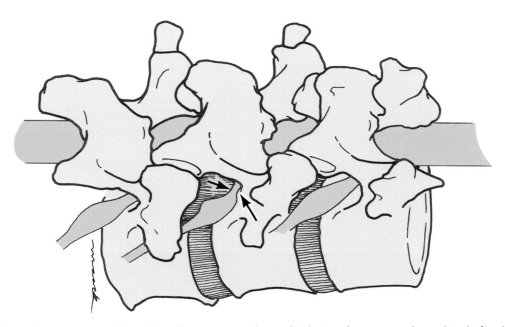

Figure 3. An extreme lateral disc herniation is shown displacing the nerve and ganglion before bone removal (the ligamentum flavum is not shown).

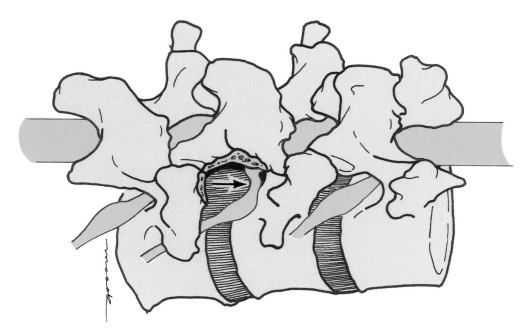

Figure 4. Exposure following bone and ligamentum flavum removal, with the underlying disc herniation shown distorting the nerve and ganglion.

cephalad margin of the foramen beneath the ligamentum flavum where it courses next to the pedicle above. The ligamentum flavum is easily separated from the pedicle. This is the location, therefore, where one should elevate the yellow ligament with a nerve hook or angled curette and visualize the nerve, then excise the ligament with rongeurs or by sharp dissection, while protecting the nerve and ganglion throughout. The ligamentum flavum is removed laterally to the intertransverse ligament, allowing full exposure of the nerve, its ganglion, and its more peripheral extent to the edge of the vertebral body and disc. There is usually an abundance of epidural fat and veins in the region. The disc herniation usually lies inferior and medial to the nerve, which is distorted posteriorly and laterally. The nerve is protected with cottonoids, and bipolar cautery is utilized if needed.

Although sequestrated fragments may be seen, more commonly the fragments of extruded disc lie beneath the posterior longitudinal ligament over the body of the vertebra cephalad to the disc space. More laterally placed herniations may indeed lie directly over or lateral to the disc space. Thus, the posterior longitudinal ligament is opened and a thorough search made for fragments, which are removed, using nerve hooks and micro-pituitary rongeurs. One must be certain to explore to the lateral edge of the vertebral body and disc as well as medially to the dural margin, in order to avoid retained fragments. The annular defect is then identified and entered with a variety of pituitary rongeurs for enucleation of the lateral por-

tion of the disc. While curettes are occasionally used to assist with enucleation, vigorous curettement is not done. The nerve is then inspected throughout its course to ensure thorough decompression (Fig. 5).

Following final inspection, the subcutaneous fat graft that was previously removed and preserved is placed over the nerve and far lateral space. Small pledgets of Gelfoam soaked in saline are occasionally used for hemostasis or in the absence of useful fat. The wound is then closed with absorbable interrupted fascial, subcutaneous, and subcuticular sutures. Steri-strips are applied to the skin followed by a light, non-adherent, breathable bandage. Drains are never used.

POSTOPERATIVE MANAGEMENT
Postoperatively the patient is ambulated briefly on the date of surgery, more frequently on the following day, and is usually discharged by the second postoperative day. Injectable narcotic analgesics are used, if necessary, on the day of surgery and oral narcotics thereafter, briefly following discharge. A mild muscle relaxant is used for incisional stiffness for about one week and a rapidly tapering prednisone regimen is used postoperatively for 5–6 days. The patient is activated progressively, including the initiation of an exercise program with aerobic exercise within three weeks following surgery.

COMPLICATIONS
The complications attendant to this procedure are common to all procedures for disc surgery. Significant

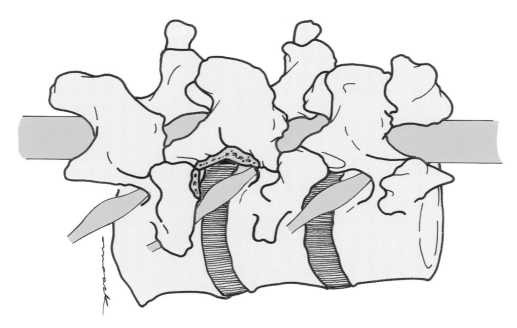

Figure 5.   The ganglion and nerve are well decompressed following excision of the disc herniation.

bleeding or infection has not occurred and should be rare if attention is paid to technique. Major vessel injury has not been encountered. Intraoperative nerve injury can be avoided with careful microdissection and with particular attention to avoid excessive manipulation of the highly sensitive ganglion. Facet pain and instability have not occurred with this procedure. Recurrent disc herniation seems to occur at a rate similar to or less than that following intraspinal disc surgery.

RESULTS AND CONCLUSIONS

Foraminal and extreme lateral disc herniations are relatively common. This technique has been used for more than six years by the author. More than 90% of patients have experienced satisfactory relief of pain, with return to usual activity. The surgeon should be prepared to deal properly with herniations in this region, adapting the technique to the patient's needs. This technique provides such an adaptation.

TENTORIAL MENINGIOMAS

LALIGAM N. SEKHAR, M.D.
ATUL GOEL, M.Ch.

INTRODUCTION

The tentorium is a tough double-layered dural wall separating the cerebral hemispheres from the cerebellum. The tentorial notch or incisura is of the shape of a necklace around the midbrain and is the only communication between the supra- and infratentorial spaces. Its dimensions are variable. The tentorium is shaped like a "tent," sloping downward from its apex at the posterior edge of the tentorial notch to its attachments anteriorly to the petrous ridge and posterolaterally to the inner surface of the occipital and temporal bones. The anatomy of the tentorium and its anterior extensions into the anterior and posterior clinoid processes has been described in the various reviews on this subject.

The problems of surgically excising tentorial meningiomas are related to the difficult access, especially with medial tentorial lesions, and the relationships to the temporal lobe, brain stem, cranial nerves, blood vessels, and venous sinuses. The relationships of the posterior cerebral and superior cerebellar arteries, the perforating arteries, the vein of Labbé, and the veins draining the brain stem are particularly important. Thus the classification of these meningiomas according to their location into medial, lateral, posterior, and falcotentorial is useful in planning surgery and comparing the results (Fig. 1). The tumors can arise from either the inferior or the superior surface of the tentorium and can extend correspondingly into the posterior fossa or supratentorially. Tentorial tumors usually have extensions in both superior and inferior compartments. Similarly, these tumors may extend into the petroclival or falcine areas.

Despite the advancements in microsurgical operative techniques and instrumentation, neuroanesthesia, radiology, and the medical management of elevated intracranial pressure, meningiomas arising from the tentorium pose a challenge for the surgeon due to the following characteristics:

1. The tentorial meningiomas are usually diagnosed when they are large in size.
2. They have a close relationship to the brain stem, the cranial nerves, important blood vessels, and the cavernous sinus.
3. The neurologic deficits are often minimal early in their presentation in spite of the location and the large size of the tumor.
4. The tumors are located deep and require the retraction of vital parts of the brain to approach them.
5. The blood supply of the tumor is derived from arteries which usually arise deep to the large tumors and are relatively difficult to obliterate early in the operation.
6. Factors relating to the tumor, such as arterial encasement, compromise of important venous structures, degree of brain stem compression, tumor vascularity, tumor consistency (soft as opposed to firm), and the presence (or absence) of a subarachnoid plane between the tumor and the brain stem are important variables which ultimately decide the course of the surgical resection and the results. Presence of scar tissue from previous surgery and prior radiation therapy are also important problems for the surgeon.

PRESENTATION AND INVESTIGATIONS

Signs of elevated intracranial pressure or dementia (due to the large size of the tumor or to hydrocephalus) are the most common forms of presentation, followed by cerebellar symptoms and pyramidal and cranial nerve involvement. Psychomotor seizures may occur if the tumor compresses the temporal lobe.

Computed tomography (CT) with soft-tissue and bone algorithms continues to remain the primary investigation for tentorial meningiomas. Magnetic resonance imaging (MRI) before and after contrast administration demonstrates the relationship of the tumor with important surrounding blood vessels better than any other investigation presently available. In addition, the presence or absence of an arachnoid plane can also be discerned from MRI. Angiography is important to delineate the extent of the vascularity of the tumor, its source of blood supply, and the degree of involvement and shifts of the blood vessels. Therapeutic embolization of the feeding tentorial arteries can be performed whenever the feeders are large and can be

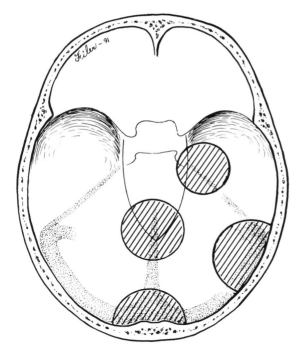

Figure 1. The common sites of tentorial meningiomas are shown.

cannulated via the internal carotid artery (ICA). When they cannot be cannulated, sometimes the ICA may be temporarily occluded with a balloon, and absolute alcohol may be infused into the feeding meningohypophyseal artery or other branches. The vertebral angiogram and MRI must be examined carefully to note the location of the basilar artery and its terminal branches in relation to the tumor.

GENERAL PRINCIPLES

Electrophysiological Monitoring
Monitoring of somatosensory evoked potentials (SSEP), brain stem evoked responses (BSER), and electroencephalogram (EEG) keeps the surgeon aware of the changes in vital functions. Cranial nerve (CN) monitoring may include CNs VI to XII.

Instrumentation
As the operation may be prolonged, the surgeon should be in a comfortable operating position during the surgery. A comfortable chair with armrests and a Zeiss Contraves microscope are usually used by the senior author. A Malis irrigation bipolar forceps is useful for tumor dissection and fine work, whereas Aesculap bipolar equipment is useful for rapid tumor removal. CO_2 and neodymium-yttrium-aluminum-garnet (Nd-YAG) lasers and a Cavitron ultrasonic aspirator are useful for debulking the tumor in selected

situations. In addition to standard microsurgical instrumentation, the surgeon should also have available instruments for the repair of small and large vessels.

Brain Retraction and Tumor Exposure
Brain retraction should be minimized as much as possible. Adequate basal bone removal and wide exposure, the opening of appropriate cisterns and fissures, the drainage of cerebrospinal fluid (CSF), and sometimes the judicious resection of noneloquent areas of brain are useful in avoiding excessive retraction. The use of osmotic diuretics, moderate hyperventilation, low-dose barbiturate infusion, appropriate anesthetic agents, steroids, and the replacement of volume loss with colloids rather than crystalloids helps in maintaining optimum brain relaxation.

Tumor Removal
All dissections must be carried out under direct vision. Use of a monopolar nerve stimulator can help in the identification of cranial nerves, some of which may be very thin and splayed over the tumor. With lateral tentorial meningiomas, the major technical problem is the involvement of the venous sinuses. Medial tentorial lesions are technically more difficult considering their relationships.

The general principle of tumor resection includes early devascularization of the tumor, if possible, and reduction of tumor bulk by coring out the center of the tumor before attempting dissection from the brain. The arachnoidal planes are usually preserved around the tumor and dissection must be carried out in that plane. In cases of large tumors, however, the arachnoidal plane may be missing and in such cases efforts are made to preserve the pial plane. When critical vessels and nerves are encountered, dissection is done from the normal to the abnormal area parallel to the direction of the encased structure. Sharp dissection is preferable in the proximity of blood vessels and nerves. Dissection of the small perforating vessels, of encased and narrowed arteries, of compressed brain stem, and through scar tissue are most difficult tasks.

Total tumor removal with excision of the involved tentorium is the goal of the surgery. However, this may not be feasible with medial tentorial lesions because of tumor extension onto the petrous ridge or the cavernous sinus or because of occasional dense adherence of the tumor to important blood vessels.

OPERATIVE APPROACH
The approach to a tentorial meningioma depends upon its location on the tentorium and its size. Generally, when the tumor is small in size or extends only into the supra- or infratentorial spaces, the tumor

may be removed through an approach only on one side. Larger tumors, however, will require exposure on both sides of the tentorium.

Lateral Tentorial Meningiomas

The craniotomy is performed in the occipital or temporal area and in the posterior fossa, encircling the tumor. The tumor is removed as described. Where there is adequate collateral circulation, and when the sinus is nondominant, when the sinus is already occluded, and in younger patients, the sinus may be resected to achieve complete tumor resection. When the sinus is dominant, a trial occlusion with temporary clips is performed prior to permanent occlusion even if adequate cross circulation is present. In all patients, a reconstruction of the venous sinus is attempted, for potential long-term benefits.

Medial Tentorial Meningiomas

Small medial tentorial meningiomas may be removed by a subtemporal, transzygomatic, and transpetrous apex approach. Larger medial tentorial meningiomas require a subtemporal, presigmoid, retrolabyrinthine, or translabyrinthine approach.

Falcotentorial Meningiomas

Large falcotentorial meningiomas are removed by a combined occipital-transtentorial and suboccipital approach, with the temporary division of the transverse sinus.

Posterior Tentorial Meningiomas

Larger tumors in this area need a bilateral occipital and suboccipital craniotomy with the exposure of both transverse sinuses and the superior sagittal sinus. Unless the torcular herophili is already occluded by the tumor, a total resection of these meningiomas cannot be performed. Fortunately, most of the tumors in this area involve only a corner of a venous sinus such that the tumor can be removed and the sinus repaired.

SPECIFIC OPERATIVE APPROACHES: EXAMPLES

Posterior Subtemporal with Presigmoid Approach

A posterior subtemporal and presigmoid approach is used to resect large or giant-sized medial tentorial meningiomas. While in some patients one can proceed by a retrolabyrinthine approach, in others a translabyrinthine approach with sacrifice of ipsilateral hearing is needed. This can be done more readily if hearing is very poor in that ear. The removal of the zygomatic arch with the condylar fossa permits a further inferior mobilization of the temporalis muscle

and improves the exposure of the interpeduncular cistern area.

The advantages of this approach are:

1. There is wide and shallow exposure to difficult anteromedially placed tentorial meningiomas. The operating distance to the tumor is shortened by about 3–4 cm.
2. The retraction of the cerebellum and the temporal lobe is minimized.
3. The surgeon has reasonable access to the anterior and lateral aspects of the brain stem.
4. The continuity of the transverse venous sinus is not affected.
5. Tumor extensions into the cavernous sinus and clivus can be dealt with during the same sitting.

Operative Steps

A curvilinear scalp incision is made behind the ear extending from the retromastoid to the temporal region (Fig. 2). The ear canal is transected and reflected forward with the flap. The incision in the ear canal is made through the pinna and the skin is resutured at the end of the operation if the exposure is retrolabyrinthine. If a translabyrinthine exposure is performed, the external ear canal is divided and closed as a blind sac and covered additionally with a fascial flap. A temporal craniotomy is first performed from the pterion anteriorly to about 2 cm behind the mastoid process posteriorly. The dimensions of this flap are varied to suit the tumor. The transverse sinus is separated under direct vision and then a retromastoid craniectomy is performed, usually 2–3 cm in size. Middle fossa dura is separated from the floor.

The temporomandibular joint capsule is then opened and the meniscus is depressed from the glenoid fossa. Using a reciprocating saw, a zygomatic osteotomy is performed with its anterior limit being just behind the lateral orbit. Posteriorly, the cuts include the glenoid fossa. One should be careful while making the posterior cut and should not go beyond the confines of the glenoid fossa because of the proximity to the petrous ICA. Posteriorly lie the middle ear and the external ear canal. When the zygomatic osteotomy is carefully reapproximated at the end of the operation, no dysfunction of the temporomandibular joint is observed.

A mastoidectomy is performed next, with complete skeletonization of the sigmoid sinus. In older people, a very thin shell of bone should be left over the sigmoid sinus because it may be easily torn as a result of adhesions during attempted separation. Next, a labyrinthectomy is performed, with removal of the posterior, superior, and lateral semicircular canals. The tympanic and mastoidal segments of the facial nerve are skeletonized but not displaced. By an extradural middle fossa approach, the petrous ICA is exposed in

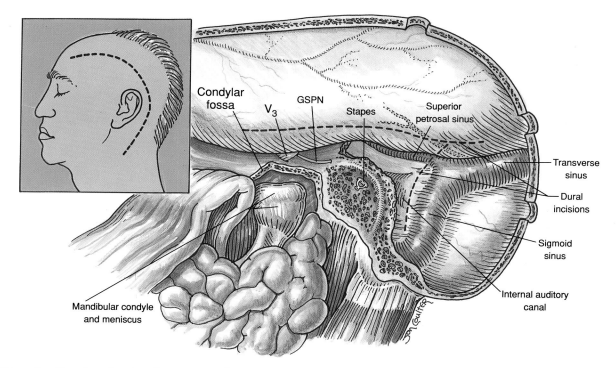

Figure 2. Drawing showing the exposure for a posterior subtemporal with presigmoid approach. The ear canal has been transected and the scalp flap reflected anteriorly. Laby-rinthectomy has been carried out and the facial nerve skele-tonized. The *dashed line* shows the site of dural incision.

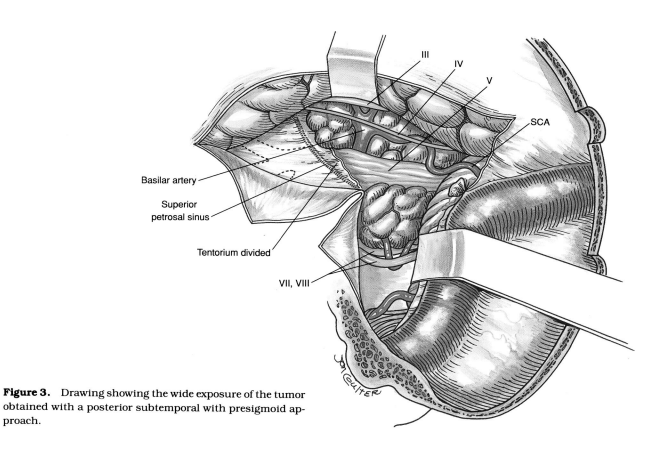

Figure 3. Drawing showing the wide exposure of the tumor obtained with a posterior subtemporal with presigmoid approach.

its horizontal segment, and a petrous apicectomy is performed if needed.

The dura is opened in the presigmoid area and also in the temporal region (Figs. 2 and 3). After suture ligation of the superior petrosal sinus, the tentorium is divided from a lateral to medial direction, posterior to the tumor. The temporal lobe and cerebellum are gently retracted, taking care to avoid injury to the vein of Labbé. Any middle fossa tumor is removed first. The lateral wall of the cavernous sinus is peeled posteriorly, and Meckel's cave is opened. These tumors often extend into Meckel's cave and the posterior cavernous sinus. Removal of the tumor from the posterior cavernous sinus may allow the tumor to be devascularized further by the division of the meningohypophyseal artery.

The tumor is then debulked centrally. Dissection from critical structures follows. These include the brain stem, basilar artery, posterior cerebral and superior cerebellar arteries, and CNs III, IV, V, and VI. With giant-sized tumors, it is usually not possible to preserve CN IV. It may be reconstructed with a graft if the proximal stump is present and by finding the distal end in the lateral wall of the cavernous sinus. As much as possible, dissection of the tumor from the brain stem must be made in the subarachnoidal plane.

Illustrative Cases

JP: This 26-year-old man experienced a single grand mal seizure. There was no neurologic deficit. Investigations (MRI and CT scan) showed a large tumor extending on both sides of the tentorium (Fig. 4, A–C). An attempt to remove the tumor at another institution was unsuccessful because the tumor was very vascular, and the subtemporal and retrosigmoid exposure was restricted by a dominant sigmoid sinus and a large vein of Labbé on the ipsilateral side. At our institution, the patient underwent a cerebral angiogram (Fig. 4D) and a balloon occlusion test of the left internal carotid artery. Absolute alcohol embolization of the tentorial branch of the internal carotid artery was then carried out. Following this procedure the patient developed a partial third nerve and a complete sixth nerve paralysis on the left side, presumably due to devascularization of these cranial nerves. The operation was performed by using the approach described above, with labyrinthectomy. A total tumor resection

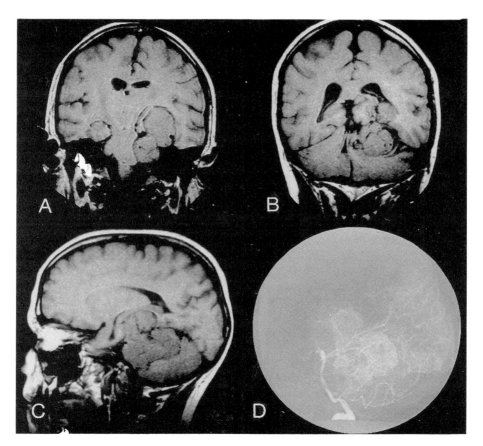

Figure 4. **A—C,** MRI scans of patient JP showing the large tentorial meningioma compressing the brain stem. **D,** a vertebral artery angiogram showing the marked vascular tumor blush.

was achieved. The patient's facial paresis and ocular nerve palsies resolved. The final pathological diagnosis was hemangiopericytoma. Adjuvant radiotherapy and chemotherapy were administered.

CG: This 44-year-old male patient presented with history of a single grand mal seizure. He was also noted to have progressive imbalance, staggering of gait, and decreased hearing on the right side. Diplopia had been present for two years and became worse in the last six months before presentation. Cranial nerve examination revealed a mild right third nerve paresis with slight ptosis, enlargement of the pupil, and restriction of upward and medial gaze. Radiologic investigations showed a large tentorial tumor also involving the cavernous sinus (Fig. 5). The tumor was excised, using a posterior subtemporal presigmoid and retrolabyrinthine approach. Postoperative cerebrospinal fluid leakage and meningitis occurred because of transient hydrocephalus. These were successfully treated. The patient suffered an abducens palsy but otherwise recovered uneventfully.

Combined Supra- and Infratentorial Approach

A combined supra- and infratentorial approach can be used for a giant falcotentorial (pineal region) meningioma. The majority of surgeons currently use either a supracerebellar infratentorial approach or an occipital transtentorial approach to the lesions situated at this site, depending on the extensions of the tumor. However, for some giant sized and extensive lesions, the two approaches can be combined by division of the tentorium and the nondominant (communicating) transverse sinus. This combined approach makes use of the advantages of both approaches, while avoiding the disadvantages. The transverse sinus is resutured at the end of the procedure to re-establish the blood circulation.

The advantages of this approach are:

1. The procedure is indicated for giant and extensive meningiomas. It provides a direct and wide exposure of the lesion. The brain stem and the vital veins of this region are widely exposed so that they can be dissected free under vision early in the operation. A large additional exposure is obtained at the depth by the section of the transverse sinus, because it is close to the surgeon's line of vision.
2. The retraction of both the cerebellum and the occipital lobe is minimized.
3. The transverse sinus is resutured at the end of the operation, especially in younger patients, to restore its patency. This maintains the natural venous communication, in case the patient develops occlusion of the contralateral venous sinus later in life.
4. The surgeon operates in a comfortable working position, without the disadvantages attendant to the patient being in a sitting position.

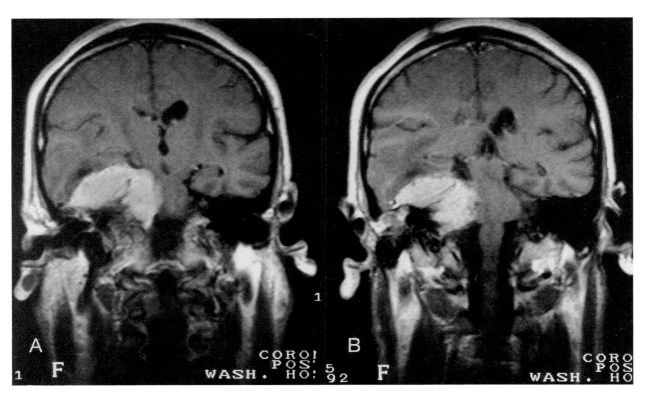

Figure 5. **A,B,** MRI scans showing the large tumor of patient CG.

Operative Steps

The patient is placed in right lateral decubitus (Sugita) position. A horseshoe-shaped incision is made starting in the suboccipital region, curving well above the lambda, and then curving back on the other side (Fig. 6). A large free bone flap is first cut in one occipital area. After separation of the sagittal sinus, a second occipital flap is elevated. After separating the transverse sinus under direct vision, the suboccipital flap is elevated. The dura covering the posterior aspects of both occipital lobes and cerebellar hemispheres and the three venous sinuses is thus exposed.

The occipital dura is opened on the side of the nondominant transverse sinus, bordering the superior sagittal sinus and the transverse sinus (Fig. 6). The dura is also opened in the suboccipital area in a linear fashion just below the transverse sinuses, and the occipital sinus is ligated. The occipital lobe is gently retracted away from the tentorium up to the tentorial notch.

Two temporary clips are placed across the nondominant (usually the left) transverse sinus approximately 1 cm lateral to the torcular herophili. After an observation period to check for possible brain swelling, the transverse sinus is divided between the two clips. The tentorium is then incised parallel to and about 1 cm from the straight sinus up to the tentorial notch (Fig. 7). There is usually significant bleeding from the venous sinuses in the tentorium, but it can be controlled with gentle packing with oxidized cellulose and with bipolar coagulation. The left half of the left transverse sinus and the tentorium are retracted away to provide a large space between the cerebellum and the occipital lobe. Very often, the occipital dura on the other side will also have to be opened to divide the tentorium on the other side, lateral to the tumor. Be-

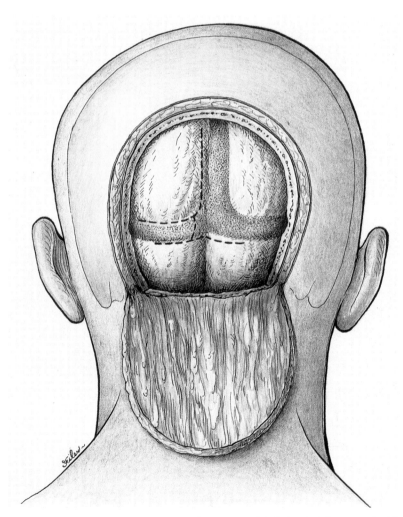

Figure 6.   Drawing showing the exposure for a combined supra- and infratentorial approach. The *dashed line* shows the site of dural incision.

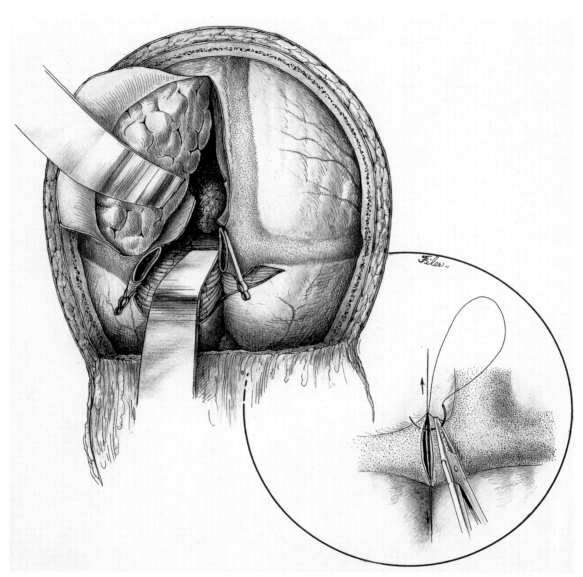

Figure 7. Drawing showing the large exposure of the tumor obtained after the combined approach. The transverse sinus has been sectioned and the two edges are held in clips. The *inset* shows the resuturing of the transverse sinus.

cause the blood supply to these tumors is derived from the tentorial arteries, the tumor is completely devascularized thus.

The tumor is then debulked with bipolar cautery and scissors or a Cavitron ultrasonic aspirator. Dissection of the tumor is performed from the cerebellum with further piecemeal excision. The upper pole of the tumor is then delivered inferiorly, and careful dissection is performed, separating the tumor from the vein of Galen and its tributaries. The tumor is then dissected away from the compressed brain stem. Finally, the dural attachment of the tumor is excised. However, a small area of the tumor attachment around the straight sinus and the entrance of the vein of Galen can only be cauterized. Reconstruction of the transverse sinus can be performed if preferred. This is done with 5-0 or 6-0 Prolene interrupted sutures (Fig. 7, *inset*).

Illustrative Case

PG: A 45-year-old man presented with a one-year history of progressive loss of balance while walking and bilateral hearing loss. Except for mild abnormality of cortical function, and difficulty in tandem walking, he had no neurologic deficit. Magnetic resonance imaging showed a large mass in the pineal region, straddling the tentorium, suggestive of a meningioma (Fig. 8). There was associated hydrocephalus. Angiography showed that the tumor was fed mainly by a large tentorial branch of the right meningohypophyseal trunk. The right transverse sinus was dominant, but there was good communication across the torcular herophili.

A combined supra- and infratentorial approach was used to resect this tumor completely. The patient made a complete recovery after a short period of reha-

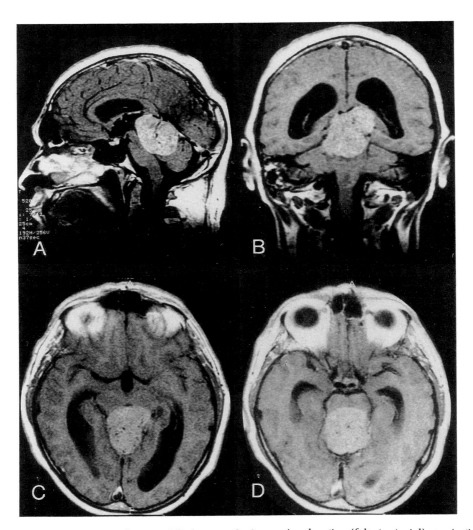

Figure 8. **A—D,** MRI scans of patient PG showing the large pineal region (falcotentorial) meningioma.

bilitation. Postoperative scans showed the absence of the tumor and the patency of the transverse sinus.

Subtemporal, Transcavernous, and Transpetrous Apex Approach

A subtemporal, transcavernous, and transpetrous apex approach (Fig. 9) is ideal in situations where there is a large anteromedial tentorial meningioma which involves the cavernous sinus. This approach is suitable for lesions in the region of the upper clivus and petrous apex area. The approach is the modification of the transpetrous apex approach described by Kawase.

The advantages of this approach are:

1. This approach is useful when there is involvement of the cavernous sinus by a small or medium sized tentorial meningioma. It may be emphasized that the dura of the superior and lateral walls of the cavernous sinus are extensions of the tentorium and hence it is involved frequently by medial tentorial meningiomas.
2. The removal of the glenoid fossa leaving the cartilage of the joint intact does not affect the function of the joint significantly.
3. Because the approach is very basal, the retraction of the brain is greatly minimized and the surgical depth of the lesion is reduced.
4. A wide working space is available for the surgeon to operate in the critical areas anterior to the brain stem.

Operative Steps

A curvilinear scalp incision is made starting in the temporal region, curving inferiorly above the pinna of the ear and extending to the preauricular area. The skin flap is reflected deep to the superficial layer of the temporal fascia to preserve the frontal branches of the facial nerve. Below the level of the zygomatic arch the scalp is reflected just over the masseteric fascia to avoid injury to the parotid gland. A temporal craniotomy is performed, with its posterior extent just above the mastoid process. This is followed by zygomatic osteotomy. The glenoid fossa of the temporomandibular joint may be included in the osteotomy if a more extensive exposure of the region is necessary.

Extradural middle fossa dissection is then performed from a lateral to medial and from a posterior to anterior direction to identify the following landmarks: tegmen tympani, arcuate eminence, the lesser and greater superficial petrosal nerves (LSPN and GSPN), the middle meningeal artery, the mandibular nerve (V₃), and the horizontal segment of the petrous internal carotid artery (if it is uncovered by bone). The GSPN may be distinguished from the LSPN by the fact that the LSPN joins the middle meningeal artery at the foramen spinosum, and by electrical stimulation of the GSPN, with observation of resulting contraction of the facial musculature on electromyography.

The dura is opened and the temporal lobe is gently

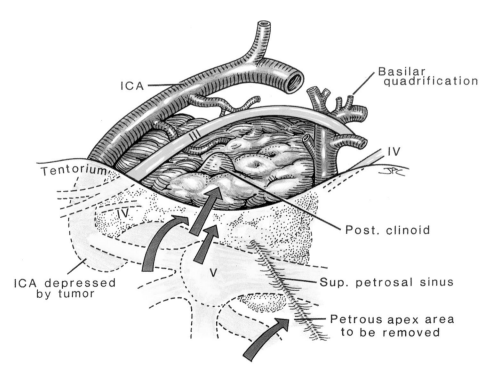

Figure 9. Drawing showing the subtemporal and transpetrous apex approach. The *arrows* indicate the directions in which the surgeon can approach the tumor after the initial exposure.

retracted after splitting the sylvian fissure widely, working with the aid of the surgical microscope. The arachnoid membrane of the perimesencephalic cistern is opened, taking care not to injure the posterior cerebral and the superior cerebellar arteries which lie immediately under the arachnoid in this area. The fourth cranial nerve is identified and the tentorium is divided well posterior to the tumor and posterior to the entrance point of the trochlear nerve. The division of the tentorium is extended posterolaterally, just posterior to the superior petrosal sinus. The tentorial division is then extended anterolaterally into the middle fossa, across the superior petrosal sinus, and opening Meckel's cave. The superior petrosal sinus is packed with oxidized cellulose. The trigeminal root is identified.

The dissection in the cavernous sinus will depend on the extent of the tumor involvement and the preoperative state of the extraocular muscle function. The lateral wall of the cavernous sinus is peeled away from a posterior to an anterior direction, exposing the trigeminal ganglion, and cranial nerves IV and V_1. If patent, some of the cavernous sinus is packed with Surgicel between cranial nerves IV and V_1. The dura is also opened all the way forward along the lower border of the trigeminal root, trigeminal ganglion, and V_3, and the lateral wall of Meckel's cave is opened completely. It may be essential to dissect the fourth cranial nerve in the lateral wall of the cavernous sinus and move it superiorly to allow the surgeon to work between cranial nerves IV and V in Parkinson's triangle. The surgeon may also work in the cavernous sinus between cranial nerves III and IV and between rootlets of cranial nerve V in Meckel's cave.

The tumor in the prepeduncular area is now exposed widely and can be dissected. For additional exposure the petrous apex bone is removed with a high-speed drill, lateral to the trigeminal root and ganglion, working intradurally. The lateral border of the removal of the petrous apex is the horizontal segment of the petrous internal carotid artery. It is often easier to do this intradurally rather than extradurally since the dura restricts the exposure of the petrous apex during extradural bone removal. The sixth cranial nerve will be identified just medial to the trigeminal root and can be followed into the cavernous sinus at this time; care has to be taken not to damage it. The surgeon may have to remove all the bone of the dorsum sellae, both posterior clinoids, the floor of the sella turcica, and any of the involved sphenoid and petrous apex bone.

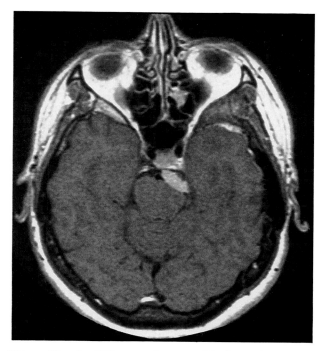

Figure 10. An MRI scan of patient PS shows the medial tentorial tumor extending into the petroclival region and the cavernous sinus.

Illustrative Case

PS: This woman had a five-year history of headache and left retro-orbital pain which recently increased in severity and a one-year history of progressive facial numbness. There was no other neurologic deficit. The investigations (CT scan and MRI, Fig. 10) revealed a petroclival meningioma extending into the ipsilateral cavernous sinus. She underwent a subtemporal, transcavernous, and transpetrous apex approach for this lesion which was totally excised. The patient had postoperative third and sixth nerve palsies which resolved completely by eight months after the operation.

COMPLICATIONS

Complications following surgery for tentorial meningiomas may be related to brain retraction, injury to the brain stem, injury to the basilar artery branches, injury to major veins or venous sinuses, CN injuries, CSF leakage, and infection. Fortunately, with adequate exposure and with the use of microsurgical technique such complications can be greatly minimized.

Index

Page numbers in *italics* denote figures; those followed by "t" denote tables